TRANSPLANTATION ETHICS

SECOND EDITION

TRANSPLANTATION ETHICS

SECOND EDITION

Robert M. Veatch & Lainie F. Ross

Georgetown University Press
Washington, DC

Library of Congress Cataloging-in-Publication Data

Veatch, Robert M., author.
  Transplantation ethics / Robert M. Veatch, Lainie Friedman Ross.—Second edition.
    pages   cm
  Includes bibliographical references and index.
  ISBN 978-1-62616-168-9 (hardcover : alk. paper) — ISBN 978-1-62616-167-2
  (pbk. : alk. paper) — ISBN 978-1-62616-169-6 (ebook)
  1. Transplantation of organs, tissues, etc.—Moral and ethical aspects.   I. Ross, Lainie Friedman, author.   II. Title.
    RD120.7.V43   2015
    174.2′97954—dc23
                                                                          2014019683

♾ This book is printed on acid-free paper meeting the requirements of the American National Standard for Permanence in Paper for Printed Library Materials.

18   17   16   15   9   8   7   6   5   4   3   2   First printing

Printed in the United States of America

Cover design by George Kirkpatrick. Cover image by Blend Images/ERproductions Ltd.

*Siblings are the most common bond
between living donors and recipients
in organ transplantation.*

In that vein, we dedicate this book to
Bruce Lee Friedman
Mark Jay Friedman (1955–1999)
William C. Veatch

CONTENTS

ILLUSTRATIONS

PREFACE

It has been fourteen years since the publication of the first edition of *Transplantation Ethics*. In the world of ethics, from before Plato and the Bible, that may be a mere moment, but in the world of transplantation, it is an eternity. During this period organ transplants have emerged from the status of a controversial, innovative therapy and have become something closer to routine.

Also during this period, however, there have been many innovations in transplants, and some of them have been controversial. We have begun to transplant faces and hands. Transplants of the uterus are in their pioneering stage. Enormous strides have been made in immunosuppression. Living donor organ swaps and chains have emerged.

In the world of transplant policy, much is different. We have just adopted a new kidney allocation formula that incorporates age as a consideration as well as expected organ quality. We have realized the important role of geography in determining who gets an organ. We have begun to understand that there are therapeutic alternatives to transplants—for example, diet for the control of liver damage in maple syrup urine disease. Living kidney donations are much more accepted, so that even strangers are stepping forward to become nondirected donors.

At the same time, it is now clear that shortages of organs for transplants are a permanent problem for society—at least until nonhuman animal transplants are successful or artificial organs are produced from stem cells or three-dimensional printers. We are more aware of the role of the media and of status in determining who gets organs. We know of sophisticated internet campaigns to get organs and of elites like Steve Jobs and Dick Cheney who appear to get advantages. A girl with cystic fibrosis was able to mount a successful legal effort to override the lung allocation formula and thus to get listed on both the adult and children's wait lists, enabling her to receive a lung transplant not available to others who appear similarly situated.

Alternatives to the donation model for transplants are now being debated much more openly. We now know of a major, legal market mechanism for procuring kidneys operating in Iran that reportedly has eliminated a wait list. We have vivid accounts of black markets for organs that often leave the destitute worse off medically as well as financially. We are beginning to see nations and areas within nations adopt policies of routine procurement without explicit consent—sometimes mistakenly called "presumed consent" policies.

This second edition introduces all these ethically controversial topics, adding chapters on the impact of the media on organ procurement; on elective transplants; and on vascular composite allografts—that is, face, hand, and uterus transplants.

The ethics of organ transplantation naturally divides itself into three general topics: deciding when human beings are dead, deciding when it is ethical to procure organs, and deciding how to allocate organs, once procured. These three topics provide the overall framework for this book. After two introductory chapters, one summarizing major religious and cultural views on transplantation and one sketching an overarching ethical framework, part I addresses the definition of death; part II, procuring organs; and part III, allocating them.

We have written this book primarily for those interested in a broad and systematic overview of the ethics of transplantation for transplant professionals, physicians, nurses, social workers, and those participating in the public policy process, including staff members of organ procurement organizations and government officials involved in the regulation of transplantation. We hope it will also be useful for students of bioethics who are seeking a systematic study of one area of applied ethics. We have tried to write the book assuming no special preparation by the reader in either the science of transplantation or the science of ethical analysis. When medical facts or ethical theory are needed, we attempt to provide enough information so that the reader not previously familiar with the literature should be able to follow the discussion. Nevertheless, several chapters journey quite far into either transplantation science or ethical theory. In particular, the chapters on the conscience clause (chapter 7), the salvaging of organs (chapter 10), and socially directed donation (chapter 23) are meant to carry the discussion to the cutting edge; for instance, chapter 23 introduces the idea that transplant policy has the potential to challenge the currently dominant philosophical theory of justice.

In general, as authors, we had little trouble agreeing on the ethical arguments and policy recommendations that we present in the chapters that follow. For instance. we endorse a modification of the definition of death—one that incorporates a conscience clause that permits people to opt for alternative definitions. The recent case of Jahi McMath, a girl who suffered the complete destruction of her brain and whose mother insisted she was still alive, epitomizes the kind of case where such a law might be relevant. For only one chapter, however, we could not agree on the ethical policy that we would recommend. Therefore, in chapter 18, where we consider whether voluntary lifestyle choices should in any way be relevant to organ allocation—for example, whether a history of alcoholism is at all relevant to allocating livers—we agree to disagree and air our long hours of debate.

The two introductory chapters provide an orientation about the views of various cultures on the key issues of this volume and the ethical framework that is used. Those not feeling a need for such an orientation should feel free to move directly to one of the three main parts of the book as their interest dictates.

The definition-of-death debate has been historically intimately linked with transplantation. The Harvard committee that put forward a brain-based definition of death was completing its work at the same that time heart transplantation was hurling itself onto the world scene. The first heart transplant took place in South Africa in December 1967, whereas the Harvard committee reported in May 1968, having worked for many months before that. Part I of the book starts with a case study involving a man in Richmond from whom a heart was taken without any advance permission or even a clear agreement that he was dead. Then the next three chapters set out the core philosophical and public policy alternatives in the definition-of-death debate: the whole-brain, circulatory (or somatic), and higher-brain definitions. We suggest that because the circulatory and higher-brain views have strong scholarly defenders, they cannot easily be set aside in favor of the whole-brain view that is the basis for the current law in much of the world. This sets the stage for our proposal for a conscience clause that would permit people to assert their dissent from some societally adopted default definition. The discussion of the need for a new definition of death is concluded in chapter 8, which sets out our proposal for a new definition of death incorporating these ideas.

The reader who is less interested in the definition of death than the explicit ethical issues of organ procurement and allocation may wish to turn directly to part II, keeping in mind that those chapters presume that some understanding of what it means to be dead has already been gained.

Part II addresses the ethics of procurement. Chapters 9, 10, and 11 have been extensively restructured from the book's first edition in order to set out, respectively, the three major options for procuring organs: donation, routine salvaging, and markets. The emergence of market mechanisms has led us to devote a new chapter to this option. Although organ procurement from infants with anencephaly was a controversial topic fifteen years ago, it has largely disappeared from the debate today, so the chapter about it was dropped. In chapter 12 we expand our discussion of living donor procurement, including much new consideration of organ swaps and chains. We show that there are hidden problems of justice in these initiatives, even if they offer great promise to increase the supply of kidneys. In chapter 13 we enlarge the discussion of organ donation by high-risk candidates—for example, those with HIV, other viral diseases, and cancer. We suggest that the combination of the increased realization of the chronic shortage of organs and the right of recipients to make informed choices should lead to a much greater availability of these high-risk organs for consenting recipients.

In chapter 14 we take up xenografts (transplants from one species to another), which could turn out to be the true solution to the organ shortage. It turns out, however, that it could also lead to a world-shaking catastrophe. We are particularly interested in taking organs from nonhuman animals for use in humans.

Finally, in part II we include the entirely new chapter 15, which considers the increasing role of the media in connecting potential organ sources to recipients and the justice issue it raises vis-à-vis one's computer and media skills.

Once we have examined the nuances of procuring organs, we can turn to deciding how to allocate them. Part III begins with a brief chapter that calls into question the assumption that doctors have difficult choices to make in allocating organs. We shall see, in fact, that if there are difficult choices, they will not need to be made by physicians at the bedside because such choices are not for physicians to make. They are the responsibility of all of us, as society; thus, they need to be made by national and state governments, by the courts, and by local organ procurement organizations governed by diverse groups.

After making sure we understand the nature of the decisions to be made, in chapter 17 we set out a general theory of organ allocation, noting that, although most transplant surgeons were nurtured on the Hippocratic Oath's ethic of doing as much good for their patients as possible, it is not at all obvious that we want to allocate organs so as to be maximally efficient in benefiting patients. The law, in fact, requires that the allocation system consider not only efficiency but also equity. Seeing how to integrate these two moral mandates is the project of this chapter.

Chapter 18 introduces the controversial issue of whether voluntary lifestyle choices that lead to the need for organs have any legitimate role in allocation. We take the history of alcoholic cirrhosis in cases of liver transplant as our primary example. We easily rule out two more extreme options—totally ignoring whether one is an active alcoholic, or completely banning patients with the history of alcoholism—and then play out our debate, as authors, about whether this history is at all relevant.

Increasingly, as grafts are rejected, some recipients are coming back for second, third, and even fourth transplants. And as we get better at managing transplants, people are stepping forward to receive more than one organ at a time—a kidney and a pancreas; a heart and lungs; or, in one case we consider, no fewer than four different organs. Inevitably, someone perceives these repeat and multiple transplants as consuming more than one's fair share of the scarce resource of organs. Chapter 19 analyzes this problem and argues that not all these "high-consumer" cases are unjustified.

Then, in chapter 20, we deal with the increasingly contentious problem of whether some people are too old or too young to receive organs and what role age ought to have in deciding priorities in allocation. It is here that we examine in detail the new kidney allocation formula. It was first considered because young, prime kidneys were being allocated to elderly recipients who would die with their well-functioning kidney intact, and old kidney donors were providing kidneys that went into young recipients. This led to controversial proposals for age matching and eventually to the newly adopted kidney allocation formula, which takes age into account in a major way. We provide arguments defending the incorporation of age into an allocation formula while also giving reasons why the new formula is ethically deficient.

This is followed by a chapter on the role of fame or status in allocation. We have been able to add two additional case studies—on the now-deceased Apple chief executive officer Steve Jobs and former US vice president Dick Cheney—to the earlier cases of the baseball hero Mickey Mantle and Pennsylvania governor Bob Casey. We try to show just how they got what appear to have been some advantages because of their status while we deflate some mistaken suspicions.

Chapter 22 takes up the increasingly contentious issue of whether where one lives unfairly influences one's likelihood of getting an organ. We suggest that, if equity is a moral requirement for organ allocation, more work must be done to eliminate the unfairness of geographical advantage. We show that even the new kidney formula failed to give adequate consideration to geography.

Chapter 23 takes up what we call socially directed donation, that is, donation with strings attached, giving in such a way that the organs can be used only for members of a certain race, religion, gender, or other sociological group. The early examples involved racially directed donation, but now we are also debating a range of other sociological groups that may be targeted, including children and the military.

Finally, we add two completely new chapters in this second edition: one dealing with elective transplants—transplants for which there is a therapeutic alternative, such as diet; and one dealing with vascular composite allografts—transplants of complex tissues making up critical body parts, including the face, hands, and the uterus.

We have had a great deal of help in preparing this volume. Chapter 10, which claims that countries often believed to have "presumed consent" laws generally make no presumption of consent at all, was originally developed with Jonathan Pitt while he was an intern at the Kennedy Institute of Ethics. For this second edition, much additional research on this chapter, as well as on many others, was done by Thomas Gerkin, to whom we express our acknowledgment and gratitude. He will see sentences from his extensive research incorporated into this volume.

Over the years both authors have also served multiple terms on the Ethics Committee of the national United Network for Organ Sharing (UNOS), which has given us an exposure to the cutting-edge debate on the moral and policy issues as they have emerged on the national scene. The various UNOS chairpersons, members, and staff have been enormously helpful and tolerant when one of us either failed to understand or pressed certain concerns too aggressively. We are particularly grateful to James F. Burdick, Jeremiah G. Turcotte, Michael Shapiro, and Alexandra Glazier, each of whom served as chairs of the UNOS Ethics Committee while we served our terms. We would also like to thank Jason Livingston, the UNOS staff liaison to the committee in recent years and an incredible resource for all UNOS policies and procedures. We have also, at various times, been on UNOS's Living Donor Committee and Vascular Composite Allograft Committee. These UNOS assignments have greatly enriched our understanding of the issues.

Individually, we have had involvement in many other activities over the years that have prepared us for writing this volume. Robert M. Veatch (hereafter, RMV) has, since 1988, been a member of the Board of Directors of the Washington Regional Transplant Community (WRTC), the organ procurement organization for the Washington metropolitan area, and he has grown to have enormous appreciation and respect for the work this group does. He would particularly like to express appreciation to Lori Brigham, the WRTC's president and chief executive officer during that entire time, for the continuing education on all matters transplant. He served as a member of the national Data Safety and Monitoring Committee for the National Institutes of Health / National Eye Institute multicenter Collaborative Cornea Transplant Study from 1986 to 1992. This study, which was working at the frontiers of tissue-typing research, provided an ideal laboratory for on-the-job training in immunology, tissue typing, and immunosuppression science. In the world of privately funded research, he served on the Data Safety Monitoring Board of the Syntex Development Research study of the immunosuppressive drug mycophenolate mofetil, an agent for preventing acute rejection in cardiac transplantation. Also, during the past decade he has been involved in the transplant programs of Georgetown University Medical Center, working on occasion with its transplant programs and growing to appreciate its leadership. He served a three-year term as the ethics consultant to the North American Transplant Coordinators Organization, which he assisted in addressing a number of issues, particularly those related to xenotransplantation. Finally, in the years when the definition-of-death debate was in its infancy, he had the privilege of falling under the wing of and then working with Henry Beecher, the chair of the Harvard Ad

Hoc Committee to Examine the Definition of Brain Death, as well as several committee members, especially Ralph Potter, first while he was a graduate student at Harvard University and then for many years when he served as the staff director of the Hastings Center's Research Group on Death and Dying. These two people, as well as the other members of that research group, provided the ideal context for collaborating and sharing stimulating ideas with some of the most creative and controversial minds in the definition-of-death debate.

Lainie Friedman Ross (hereafter, LFR) has been involved with the University of Chicago's Transplant Surgery team since 1995, when she answered a research ethics consultation phone call from Steve Woodle about the possibility of organ swapping. This led to a *New England Journal of Medicine* publication in 1996. In 1998 she was invited to give a talk about kidney paired exchanges by Bill Barrable, then director of the British Columbia Transplant Society. When the University of British Columbia decided to apply for a Health Research Training Program in Transplantation through the Canadian Institute of Health Research, she was invited to be a co-investigator, and she has visited annually since 2002 to hear progress updates, to give lectures on ethical and policy issues in organ transplantation, and to help with mentorship. She would like to thank Stephen Cheung, Alice Mui, Eric Yoshida, and many other University of British Columbia faculty members, as well as the British Columbia Transplant Society, for their interest in promoting an awareness of ethics among their trainees.

At the University of Chicago, LFR has served informally as the university's first living donor advocate—a role she took on voluntarily, before it became an institutional requirement, as part of her duties as chair of the clinical ethics consultation service. In this capacity she met some of the most generous people she ever imagined—individuals who were willing to fight institutional obstacles to risk their own health for others, despite the unwillingness of the doctors and social workers they met. She also began a long-standing collaboration with Dick Thistlethwaite, who has helped her understand the science and practice of organ transplantation from a surgeon's perspective.

Over the years LFR has participated in several national conferences related to transplantation. She was a member of the working group on assigning priority on the wait list for the National Conference to Analyze the Wait List for Kidney Transplantation, in March 2002; of the Women's Health Committee of the American Society of Transplantation, Reproduction, and Transplantation, in March 2003; of the Workshop on Children with Disabilities and Organ Transplantation, sponsored by the Stanford Center on Biomedical Ethics and the Greenwall Foundation, in August–September 2006; and of the Consensus Conference on Best Practices in Live Kidney Donation, in June 2014.

To the literally hundreds of transplant professionals, bioethics colleagues working in transplantation, transplant recipients, living donors, and donor families we have met while doing research, we express our gratitude for their insights, shared experiences, and stimulation during the many years we have together pursued the issues explored in this volume. It is often when we have fought most intensely that we have learned the most. Those with whom we have done intellectual battle will be only too happy to confirm that they are not responsible for the views expressed here; but at the same time, we are grateful to the many people whose ideas we have borrowed and transformed into this book.

Finally, we are grateful to Richard Brown, the director of Georgetown University Press—an admired editor, academic, and lover of books for many years—for the opportunity to place this volume in the Press's bioethics series.

Robert M. Veatch, Washington
Lainie Friedman Ross, Chicago

Chapter 1

Religious and Cultural Perspectives

Although fantasies about replacing body parts date from ancient times, the modern bioethical debate over organ transplants does not go back much further than the first kidney transplant in 1954—only a moment in time in the history of the world's religions and cultures. The current generation of controversy, however, is even more recent. It can be dated from December 3, 1967, when a South African physician, Christiaan Bernard, transplanted the first human heart into the chest of Louis Washkansky. It is thus necessarily difficult to determine what the great religious and cultural traditions might have thought about such a project.

We can imagine someone seeing such an enterprise as "tampering" with God's creation. Conversely, Judeo-Christianity, one of the world's great religious traditions, has long taught that the human was created with the command to have dominion over the Earth and subdue it—to use the God-given faculties of reason and observation to overcome illness and heal the afflicted. Although some sectarian religions might see all of modern medical science as reflecting a lack of adequate faith in divine power, the mainstream Western religious traditions have supported the use of medical science. Their members have run hospitals, trained physicians and nurses, and contributed countless sums attempting to overcome disease.

Before pursuing the more specific issues of the ethics of transplants, however, it is helpful to look at the positions of the major religious and cultural traditions to see how they incorporate this very new issue into their ancient ethical frameworks. The contemporary bioethical debate over organ transplantation contains two issues that can be considered preliminary and two issues that are central or core. The ethics of the definition of death, which is the focus of part I of this volume, and the potential controversy over intervening in a dead body for the removal of cadaver organs can be thought of as preliminary. The justification for procuring organs, which is the subject of part II, and the distribution of organs once procured, which are explored in part III, are central.

Defining Death and Desecrating the Corpse: Two Preliminary Issues

We first consider the two preliminary issues: defining death and removing organs from dead bodies. Both are addressed, at least indirectly, by many of the world's religions.

1

Defining Death

All the major religious traditions reveal some differences of opinion over a shift to the use of a brain-oriented definition of death, a shift that is important if organ procurement is to be facilitated. Let us briefly consider their views.

Judaism

Within Judaism, there has been considerable resistance to shifting to a brain-oriented definition of death. Rabbi David Bleich, a philosopher at Yeshiva University, for example, opposes any shift, saying that "the patient cannot be pronounced dead other than upon the irreversible cessation of both cardiac and respiratory activity."[1] This interpretation was confirmed recently by the United Kingdom's chief rabbi, Jonathan Sacks, who issued an edict indicating that Judaism can only accept the traditional halachic definition based on cardiorespiratory failure.[2] Conversely, other rabbis from the Conservative and Reformed traditions have endorsed the use of brain criteria for death pronouncements.[3] The Orthodox Rabbinical Council of America takes no stand on whether brain-based death pronouncement conforms to halachic teaching.[4]

Roman Catholicism

Among Catholics, Pope Pius XII opened the door for a shift in the definition of death in 1957, saying, "It remains for the doctor, and especially the anesthesiologist, to give a clear and precise definition of death and the moment of death of a patient who passes away in a state of unconsciousness."[5] In the United States, the most recent statement of the Conference of Catholic Bishops continues to imply that "commonly accepted scientific criteria" provide a basis for determining death.[6] There have never been any principled theological objections to a brain-oriented definition of death among Catholics, although occasionally conservative Catholics, often those most militantly associated with right-to-life positions, have expressed the fear that endorsing the view that an individual is dead when the brain is dead might indirectly lessen respect for those who are still living.[7] Recently, a few Catholic commentators have criticized brain-based death pronouncements, but a September 2006 meeting convened by the Pontifical Academy of Sciences reaffirmed the papal position that a human dies when brain function is lost irreversibly.[8]

Protestantism and Eastern Orthodoxy

Protestant theologians and Protestant groups, when they have spoken on the subject, have almost uniformly favored some brain-oriented definition of death, whether they represent more conservative (Paul Ramsey) or liberal (Joseph Fletcher) perspectives.[9] Major Protestant communions support its use, including Anglicans, Lutherans, Methodists, and the Reformed traditions.[10] The same can be said for Eastern Orthodox groups.[11]

Thus, though there is some concern about the use of a brain-oriented definition of death, at least some responsible members of all major Judeo-Christian religious traditions accept it theologically and find it appropriate as a basis for procuring organs from deceased donors. Most have not pursued the more recent distinction, made in part I of this book, between whole-brain and higher-brain views, although some who have worked in both the Catholic and Protestant communities have moved on to endorse the higher-brain view. Almost all in these traditions also accept organ procurement from people pronounced dead by traditional circulatory criteria.

Other Major Religions

Most of the other major religions of the world also have members who have come to accept death pronouncement based on brain criteria. Let use briefly examine each one.

ISLAM

The 1981 Islamic Code of Medical Ethics of the International Organization of Islamic Medicine is vague on the subject of the definition of death. In language reminiscent of Pius XII, it said, "To declare a person dead is a grave responsibility that ultimately rests with the Doctor."[12] It says nothing against the use of brain criteria for death pronouncement, but does not explicitly endorse them either. Initially, there were reservations among Muslims about death defined as lack of brain activity rather than the conventional definition of respiratory and circulatory arrest. These issues were discussed at a seminar titled "Human Life: Its Inception and Its End as Viewed by Islam."[13] The report of this meeting concluded that the Quran does not define death. The participants came to the conclusion that when the area of the brain responsible for vital body functions is lifeless, the patient can be said to have died. This they identified with the brain stem.[14] They concluded that while the brain stem is still alive, all efforts must be made to revive the person. If the brain stem is dead, even when signs of activity are still visible in the bodily organs, and if there is no hope of reviving the patient, then the patient is "considered to have withdrawn from life," and behaviors associated with the dead—including procuring of organs—are permitted.[15] A similar conclusion was reached at the Third International Conference of Islamic Jurists meeting in Amman in October 1986, where they endorsed the view that a person may be declared dead either based on heart criteria or if there is "complete stoppage of all the vital functions of the brain, and the doctors decide it is irreversible, and the brain has started to degenerate."[16] Some Islamic countries, such as Turkey, have an explicit law defining death in terms of irreversible loss of brain function.[17] Iran accepted this view by law in 2000, and its Cabinet Council established bylaws governing brain-based death pronouncement in 2002.[18]

HINDUISM

Traditionally, Hindu texts associated death with respiratory failure. However, a physician, Prakash Desai, who is a specialist in Indian medical ethics, claims to see a basis for support of brain death in the notion from folklore that at death the *prana* (breath) escapes from the brain.[19] Suffice it to say that there appears to be no formal resistance to death pronouncement based on brain function criteria in Hinduism.

CONFUCIANISM/TAOISM

In China traditional religious and cultural systems of thought are still influential, although it is often hard to draw direct links between traditional views and contemporary biomedical practices. Because "brain death" was not explicitly recognized in ancient times and traditional Chinese religious thought has not received much attention in contemporary Marxist China until very recently, it is hard to know exactly what the major Chinese systems of belief and value would think about it. There is nothing explicit to which one could point to identify resistance to brain-based concepts of death in either Confucian or Taoist thought, but there are reports that there is a "lack of widespread acceptance of 'brain death' criteria in China."[20]

Buddhism and Shintoism

In addition to the traditions already mentioned, India and China—as well as many other Asian countries—are influenced by Buddhism. Buddhism is decidedly ambivalent about organ transplantation, and especially about efforts to redefine death that are linked to facilitating transplants. As with the other major religious traditions, Buddhism comes in many different varieties, and its expression varies from one country and group to the next.

Japan is particularly well known for its resistance to brain-oriented definitions of death, and this resistance is often attributed either to Buddhist influences or to the indigenous Japanese belief system that Westerners call Shintoism. Buddhism does not directly oppose brain-oriented definitions of death, but it has sometimes suggested skepticism. A 1990 report from the Japanese Association of Indian and Buddhist Studies could only state the opinion that "Buddhists should resolve the issue of brain death and organ transplantation," expressing the confusion found in Pope Pius XII and other Western thinkers that this is a question for physicians to resolve. It said in somewhat nonsyntactic English, "We Buddhists ask the medical world to make a consensus among medical doctors."[21]

Some Buddhist scholars find a brain-based concept of death compatible with their traditional concept of death. The Buddhist concept of *prana*, variously translated "breath" or "life," is associated with brainstem functioning by the Thai monk Bhikkhu Mettananda.[22] This conclusion is shared by other Buddhist scholars, even though they would clearly reject a higher-brain view.[23] One Western analyst goes further, associating death in Buddhist thought with the loss of consciousness.[24] In 1995 Soka Gakkai, Japan's largest lay Buddhist organization, endorsed support for brain-based criteria for death pronouncement once the medical community supports such efforts.[25]

Nevertheless, some Buddhist scholars find themes in Buddhism that lead them to conclude that pronouncing death based brain criteria requires viewing the body as an "assemblage of organs." As Masao Fujii, a professor of religious studies at Taisho University, a private Buddhist university located in Nishi-Sugamo, northwest Tokyo, puts it: "Brain death . . . seems unequivocally opposed to Buddhist ideals. For brain death regards the body simply as an assemblage of organs, of which the brain is the critical one. Thus, if the brain dies, one is to disregard the fact that other organs are still functioning, and declare the whole body and the whole person dead. In this respect, the cycle of birth and death is broken; one is permitted to explant particular organs whose cells are alive from a body [whose] brain is [dead]. This way of thinking is incompatible with the Buddhist ideal of the "oneness of birth and death."[26]

The same Western analyst who associates Buddhist notions of death with the loss of consciousness suggests that Buddhists will not localize this consciousness in the brain, and also notes that this consciousness may reside within the body for up to a week after the dying process would be considered completed by Westerners. He ends up concluding that Buddhism actually opposes brain-based concepts of death.[27] The most reasonable conclusion seems to be that there is sufficient ambiguity within Buddhist thought that brain-based definitions of death can be both defended and opposed.[28]

It is possible that the uniquely Japanese resistance to brain-based definitions of death should be traced more to the indigenous religious beliefs that Westerners call Shintoism. Two themes are particularly important. First, Shinto thought resists a rigid separation of the body and the soul, making the association of death with a particular organ difficult. One wise Japanese medical professional once told one of us, "You Westerners believe that the soul resides in the brain. We Japanese think the soul exists throughout the body." In this observation, she was reflecting a classical Shinto insight. Second, Shinto thinkers have held unique beliefs about the newly dead body, maintaining that there is a period of some forty-nine days when the soul is considered polluted by death in which the person is considered not yet fully dead.[29]

Given these reservations based on traditional religious views, it is not surprising that Japan has been one of the last countries of the developed world to adopt a brain-oriented definition of death. After a decades-long national debate, in 1997 it adopted a very narrowly focused law authorizing death pronouncement based on brain criteria, but only if the intent is to procure organs, and then only if the deceased has consented in advance to both organ procurement and the use of brain-criteria and only if the family also agrees.[30] Even so, many Japanese continue to resist brain-based death pronouncement.

Desecrating the Corpse

The second preliminary topic is the cultural views about desecrating the corpse in the major religious traditions. Even if one concludes that the body is dead, an ethical judgment still needs to be made about the legitimacy of removing organs.

Judeo-Christianity

In the Jewish and Christian traditions, we first briefly describe the teachings of Catholic and Protestant groups. Then we discuss the teachings of Judaism, Fundamentalist Protestantism, and African American Christianity.

Catholic and Protestant Groups

Substantial ethical agreement also exists on the second preliminary ethical question, the ethics of intervening into the dead body in order to remove organs for transplanting. Objections to the removal of organs for lifesaving purposes from human bodies once it is established that they are dead are rare among either the secular or religious bioethical community. Protestants and Catholics have raised no serious questions about cadaver organ removal, provided that appropriate respect is shown for the deceased and appropriate permissions are obtained.[31] In fact, these groups have generally endorsed such a lifesaving gift giving as a noble act. They have also tended to support the xenotransplantation of organs from nonhuman animals. Undoubtedly, these views are related to the religious view of creation that places the human in a privileged position, considering the "lower animals" to have a subordinate status over which humans should have dominion.

JUDAISM

Jewish thought poses a more serious question because in Judaism there are religious obligations to bury the dead with organs intact.[32] However, this obligation is superseded when a cadaver organ can be removed for the purpose of saving the life of another identified person in need. Thus the dominant American religious traditions accept the legitimacy of removing cadaver organs for lifesaving transplantation. Some may insist on more conservative heart-and-lung-oriented criteria for death and some, especially Orthodox Jews, may object to organ removal for research or educational purposes, but the two preliminary ethical problems pose no insurmountable obstacles for cadaver organ procurement. In fact, Judaism, Catholicism, and the major Protestant denominations all place a high value on the saving of human life so that, though the state may not be authorized to salvage organs routinely, individuals bear at least a moral obligation to facilitate organ procurement for lifesaving purposes.[33]

FUNDAMENTALIST PROTESTANTISM

One religious doctrine potentially poses a problem for members of more fundamentalist Protestant groups. Christianity is a religion that affirms a bodily resurrection. For certain fundamentalist groups, this doctrine plays a very central role. The resurrection in bodily form is a vivid hope for the oppressed and a near-constant source of solace for those who have been separated from loved ones. This is an otherworldly spiritualism that takes the biblical vision of a new heavenly life quite literally. For such believers, the thought of a resurrection without some of their vital organs must be quite horrifying, and such an image has undoubtedly produced some resistance to organ donation.

This turns out to be an overly simplistic theological interpretation. Concern about disease or a damaged physical body has been voiced by Christian theologians since the middle ages. After all, deaths have always occurred with painful, debilitating diseases; and deaths involving immolation in fires or in body-crushing accidents would have always posed a serious concern for believers in a bodily resurrection. A more nuanced understanding of church teaching, however, reveals that the medieval theologians held the doctrine of the "new" of "perfect" body. They held that the saved would regain life in bodily form, but the body would be in a new and perfected form. It would have the same physical appearance as one's earthly body, but without any of its flaws, diseases, or damage. They had seen skeletal remains of deceased humans and knew that flesh deteriorates, but have long had a theological solution to this problem. The idea of the new body is well-known in contemporary fundamentalist Christianity. Consider, for example, the very popular gospel song, "I'll Have a New Body," recorded by Hank Williams (senior), the greatest country singer of all time:

> When 'ol Gabriel blows his trumpet and we walk the streets of gold
> I'll have a new body, praise the Lord I'll have a new life
> No more pain, worry, sorrow in this wicked world of sin
> I'll have a new body praise the Lord I'll have a new life!

Never let it be said that those country singers did not know their medieval theology. Thus, fundamentalist Christians who really understand their church's doctrine should not have any problem with organ donation as far as belief in a resurrection of the body is concerned.

AFRICAN AMERICAN CHRISTIANITY

African American culture is heavily influenced by the black church, which is often Protestant. Its power cannot be overemphasized. As with the more fundamentalist white Protestant church, which was often historically the source of black denominations, concern about the body and its resurrected condition has often been great. Much attention has been given to the reasons why African Americans are less inclined to donate organs for transplant. This is a particular problem because hypertension rates are much higher among blacks, and therefore kidney failure is a significant problem, generating the need for organs that are histocompatible with black recipients.

Clive Callender, professor of surgery and director of the Transplant Center at Howard University in Washington, has conducted research attempting to determine the reasons for the low donation rate among blacks. He has identified eight reasons, including a perception among blacks that organs are inequitably distributed, distrust of the white-dominated health care system, and fear that signing donor cards will lead to premature declaration of death. He also lists several social and educational reasons: suboptimal use of the community as a change agent, inadequate involvement of the community in decision making, a lack of transplant awareness, and an inadequate emphasis on behavior modification toward health promotion and disease prevention. However, one of the reasons he identifies is "religious myths and misperceptions."[34]

As one African American clergyman put it, "On their great getting-up morning, blacks don't want to go to the pearly gates without organs; . . . they want to go to Jesus whole."[35] A very insightful and sensitive analysis of the relation between the African American church and organ donation is provided by Howard Divinity School professor Cheryl Sanders.[36] She acknowledges that the black church has sometimes endorsed views about the resurrection that have made African Americans resistant to donation, but she is critical of those who would simply ridicule these beliefs as superstition and "myth" (in the pejorative sense). She, however, "revisits" the religious considerations in an effective attempt to show that black theology can provide a basis for supporting organ donation. She reviews the arguments leading to the conclusion that the resurrection of the body cannot be contingent upon the condition of the bodily remains, pointing to the effect on the corpse of embalming practices that remove blood as potentially posing similar problems for those concerned about a resurrected body that was damaged during earthly life.[37] She concludes that "it may well be that the individual whose body has been mutilated as a result of a decision to donate based upon the practice of [the Christian virtues of] faith, hope, and love will fare much better in the final judgment than the one whose body parts remained intact because of a refusal to take steps to provide the gift of life for someone else."[38]

Sanders suggests, based on the doctor of ministry dissertation of Father George Ehusani, an African who is a Roman Catholic priest, that African American religious concerns about preserving the body intact may have roots that are deeper than the fundamentalist Protestant theology taught by Caucasians.[39] Ehusani, describing the beliefs of his own Ebira of Nigeria, indicates that African culture attributes sacredness to the entire human body, viewing each part or organ as a microcosm of the whole person and thus leading to the practice of carefully disposing of hair and hair and nail clippings because of the spiritual power associated with any human body parts. Sanders observes that "a people who discern spirit identity in hair and nail cuttings would necessarily be skeptical of the practice of removing and transplanting vital bodily organs such as the kidney and the heart."[40] Thus African American resistance to organ donation may reflect lingering hints of a deeply embedded belief system that will need to be considered by programs designed to promote organ donation in this community.

Other Major Religions

Similar concerns about taking organs from the dead body arise in other religions. Islam is one tradition to consider. Then we also discuss Hinduism and Buddhism.

ISLAM

Muslims hold that the body is sacred—entrusted to one's care on Earth. They maintain that harm must not be done to it, in life or in death. Arab countries generally agree with organ procurement, whereas Muslims on the Indian subcontinent usually do not. For example, it is reported that many Muslim jurists in Pakistan have concluded that organ donation is not acceptable.[41] Nevertheless, in recent years, Pakistani leaders have reviewed the fatwas and substantiated their legitimacy, and have passed legislation to ensure correct transplantation norms.[42] The general population also tends to feel positively toward donation.[43] But guidelines set limits, including that transplants occur only when no other treatment is available, that the procedure has a good chance of success, that voluntary consent is obtained from either the donor or the next of kin to procure the organs, and that death has accurately been pronounced. Live organ donation is considered to be a risk to the body and is only permitted when it is a lifesaving procedure. But as part of a collective society, it is a Muslim's duty to aid others through organ donation if life is at stake.[44]

Although considerable debate has taken place within various Islamic societies, generally, procurement by donation has been considered acceptable to many Muslims. In fact, in ways similar to Judaism, the donation of organs in Islam is seen as a duty to one's fellow human beings. According to the Islamic Code of Medical Ethics: "The individual patient is the collective responsibility of Society, that has to ensure his health needs by any means inflicting no harm on others. This comprises the donation of body fluids or organs such as blood transfusion to the bleeding or a kidney transplant to the patient with bilateral irreparable renal damage. This is another 'Fardh Kifaya', a duty that donors fulfill on behalf of society."[45]

The physician and medical ethicist Hassan Hathout further explicates the Islamic community's position, citing other authoritative meetings. He cites two juridical rules: first, that "necessities overrule prohibitions"; and, second, that "the choice of the lesser of two evils" is morally preferred.[46]

Hinduism

In the early years of transplants, deceased donor organ transplantation was reported to be rare in India.[47] Although the first deceased donor renal transplant was performed in 1965, even up to the late 1980s, only three states in India had passed legislation to permit deceased donor procurement.[48] In 1994 India passed the Transplantation of Human Organ Act (THOA), which was adopted in all the country's states except Jammu and Kashmir and Andhra Pradesh, which have enacted their own legislation; but few deceased donor transplants occurred.[49] THOA permitted living donation between first-degree relatives and spouses and proposed civil and criminal penalties for other live donations unless reviewed by an authorization committee, and yet living organ trafficking persisted. THOA was revised in 2008 and 2011, and it is now mandatory that hospital staff request deceased donation from family members of a brain-dead patient.[50] The revisions expand the definition of "near relatives" to include grandparents and grandchildren, and propose criminal and civil penalties for falsifying documents.[51] But the evidence of any religiously based objection is complex. The fact that organs are regularly procured from living sources (donor is not the right word, as we shall see below) suggests that there is no principled objection either to organ procurement or to transplantation itself. Recent reviews support this conclusion.[52] The great expense of transplantation and the relatively small numbers of people that it benefits suggest that India may simply have other priorities.

Wendy Doniger points out that the Hindu religious imperative to reduce the body to ashes and the belief that a dead body is literally untouchable may account for Hindus' disinclination to donate their organs.[53] Conversely, she traces Hindu as well as Buddhist myth that treats the giving of eyes and other body parts as virtuous behavior.[54] Prakash Desai cites these myths as a basis for his claim that organ transplants are well received when they are available.[55] That these myths involve living donors is probably not irrelevant to current live donor and live vendor practices in India.

Doniger also sees significance in the Hindu doctrine of karma, which holds that the action one engages in this world affects how one will be reborn. This creates what she calls a "boundary" problem.[56] Karma can be transferred in intimate exchanges with others. This affects the Hindu understanding of the sharing of food and sexual relations. It surely would also have a bearing on organ exchanges. Depending on whether good or bad karma is being transferred, a Hindu may be more or less inclined to donate or receive the organs of others. Citing the work of E. Valentine Daniell, she summarizes, "The fluidity of bodies in India makes you more, rather than less, nervous about sharing body parts."[57]

Relatively little information is available about the medical and ethical views of the Sikhs, a modern movement with roots in Hinduism that is monotheistic and rejects the Hindu caste system. Black reports that Sikhs also accept organ transplants.[58] More recent surveys support this conclusion.[59]

Confucianism/Taoism

As noted above, there is relatively little information available in the West regarding Chinese ethical views on transplantation.[60] Aside from the reported resistance to the use of brain criteria for death pronouncement, there appears to be no principled objection to organ procurement for transplantation. Kidney transplantation has been performed in China for many years. The main resistance seems to be one of economic priority. There is a clear preference for using scarce resources for prevention and early-stage treatment. Ren-Zong Qiu, the leading biomedical ethicist in China today, says that "the emphasis should be put on prevention, early treatment, treatment of pre-end-stage renal diseases, and nondialysis treatment."[61] Nevertheless, large numbers of transplants now take place in China, although there has been some decline because commitments have been made to restrict the procurement of organs from executed prisoners. This was formerly a large source of organs, but a commitment exists to develop a system of organ donation and to stop using prisoners in 2014.[62]

These attitudes seem compatible with traditional Confucian views that are more accepting of the inevitability of death than Western religious traditions.[63] Conversely, Taoism has tended toward more aggressive pursuit of the prolongation of life, an attitude that could fuel support for organ transplants.[64]

BUDDHISM

Buddhism, the other great religious tradition of Asia, is somewhat more ambivalent about transplantation. One scholar noted that by his writing in 1988 the Sangha, the organization of Buddhist followers, has taken no absolute position on organ transplantation.[65] Buddhist scholars generally praise donation of organs as a compassionate and praiseworthy gesture. Scholars of Buddhism, writing about transplantation, have pointed to the teaching of Buddha encouraging dedication to the benefit of others through giving, including admiration of self-immolation, which is seen as relevant to donation of body parts.[66] In fact, they give this generosity such prominence that they are not always greatly concerned about whether death has been firmly established before organs are procured.[67] Moreover, Buddhism deemphasizes the importance of the body, and its embrace of cremation is taken by Buddhist scholars as evidence that the body is unimportant for any future life.

Conversely, though there is no direct proscription on transplants in Buddhism, there are tenets within the tradition that might discourage it. For one, Buddhism opposes an "unseemly attachment to life as well as disruption of the dying process."[68] This leads Masao Fujii to conclude that "Buddhism affirms the idea of giving one's internal organ to others, but the idea that a recipient would receive an organ with the desire to prolong his own life is not supported."[69] Any uncertainty about whether the still-respiring body is really dead could be exacerbated by these concerns. According to the anthropologist Margaret Lock, most Japanese remain aware that in Buddhism, "the process of dying is not complete until services held on the seventh and forty-ninth days are performed."[70] This surely could create an environment in which a family would be reluctant to support procurement of organs from the body.

Nolan, after considering the claim that Japanese resistance to organ transplant can be traced to Buddhist beliefs about reincarnation, concludes that "concerns about survival in the afterlife and bodily reincarnation actually fit more closely with Confucian and Shinto beliefs about the unity of body and spirit than with Buddhist notions of rebirth.[71]

Shintoism

In addition to the indigenous Japanese religious beliefs about the unity of body and spirit, Shintoism traditionally has considered all contact with the dead body as ritually polluting.[72] Moreover, Shintoism centers on the religious significance of the spirits of the ancestors. Not only does this lead to skepticism about the use of brain criteria for pronouncing death, but also to pervasive doubt that procuring organs is an appropriate way to show respect for one's future ancestors.[73] Helen Hardacre, in a review of Buddhist and Shinto views on brain death and organ transplants, concludes that Shinto writers are either clearly opposed to organ transplants or extremely cautious.[74]

The Two Central Ethical Issues

This brings us to the two central issues: procurement and allocation. We consider procurement first, and then allocation.

Donation versus Routine Salvaging

This brings us to the two more critical and controversial core ethical issues that are the primary foci of this book. First, there is the controversy over donation versus the routine salvaging of organs, which is the topic of part II. It has been recognized for years that there are two basic alternatives for organ procurement: donation and salvaging. A more detailed examination of these two major alternative models for organ procurement will be given in chapters 9 and 10. (A third option, the use of market mechanisms, will be explored in chapter 11.) Here, we want simply to see how the major religious and cultural traditions approach this central choice.

One of the earliest plans for the systematic procurement of organs was offered in 1968 by a lawyer, Jesse Dukeminier, and a physician, David Sanders. They proposed that organs from the deceased be routinely "salvaged"—that is, taken without any formal consent when they are needed as a social resource.[75] The dead body would simply be presumed to be the property of the state when it could serve a useful purpose. Normally, advocates of salvaging would permit individuals to object in writing while living or even permit relatives to object in cases where the individual has not expressed his or her wishes to the contrary.

The other alternative relies on donation. The assumption is that an individual has rights over and against the state, including the right to bodily integrity. Holders of this view insist that these rights do not cease upon death. Although the state possesses certain rights to protect society from infectious diseases and to perform an autopsy when foul play is suspected, it does not automatically have the right to appropriate body parts. Under this approach, the deceased retains some right of control over how his or her body is treated, even after death. Some advocates of this view believe that this property right includes the option of selling body parts, not just donating them. Hence, arrangements to transfer organs through the use of markets and incentives can be seen as a variant of the donation model. Both rely on the belief about some level of right to control access to the dead body.

Relatives or people designated by the deceased when he or she was still alive may acquire a limited quasi–property right to make certain decisions about disposition (within the framework of the deceased's own wishes). These rights may be limited not only by constraints on the taking of valuable consideration but also by the duty to dispose of the bodily remains respectfully and properly. Thus others with authority to speak for the deceased may acquire a right to make the decision whether to permit organs to be procured (within the constraints of the deceased's own wishes).

Judeo-Christianity

It is this second alternative that has been favored by virtually every writer within the Judeo-Christian tradition and by every religious group speaking on the subject.[76] The reason is fundamentally that according to the Judeo-Christian tradition, respect for the individual and the rights associated with that individual do not cease at death. Obligations of respect—for the wishes of the deceased and the integrity of his or her earthly remains—must continue. In the Judeo-Christian tradition, as opposed to much pagan Greek thought, the body is affirmed to be a central part of the total spiritual being. Any approach that abandons the mode of donation in favor of viewing the cadaver as a social resource to be mined for worthwhile social purposes will directly violate central tenets of Christian thought and will also create serious problems for Jews. It will predictably produce vociferous, agitated opposition, although probably less dramatic than the street riots sparked in Israel after the passage of autopsy laws permitting routine violation of the corpse.[77] Markets for organs have generally been rejected, at least in part due to their perceived infringing on obligations to the newly deceased.

At the same time there is uniform support in all major traditions not only for the ethical acceptability of donation but also for the actual moral obligation to take organ donation seriously. In fact, Judaism has been interpreted as imposing a positive duty to provide organs for transplant if an identifiable life can be saved. This suggests that, though Judeo-Christianity would oppose routine salvaging by the state and would be skeptical of any financial compensation for organs, these traditions would look favorably upon public policies to make donation as easy as possible. Given the fact that these religious traditions all support organ donation in at least some circumstances, and in fact consider it a morally weighty obligation, they would favor public policies making it as easy as possible to express a willingness to donate organs for lifesaving purposes.

Israel passed the Organ Transplant Act 2008, which came into effect in January 2010. This act gives bonus allocation priority points to individuals waiting for a deceased donor organ if (1) the individual signs a donor card, (2) the individual's family members sign donor cards, and (3) the individual consents to the donation of organs of deceased first-degree relatives.[78] Although the law raises questions of justice and fairness, and there are concerns that individuals will "game" the system, the law makes Israel the first country to implement a system to give priority points to those willing to donate, a concept that has been proposed in the United States for a number of years.[79]

The public policy implication is that the correct solution to the donation-versus-salvaging controversy is maximum encouragement to facilitate donation, provided this does not subtly coerce those unwilling to donate and does not trick them into donating unintentionally. Donor registries, such as those at state departments of motor vehicles, would seem reasonable. In addition, questions on federal documents, especially those already computerized for easy retrieval, such as income tax returns or social security records, might also be appropriate. This is a proposal we consider more formally in chapter 11.

Other Major Religions

Similar concerns arise in the other major religious traditions. Islam is considered first, and then Hinduism, Confucianism/Taoism, and Buddhism and Shintoism.

ISLAM

Islamic documents stress that organ procurement must be by voluntary donation, either from the deceased, through an advance gift, or from the family. According to the Islamic Code, "Organ donation shall never be the outcome of compulsion, family embarrassment, social, or other pressure or exploitation of financial need."[80] There is also a stricture that the donation "not entail the exposure of the donor to harm," a requirement easily met in the case of cadaver donation, but presumably difficult to satisfy in the case of living donation.[81] However, because the code speaks clearly of developing regulations for the live donation of organs, some level of harm greater than that of live donor organ procurement must be implied. Even in the face of the commitment that saving another's life is morally imperative, still, according to Islamic scholars, no organ should be taken by coercion or even pressure. In Singapore a law permitting organ procurement without explicit donor consent originally excluded Muslims, who had to opt in to become donors. That law was amended in 2008 so that Muslims also could have organs taken without explicit consent because Singapore's Fatwa Committee, under the leadership of its highest Islamic authority, Mufti Syed Isa Semait, had determined that Muslims had sufficient opportunity to opt out of procurement.[82] Markets in human organs are proscribed by key fatwas (legal rulings), although some opening to markets may be implied by the maxim that necessity makes prohibited behavior acceptable.[83] A limited government-controlled market to buy kidneys from willing citizens exists in Iran.[84]

HINDUISM

Although many cultures debate the differences between organ donation and routine salvaging, some theoreticians propose markets for organs, in which those needing organs who are able and willing to pay will buy a kidney from someone who would rather have the money than the organ.[85] One culture where such markets are known to have existed was India.[86] A surgeon, K. C. Reddy, brokered transactions in which those desperate for money sold one of their kidneys to those willing to pay.[87] The relation with Hinduism is difficult to establish. Prakash Desai, a respected physician and interpreter of bioethics in India, and C. M. Francis, the director of Saint Martha's Hospital in Bangalore, condemn the practice.[88] Nevertheless, even though there are many critics and though buying and selling organs in India is illegal, something in Indian culture makes a market for organs thinkable in a way that it is not in other societies. Some of these reasons are undoubtedly socioeconomic. The poverty of large masses in India makes their situation desperate. Even modest payments from wealthy elites from India or elsewhere provide multiples of yearly incomes for the destitute. It is very hard for people from other cultures to understand the economic pressures and even harder to be critical of a mother who decides to sell her kidney in order to feed her children.

The tougher question is whether there is something in Indian culture—perhaps particularly in Hinduism—that contributes to this complex and tragic situation. The Hindu doctrine of karma suggests that people are reborn into this world into positions determined by their previous life. Those who are born into lower socioeconomic strata (reflecting a traditional caste system grounded in Indian religion and culture) may be said to deserve what they get. Perhaps that contributes to an indifference that helps make a market for organs possible.[89]

Confucianism/Taoism

Traditional Confucian ideals isolate the practice of medicine from the business of medicine. In fact, the norm was to strive to practice medicine within the family rather than having to make do with a "mere professional" physician.[90] There are still signals of moral preference for the donation of organs and opposition to commercialization.[91] Nevertheless, recent reports from China suggest compromises—first with reports of markets for organs; and second with what appears to be a widespread practice of organ procurement from condemned prisoners (albeit with the formal requirement of consent).[92] However, this situation may be evolving. During a conference in March 2012, Huang Jiefu, China's vice minister of health, announced that China will ban the transplantation of human organs from executed prisoners in three to five years.[93]

Buddhism and Shintoism

Buddhism also places great emphasis on organs being donated freely. Nolan quotes the Tibetan meditation master Sogyal Rinpoche: "Masters whom I have asked . . . agree that organ donation is an extremely positive action, because it stems from a genuine compassionate wish to benefit others. So, as long as it is truly the wish of the dying person, it will not harm in any way the consciousness that is leaving the body. On the contrary, this final act of generosity accumulates good karma."[94]

In Japan the explicit consent of both the donor and the donor's family is required by the new transplantation law, a policy that has been grounded in the Buddhist affirmation of giving.[95] Routine salvaging seems unlikely, and buying and selling organs is illegal.[96] If organs were obtained by any intervention other than one based on donation, the act would manifest "little or no virtuous benefit."[97] In 1992, presumably relying on the traditional cardiac definition of death, a physician who is also a Buddhist priest turned off the respirator of a comatose woman and removed the kidneys and corneas. He did so based on the specific gift of the donor and the consent of the family.[98] Conversely, Japanese culture includes patterns that would make obtaining such a donation difficult. Asking for the gift is something physicians are reluctant to do. Moreover, the gift-giving ritual in Japan is extremely complex and normally requires reciprocity, something the organ recipient would not be able to provide to the deceased. Finally, though markets for organs are prohibited, it is a common practice for the Japanese to give gifts to their physicians and surgeons. This could potentially lead to associating reward to surgeons with the provision of the transplant, which could leave the borders between gift giving and payment ambiguous.[99]

The Distribution of Organs

This brings us to the other critical question that this book considers: the distribution of organs once they are procured. The primary moral tension in allocating organs among those waiting for them is the conflict between their efficient use and fair distribution. It turns out that sometimes distributing organs to those who will predictably get the most benefit from them—the most years of expected organ and patient survival, for example— will mean they are distributed in ways that most people would consider unfair. There are also issues related to the ethical principle of autonomy. These issues are addressed in part III of this book, but a preliminary summary of the views of the major religious traditions is appropriate here.

Judeo-Christianity

The Judeo-Christian tradition is deeply committed to distribution on the basis of need. The single dominant theme of both Jewish and Christian ethics has been the responsibility to those in need—the lame, the halt, the blind, and those in need of organs. Any allocation system that permits other variables—such as ability to pay or judgment about how socially useful a recipient will be—is uniformly opposed by all commentators working from within these traditions.

Some unfair allocation systems may not seem as blatant as direct market mechanisms to buy organs. In the early years of transplants, Medicare policy prohibited the funding of heart transplants under government health insurance, a policy that had a similar impact of discriminating against the needy. Spokespeople for religious groups and theologians writing within these traditions are realists. They recognize that the government cannot make a commitment to pay for all possible medical care. They do, however, share with the President's Commission for the Study of Ethical Problems in Medicine and Biomedical and Behavioral Research the conviction that there should be some floor level of health care under which no one ought to fall. In the allocation of scarce organs for transplants—at least in cases such as hearts, kidneys, and livers, where the organs are literally lifesaving—allocation is simply unfair if it is based on the potential recipient's ability to pay. If anyone has access, all should have an equal chance—by some lottery system, a random assignment of organs to those in equal need, or by the randomness of having each person wait in line for the needed organs. This is the conclusion reached by virtually every theologian writing in the Judeo-Christian tradition.

The Other Major Religious Traditions

We now turn to the other major religious traditions. There is considerable ambiguity here.

ISLAM

Little is said in the Islamic medical ethical literature about the specific principles of allocation of organs for transplanting, but the implications of more general statements about the duty of society to protect the individual seem clear. In the section quoted above of the "Islamic Code of Medical Ethics," dealing with modern biomedical advances—which deals primarily with organ transplants—the collective responsibility of the community is stated directly: "The individual patient is the collective responsibility of the Society."[100] Although this literature offers no explicit injunction to allocate scarce organs equitably, this conclusion seems evident from the emphasis on collective responsibility. If one member suffers an ailment, all others "rally in response." In a section focusing on equitable access to health care, Gamal Serour emphasizes that the ethical principle of justice in Islam implies that all people should have equitable access.[101] Nevertheless, at least one source suggests that when it comes to a Muslim accepting an organ, it should come from a non-Muslim only if none is available from a Muslim.[102]

HINDUISM

Traditional Hinduism is well known to have embraced a caste system that places socioeconomic status on a deep-seated religious basis. The idea that one's future lives will be affected via the doctrine of karma by the life one is presently leading permeates a Hindu sense that people "get what they deserve." This is reflected in medicine and attitudes about the allocation of medical resources. For example, the Caraca Samhita, the best-known ancient code of ethical conduct for physicians from the Vedic scriptures, contains the following: "No persons, who are hated by the king or who are haters of the king or who are hated by the public or who are haters of the public, shall receive treatment. Similarly, those who are extremely abnormal, wicked, and of miserable character and conduct, those who have not vindicated their honor, those who are on the point of death, and similarly women who are unattended by their husbands or guardians shall not receive treatment."[103]

Of course, not all modern Hindus subscribe rigidly to this ancient doctrine, but such a stance cannot help but provide a background for contemporary theories of the allocation of organs. One suspects that this ancient religious doctrine shapes both the enormous differences in income levels in modern India and the willingness of many of its people to tolerate such practices as markets for organs. If the poor and wealthy are in their divergent positions because of their own past actions, toleration of great inequities is easier. That karma may be exchanged in the process of a transplant provides even further reason why there may be tendencies to want to match castes when organs are transplanted. Similar inclinations have been reported in the case of semen donation.[104]

CONFUCIANISM/TAOISM

Traditional Confucian thought was concerned about equality of treatment in its medical ethics. The late-sixteenth-century Confucian scholar Chu Hui-ming says, "In antiquity it was said: 'There are no two kinds of drugs for the lofty and the common: The poor and the rich receive the same medicine.' "[105] This egalitarianism is a common theme in Confucian medical ethics. By contrast, Ren-Zong Qiu sees a much more social utilitarian view in contemporary China. He says the watchword is "profit," a term interconnected in Chinese thought with "benefit" and "utility." He reflects contemporary attitudes about organ allocation, giving emphasis to those whose lives can be considerably improved and who "will probably make potential contributions to society and/or mankind."[106] He suggests that though these may often be people "in higher rank cadres or on the higher grade on the wage scale," this will not necessarily be the case. He specifically rejects choosing patients for transplantation by first come, first served, or by lottery, seeing this approach only as a secondary principle if other conditions are the same for two patients. He asks, rhetorically, "Is this unjust to those patients who are barred from dialysis or transplantation for financial reasons or shortage of machines or organs?" His response is, "Yes, in the sense that their condition dictates treatment. . . . But under the present conditions, we cannot avoid all unfortunate events, and sometimes we have to choose the lesser of two evils."[107] Apparently, both the traditional Confucian ideal and the ideology of Marxism are tempered by contemporary reality.

BUDDHISM AND SHINTOISM

Because Buddhism and Shintoism have been so ambivalent about organ transplants and thrive in countries that for either economic or cultural reasons have not pursued transplants, they have had little opportunity to develop an explicit ethical position on how organs should be allocated among potential recipients. Live donation has taken place, primarily among family members, foreclosing the problem of deciding who among a long list of potential recipients has the first claim on organs.

This situation forces us to examine more general works on Buddhist and Shinto ethics to glean some hint of how Buddhist and Shinto scholars would allocate organs. In particular, we would like to know how these traditions would respond if a society must choose between an allocation to the one who predictably will get the most benefit and to the one who has the greatest need.

Unfortunately, these are not major themes in the more general ethical writings of these traditions either.[108] For example, no discussion of justice or resource allocation occurs in Damien Keown's book-length treatment *Buddhism & Bioethics*.[109] Fujii suggests that Theravada Buddhism (the branch of Buddhism dominant in Sri Lanka, Myanmar, Thailand, Laos, and Cambodia) has borrowed its social ethics from the Brahmanic tradition of Hinduism—a tradition that is notoriously hierarchical and not inclined toward concerns about justice for the most needy. Conversely, Mahayana Buddhism—which is more influential in Tibet, Mongolia, China, Vietnam, South Korea, and Japan—is not as closely tied to Hinduism. However, the available literature from these countries does not provide much guidance on the ethics of the allocation of resources either.

Conclusion

Our conclusion is that no major religious or cultural group completely opposes organ transplantation. They all have resources within them that endorse brain-based criteria for death pronouncement—although some, such as Shinto and Buddhist beliefs, provide considerable resistance. None offer explicit, principled objection to cutting the corpse when it can be lifesaving to do so. Some, such as Judaism, actually view transplantation as an affirmative moral duty when it will save a life. Other traditions, including some Buddhists and Hindus along with Native Americans, hold beliefs that can arouse suspicion about the value of merely extending biological existence in this world, but at least some within these traditions support organ transplants. Some forces within the black American and fundamentalist Protestant cultures are skeptical not only about theological matters related to a belief in the bodily resurrection but also about the fundamental fairness of the transplant system. Nevertheless, all these groups participate in organ transplants, sometimes enthusiastically, and none offers formal objection to them. Worldwide, the preference has been for the "donation" model of procuring organs. Only occasional proponents of the market-based selling and buying of organs have surfaced, and then primarily from secular thinkers. Although, as we shall see in the chapters that follow, some cultures, particularly those that stress community solidarity, have accepted laws that procure organs without explicit consent, even those tend to favor the right of individuals who record their opposition to opt out of the procurement of their organs. This tension between donation and salvaging useful body parts without explicit consent is the focus of part II of this book. Finally, all the major religious and cultural traditions reveal strong commitments to allocating organs in ways that stress justice or equity. The tension between maximizing the benefits of the transplant program and distributing organs equitably is the focus of part III.

Notes

1. Bleich JD, "Neurological death and time-of-death statutes," in *Jewish bioethics*, ed. Rosner F, Bleich JD (New York: Sanhedrin Press, 1979), 310.

2. "Religion, organ transplantation, and the definition of death," *Lancet* 2011;337: 271.

3. Rosner F, "Organ transplants: The Jewish viewpoint," *Journal of Thanatology* 1975;3: 233–41; Grodin MA, "Religious exemptions: Brain death and Jewish law," *Journal of Church and State* 1994;36 (2): 357–72.

4. Rabbinical Council of America, "Brain stem death and Jewish law," Jan. 7, 2011, www .rabbis.org/news/article.cfm?id = 105607.

5. Pius XII, "The prolongation of life: An address to an International Congress of Anesthesiologists on November 24, 1957," *The Pope Speaks* 1958;4: 396.

6. US Conference of Catholic Bishops, *Ethical and religious directives for Catholic health care services*, 5th ed. (Washington, DC: US Catholic Conference of Catholic Bishops, 2009), 32, www .usccb.org/issues-and-action/human-life-and-dignity/health-care/upload/Ethical-Religious-Directives -Catholic-Health-Care-Services-fifth-edition-2009.pdf.

7. Byrne PA, O'Reilly S, Quay PM, "Brain death: An opposing viewpoint," *Journal of the American Medical Association* 1979;242: 1985–90.

8. Glatz C, "Vatican resuscitates issue of whether brain death means total death," Catholic News Service, Sept. 15, 2006, www.catholicnews.com/data/stories/cns/0605285.htm.

9. Ramsey P, "On updating procedures for stating that a man has died," in *The patient as person*, by Ramsey P (New Haven, CT: Yale University Press, 1970), 59–112; Fletcher J, "Cerebration," in *Humanhood: Essays in Biomedical ethics* (Buffalo: Prometheus Books, 1979), 159–65.

10. For Anglicans, see Granbois JA, Smith, DH, "The Anglican Communion and bioethics," in *Bioethics yearbook, volume 5: Theological developments in bioethics, 1992–1994*, ed. Lustig BA (Dordrecht: Kluwer Academic Publishers, 1997), 93–119. For Lutherans, see Nelson P, "Lutheran perspectives on

bioethics," in *Bioethics yearbook, volume 3: Theological developments in bioethics, 1990–1992*, ed. Brody BA, Lustig BA, Engelhardt HT, McCullough LB (Dordrecht: Kluwer Academic Publishers, 1993), 178–80. For Methodists, see Shelton RL, "Biomedical ethics in Methodist traditions," in *Bioethics yearbook, volume 3*, ed. Brody et al., 228–29. And for the Reformed tradition, see Vaux KL, *Health and medicine in the Reformed tradition: Promise, providence, and care* (New York: Crossroad, 1984), 38.

11. Harakas SS, "Eastern Orthodox bioethics," in *Bioethics yearbook, volume 3*, ed. Brody et al., 119–20.

12. International Organization of Islamic Medicine, *Islamic code of medical ethics* (Brandon, FL: International Organization of Islamic Medicine, 1981), 67.

13. Mazkur, K, et al., eds., *Human life: Its inception and its end as viewed by Islam*, trans. M. M. S. Asbahi, Islamic Organization for Medical Sciences, and Kuwaiti Foundation for the Advancement of Science, Kuwait, as summarized by Hathout H, "Islamic concepts and bioethics," in *Bioethics yearbook, volume 1: Theological developments in bioethics, 1988–1990*, ed. Bole, TJ (Dordrecht: Kluwer Academic Publishers, 1991), 112–14.

14. This is also the position of many in Britain and in the Commonwealth countries. Because the death of the brain stem is closely associated with the death of the entire brain, the significance of the difference between brain stem death and whole-brain death is minimal. In a later review, Hathout actually refers to this position as "total brain death," implying that he does not see a significant difference between the two. See Hathout H, "Bioethical developments in Islam," in *Bioethics yearbook, volume 3*, ed. Brody et al., 133–48.

15. Hathout, "Islamic Concepts," 103–18; for a similar conclusion, see Rispler-Chaim V, "Islamic medical ethics in the 20th century," *Journal of Medical Ethics* 1989;15: 203.

16. Cited by Daar AS, "Islam," in *Organ and tissue donation for transplantation*, ed. Chapman JR, Deierhoi M, Wight C (New York: Oxford University Press, 1997), 29–33, at 32.

17. For a somewhat more cautious account, including descriptions of scholars continuing to support cardiovascular definitions of death, see Serour GI, "Islamic developments in bioethics," in *Bioethics yearbook, volume 5*, ed. Lustig, 171–88.

18. Akrami, SM, Osati Z, Zahedi, F, Raza M, "Brain death: Recent ethical and religious considerations in Iran," *Transplantation Proceedings* 2004;36: 2885.

19. Desai P, "Medical ethics in India," *Journal of Medicine and Philosophy* 1988;13: 240.

20. Qiu, RZ, Jin, DJ, "Bioethics in China: 1989–1991," in *Bioethics yearbook, volume 2: Regional developments in bioethics, 1989–1991*, ed. Lustig, BA, et al. (Boston: Kluwer Academic Publishers, 1992), 355–77; Qiu, RZ, "Ethical problems in renal dialysis and transplantation: Chinese perspective," in *Ethical problems in dialysis and transplantation*, ed. Kjellstrand CM, Dossetor JB (Boston: Kluwer Academic Publishers, 1992), 227–28.

21. Japanese Association of Indian and Buddhist Studies Committee for Inquiry on Brain Death and Organ Transplantation, September 1990, text reprinted by Fuji M, "Buddhist bioethics and organ transplantation," *Okurayama Bunkakaigi Kenkyunenop* 1991;3 (2): 1–11.

22. Mettananda B, "Buddhist ethics in the practice of medicine," in *Buddhist ethics and modern society: An international symposium*, ed. Fu CW, Wawrytho SA (New York: Greenwood Press, 1991), 195–213.

23. Ikeda D, "Thoughts on the problem of brain death (1): From the viewpoint of the Buddhism of Nichiren Daishonin," *Journal of Oriental Studies* 1987;26: 193–216; Keown D, *Buddhism and bioethics* (London: St. Martin's Press, 1995), 153–58.

24. Lecso PA, "The Bodhisattva ideal and organ transplantation," *Journal of Religion and Health* 1991;30 (1): 39.

25. Ross C, "Towards acceptance of organ transplantation: Tokyo perspective," *Lancet* 1995;346 (8966): 41.

26. Fujii M, "Buddhism and bioethics," in *Bioethics yearbook, volume 1*, ed. Bole, 67.

27. Lecso, "Bodhisattva ideal," 39. See also Hardacre H, "Response of Buddhism and Shinto to the issue of brain death and organ transplant," *Cambridge Quarterly of Healthcare Ethics* 1994;3: 595.

28. Nolan K, "Buddhism, Zen, and Bioethics," in *Bioethics yearbook, volume 3*, ed. Brody et al., 204–5.

29. Feldman EA, "Defining death: Organ transplants, tradition and technology in Japan," *Social Science and Medicine* 1988;27 (4): 341.

30. Law Concerning Human Organ Transplants (Law No. 104, in 1997). For accounts of the protracted controversy, see Kimura R, "Japan's dilemma with the definition of death," *Kennedy Institute of Ethics Journal* 1991;1: 123–31; Watanabe Y, "Why do I stand against the movement for cardiac transplantation in Japan?" *Japanese Heart Journal* 1994;35 (6): 701–14; Feldman EA, "Culture, conflict and cost: Perspectives on brain death in Japan," *International Journal of Technology Assessment in Health Care* 1994;10 (3): 447–63; and Hoshino K, "Legal status of brain death in Japan: Why many Japanese do not accept 'brain death' as a definition of death," *Bioethics* 1993;7 (2–3): 234–38.

31. Ramsey P, "Giving or taking cadaver organs for transplant," in *Patient as person*, by Ramsey, esp. 205–9; Department of Health Affairs, US Catholic Conference, *Ethical and religious directives for Catholic health facilities*, Directive 30 (Washington, DC: US Catholic Conference, 1971), 8; reaffirmed in *Ethical and religious directives*, 2009 edition, Directive 63, 32.

32. Freund P, "Organ transplants: Ethical and legal problems," *Proceedings of the American Philosophical Society* 1971;15: 276; Rosner F, "Organ transplantation in Jewish law," *Jewish bioethics*, ed. Rosner and Bleich, esp. 360.

33. For Judaism, see Dorff EN, "Choosing life: Aspects of Judaism affecting organ transplantation," in *Organ transplantation: Meanings and realities*, ed. Youngner SJ, Fox, RC, O'Connell, LJ (Madison: University of Wisconsin Press, 1996), 168–93. For Catholicism, see Spagnolo AG, Sgreccia E, "The Roman Catholic Church," in *Organ and tissue donation for transplantation*, ed. Chapman JR, Deierhoi M, Wight C (New York: Oxford University Press, 1997), 27–29. For the major Protestant denominations—e.g., the Church of England—see Habgood J, "The Church of England," in *Organ and tissue donation for transplantation*, ed. Chapman, Deierhoi, Wight, 25–27.

34. Callender C, " 'Testimony of Group 13: Increasing organ donation liver allocation, December 10, 11, 12, 1996," Natcher Center, National Institutes of Health, Bethesda, MD. Callender groups these into five categories, including religious reasons; see Callender CO, "Organ donation in blacks: A community approach," *Transplantation Proceedings* 1987;19: 1551.

35. Abraham L. Surgeon preaches the need for organ donation; see *American Medical News*, October 2, 1987, cited by Sanders C, "African Americans and organ donation: Reflections on religion, ethics, and embodiment," in *Embodiment, morality, and medicine*, ed. Cahill LS, Farley MA (Boston: Kluwer Academic Publishers, 1995), 145.

36. Sanders, "African Americans," 141–53.

37. Ibid., 148.

38. Ibid., 141–53.

39. Ehusani GE, *An Afro-Christian vision* (Lanham, MD: University Press of America, 1991), cited by Sanders, "African Americans," 146.

40. Ibid., 147.

41. Gatrad AR, "Muslim customs surrounding death, bereavement, postmortem examinations, and organ transplants," *British Medical Journal* 1994;309: 523. It is probably because most Muslims living in Britain come from Asian countries such as Pakistan and Bangladesh that Black reports that transplantation is rarely permitted among them. Black J, "Broaden your mind about death and bereavement in certain groups in Britain [Hindus, Sikhs, Moslems]," *British Medical Journal* 1987;295: 538.

42. Bile KM, Qureshi JARH, Rizvi SAH, Naqvi SAA, Usmani AQ, Lashari KA, "Human organ and tissue transplantation in Pakistan: When a regulation makes a difference," *Eastern Mediterranean Health Journal* (*La Revue de Sante de la Mediterranee orientale*) 2010;16: S159–66.

43. Rispler-Chaim V, "Islamic medical ethics in the 20th century," *Journal of Medical Ethics* 1989;15: 203–8; Daar AS, "Islam."

44. Gatrad, "Muslim customs," 309.

45. International Organization of Islamic Medicine, *Islamic code*, 81, 84.

46. Hathout, "Islamic Concepts," 115. These are also taken from the Islamic Code of Medical Ethics.

47. Francis CM, "Ancient and modern medical ethics in India," in *Transcultural dimensions in medical ethics*, ed. Pellegrino ED, Mazzarella P, Corsi P (Frederick, MD: University Publishing Group, 1992), 194.

48. Agarwal SK, Srivastava RK, Gupta S, Tripathi S, "Evolution of the Transplantation of Human Organ Act and law in India," *Transplantation* 2012;94: 110–13.

49. Ibid., citing Transplantation of Human Organ Act, 1994.

50. Ibid., citing *Gazette* notification "Transplant of Human Organs Act and rules 2008 and the Transplantation of Human Organs (Amendment) Bill," 2011.

51. Ibid.

52. Oliver M, Woywodt A, Ahmed A, Saif I, "Organ donation, transplantation and religion," *Nephrology, Dialysis, Transplantation* 2011;26: 440.

53. Doniger W, "Transplanting myths of organ transplants," in *Organ transplantation*, ed. Youngner et al., 200.

54. Ibid., 200–202.

55. Desai, "Medical ethics," 245. Black reports a similar conclusion for Hindus in Britain. See Black, "Broaden your mind," 537.

56. Doniger, "Transplanting myths," 210–12.

57. Ibid., 212.

58. Black, "Broaden your mind," 537.

59. Oliver et al., "Organ donation, 12–13.

60. Qiu and Jin, "Bioethics," 366.

61. Qiu, "Ethical problems," 230.

62. Juan S, "New system to boost number of organ donors," *China Daily*, Apr. 10, 2010, www .chinadaily.com.cn/china/2010-04/10/content_9711027.htm; Hui L, Blanchard B, "China to end use of prisoners' organs for transplants in mid-2014," Reuters, Nov. 2, 2013, www.reuters.com/article/2013/ 11/02/us-china-organs-idUSBRE9A011N2 0131102.

63. See Veatch RM, *A theory of medical ethics* (New York: Basic Books, 1981), 66. Also see Lo P, *Confucian views on suicide*, Hong Kong Baptist University Occasional Paper (Hong Kong: Centre for Applied Ethics, 1997).

64. Girardot NJ, "Taoism," in *The encyclopedia of bioethics*, vol. 1 (New York: Free Press, 1978), 1631–38, esp. 1636.

65. Tsuji KT, "The Buddhist view of the body and organ transplantation," *Transplantation Proceedings* 1998;20 (1 Suppl): 1076.

66. Fujii M, "Buddhist bioethics and organ transplantation," *Okurayama Bunkakaigi Kenkyunenop* 1991;3 (2): 5; Lecso, "Bodhisattva ideal," 37.

67. Nolan, "Buddhism," 206.

68. Ibid., 205; Lecso, "Bodhisattva ideal," 36.

69. Fujii, "Buddhist bioethics," 8; Fujii, "Buddhism and bioethics," 66.

70. Lock M, "Deadly disputes: Ideologies and brain death in Japan," in *Organ transplantation*, ed. Youngner et al., 157.

71. Nolan, "Buddhism," 205.

72. Lock, "Deadly disputes," 342.

73. Feldman, "Defining death," 342.

74. Hardacre, "Response," 598.

75. Dukeminier J, Sanders D, "Organ transplantation: A proposal for routine salvaging of cadaver organs," *New England Journal of Medicine* 1968;279: 413–19.

76. Veatch R, "A policy for obtaining newly dead bodies and body organs," in *Death, dying, and the biological revolution* (New Haven, CT: Yale University Press, 1976), 266–76. For Roman Catholicism, see US Conference of Catholic Bishops, *Ethical and religious directives*, 2009, Directive 63, 32. The use of organs and tissues of deceased infants with the consent of parents or guardians is endorsed in Directive 65.

77. Rosner F, "Autopsy in Jewish law and the Israeli autopsy controversy," in *Jewish bioethics*, ed. Rosner and Bleich, 343.

78. Organ Transplant Law 5678-2008, Israeli Book of Laws (English translation provided by the Israeli Ministry of Justice), as cited by Quigley M, Wright L, Ravitsky V, "Organ donation and priority points in Israel: An ethical analysis," *Transplantation* 2012;93: 970–73.

79. Ibid. See also Guttman N, Ashkenazi T, Gesser-Edelsburg A, Seidmann V, "Laypeople's ethical concerns about a new Israeli organ transplantation prioritization policy aimed to encourage organ donor registration among the public," *Journal of Health Politics, Policy and the Law* 2011;36 (4): 691–716.

80. International Organization of Islamic Medicine, *Islamic code*, 81.

81. Ibid.

82. Human Organ Transplant Act 1987 [of Singapore], http://statutes.agc.gov.sg/aol/search/display/view.w3p;page=0;query=DocId%3A%22db05e985-f8a0-4d61-a906-9fd39f3b5ac9%22%20Status%3Apublished%20Depth%3A0;rec=0#pr5-ps2-p1f-; "Singapore Muslims in donor ruling," BBC News, July 27, 2007, http://news.bbc.co.uk/2/hi/asia-pacific/6919879.stm.

83. Daar, "Islam," 32.

84. Ghods AJ, Shekoufeh S, "Iranian model of paid and regulated living-unrelated kidney donation," *Clinical Journal of the American Society of Nephrology* 2006;1 (6): 1136–45; Bagheri A, "Compensated kidney donation: An ethical review of the Iranian model," *Kennedy Institute of Ethics Journal* 2006;16: 269–82.

85. Peters DA, "Marketing organs for transplantation," *Dialysis & Transplantation* 1983;13: 40–41; Peters TG, "Financial incentives in organ donation: Current issues," *Dialysis & Transplantation* 1992;21 (5): 270–73; Peters TG, "Life or death: The issue of payment in cadaveric organ donation," *JAMA* 1991;265: 1302–5; cf. Harvey J, "Paying organ donors," *Journal of Medical Ethics* 1990;16: 117–19; American Medical Association, Council on Ethical and Judicial Affairs, "Financial incentives for organ donation," *Archives of Internal Medicine* 1995;155: 581–89.

86. There are reports of such practices in other countries such as the Philippines and Turkey, but they are not well documented. See Mani MK, "The argument against the unrelated live donor," in *Ethical problems in dialysis and transplantation*, ed. Kjellstrand CM, Dossetor JB (Boston: Kluwer Academic Publishers, 1992), 163–68; and Francis, "Ancient and modern medical ethics," 193.

87. Reddy KC, "A perspective on reality," in *Ethical problems*, ed. Kjellstrand and Dossetor, 155–61. Also see Francis, "Ancient and modern medical ethics," 193; Colabawala BN, "Kidneys for a price," *Indian Post*, Feb. 23, 1989; and "Cover story: The organs bazaar," *India Today*, July 31, 1990, both cited by Desai, "Medical ethics," 55.

88. Desai, "Medical ethics," 55; Francis, "Ancient and modern medical ethics," 175–96.

89. For further discussion of Indian culture and the impact of its Hindu roots, see ibid.; and Desai, "Medical ethics," 55.

90. Unschuld PU, "Confucianism," in *Encyclopedia of Bioethics*, ed. Reich WT (New York: Free Press, 1978), 200–204.

91. Qiu and Jin, "Bioethics," 366.

92. Rothman DJ, et al., "The Bellagio Task Force report on transplantation, bodily integrity, and the international traffic in organs," *Transplantation Proceedings* 1997;29: 2739–45; Rothman DJ, "Body shop," *The Sciences* 1997;37 (6): 17–21; Sun, LH, "China's social changes spur more executions: Families don't see the body, but they pay for the bullet," *Washington Post*, March 27, 1994.

93. Bradsher K, "China moves to stop transplants of organs after executions," *New York Times*, March 23, 2012, www.nytimes.com/2012/03/24/world/asia/china-moves-to-stop-transplants-of-organs -after-executions.html?pagewanted-all&_r = 0.

94. Rinpoche S, *The Tibetan book of living and dying* (San Francisco: HarperSanFrancisco, 1992), 376, cited by Nolan, "Buddhism," 206.

95. Lecso, "Bodhisattva ideal," 37.

96. Lock, "Deadly disputes," 148.

97. Lecso, "Bodhisattva ideal," 40.

98. "Sai josei 'sengensho' ikasu" (Written declaration of 53-year-old woman restores life), *Yomiuri Shinbun*, October 18, 1992, cited by Lock, "Deadly disputes," 149.

99. Lock, "Deadly disputes," 158.

100. International Organization of Islamic Medicine, *Islamic Code*, 81. Also see the emphasis on justice by Nanji AA, "Medical ethics and the Islamic tradition," *Journal of Medicine and Philosophy* 1988;13: 257–75, esp. 268–69.

101. Serour, "Islamic developments," 181.

102. Gatrad, "Muslim customs," 523.

103. Menon A, Haberman, HF, "Oath of initiation (from the *Caraka Samhita*)," *Medical History* 1970;14: 295–96.

104. Desai, "Medical ethics," 247.

105. Chu Hui-ming, *Tou-chen ch'uan-hsin lu*, chap. 16, 1b–3b, 5a–5b, cited by Ch'eng Yung-p'ei, *Liu-li chai i-shu shih-chung*, reprinted in English translation by Unschuld, "Confucianism," 63.

106. Qiu, "Ethical problems," 232–33.

107. Ibid., 233.

108. Nolan, "Buddhism," 203.

109. Keown, *Buddhism.*

Chapter 2

An Ethical Framework

General Theories of Ethics

W*hat is needed* is a general, overall ethical theory in which to ground an ethic for transplantation. In order to know how to procure and allocate organs ethically, one needs to know first what it means to act ethically in the generic sense. The approach taken in this book is to first—in the present chapter—provide a brief sketch of what we know about general theories of normative ethics and then—in the remainder of the book—spell out what these theories mean for organ procurement and allocation. After examining the definition-of-death controversy in part I, we tease out the implications for organ procurement in part II and for organ allocation in part III.

It stands to reason that a theory for the ethics of organ procurement and allocation would somehow be related to more general ethical theories. In fact, the position one takes on important transplant issues should be determined by one's position on the classical controversies in ethics. It is only reasonable that a Marxist will procure and allocate differently than one who subscribes to classical liberal political philosophy; a utilitarian differently than a Kantian. The proper way to resolve the efficiency-versus-equity debate in organ allocation must be dependent on how one resolves these conflicts more generally. Each major normative theory of ethics should have its own implications for organ procurement and allocation. In this sense, the ethics of medicine, or a branch of medicine, does not have its own ethic "internal to medicine."[1] Rather, the ethics of medicine is dependent on broader, more fundamental foundations. There will be as many ethics for medicine as there are ethical systems in the world, one medical ethic per system of belief and value; and likewise, one medical ethic per religious or philosophical worldview.

Religious Ethical Approaches

One major group of approaches to ethics is those of the major world religions. As we have seen, no major world religion actively opposes organ procurement. Each religion, however, has positions regarding ethical norms that would shape the way organs are procured and allocated. Judaism and Christianity, for example, are religions of social justice. Moreover, they have particular interpretations of what a just world would look like. They give priority to those among us who have the greatest need: the lame, the halt, the blind, and, presumably, those in most serious organ failure. Conversely, some more otherworldly versions of Christianity are committed to recognizing the limits of human existence. Many Catholic theologians, for instance, have been critical of experimental multi-organ transplants for people who have such severe medical problems that survival is unlikely. They see such efforts as placing too much emphasis on survival in bodily form in this world and not enough on the "final ends" of human existence that are more otherworldly. Some interpretations of the Hindu doctrine of karma may imply that some people with severe, chronic organ failure may be reaping the rewards of evils in a previous life.

Anyone deeply committed to a religious perspective will draw on that tradition's ethical framework in deciding how organs should be allocated. For purposes of public policy, however, particular religious ethics will have only an indirect impact. The competing secular ethical theories will be more central to the public formulation of an allocation system.

Secular Ethical Approaches

Secular normative ethical theory has been a lively field in recent decades. Old debates have run their course; new theoretical approaches are emerging, some of which have very definite implications for organ allocation.

Virtue Theories

Several approaches to ethics historically focused on the virtues. Virtue theories focus on the character of people rather than the rightness or wrongness of their behavior. A *virtue* is a character trait or a "persistent disposition" to act in a certain way. Classical Greek ethics, particularly the ethics of Aristotle, was an ethics of virtues.[2]

Classical Virtue Theories

The classical Greek virtues were wisdom, courage, temperance, and justice. People were considered virtuous to the extent that they manifested these character traits in their daily lives. There has been a recent resurgence in virtue theory, particularly in medical ethics.[3] Virtue theory is unique in that it focuses on the character of actors rather than the morality of actions. The key question is, "Was the disposition of the actor in accord with certain key virtues?"; it was not, "Was the behavior morally the right behavior?" The implication for transplants, however, is remote. Although some have spoken of the "virtues" of institutions, almost all virtue theory focuses on the character of individual humans. Because the organ allocation system is a practice that is grounded in an institution, asking what the character traits of individuals should be may turn out to be a question of only secondary importance. Moreover, focusing on the character of actors tends to ignore or minimize the question of what the ethically proper allocation should be. An ethical system that tells us to be courageous or temperate does not directly tell us whether organs should go to the sickest recipient or the one who is expected to have the longest graft survival. Virtue theory, no matter how important for shaping the character of individuals, is not promising as a basis for developing a theory of organ allocation.

Feminist Theories

Recent developments in biomedical ethics also include a major movement under the label of *feminist theory*.[4] There is a great deal of work going on in biomedical ethics, particularly nursing ethics, in what is called *care theory*, which is closely allied with feminist theory.[5] Some interpret this work as a kind of virtue theory.[6] To the extent that care is a virtue, it describes a character trait that many consider important in practicing good medicine or good nursing. It is closely related to the virtues of compassion, humaneness, and benevolence. Certainly, we would very much want our organ procurement, allocation, and implantation personnel to manifest these virtues. It is less clear, however, how these virtues would provide guidance for when organs should be procured or on what basis they should be allocated. This cluster of virtues is more often associated with the clinical professions rather than the institutional and administrative groups that are responsible for organ procurement and allocation. To say that one should be caring or compassionate or humane in procurement or allocation does not really tell us very much about whether it is acceptable to procure organs from an HIV-positive donor or from someone who insists the organs go only to members of a certain race. These virtues do not tell us whether we should allocate organs to those who will get the most benefit or to those who need the organs the most. In fact, these virtues manifest in clinical professionals—including transplant surgeons, nurses, and social workers—can easily lead to advocacy for one's own patients, a commitment that can only distort the perspective of those concerned with how to procure and allocate organs ethically.

Hippocratic Ethics

The clinical focus on care and other virtue theories is often in creative tension with the classical ethical system of the health professions: the ethic based on the Hippocratic Oath. Although some people have viewed the Hippocratic ethic as a kind of timeless, all-purpose ethic for physicians and other health professionals, in fact it is only one among many possible ethics for medicine.

Its Origins

The Hippocratic ethic has its roots in one particular kind of Greek medicine, sometimes called the Hippocratic school. The ethics reflected in the Hippocratic Oath is closely related to Pythagoreanism.[7] The Hippocratic ethical tradition is, at least indirectly, the perspective into which many organ transplant personnel have been socialized. In theory, we could develop an allocation system that reflects the Hippocratic ethic. It is puzzling, however, why health professionals or the general public would want to run an allocation program based on a system of ethics from an ancient Greek cult that functioned with a set of values quite alien to our present ones.

Its Characteristics

The Hippocratic ethic includes a virtue element. The original Oath included *purity* and *holiness*. For the Florence Nightingale Pledge for nurses, the equivalent is *purity* and *faithfulness*. These are virtues that do not resonate with many moderns. The contemporary equivalents in the American Medical Association's Principles of Ethics are *compassion* and *respect for human dignity*.[8] The American Nurses Association refers to *respect for human dignity and the uniqueness of the client*. Although these virtues seem uncontroversial, the problem is that they really do not tell health personnel how to procure or allocate organs.

In addition to its virtue component, Hippocratic ethics includes some important normative commitments that are not necessarily friendly to or useful for organ allocation. The core ethical principle is that the physician pledges to "benefit the patient according to my ability and judgment." Logically, this would require every clinical professional to work the system for the best interests of his or her patient. This could mean each surgeon lobbying for organs for his or her patients. At its worst it would require "gaming" the system (e.g., by stretching the facts of a diagnosis so that a patient who will eventually need a transplant can get listed sooner) so that one's own patients beat out others to get scarce organs. This Hippocratic principle has two characteristics that are particularly controversial. It can be described as individualistic and consequentialistic.

First, let us consider individualism. Often in ethics there are conflicts between one's duties to an individual (e.g., a patient) and duties to society. This is a major problem in using human subjects for medical research. It is a problem in certain confidentiality cases, and it is a critical problem when it comes to allocating scarce resources. Imagine that we could align all ethical systems along a continuum, from those that focus more on the duties to the individual to those that focus on the duties to society. Marxism might be seen as being at the societal end. So would social utilitarianism. They hold that it is morally necessary when there is a conflict to sacrifice the individual for the good of society. Others line up much more at the end of the spectrum at which society's interests are subordinated to one's duties to the individual.

The Hippocratic ethic is at the extreme individualist end of the spectrum. The physician's exclusive loyalty is to the individual patient. Taken literally, the Hippocratic ethic would never accept a physician using his or her patients for so-called nontherapeutic research. In such research, the purpose is to gain knowledge for the benefit of society. Even though the risk to the subject may be very small, what is done is not for the patient's benefit. A purely Hippocratic physician could not participate because he or she would not be working solely for the benefit of the patient.

Any ethic of resource allocation must look beyond the good of the individual patient. For these reasons, we claim in chapter 16 that Hippocratic clinicians would make particularly bad allocators of organs. They would feel duty-bound to do what was necessary to benefit their patient at the expense of others.

Second, let us consider consequentialism. The second characteristic of the Hippocratic ethic is that it focuses exclusively on consequences. The duty of the physician is expressed in terms of benefiting the patient and protecting him or her from harm. By contrast, other ethics judge the rightness or wrongness of actions by considerations other than consequences. These ethics are sometimes called *deontological*. The term comes from the Greek word meaning duty. The general idea is that there are certain behaviors that are simply one's duty, regardless of the consequences. Anyone who believes it is wrong to tell a lie or break a promise, regardless of the consequences, understands that there can be more to ethics than merely calculating consequences. In bioethics, many people now hold that it is the physician's duty to respect the autonomous choices of their patients to refuse treatment, even if they know that the consequences would be better if the physician treated against the patient's wishes.

To see why simply striving to produce consequences that are as good as possible is ethically suspect, we consider in chapter 12 whether it would be wise for the members of a group of people who each are near death from need of an organ (e.g., a heart, liver, lung, or pancreas) to come together and sign a binding contract to hold a lottery of which the loser would be sacrificed (i.e., killed) so that his or her good organs could save the others. With such a lottery, perhaps four or five people would live who would otherwise die; whereas without the lottery, all would die. (Because procured lungs, liver, and pancreata could potentially be divided, there might be more beneficiaries than one would expect. Conversely, presumably most kidney patients would not enter because they can be maintained on dialysis.) If ethics is nothing more than a matter of maximizing good consequences, it is hard to see why this lottery would not be ethically acceptable. But if ethics involves something more—for example, an intrinsic duty not to kill—the lottery may pose serious problems.

Many of the most sophisticated ethical systems of the world insist that ethics is more than consequence maximizing. These systems are deontological in character; that is, they include duties that go beyond consequences. The best-known is the ethic of Immanuel Kant.[9] He held that ethics is a matter of doing one's duty, independent of consequences.

Many twentieth-century ethical theories fall somewhere in the middle of the continuum between an exclusively consequence-oriented ethic and one that is totally nonconsequentialistic. W. D. Ross, for example, held a theory that includes both kinds of considerations.[10] Many ethicists doing contemporary work in bioethics position themselves similarly in the middle of this continuum. Some—for example, Tom Beauchamp and James Childress, in *Principles of Biomedical Ethics*—claim that one must balance the concern about consequences with concerns about other principles, such as distributing goods fairly and respecting autonomy.[11] The point here is that the Hippocratic ethic is exclusively consequentialistic. It has no principle of respecting autonomy and no notion of fairness or equity, as called for in current American transplant policy. It looks only at benefits and harm, trying to maximize the benefit and minimize the harm.

Mainstream Theories of Right Action

Most modern normative moral theories that focus on the morality of actions rather than the morality of character can be described in terms of two characteristics: the individualism/society dichotomy, and the consequentialist/deontological dichotomy. Essentially, no respectable contemporary ethical theory would do what the Hippocratic theory does— totally ignore duties unrelated to consequences and duties that are more social: the allocation of resources, conflicts between the individual and society, and the like. How one resolves the controversies over these matters of general theory could have a major influence on one's theory of organ procurement and allocation. Two major views have dominated, which we now summarize.

The Social Utilitarians

The first major view, called *social* or *classical utilitarianism*, is the view of philosophers like Jeremy Bentham and John Stuart Mill.[12] Social utilitarians hold that the only considerations that count in morality are consequences; but unlike Hippocratic consequentialists, social utilitarians consider consequences for all affected parties. They hold that the course of action that produces the best net consequences is the morally right course, but they first determine the net of benefits minus harms for each individual and then add up the net benefits for each party getting an aggregate sum. We refer to them as "aggregate maximizers." For example, in allocating organs, a social utilitarian would opt for the allocation that maximizes the aggregate good consequences, measured by some criterion such as years of graft survival.

The Deontologists

The second major view is that of the *deontologists*, such as Kantians, who by definition consider features of actions other than consequences to be relevant to deciding what the moral course of action is. They differ among themselves as to exactly which features are morally important. Just as the consequentialists vary in their emphasis on the individual and the social dimensions of actions, so the deontologists do as well. The principles of action at the individual level that they sometimes emphasize are respect for autonomy, fidelity (promise keeping), veracity (truth telling), and the duty to avoid killing.[13] Collectively, these principles are sometimes referred to as "respect for persons."

These deontologists insist that we show respect for persons by not infringing on choices made according to a substantially autonomous life plan, following the principle of autonomy. Also, we must show respect by keeping promises made and avoiding lying. Finally, some deontologists believe that, if we respect persons, we can never kill them—even when they are suffering so badly that a case could be made that the consequences would be better if they were dead. These are all principles that could be applied in one's actions toward a single individual. And they all present alternatives to the Hippocratic way of treating an individual. Most of the conflicts in medical ethics of the 1970s were conflicts at this individual level. The holders of these "respect-for-persons" views challenged traditional Hippocratic assumptions about how to treat the individual patient. The challengers said that we must respect autonomy, keep promises, avoid lying, and perhaps avoid killing as well, even though the results might be better for the patient if we were more Hippocratic.

Almost everyone now believes that over the past thirty years, the deontologists have won this fight with the Hippocratists. At least the law requires that autonomy be respected. It generally requires that promises, such as the promise of confidentiality, be kept—even if the clinician believes the patient would be better off if these principles were rejected. The American Medical Association has revised its code of ethics, generally removing Hippocratic paternalism in favor of more respect for patients, and it has a much more acceptable code because of it.[14]

Deontologists also differ from utilitarians at the social level. The key is understanding how each one would handle the problem of distributing scarce resources. Although social utilitarians will resolve conflicts among the interests of parties in a social setting by summing up the net consequences of alternative courses of actions and opting for the choice that maximizes aggregate utility, deontologists may appeal to some other feature or features of the distribution. Thus, for example, if there are many more people waiting for livers than there are livers available, the social utilitarian will place the organs where they will do the most good. Those deontologists committed to the principle of justice, however, will recognize that the ones who need the organs the most may not be the same people who will predictably get the most benefit from them. For instance, those in greatest need may be so ill that the chance of a successful graft is less. Those committed to the principle of justice may focus on the potential recipients' need rather than the amount of good that will be done.

In general, those whose ethic of allocation concentrates on justice look at "patterned end states," that is, the pattern in the way that goods end up being distributed. For example, they may insist that people of all races have an equal chance at getting an organ, even though statistically members of one racial group may be expected to do somewhat better (because they match the donor pool better or for some other reason). The morally correct pattern—in this case, a pattern of equal access—is usually referred to as a *just* distribution. The principle holding that the action is right that leads to a distribution matching this pattern is called the *principle of justice*. Because there are many different notions of exactly what constitutes the right pattern of distribution, there are many different versions of the principle of justice.

Aristotle recognized that justice as a principle of distribution could have many different criteria. He considered distributing according to whether one was of "free birth," whether one was of "noble birth," or whether one was an aristocrat. These, apparently, were the only patterns of distribution that he could think of.

Modern justice theorists often are *egalitarians*. They are concerned about the pattern of distribution of the good, but the pattern that they consider to be right is the one that gives people opportunities for equality. There is an endless dispute among egalitarians over exactly what this means. Some seek end-state outcomes with the goal that people are equal in their welfare. Others have more sophisticated views. One of these holds that what is really needed is a distribution in which there is equality of resources, leaving individuals to make decisions about what they want to do with their resources.[15] If, when considering resources, they include people's biological resources—mainly, their genetic makeup, and their propensity for disease—giving people equality of resources could be the basis for an egalitarian health policy that focuses on giving those with poor health states opportunities to be normally healthy, insofar as this is possible. This view of the equality of resources, combined with the right of people to choose how they use their resources, will accept inequalities of outcomes, provided the differences result from the different choices that people make.

One important version of a justice theory is called the "maximin." It is defended by the philosopher John Rawls.[16] Although it is a very complex, sophisticated theory, one of its features is that for a practice to be just, it must redistribute goods so as to achieve the maximum advantage for the worst-off persons or groups. (The allocation is designed to *maxi*mize the *min*imum good that persons have, hence "maximin.") This can differ from simply making everybody equal, a distinction that will prove important in our consideration of the ethics of socially directed donation in chapter 23.

The one thing that all these deontological justice theorists agree on is that distributing resources is not merely a matter of maximizing the aggregate good consequences. In *The Foundations of Justice*, one of us (RMV) has argued that a patterned, end-state theory of justice has moral priority over the maximizing of aggregate net utility. Many other, but not all, theorists have reached this same conclusion. So, too, do those who articulate the basic principles of liberal political traditions.

An ethic limited to maximizing good consequences has implications that are strongly counterintuitive. It would justify slavery—if only the sum of the consequences to the advantaged majority exceeded the burdens to the enslaved. It would justify the compulsory conscription of a minority into dangerous medical research, if only the anticipated benefits to the population as a whole were large enough. It would even justify the forced procurement of organs from some in order to benefit others, provided the benefit to the recipients exceeded the harm to the one whose organs were commandeered—an outcome easy to imagine if several could live for each person selected for death.

Consider a plan to pick a small group of people, perhaps those who are not very useful to society, who are mentally depressed to the point that they have only a slight preference for living. Killing one of them and taking his or her organs could save several lives of people who are desperate to live, while generating only a modest burden for the one person killed. It seems obvious that, if done carefully, the lifesaving benefit multiplied by the number of people receiving the life-prolonging organs could easily exceed the burden to the one person killed. Yet almost everyone would think it obvious that such a policy would be morally wrong—indeed, an outrage. Why is such a policy so obviously wrong, if the expected benefits seem large in comparison with the burdens?

This policy is wrong because it violates several of the basic principles we have identified. It violates respect for persons by violating the autonomy of the one selected to be killed. It violates this respect by treating the one who is killed as a mere means to the benefit of others. It violates it by intentionally killing. Finally, it distributes the benefits and burdens in a very unequal way. The benefits all go to one group; the harm entirely to someone else. Not only militant egalitarians, but just about everyone, recognizes the unfairness of such a foul distribution of burdens and benefits. There is a sense that something is terribly wrong with assigning all the burdens to one and all the benefits to others. This moral sense, sometimes called a "sense of justice," appears commonly in our moral deliberations. It is not suppressed by the recognition that the aggregate social good would be greater, much greater, if we followed only the principle of social utility maximizing.

Our public policies depend on how we compare the moral force of the principles of utility maximizing and justice. We are convinced that justice—striving for opportunities for equality of well-being—takes absolute priority over maximizing aggregate social utility and, at the level of the individual, that the principles grouped under the rubric of respect for persons take precedence over net utility as well. We argue that there is no clear priority among the deontological principles (e.g., between respecting autonomy and promoting justice), so that, when these principles conflict, the claims of each must be balanced to determine which one is more weighty. Conversely, once these deontological principles have been balanced against one another, the resulting moral imperative takes absolute precedence over considerations of consequences.[17]

Considerations of utility, in this view, are not irrelevant, but they play a much smaller role than in utilitarian theory. Utility would merely break ties when two or more deontological principles are so evenly balanced that neither carries the day. Moreover, it is the nature of many of the deontological principles, especially those subsumed under the rubric of respect for persons, that they can often be fully satisfied rather easily. We can go through an entire day without lying, breaking a promise, or killing anybody. We can even go through the day without violating another's autonomy. When the requirements of the deontological principles are satisfied, then utility maximizing can take its place center stage as the guiding principle for both public policy and the individual moral life.

In the chapters that follow, our analysis of organ procurement and allocation incorporates this view that these principles we have called "deontological" have priority over consequences. Yet it is clear that some consequentialists (both Hippocratists and social utilitarians) participating in the policy discussion are seriously committed to morally proper allocation.

It is in this context that we must understand the federal law mandating that the United States' organ allocation system be based on both efficiency and equity. *Efficiency* is a term signaling concern about maximizing net benefits; *equity* requires that we pay attention to the patterns in the distribution—to the principle of justice. The law requiring both efficiency and equity in a national transplant program is, in effect, a law requiring that neither a purely utilitarian (consequence-maximizing) nor a purely deontological approach prevail.

The task for ethical analysis in public policy is to work out the implications of this mandate for organ procurement and allocation while keeping in mind that certain individuals will be committed to personal religious or secular ethics that focus exclusively on consequence maximizing or on some deontological principle—such as respect for autonomy and self-determination or justice in allocating organs. Our goal is to provide a moral framework for thinking about transplantation as a matter of public policy, that is, when both consequences (efficiency) and just allocation (equity) are taken into account.

Notes

1. For the contrasting view, see Pellegrino ED, Thomasma DC, *For the patient's good: The restoration of beneficence in health care* (New York: Oxford University Press, 1988), 115; Brody H, Miller FG, "The internal morality of medicine: Explication and application to managed care," *Journal of Medicine and Philosophy* 1998;23: 384–410; and Pellegrino ED, "The goals and ends of medicine: How are they to be defined?" in *The goals of medicine: The forgotten issue in health care reform*, ed. Hanson M, Callahan D (Washington, DC: Georgetown University Press, 1999).

2. Aristotle, *Nicomachean Ethics*, trans. Ostwald M (Indianapolis: Bobbs-Merrill, 1962).

3. MacIntyre A, *After Virtue* (Notre Dame, IN: University of Notre Dame Press, 1981).

4. Holmes HB, Purdy LM, eds., *Feminist perspectives in medical ethics* (Bloomington: Indiana University Press; 1992); Sherwin S, *No longer patient: Feminist ethics and health care* (Philadelphia:

Temple University Press, 1992); Little MO, "Feminist perspectives on bioethics," special issue of *Kennedy Institute of Ethics Journal* 1996;6: 1–103.

5. Noddings N, *Caring: A feminine approach to ethics and moral education* (Berkeley: University of California Press, 1984); Bishop AH, Scudder, JR, *Nursing ethics: Therapeutic caring presence* (Boston: Jones and Bartlett, 1996); Carse AL, "The 'voice of care': Implications for bioethical education," *Journal of Medicine and Philosophy* 1991;16 (1): 5–28; Reich WT, "Care, II: Historical dimensions of an ethic of care in health care," in *Encyclopedia of bioethics*, rev. edition, ed. Reich WT (New York: Simon & Schuster, 1995), 331–36; Jecker NS, Reich WT, "Care, III: Contemporary ethics of care," in *Encyclopedia*, ed. Reich, 336–44; Sharpe VA, "Justice and care: The implications of the Kohlberg-Gilligan debate for medical ethics," *Theoretical Medicine* 1992;13 (4): 295–318.

6. Knowlden V, "The virtue of caring in nursing," in *Ethical and moral dimensions of care*, ed. Leininger MM (Detroit: Wayne State University Press, 1990), 89–94; Salsberry PJ, "Caring, virtue theory, and a foundation for nursing ethics," *Scholarly Inquiry for Nursing Practice* 1992;6 (2): 155–67; Curzer HJ, "Is care a virtue for health care professionals?" *Journal of Medicine and Philosophy* 1993;18: 51–69; Veatch RM, "The place of care in ethical theory," *Journal of Medicine and Philosophy* 1998;23: 210–24.

7. Edelstein, L, "The Hippocratic Oath: Text, translation and interpretation," in *Ancient medicine: Selected papers of Ludwig Edelstein*, ed. Temkin O, Temkin CL (Baltimore: Johns Hopkins University Press, 1967), 3–64.

8. American Medical Association, Council on Ethical and Judicial Affairs, *Code of Medical Ethics: Current Opinions with Annotations, 1998–1999 Edition* (Chicago: American Medical Association, 1998).

9. Kant I, *Groundwork of the metaphysic of morals*, trans. Paton HJ (New York: Harper & Row, 1964).

10. Ross WD, *The right and the good* (Oxford: Oxford University Press, 1930).

11. Beauchamp TL, Childress, JF, eds., *Principles of biomedical ethics*, 4th ed. (New York: Oxford University Press, 1994).

12. Bentham J, "An introduction to the principles of morals and legislation," in *Ethical theories: A book of readings*, ed. Melden AI (Englewood Cliffs, NJ: Prentice Hall, 1967), 367–90; Mill JS, "Utilitarianism," in *Ethical theories*, ed. Melden, 391–434.

13. For a much fuller discussion of these principles, see Veatch RM, *A theory of medical ethics* (New York: Basic Books, 1981).

14. American Medical Association, Council on Ethical and Judicial Affairs, *Code*.

15. Dworkin R, "What is equality? Part 1: Equality of welfare," *Philosophy and Public Affairs* 1981;10: 185–246; Dworkin R, "What is equality? Part 2: Equality of resources," *Philosophy and Public Affairs* 1981;10: 283–345. For a fuller discussion, see my book-length treatment of the issues: Veatch, RM, *The foundations of justice: Why the retarded and the rest of us have claims to equality* (New York: Oxford University Press, 1986).

16. Rawls J, *A theory of justice* (Cambridge, MA: Harvard University Press, 1971).

17. Veatch, *Theory*; Veatch RM, "Resolving conflict among principles: Ranking, balancing, and specifying," *Kennedy Institute of Ethics Journal* 1995;5: 199–218.

PART I

Defining Death

Chapter 3

The Dead Donor Rule and the Concept of Death

On May 25, 1968, at the beginning of the era of transplantation, Bruce Tucker was brought to the operating room of the hospital of the Medical College of Virginia in Richmond. Tucker, a fifty-six-year-old black laborer, had suffered a massive brain injury the day before in a fall. He had sustained a lateral basilar skull fracture on the right side, a subdural hematoma on the left side, and brain stem contusion. The case revealed the complexities of procuring organs and eventually ended up in the Virginia courts.

According to a timetable summarized by Judge A. Christian Compton, who eventually heard the case when it came to court, Tucker was admitted to the hospital at 6:05 pm, and an emergency right temporoparietal craniotomy was performed with a right parietal burr hole drilled.[1] He was placed on a respirator, which kept him "mechanically alive." The treating physician noted that his "prognosis for recovery is nil and death imminent." By 1:00 pm the next day, the neurologist called to obtain an electroencephalogram (EEG), with the results showing "flat lines with occasional artifact. He found no clinical evidence of viability and no evidence of cortical activity."

At 2:45 pm Tucker was taken to the operating room. From then until 4:30 pm, "he maintained vital signs of life, that is, he maintained, for the most part, normal body temperature, normal pulse, normal blood pressure and normal rate of respiration." At 3:30 pm the respirator was cut off, and the patient was pronounced dead. His heart and kidneys were removed for transplanting.

The Tucker case was to become the first widely publicized controversy about the question of when a person is dead. Many interpret the case as establishing a brain-oriented definition of death for the state of Virginia, but it could equally be viewed as the first case where a ventilator was disconnected for the purpose of causing the death of the patient, by traditional heart criteria, in order to procure organs for transplant.

Tucker's brother, William Tucker, apparently saw it in this way. He sued for $100,000 in damages, charging that the transplant team was engaged in a "systematic and nefarious scheme to use Bruce Tucker's heart and hastened his death by shutting off the mechanical means of support." Moreover, the organs were apparently procured with only minimal effort to locate the next of kin to obtain permission either to stop the respirator or procure the organs. There were insinuations that the transplant team was quicker to act because the patient was black (and it does not help that the recipient was white). It might be worth noting that William Tucker's attorney was a young black Virginia state senator, L. Douglas Wilder, who was later to become governor and a nationally known Democratic politician. The result of the legal case was ambiguous. The doctors were exonerated, but it is unclear whether the court held that the doctors had the authority to turn off the ventilator on a still-living patient in these circumstances or whether it held that Tucker was already dead based on brain criteria. The Virginia definition of death did not change as a result of the case.

In those early years of the definition-of-death debate and the organ transplant controversy, this case was one of the most complicated and significant. Whether it should, in fact, be treated as a "brain death" case is unclear, but certainly that is the way the principals in the case and the press handled it. The Internal Medicine News Service headed its report "'Brain Death' Held Proof of Demise in Va. Jury Decision."[2] The *New York Times*'s headline said, "Virginia Jury Rules That Death Occurs When Brain Dies."[3]

The surgeons who removed Bruce Tucker's heart evidently also interpreted it as a case of deciding when a patient is dead. David Hume, the assisting surgeon in the case, is quoted as saying that the court's decision in favor of the physicians "brings the law up to date with what medicine has known all along—that the only death is brain death."

Most people assumed that, asked to decide whether the physicians were guilty of causing the death of the heart donor, the jury in the Tucker case was in effect being asked to make a public policy judgment about whether the irreversible loss of brain function is to be equated for moral, legal, and public policy purposes with the death of an individual. Because almost all organs for transplant except for those from living kidney donors come from the bodies of the newly deceased and getting those organs in a viable condition is usually assumed to require getting them as soon after death as possible, it is critical to be clear on exactly what it means for a human to be dead.

It is possible that the court found the physician behavior acceptable because it believed that Tucker's brain had irreversibly stopped functioning and that this "death" of the brain should, contrary to what was then Virginia law, be the basis for pronouncing the person dead. It is also possible, however, that the members of the jury approved of the physicians' behavior because they believed that it was acceptable to stop the ventilator and let him die (based on the stopping of heart function). He would then be what we now would call a donation after circulatory death case.

The case leaves many questions unanswered in addition to the issues related to the lack of consent for procuring organs. Why, for example, should a single, flat-line EEG reading be taken as evidence of the irreversible loss of brain function? These events occurred days after the publication of the famous report by the Harvard Ad Hoc Committee that proposed the first peer-reviewed criteria for measuring the death of the brain.[4] A single flat EEG reading would not be sufficient by Harvard committee standards or any set of criteria published since then. Also, if Tucker was believed to be dead based on brain function loss sometime before 3:30 pm, why was the respirator turned off at that time? Unless one feels a need to pronounce death based on heart function loss, it makes no sense to turn off the respirator on a man who is a candidate for organ procurement. Based on brain function loss, he would already be dead before the respirator was stopped.

This case shows how confusing the early days were for pronouncing the deaths of severely brain-injured patients who were potential sources of organs for transplant. It reveals that we needed to do a great deal of work to understand precisely what it means to be dead in a context where someone envisions medical use of a body and when that use is only acceptable once the individual is considered deceased. Part I of this book focuses on this question, which is crucial for almost the entire organ transplant endeavor.

The task of defining death is not a trivial exercise in coining the meaning of a term. Rather, it is an attempt to reach an understanding of the philosophical nature of the human being and what it is that is essentially significant to humans that is lost at the time of death. When we say that an individual has died, there are appropriate behavioral changes: We go into mourning, perhaps cease certain kinds of medical treatment, initiate a funeral ritual, read a will, or, if the individual happens to be president of an organization, elevate the vice president to the presidency. According to many, including those who focus on the definition of death as crucial for the transplant debate, it is appropriate to remove vital, unimpaired organs after, but not before, death. This is what is usually called the "dead donor rule." So there is a great deal at stake at the policy level in the definition of death. We can start by examining this rule.

The Dead Donor Rule

The dead donor rule holds that a human being must be dead before life-prolonging organs (e.g., the heart, liver, or lungs) can be procured for transplant or other purposes. This would exclude procuring a single kidney or a lobe of the liver, either of which would not be expected to end the life of the one from whom the part was taken. The dead donor rule has been discussed in the organ procurement literature for at least the past twenty-five years.[5]

The Standard View

At least until recently, almost everyone accepted this rule. People might have disagreed about exactly what it means to be dead, but there has been a widespread consensus that life-prolonging organs can only be procured once death has occurred. Otherwise, the one procuring these organs would cause the death of the one who is the source of the organs. The organ provider would be killed by means of organ procurement. And the intentional killing of an innocent human, even for the good cause of saving the lives of others, has been almost universally viewed as both unethical and illegal. Some with more radical views would even extend the prohibition on killing to cases of war and self-defense, but almost everyone has assumed that innocent people should not be killed intentionally. This includes the killing of those near an inevitable death, even if they give their permission. Just as the intentional killing of another for mercy has almost universally been unacceptable in medicine, so, too, killing for purposes of procuring organs has been condemned.

The Challenge

Recently, a number of critics have challenged the dead donor rule. Some are concerned that organs will deteriorate unnecessarily if the person who is to be the source of the organs has a respirator stopped or otherwise goes through a process whereby the procurement team waits for the death to occur before intervening. Most of the critics argue a more principled case. They claim that it ought not to be considered immoral to kill patients under certain circumstances, particularly when they are terminally ill and give their permission to have their lives terminated.

This is essentially the position of those who, outside the context of organ procurement, are now defending active, intentional killing—often called euthanasia or physician-assisted suicide. It stands to reason that those who favor euthanasia would be open to killing by means of organ removal in cases where they found other means of euthanasia acceptable. A group of scholars and activists have, during the past two decades or more, been pressing their case for the morality, and sometimes even the legalization, of such killings.[6] For now, however, professional groups, academics, and religious bodies have for the most part remained opposed to these efforts.[7]

Recently, however, a small group of serious scholars has endorsed the procurement of organs without waiting for death to be pronounced, though not necessarily taking a position on the broader question of intentional killings for mercy.[8] Robert Truog, as a coauthor with Franklin Miller and Dan Brock, has provided arguments that he and his colleagues believe support procurement before death pronouncement in cases where the patient has consented to withdrawal of life support and has agreed to donate organs.[9] They first claim, correctly, that even with the withdrawal of life support, the physician who withdraws the life-supporting intervention plays a role in the causal chain leading to the patient's death.

They then claim that if a valid consent is obtained, there is no substantial difference between death from support withdrawal and death by active intervention (including the intervention of removing vital organs). This claim is controversial, and there have been two distinct challenges to their position. One objection focuses on the right of individuals to noninterference. The autonomous refusal of life support, whether by requesting the withholding or the withdrawing of life support, must be respected, lest physicians be liable for battery or assault. But competent patients cannot demand treatments, and as such, they cannot demand the removal of a vital organ that is not clinically indicated. A second objection is based on the doctrine of double effect. This doctrine holds that an evil effect (e.g., death) can be morally tolerable if it is a side effect of an action undertaken with a good intention, if the evil effect is not a means to the good one, and if the harm is proportional to the good effect.[10] This is a widely held view first developed by Roman Catholic theologians but later adopted by many secular thinkers, the American Medical Association, the American courts, and (with qualifications) an important President's Commission.[11] The mainstream of Western thinking relies on the doctrine of double effect or on other related arguments in order to assert the position that forgoing life support can be morally tolerable when the treatment is useless or gravely burdensome, considering the circumstances. By contrast, removing organs and the ensuing death cannot be considered a "side effect," but rather is a means to the good effect of benefiting those who receive the transplants. Hence, the mainstream of Western thinking has consistently rejected Miller and Truog's position that killing to procure organs is no different from withdrawing life support.[12] Even Miller and Truog, however, concede that such procurement is not only presently illegal, but is not likely to be legalized in the foreseeable future.[13]

Candidates for a Concept of "Death"

As long as ethically and legally legitimate organ procurement for transplanting life-prolonging organs is so closely tied to death—that is, as long as we accept the dead donor rule—it becomes crucial to understand with clarity and precision what it means to be dead. But answering this question is not as simple as it might seem.

Four Concepts of Death

There are several plausible candidates for a concept of death. All are attempts to determine that which is so significant to a human being that its loss constitutes the ultimate change in the moral and legal status of the individual. Here, we focus on four main concepts of death. First, the traditional religious and philosophical view in Western culture was that a human died at the time when the soul left the body. This separation of body and soul is difficult to verify scientifically and is best left to the religious traditions, which in some cases still focus upon this soul-departure concept of death.

Traditional secular thinkers have held a second concept of death, one that focused on the cessation of the flow of the vital body fluids, blood and breath; thus, when the circulatory and respiratory functions cease irreversibly, the individual is dead. This is a view of the nature of the human being that identifies the human essence with the flowing of fluids in the animal species. Variations on this view are still held by some, including those who oppose organ procurement before death and also some who are prepared to abandon the dead donor rule.

There are also two new candidates for a concept of death. One of these is that death occurs when there is a complete loss of the body's integrating capacities, which have, until the very recent discussion of the inclusivity of brain functions vis-à-vis death, been signified by the activity of the central nervous system. This third candidate for a concept of what it means to be dead has for the past half century been closely associated with what is popularly, if ambiguously, called "brain death." However, recently in the literature, some have begun to question the adequacy of this notion of death, claiming either that it is too inclusive, by including brain functions that are not critical, or that it is not inclusive enough, because it omits integrative functions that are not brain based. Some ask why is it that one must identify the entire brain with death; is it not possible that we are really interested only in certain more important brain functions? For example, the now-standard definition of death based on brain function loss considers the presence of lower-brain reflexes, such as the gag reflex, as evidence of brain function. Therefore, an individual who has lost all brain functions except for the gag reflex would need to be classified as alive because he or she has not lost all functions of the entire brain. Because they consider someone with any brain function as alive, definitions based on the loss of all functions of the entire brain are now sometimes called *whole-brain-death* definitions. We explore these whole-brain definitions in the next chapter. Some critics, however, now insist that important integrative functions of the body—including circulation, excretion, and reproduction—can be present even in the absence of any brain functions. This has led some to revert to a definition of death that places critical importance on circulation, a view we explore in chapter 5.

Those who reject the idea that literally any function of the brain counts as evidence of a living human being believe that only certain more important brain functions should count. For example, human consciousness—the ability to think, reason, feel, experience, interact with others, and control body functions consciously—might be considered necessary. Because these functions are generally associated with the cerebral cortex, the anatomically and evolutionarily higher portion of the brain, this fourth view is sometimes called the *higher-brain-death* definition. In chapter 6 we sketch the arguments related to this higher-brain view. First, however, we need to clarify two issues that have an impact on any definition of death, and then we can identify the public policy issues at stake in the definition-of-death debate.

Moral, Not Technical

The debate about the meaning of death involves a choice among these candidates for death and other variants we shall encounter in succeeding chapters. The Harvard Ad Hoc Committee to Examine the Definition of Brain Death, a committee at Harvard Medical School made up of physicians, lawyers, theologians, and social scientists, established four operational criteria for what it called an irreversible coma, based on what was then taken to be very sound scientific evidence. These four criteria are (1) unreceptivity and unresponsivity, (2) no movements or breathing, (3) no reflexes, and (4) a flat electroencephalogram ("of great confirmatory value").[14]

What the committee did not do, however, and what it was not capable of doing, was to establish that patients in an irreversible coma are "dead"—that is, that we should treat them as if they were no longer living human beings who possess the same moral rights and obligations as other living people. Although it may be the case that patients in an irreversible coma, according to the Harvard criteria, have shifted to that status where they are no longer to be considered living, the decision that they are "dead" cannot be derived from any amount of scientific investigation and demonstration of the status of the brain. The choice among the many candidates for what is essential to the nature of the species, and, therefore, the loss of which is to be called "death," is a philosophical or moral question, not a medical or scientific one.

Thus, in the definition-of-death debate we encounter a fundamental fact/value issue. There are two more or less separate questions at stake—one normative, the other scientific. The normative question is "What change in a human being is so fundamental that we can say the individual is no longer with us as a member of the human community bearing rights such as the right not to be killed?" The answers involve some irreversible change—in the flowing of vital fluids (blood and breath), in the integration of the organism under the control of the brain, or perhaps in the dissociation of consciousness from organic (bodily) function. Choosing the point at which we should treat humans the way we treat dead people turns out to be a normative issue, not a scientific one. Expertise in neurology or cardiology does not prepare one to provide an answer. Any layperson can form an opinion.

Once we have answered the normative question, we can then move on to ask the scientific question, "How do we know that some element critical for human status—the flowing of fluids, the integrative activity of the brain, or the capacity for consciousness—has been lost irreversibly?" This second question should be largely the domain of medical science. Laypeople lack the expertise to play a direct role in providing an answer. The first question, however—that is, the normative question—is one that laypeople play a central role in answering. No amount of expertise in medical science can tell us whether fluid flow, integrative brain function, or capacity for consciousness is the normatively critical function for assigning the moral and legal status to a human as a living member of the human community.

The Irreversibility Problem

There is a second issue that has an impact on the definition of death. It arises no matter which definition of death one chooses: Must the function loss be irreversible and, if so, what does this mean? Most standard definitions of death include the requirement that the critical function loss, whatever that may be, must be irreversible. Thus, a mistake, potentially a serious mistake, is made if a patient who has suffered cardiac arrest and is then successfully resuscitated is described as having "died and been brought back to life." Other equally confusing and misleading terminology is sometimes used; for example, the patient may be said to have suffered "clinical death."

THE LANGUAGE OF DEATH

If death is, by definition, irreversible, then these accounts of such occurrences as "clinical death" logically must be wrong. One cannot suffer "death" and be brought back to life. "Clinical death" is a meaningless term and is used erroneously if it is made a synonym for suffering cardiac arrest. At no time during an episode of cardiac arrest followed by a successful resuscitation that restores cardiac function was the patient ever dead.

There are very practical issues related to this linguistic point. When one dies, many important social and psychological events occur. One is obviously no longer covered by health insurance; life insurance, conversely, pays off to the beneficiary. One's spouse becomes a widow or widower and is free to remarry. The preparation for burial begins in a way that was not appropriate when the person's loved ones merely anticipated that death was imminent. For the purposes of transplants, one can, with proper authorization, remove vital organs.

It would be a disaster if one triggered any of these behaviors by calling someone dead if the patient's condition were reversible—if, say, cardiac arrest or a loss of brain function could be reversed.[15]

LEGAL VERSUS PHYSIOLOGICAL IRREVERSIBILITY

Assuming that dying is an irreversible event, some ambiguity nonetheless remains. In particular, how ought we understand the moral and legal status of someone whose function loss could be reversed, but will not be? This problem could arise, for example, if someone suffers cardiac arrest in a nursing home or small hospital that lacks the equipment to intervene to reverse the arrest. It might arise if the arrest could be reversed because a physician or someone trained in advanced lifesaving skills was on the scene, but no such person is around. Should we say that such a person is dead as long as the loss will not be reversed, even though it could be reversed if only the proper personnel or equipment were available, or should we wait until the loss could not be reversed under any circumstances?

There is an even more important variation on this problem. Should we call someone dead whose function loss could be reversed, but will not be because that person (or that person's legally authoritative surrogate) has refused life support using an advance directive or other mechanism to refuse consent to resuscitation? What if the patient's function loss could be reversed, but will not be because a refusal of consent for cardiopulmonary resuscitation would make intervention illegal and presumably unethical?

If we say that such people are not really dead as long as they could be resuscitated (even though it would be illegal to do so), we face a serious issue in the routine clinical care of the terminally ill. Consider an elderly, terminally ill patient with metastatic cancer who has refused all further life support. This person will eventually suffer cardiac arrest. At such time, a physician on the scene could potentially restart the heart, but obviously will not. Instead, the physician would plausibly note that the patient has died and pronounce the death to have occurred. The time of cardiac arrest would plausibly be listed as the time of death, not the time several minutes later when resuscitation would be physiologically impossible.

Some commentators have described this distinction as the difference between physiological irreversibility and legal or moral irreversibility. At the time of the arrest, or very soon thereafter, legal or moral irreversibility has occurred. It can be said with certainty that function loss is irreversible, in the sense that we know functions will not resume. We say "very soon thereafter" because—as we shall see when we discuss organ procurement following circulatory arrest—we need to wait long enough to rule out a spontaneous restarting of the heart, what is called *autoresuscitation*. We pronounce death in such cases even though, physiologically, a skilled medical professional could still likely restart the heart function. If this is what we mean by irreversibility, then death can be said to occur when function loss is legally or morally irreversible, even though, physiologically, the process could possibly be reversed.

Some more conservative commentators, such as Don Marquis, have resisted this interpretation of irreversibility.[16] They believe that someone should not be called "dead" if the critical function loss could be reversed, even though it will not be. Those who see the concept of death in biological terms believe that organisms whose function could be restored should not be called dead even though the function is permanently lost.

Marquis and others are now sometimes explicating this situation by distinguishing between "permanent" and "irreversible" loss, where permanent means more or less the same thing as "legally or morally irreversible." Because the laws defining death specify that death is an irreversible event, limiting the word "irreversible" to physiological irreversibility has important practical and legal significance. Loss that is merely permanent, but is not physiologically irreversible, is not death at all. Conversely, those willing to treat as dead those people who have lost function and will not have it restored (i.e., those who equate death with permanent loss) are more likely to use permanence and legal irreversibility interchangeably, thus making such loss consistent with definition-of-death statutes that ambiguously require "irreversibility" without specifying which kind.

Thus, unless we overturn the dead donor rule, an action that would require a major change in the law as well as revision of the cultural consensus, we may procure life-prolonging organs only from dead people. And now, for public policy purposes—including organ procurement—we therefore need to understand precisely what it means to say that someone is dead.

The Public Policy Question

The public policy discussion of how to define death began in earnest in the late 1960s, not long before surgeons were confronted by Bruce Tucker's case. Now, a half century later, we are still unclear about exactly what it means to be dead. The 1960s debate began in the context of a world that had in the previous decade seen the first successful transplantation of an organ from one human being to another. By 1967 we had seen the first transplant of a human heart. It cannot be denied that this sudden infatuation with the usefulness of human organs was the stimulus for the intense debate about the real meaning of death. What many thought would be a rather short-lived debate, resolved by the combined wisdom of the health professionals and the nonscientists on the Harvard Ad Hoc Committee to Examine the Definition of Brain Death, has lingered as an intractable morass of conflicting technical, legal, conceptual, and moral arguments. Much of this confusion can be avoided, however, by focusing exclusively on the public policy dimensions of the debate about when death occurs.

Focusing on public policy means avoiding a full linguistic analysis of the term "death." Although that may be an important philosophical project, and many have undertaken it, such an analysis would be of only indirect importance for public policy questions, including the organ transplant questions that are the subject of this book.[17] Likewise, we need not provide a detailed theological account of the meaning of death. Such studies are numerous, but they are not of immediate concern for the formation of secular public policy.[18] Nor are we concerned about the ontological question of when an entity ceases to be human. Some philosophers have tried to turn the definition-of-death debate into such a deep philosophical exploration.[19] Most significantly, it is not necessary to give a scientific description of the biological events in the brain at the time of death. Of course, this description is of crucial importance for the science of neurology, and a vast literature is available giving such an account.[20] But the scientific, biological, and neurological descriptions of precisely what takes place in the human body at the point of death are not a matter that need directly concern makers of public policy.

Instead, what we are interested in is the answer to one key public policy question: When should we begin treating an individual the way we treat the newly dead? Is it possible to identify a point in the course of human events at which a new set of social behaviors becomes appropriate—at which, because we say the individual has died, we may justifiably begin to treat him or her in a way that was not previously appropriate, morally or legally? In short, what we are interested in is a social system of *death behaviors*.

Social and cultural changes take place when we label someone as dead. Perhaps, some medical treatments may be stopped when an individual is considered dead that would not be stopped if the individual were alive—even if the living individual were terminally ill. This, of course, does not imply that there are treatments that should not be stopped at other times, either before or after the moment when we label someone as dead. Many treatments are stopped before death for technical reasons. Other treatments, including some that prolong life, may justifiably be stopped before death because they are no longer appropriate, because they either no longer serve a useful purpose or are too burdensome. In other cases, if the newly dead body is to be used for research, education, or transplant purposes, it is possible to continue certain interventions even after death has been declared. Many have held that this is morally acceptable.[21] However, it appears that, at least traditionally, some treatments have been stopped when and only when we have decided that it is time to treat the individual as dead.

Other behaviors, some of which were described earlier in this chapter, also have traditionally taken place at the time we consider the individual dead—behaviors such as mourning in a pattern that is not appropriate for mere anticipatory grief, beginning the process that will lead to reading the person's will, burying or otherwise disposing of what we now take to be the person's "mortal remains," and assuming the role of widowhood or widowerhood.[22] Perhaps of most immediate relevance to the concern that generated the definition-of-death debate, we change the procedures and justifications for obtaining organs from the body. Assuming we continue to accept the dead donor rule, before death, organs can only be removed in the interests of the individual, or perhaps in procurements that are not expected to lead to the individual's death, with the consent of the individual or his or her legal guardian.[23] (These issues involving "living donors" are the subject of chapter 12.) At the moment we decide to treat someone as dead, an entirely different set of procedures is called for.

For the United States the procedures were originally designated in the Uniform Anatomical Gift Act, which was drawn up in 1968 and more recently has been refined in several proposed revisions.[24] At this point, if one has agreed while alive to donate organs after one has died, they may be removed according to the terms of the donation without further consideration of the interest of the former individual or the wishes of his or her family members. If the deceased has not expressed his or her wishes to donate, but has also not expressed opposition to donation, the next of kin or other legitimate guardian in possession of the body assumes both the right and the responsibility for the disposal of the remains and may donate the organs.

It is clear that at least in Anglo-American law, the person with such a responsibility cannot merely dispose of the body capriciously in any way he or she sees fit, but bears a responsibility to treat the new corpse with respect and dignity.[25] This, however, has been taken both in law and in morality as permitting the donation of body parts by the one with this responsibility, except when an explicit objection was expressed by the now-deceased during his or her life. (The issues surrounding the "donation" model and the alternatives to donation are explored in part II of this book.)

In short, traditionally there has been a radical shift in moral, social, and political standing when someone has been labeled as dead. Until the 1960s there was not a great deal of controversy over exactly when such a label should be applied. There were deviant philosophical and theological positions and substantial concern about the erroneous labeling of someone as dead, but there was very little real controversy about what it meant to be dead in this public policy sense.

Now, for the first time, there are matters of real public policy significance in deciding precisely what we mean when we label someone dead. In an earlier day, all the socially significant death-related behaviors were generated at the time of death pronouncement. Very little was at stake if we were not precise in sorting out the various indicators of the time when this behavior was appropriate. Virtually all the plausible events related to death occurred in rapid succession, and none of the behaviors was really contingent upon having any greater precision.

But matters have changed in two important ways. First, several technologies have greatly extended our capacity to prolong the dying process, making it possible to identify several different potential indicators of what we should take to be the death of the individual as a whole, and have separated these points dramatically in time. Second, the usefulness of human organs and tissues for transplantation, research, and education makes precision morally imperative. In an earlier day, the most that was at stake was that an individual could for a few seconds or moments be falsely treated as alive when in fact he or she should have been treated as dead, or vice versa. Of course, it is crucial, out of our sense of respect for persons, that we not confuse living individuals with their corpses, so in theory it has always been important that we be clear about whether someone is dead or alive. Yet, traditionally, the very short time frame for the entire series of events meant that there was very little at stake as a matter of public policy. We could pronounce death based on the rapid succession of an inevitably linked series of bodily events—heart stoppage, stoppage of respiration, or the death of the brain—without determining exactly which event was critical.

As we extend the period of time during which these events can occur, which in turn permits much more precision in identifying what in the human body signifies that it should be treated as dead, we must ask the question: Can we continue to identify a single, definable point when all the social behaviors associated with death should begin? It may turn out that as the dying process is extended, all these behaviors will find their own niches and that it really will cease to be important to label someone as dead at a precise moment in time. This has been called "disaggregation."[26] Life-sustaining treatment could then be stopped at one moment, mourning begun at another, and life insurance payoffs and funeral preparations made or started at still others. In this new context, organ procurement could take place at its own special moment, independent of exactly when death is pronounced. If so, death itself, and also dying, could begin to be viewed as a process.[27]

However, it seems likely that this will not happen. Rather, we may want to continue to link at least many of these social events, so we shall continue to say that there is a moment when it becomes appropriate to begin the entire series of death behaviors—or at least many of them. If so, then the death of an individual as a whole will continue to be viewed as a single event, rather than as a process.[28] There are several plausible candidates for this critical point where we can say that the individual as a whole has died—including the time when circulatory function ceases; the time when all brain functions cease; and the time when certain important brain functions, such as mental function, cease.

The question is therefore not precisely the same as the one the philosopher asks when he or she asks the question of the endpoint of personhood or personal identity.[29] Analyses of the concept of personhood or personal identity suggest that there may be an identifiable endpoint at which we should stop thinking of a human organism as a *person*. This analysis by itself, however, never tells us whether it is morally appropriate to begin treating that human the way we have traditionally treated the dead, unless personhood is simply defined with reference to death behavior, which it often is not.

Under some formulations, such as those of Michael Green and Daniel Wikler, it is conceptually possible to talk about a living individual in cases where the person no longer exists.[30] (This would be true, for example, if we said that living humans were persons only when they possessed self-awareness or the ability to distinguish themselves from others.) Some human individuals could then be alive, but not persons. Logically, we would then be pressed to the moral and policy question of whether these living bodies that are no longer persons are to be treated differently from the way we are used to treating living persons.

Fortunately, for matters of public policy, if not for philosophical analysis, we need not take up the question of personhood or personal identity, but can directly confront the question of whether we can identify a point where this series of death behaviors is appropriate. In this way death comes to mean, for public policy purposes, nothing more than the condition of some group of human beings for whom death behavior is appropriate.[31] Can we identify this point? If we can, then, for purposes of law and public policy, we shall label this point as the moment of death. The laws reformulating the definition of death do not go so far as to say that they are defining death for all purposes—theological, philosophical, and personal. Some explicitly limit the scope, saying that the law defines death "for all *legal* purposes."

We now recognize that this point at which a group of *death behaviors* is considered appropriate may not exactly match the endpoint of biological life, or even the point at which the integrated functioning of an organism ceases. Thus, the word *death* may have come to have more than one meaning. The endpoint of the organism's integrated functioning may not be the same as the point where society calls the individual dead for legal and public policy purposes. If the term *death* takes on multiple meanings, it will have many similarities to the word *person*.

The term *person* now has both nonmoral and moral meanings. The nonmoral meaning equates persons with self-aware beings; the moral meaning equates persons with beings who are the bearers of human rights (e.g., the right not to be killed). Thus, conservatives on abortion can argue for a constitutional amendment specifying that humans are "persons" from the moment of conception, without implying that the preembryo is a self-aware being. By this same bit of linguistic ambiguity, it is possible that some may be dead for public policy purposes even though biological functions remain.

In the past decade, as we have discovered the increasing complexity of the concept of death, we have been facing a linguistic choice. As it becomes increasingly clear, for example, that individuals who have irreversibly lost all functions of the entire brain may nevertheless retain many biological functions that make the body function as an integrated whole, we could insist that the word *death* retain its traditional biological meaning and claim that those with dead brains may not necessarily be dead people. In retrospect, that may have been the simpler use of terms. However, in the decades since the original proposal for brain-based concepts of death, laws and public discourse have established the pattern of also using the term *death* to refer to those beings who should be treated the way we treat the dead. The term *death*, then, like the term *person*, has taken on a second meaning—a moral as well as a biological meaning. One approach is to ask, for public policy purposes, which beings should be treated the way we treat dead people, and call those people "dead." That is the current usage. Laws in all US jurisdictions (and in most other countries of the world) affirm that individuals who have irreversibly lost certain functions shall be treated as dead, even though some biological functions, such as circulation, remain. The question for the following chapters is when, for public policy purposes, should we treat human beings the way we treat the dead—when should we call them "dead" in this second sense of the term?

In the next three chapters, omitting the religious concept involving the departure of the soul, we examine the three major answers (or groups of answers) to this question. We look first at what we call the whole-brain answers; then at the circulatory, or somatic, answers; and finally at the higher-brain answers.

Notes

1. *Tucker v. Lower*, No. 2831 (Richmond, VA, L & Eq. Ct., May 23, 1972; Frederick RS, "Medical jurisprudence: Determining the time of death of the heart transplant donor," *North Carolina Law Review* 1972;51: 172–84.

2. "'Brain death' held proof of demise in Va. Jury decision," *Internal Medicine News*, July 1, 1992, 1, 19.

3. "Virginia jury rules that death occurs when brain dies," *New York Times*, May 27, 1972.

4. Harvard Medical School, "A definition of irreversible coma: Report of the Ad Hoc Committee of the Harvard Medical School to Examine the Definition of Brain Death," *JAMA* 1968;205: 337–40.

5. Robertson JA, "Relaxing the death standard for organ donation in pediatric situations," in *Organ substitution technology: Ethical, legal, and public policy issues*, ed. Mathieu D (Boulder, CO: Westview Press, 1988), 69–76; Fost N, "Organs from anencephalic infants: An idea whose time has not yet come," *Hastings Center Report* 1988;18 (5): 5–10.

6. On the morality of intentional killings, see Rachels J, "Active and passive euthanasia," *New England Journal of Medicine* 1975;292: 78–80; Quill T, *Death and dignity: Making choices and taking charge* (New York: W. W. Norton, 1993); Beauchamp TL, *Intending death: The ethics of assisted suicide and euthanasia* (Upper Saddle River, NJ: Prentice Hall, 1996); Battin MP, *Ending life: Ethics and the way we die* (New York: Oxford University Press, 2005). On the legalization of intentional killings, see *Quill et al. v. Vacco et al.*, Docket No. 95-7028, US Court of Appeals for the Second Circuit; *Compassion in Dying v. Washington*, No. 94-35534 D.C. No. CV-94-119-BJR, US Court of Appeals for the Ninth Circuit.

7. On the positions of professional groups, see American Medical Association, Council on Ethical and Judicial Affairs, *AMA's Code of Ethics*, opinion 2.21, issued June 1994, www.ama-assn.org/ama/pub/physician-resources/medical-ethics/code-medical-ethics/opinion221.page?. On the positions of academics, see Foot P, "Active euthanasia with parental consent," *Hastings Center Report* 1979;9 (5): 20–21; Gaylin W, Kass L, Pellegrino E, Siegler M, "Doctors must not kill," *JAMA* 1988;259: 2139–40; Pellegrino ED, "Doctors must not kill," in *Euthanasia: The good patient*, ed. Misbin RI (Frederick, MD: University Publishing Group, 1992), 27–42; Kamisar Y, "Are laws against assisted suicide unconstitutional?" *Hastings Center Report* 1993;23 (3): 32–41. On the positions of religious bodies, see US Conference of Catholic Bishops, *Ethical and religious directives for Catholic health care services*, 5th ed. (Washington, DC: US Catholic Conference, 2009), www.usccb.org/issues-and-action/human-life-and-dignity/health-care/upload/Ethical-Religious-Directives-Catholic-Health-Care-Services-fifth-edition-2009.pdf.

8. Fost N, "The unimportance of death," in *The definition of death: Contemporary controversies*, ed. Youngner SJ, Arnold RM, Schapiro R (Baltimore: Johns Hopkins University Press, 1999), 172–74; Koppelman ER, "The dead donor rule and the concept of death: Severing the ties that bind them," *American Journal of Bioethics* 2003;3 (1): 1–9; Rodríguez-Arias D, Smith MJ, Lazar NM, "Donation after circulatory death: Burying the dead donor rule," *American Journal of Bioethics* 2011;11 (8): 36–43.

9. Truog RD, Miller FG, "The dead donor rule and organ transplantation," *New England Journal of Medicine* 2008;359: 674–75; Miller FG, Truog RD, *Death, dying, and organ transplantation* (New York: Oxford University Press, 2012); Miller FG, Truog RD, Brock DW, "The dead donor rule: Can it withstand critical scrutiny?" *Journal of Medicine and Philosophy* 2010;35 (3): 299–312.

10. McCormick RA, Ramsey P, eds., *Doing evil to achieve good: Moral choice in conflict situations* (Chicago: Loyola University Press, 1978); Graber GC, "Some questions about double effect," *Ethics in Science and Medicine* 1979;6 (1): 65–84; Marquis DB, "Four versions of double effect," *Journal of Medicine and Philosophy* 1991;16: 515–44; Pellegrino ED, "Intending to kill and the principle of double effect," in *Ethical issues in death and dying*, 2nd edition, ed. Beauchamp TL, Veatch RM (Englewood Cliffs, NJ: Prentice Hall, 1995), 240–42.

11. President's Commission for the Study of Ethical Problems in Medicine and Biomedical and Behavioral Research, *Deciding to forgo life-sustaining treatment: Ethical, medical, and legal issues in treatment decisions* (Washington, DC: US Government Printing Office, 1983), 80–82.

12. On Western thinking, see Veatch RM, "The dead donor rule: True by definition," *American Journal of Bioethics* 2003;3 (1): 10–11; McCartney JJ, "The theoretical and practical importance of the dead donor rule," *American Journal of Bioethics* 3 (1): 15–16; Vernez SL, Magnus D, "Can the dead donor rule be resuscitated?" *American Journal of Bioethics* 2011;11 (8): 1; and Chen Y, Wen-Je K, "Further deliberating burying the dead donor rule in donation after circulatory death," *American Journal of Bioethics* 2011;11 (8): 58–59. For Miller and Truog's position, see Miller, Truog, *Death*, 14–18.

13. Ibid., 151.

14. Harvard Medical School, "Definition."

15. There exists in the philosophical literature pertaining to the definition of death a minority view holding that "death" is indeed a reversible event and that those who suffer a cardiac arrest and are resuscitated are properly said to have died and been brought back to life. This usage is overwhelmingly rejected, however, in favor of insisting that if the arrest is reversed, death never occurred, only a cardiac arrest that would have led to death had not the arrest been reversed. See Cole DJ, "The reversibility of death," *Journal of Medical Ethics* 1992;18: 26–30; and Cole D, "Statutory definitions of death and the management of terminally ill patients who may become organ donors after death," *Kennedy Institute of Ethics Journal* 1993;3: 145–55. Cf. Lamb D, "Reversibility and death: A reply to David Cole," *Journal of Medical Ethics* 1992;18 (1): 31–33; and Tomlinson T, "The irreversibility of death: Reply to Cole," *Kennedy Institute of Ethics Journal* 1993;3: 157–65.

16. Marquis D, "Are DCD donors dead?" *Hastings Center Report* 2010;40 (3): 24–31. Even some commentators who hold very liberal views regarding organ procurement have taken the position that mere permanent function loss should not count as death. See Miller, Truog, *Death*, 106–7.

17. Becker LC, "Human being: The boundaries of the concept," *Philosophy and Public Affairs* 1975;4: 334–59; Cole, "Reversibility"; Green MB, Wikler D, "Brain death and personal identity," *Philosophy and Public Affairs* 1980;9 (2): 105–33. Lamb, "Reversibility"; Mayo D, Wikler, D, "Euthanasia and the transition from life to death," in *Medical responsibility: Paternalism, informed consent, and euthanasia*, ed. Robinson W, Pritchard MS (Clifton, NJ: Humane Press, 1979); Veatch RM, *Death, dying, and the biological revolution*, rev. ed. (New Haven, CT: Yale University Press, 1989); Veatch RM, "The definition of death: Unresolved controversies," in *Pediatric brain death and organ/tissue retrieval*, ed. Kaufman HH (New York: Plenum, 1989), 207–18; Wikler D, Weisbard AJ, "Appropriate confusion over 'brain death,'" *JAMA* 1989;261 (15): 2246; Youngner SJ, Landefeld CS, Coulton CJ, Juknialis BW, Leary M, "'Brain death' and organ retrieval," *JAMA* 1989;261: 2205–10.

18. Bleich JD, "Neurological criteria of death and time-of-death status," in *Jewish bioethics*, ed. Bleich JD, Rosner F (New York: Sanhedrin Press, 1979), 303–16; Bleich, JD, "Of cerebral, respiratory, and cardiac death," *Tradition: A Journal of Orthodox Jewish Thought* 1989;24 (3): 44–66; Fletcher J, "Our shameful waste of human tissue," in *Updating life and death*, ed. Cutler DR (Boston: Beacon Press, 1969), 1–27; Haring B, *Medical ethics* (Notre Dame, IN: Fides Press, 1973); Hauerwas S, "Religious concepts of brain death and associated problems," in *Brain death: Interrelated medical and social issues*, ed. Korein J (New York: New York Academy of Sciences, 1978), 329–38; Pope Pius XII, "The prolongation of life: An address of Pope Pius XII to an International Congress of Anesthesiologists," *The pope speaks* 1958;4: 393–98; Ramsey P, *The patient as person* (New Haven, CT: Yale University Press, 1970), 59–164.

19. Green, Wikler, "Brain death," 105–33; cf. Gervais KG, *Redefining Death* (New Haven, CT: Yale University Press, 1986).

20. Ashwal S, Schneider S, "Brain death in children, I, II," *Pediatric Neurology* 1987;3: 5–10, 69–78; Black PM, "Brain death," *New England Journal of Medicine* 1978;299: 338–44, 393–401; Collaborative Study, "An appraisal of the criteria of cerebral death: A summary statement," *JAMA* 1977;237: 982–86; Cranford R, et al., "Uniform Brain Death Act," *Neurology* 1979;29: 417–18; Harvard Medical School, "Definition"; O'Brien MD, "Criteria for diagnosing brain stem death," *British Medical Journal* 1990;301: 108–9; "Report of the Medical Consultants on the Diagnosis of Death to the President's Commission for the Study of Ethical Problems in Medicine and Biomedical and Behavioral Research," in *Defining death: Medical, legal and ethical issues in the definition of death*, ed. President's Commission for the Study of Ethical Problems in Medicine and Biomedical and Behavioral Research (Washington, DC: US Government Printing Office, 1981), 159–66; Shewmon DA, "Commentary on guidelines for the determination of brain death in children," *Annals of Neurology* 1988;24: 789–91; Task Force for the Determination of Brain Death in Children, "Guidelines for the determination of brain death in children," *Neurology* 1987;37: 1077–78.

21. Haring, *Medical ethics*; Ramsey, *Patient*, 59–164.

22. Fulton R, Fulton J, "Anticipatory grief: A psychosocial aspect of terminal care," in *Psychosocial aspects of terminal care*, ed. Schoenberg B, Carr AC, Peretz D, Kutscher AH (New York: Columbia University Press, 1972), 227–42.

23. Fellner CH, "Selection of living kidney donors and the problem of informed consent," *Seminars in Psychiatry* 1971;3: 70–85; Mahoney J, "Ethical aspects of donor consent in transplantation," *Journal of Medical Ethics* 1975;1: 67–70; Robertson JA, "Organ donations by incompetents and the substituted judgment doctrine," *Columbia Law Review* 1976;3: 48ff; Simmons RG, Fulton J, "Ethical issues in kidney transplantation," *Omega* 1971;2: 179–90.

24. National Conference of Commissioners on Uniform State Laws (NCCUSL), *Uniform Anatomical Gift Act* (Chicago: NCCUSL, 1968); NCCUSL, *Uniform Anatomical Gift Act (1987)* (Chicago: NCCUSL, 1987); NCCUSL, *Revised Uniform Anatomical Gift Act* (Chicago: NCCUSL, 2006).

25. May WF, "Attitudes toward the newly dead," *Hastings Center Studies* 1973;1 (1): 3–13.

26. Halevy A, Brody, B, "Brain death: Reconciling definitions, criteria, and tests," *Annals of Internal Medicine* 1993;119: 519–25; Truog RD, "Is it time to abandon brain death?" *Hastings Center Report* 1997;27 (1): 29–37. See also Veatch RM, "The death of whole-brain death: The plague of the disaggregators, somaticists, and mentalists," *Journal of Medicine and Philosophy* 2005;30: 353–78.

27. Morison R, "Death: Process or event?" *Science* 1971;173: 694–98.

28. Kass L, "Death as an event: A commentary on Robert Morison," *Science* 1971;173: 698–702.

29. Tooley M, "Decisions to terminate life and the concept of person," in *Ethical issues relating to life and death*, ed. Ladd J (New York: Oxford University Press, 1979), 62–93.

30. Green, Wikler, "Brain death."

31. One of us has argued this claim; see Veatch RM, "The dead donor rule: True by definition," *American Journal of Bioethics* 2003;3 (1): 10–11.

Chapter 4

The Whole-Brain Concept of Death

The concept of death that emerged in the second half of the twentieth century, the concept closely connected to the procurement of organs for transplant, is often simply referred to as "brain death." It holds that an individual has died (and should be treated the way we treat dead people) when there is an irreversible loss of all functions of the entire brain. Those proposing such a concept make clear that it is all functions of the brain—including the brain stem—that must be lost, and they must be lost irreversibly. Because it is the functions of the entire brain that must be lost, sometimes this is referred to as the "whole-brain" concept of death.

Unfortunately, the term *brain death* has emerged in the debate over the definition of death. This is unfortunate, in part because we are not interested in the death of brains; we are interested in the death of organisms as integrated entities subject to particular kinds of public behavior and control. In contrast, the term *brain death* is systematically ambiguous. It has two potential meanings. The first is not controversial; it simply means the destruction of the brain, leaving open the question of whether people with destroyed brains should be treated as dead people (more precisely, as "dead former persons"). It is better to substitute the phrase "destruction of the brain" for brain death in this sense. It makes clear that we are referring only to the complete biological collapse of the organ or organs we call the brain. Exactly how that is measured is largely a neurological question.

Confusingly, *brain death* has also taken on a second, very different, and much more controversial meaning. It can also mean the death of the individual as a whole, based on the fact that the brain has died. The problem is illustrated in the original report of the Harvard Ad Hoc Committee, which became the most significant technical document in the early stages of the American debate.[1] The title of that 1968 document is "A Definition of Irreversible Coma." The article sets out to define "characteristics of irreversible coma" and produces a list of technical criteria that purport to predict that an individual is in a coma that is irreversible. The name of the committee, however, is the "Harvard Ad Hoc Committee to Examine the Definition of Brain Death." The presumption apparently was that an irreversible coma and brain death were synonymous.

We now realize that this is not precisely true. An individual can apparently be in an irreversible coma and still not have a completely dead brain. To be even more precise, people can be either in an irreversible coma or in a persistent or permanent vegetative state (PVS) and still not have a completely dead brain. PVS is further differentiated from an irreversible coma in that those in an irreversible coma are in a sleep-like state, whereas those in PVS go through sleep–wake cycles and may appear to be alert, even though, by definition, they have no conscious experience. Some famous cases of patients in PVS have included Karen Quinlan and Terri Schiavo. We now know that neither an irreversible coma nor PVS involves complete loss of all brain functions, even though they are permanent states of unconsciousness.

In any case, the title of the report and the name of the committee, taken in the context of what the committee did, imply that the objective of the committee was to describe the empirical measures of a destroyed brain. The opening sentence of the report, however, says, "Our primary purpose is to define irreversible coma as a new criterion for death." It does not claim to be defining the destruction (death) of the brain, but death simpliciter, whereby everyone, including the committee members, meant the death of the individual for purposes of death behaviors, clinical practice, and public policy—including, of course, the procurement of life-prolonging organs in a way consistent with the dead donor rule. Yet the report contains no argument that the destruction of the brain (measured by the characteristics of an irreversible coma) should be taken as a justification for treating the individual as a whole as dead. The members of the committee and many others believed that this should be so, possibly with good reason, but the reasons were not stated.

Because the term *brain death* has these two radically different meanings, there is often confusion in public and professional discussions of the issues related to it. For instance, neurologists can claim that they have real expertise on brain death, meaning, of course, expertise in measuring the destruction of the brain. Others claim, however, that brain death is exclusively a matter for public policy consideration, meaning that the question of whether we should treat an individual as dead because the brain tissue is dead is really one outside the scope of neurological expertise. A far better course would be to abandon that language entirely, substituting precise and explicit language that either refers to the destruction of the brain or to the death of the individual as a whole based on brain criteria.

Debate over the past fifty years between holders of concepts of death that focus on the brain and those that focus on the more traditional heart and lungs has created a situation whereby defenders of the neurological concepts of death have not been forced to be particularly precise in specifying the meaning of terms. The seemingly endless prolongation of cellular and organ functioning (in what can be appropriately called human corpses) has been brought about by new death-assaulting technologies, giving rise to a new and inhuman form of existence. Although the potential use of human organs for therapeutic transplantation should never justify the adoption of a new understanding of what is essentially significant to human life and death, it may require a philosophically responsible clarification of an imprecise use of these terms, which were adequate only in a time when little that was morally critical was at stake. These developments have led to an infatuation with neurologically oriented concepts, which have made the more traditional heart-and-lung definition of death appear inadequate and outmoded. The thesis of this chapter, however, is that the time has come when crude formulations of the so-called brain definition of death can no longer be tolerated.

Holders of the whole-brain-oriented concept of death would probably grant that the only practical problem with the more traditional concept, which focuses on the heart and lungs, is that it will on special occasions produce false positive tests for human life. In these rare cases, individuals who should be considered dead are labeled alive because their heart and lung functions continue, even though brain function may have permanently and irreversibly ceased. Traditional moralists, however, or at least those who tend to hold a more rigorous, life-preserving position regarding moral obligations to an individual human being, have followed the principle of erring in the direction of following the morally safer course. Thus, Hans Jonas, one of the key players in the early definition-of-death debate, argued that unless one can be certain of the philosophical (technical uncertainty is not being considered here) foundations of the more limited brain-oriented concept, one should opt for the false positive judgment of continuing life, rather than running the moral risk of a false pronouncement of death.[2]

The risk, then, is that of considering individuals with no brain function to be dead when in fact they are alive. Those who hold the brain-oriented concept of death have apparently satisfied themselves that there is no significant risk of this mistake being made.

The Case for the Whole-Brain Concept

In chapter 3 we introduced the distinction between the concept of death, which raises philosophical and normative questions, and the scientific criteria for death, the tests for the loss of what is so significant about human life that its loss constitutes death. The significance of this distinction can be seen if one begins with a completely formal definition of death: "Death is the irreversible loss of that which is essentially significant to its nature."

Such a formal definition of death can be given substantive content only through further philosophical analysis. It is necessary to reach some understanding about what is essentially significant to the nature of the human. This can never be determined by biological investigation, but only by philosophical or theological reflection.

Although the Harvard Ad Hoc Committee did not offer any argument for a new brain-based concept of death, that project was nonetheless pursued over the following decade. The Research Group on Death and Dying of the Institute of Society, Ethics and the Life Sciences (now called the Hastings Center) took up the question in its 1972 review of the Harvard criteria.[3] This group, which included the chair of the Harvard Ad Hoc Committee, Henry Beecher, as well as a number of philosophically sophisticated thinkers such as Paul Ramsey, William May, and Daniel Callahan, recognized that there were problems in articulating a concept of death, problems not addressed by the Harvard committee. Its work pointed us in the direction of the consensus that was to emerge in the late twentieth century.

By 1981 a report titled *Defining Death* by the US President's Commission for the Study of Ethical Problems in Medicine and Biomedical and Behavioral Research clearly addressed the question.[4] It adopted a concept of death based on the irreversible loss of the body's integrating capacity: "Death is that moment at which the body's physiological system ceases to constitute an integrated whole. Even if life continues in individual cells or organs, life of the organism as a whole requires complex integration, and without the latter, a person cannot properly be regarded as alive."[5]

At about the same time, others were defining death as the "permanent cessation of functioning of the organism as a whole."[6] Often, a distinction was made between the "whole organism" and "the organism as a whole." The general belief was that the whole brain, not just the cerebrum, was the primary regulator of the functioning of the organism as a whole and that, therefore, the irreversible loss of all the functions of the entire brain constituted the death of the organism.

Thus, one candidate for the concept of death in humans is the irreversible loss of the capacity of the body to function as an integrated whole. If we are speaking of the death of the organism as a whole—and not simply the death of isolated cells, organs, or organ systems—it at first seems plausible to consider the complex integrating capacity of an organism as that which is essential to it. If this is the case, then the loss of this integrating capacity could appropriately be equated with the organism's death. At the end of the twentieth century it was accepted as common wisdom that the brain was the locus of this capacity. To be sure, the spinal cord and peripheral nerves are also important, but these do not really provide significant integration. The spinal reflex at most provides a primitive and pale imitation of integrating function. The mysterious integrating capacity of the nervous system, which has fascinated humans and been conceptualized so influentially by Claude Bernard, is, by comparison, so much grander as to constitute the difference between a simple animal and the human organism.

It seemed reasonable from what we thought we knew about the brain to relate this concept of integrating capacity to the whole brain. If this is what is seen as essentially significant to the human, then the examination of the whole brain for signs of functioning is a plausible test of the death of the individual.

On the basis of these views, the President's Commission in 1981 endorsed the "Uniform Determination of Death Act" as containing the legal definition of death proposed by the American Bar Association, the American Medical Association, and the National Conference of Commissioners on Uniform State Laws. This act reads: "An individual who has sustained either (1) irreversible cessation of circulatory and respiratory functions; or (2) irreversible cessation of all functions of the entire brain, including the brain stem, is dead. A determination of death must be made in accordance with accepted medical standards."[7] These "accepted medical standards" have been debated over the years, giving rise to various sets of what are sometimes referred to as criteria for death based on brain function loss.

Criteria for the Destruction of All Brain Functions

In the years since 1968 several sets of criteria have been proposed to measure the irreversible loss of all functions of the brain. In Europe it is common to rely on cerebral angiography.[8] In the United States the report of the Harvard Ad Hoc Committee provided the first widely accepted criteria set.

The Harvard Criteria, 1968

The Harvard report proposed four criteria:[9]

1. Unreceptivity and unresponsivity,
2. No movement or breathing,

3. No reflexes, and

4. A flat electroencephalogram (EEG).

The fourth criterion, a flat EEG, was presented as being "of great confirmatory value" but as not necessary. Presumably, if the first three criteria were met, then the claim was that the EEG would need to be isoelectric, and that an isoelectric EEG would necessarily require that the first three criteria were satisfied. The criteria set specifies that the EEG should be isoelectric when the gain is set at 5 microvolts per millimeter. This may be more controversial than it appears, because it implies that very small amounts of electrical activity coming from the brain tissue can be ignored. Some activity could be from tissues surrounding the brain or from an artifact, but if there are even small amounts of electrical activity from the brain itself, this implies that the tissue is not really dead.

These tests were to be repeated at least 24 hours later with no change in findings. Two medical conditions, hypothermia and central nervous system depressants, had to be excluded.

The Minnesota Criteria, 1971

In 1971 a similar set of criteria was proposed by Mohandas and Chou, writing in the *Journal of Neurosurgery*.[10] They refined the reflex tests, excluding spinal reflexes, and extended the time period for the apnea testing from 3 to 4 minutes. They shortened the time period for repeat testing to 12 hours. They specifically rejected the need for an EEG.

National Institute of Neurological Diseases and Stroke, 1977

The National Institute of Neurological Diseases and Stroke formed a panel that developed further variations on the criteria set.[11] It added cardiovascular shock and remedial lesions to the list of exclusions and called for repeating tests 6 hours later. The EEG should show no activity greater than 2 microvolts per millimeter. It endorsed cerebral blood flow tests for confirmation.

Minnesota Medical Association Criteria, 1978

The Minnesota Medical Association endorsed a criteria set in 1978 that added intoxication as an exclusion criterion.[12] It accepted the 3-minute apnea test and a 12-hour period of repeat testing. It considered an EEG or angiography to be optional.

Medical Consultants to the President's Commission, 1981

The US President's Commission for the Study of Ethical Problems in Medicine and Biomedical and Behavioral Research established a group of medical consultants whose members presented their consensus criteria set as an appendix to the *Defining Death* report.[13] They modified the Harvard criteria by adding neuromuscular blockade, cardiovascular shock, and metabolic disturbances to the exclusions, and also excluded the use of the criteria in children below the age of five years. They extended the period of apnea testing to 10 minutes and supported EEG or cerebral blood flow for confirmation. They proposed a more complex time period for repeating the tests: 6 hours with confirmatory tests, 12 hours without, and 24 hours desirable for anoxic brain damage. Furthermore, they required the cause of coma must be established.

American Academy of Pediatrics, 1987

The exclusion of children under the age of five years from the medical consultants report to the President's Commission led to a Special Task Force of the American Academy of Pediatrics (AAP) to develop guidelines for the determination of brain death in children in 1987. The AAP affirmed the definition of death and what was required for its determination, noting that there were no unique legal issues, but only medical ones. Noting that that the newborn is difficult to evaluate clinically after perinatal insults, the task force stated that the current criteria were valid in term newborns (greater than 38 weeks' gestation), seven days after the neurologic insult. From seven days to two months, the task force recommended two examinations and EEGs separated by at least 48 hours. From two months to one year, the task force recommended two examinations and EEGs separated by at least 24 hours, although the second examination and EEG were not necessary if a concomitant cerebral radionuclide angiographic study demonstrated no visualization of cerebral arteries. For children older than one year, laboratory testing was not required when an irreversible cause existed, and the task force recommended an observation period of at least 12 hours. For some conditions, like hypoxic-ischemic encephalopathy, where it was difficult to assess the extent and reversibility of brain damage, the task force recommended a more prolonged period of at least 24 hours of observation, which could be reduced if the EEG demonstrated electrocerebral silence or the cerebral radionuclide angiographic study did not visualize cerebral arteries. Other ancillary tests were being developed but not yet ready for inclusion in the guidelines.

American Academy of Neurology, 1995

Responding to a perceived variability in the practice of diagnosis, in 1995 the American Academy of Neurology (AAN) published a set of practice parameters for diagnosing brain death.[14] Its criteria were similar to the 1981 criteria endorsed by the medical consultants to the President's Commission. It specified that the proximate cause of the brain pathology must be known and demonstrably irreversible. It also added electrolyte, acid-base, and endocrine disturbances to the list of medical conditions that must be excluded as a prerequisite of brain death, reduced the apnea test to 8 minutes from the President's Commission's required 10 minutes, and reduced the time period for repeat testing to 6 hours.[15] It did not require confirmatory tests, such as an EEG and tests of cerebral blood flow, though it recommended such tests when other components of clinical testing could not be reliably performed or evaluated.

UK Academy of Medical Royal Colleges, 2008

In 2008 the Academy of Medical Royal Colleges in Great Britain provided a report titled *A Code of Practice for the Diagnosis and Confirmation of Brain Death*.[16] Its criteria resembled the various American sets (a feature worth noting because, as we shall see below,

Great Britain generally claims to be diagnosing only brain-stem function loss). It excluded the presence of depressant drugs; potentially reversible circulatory, metabolic, and endocrine disturbances; and neuromuscular blocking agents as causes of unconsciousness, along with primary hypothermia. It required testing for reflexes including pupillary light reflexes, oculovestibular reflexes, the corneal reflex, and the gag reflex. Apnea testing should last 5 minutes, and formal testing of brain-stem reflexes was usually carried out twice, 12 to 24 hours apart, by two experienced clinicians.

American Academy of Neurology, 2010

Addressing developments in technology and seeking research-based answers to outstanding questions, the AAN issued an update in 2010.[17] The apnea test was changed from 8 minutes to 8–10 minutes. Although it had recommended a 6-hour interval for retesting in 1995, in 2010 the AAN claimed that there was insufficient evidence to determine the minimally acceptable observation period, and it included no recommendation as to a retest interval. Ancillary tests, including EEG, nuclear scan, and cerebral angiogram, remained options whose use was suggested when there was uncertainty about other parts of the clinical evaluation.

American Academy of Pediatrics, Society of Critical Care Medicine, and Child Neurology Society, 2010

In 2010 the AAP Section on Critical Care, in conjunction with the Pediatric Section of the Society of Critical Care Medicine and the Child Neurology Society, revised and updated their guidelines for the establishment of brain death in children. These guidelines only held for newborns (greater than 37 weeks gestational age) and older infants and children. Until thirty days of age, the guidelines recommended a 24-hour observation period for infants and 12 hours for children older than thirty days to eighteen years. As with the adult studies, ancillary studies were not necessary unless (1) the apnea test could not be completed safely due to the condition of the patient; (2) there was uncertainty about the results of the neurologic examination; (3) if a medication effect could be present; or (4) to reduce the interexamination observation period.[18] The guidelines stated that four-vessel cerebral angiography was the gold standard for determining absence of cerebral blood flow but acknowledged that it was difficult to perform in infants and small children, could not be readily available, and required moving the patient to the angiography suite. EEG and use of radionuclide cerebral blood flow determinations to document the absence of cerebral blood flow remained the most widely used methods to support the clinical diagnosis. Other ancillary studies—such as trancranial Doppler study, CT angiography, CT perfusion using arterial spin labeling, nasopharyngeal somatosensory evoked potential studies, MRI-MR angiography, and perfusion MRI—had not been studied sufficiently nor validated in pediatrics at that time.

The Fact/Value Distinction Revisited

These criteria sets represent the consensus of medical experts for diagnostic criteria that identify brains that have irreversibly ceased to function. Recalling the distinction between scientific questions of the measurement of brain function and the more policy-oriented question of when someone should be treated as dead, almost everyone would recognize these criteria sets as scientific. They purport to be the best determiners of when a brain has irreversibly lost all its functions. (We shall see in chapter 5 that, in fact, certain brain functions—such as neurohormonal regulation and some electrical evoked potentials—may remain, even though the criteria represented in these tests are met.) Although it is true that these criteria are grounded in neurological science, in them we discern some messy overlap between facts and value judgments.

Is the choice of criteria really a scientific question? In addition to the brain functions that are known to be compatible with patients who satisfy these criteria sets, some other assumptions are made that require normative judgments. For example, Henry Beecher was aware that some neurological integrative functions occurred in the spinal cord. These spinal reflexes are not greatly different from simple brain-stem reflexes, but he felt comfortable excluding spinal cord reflexes as insignificant.

Another example where value judgments impinge on statements of science is seen in how the different criteria sets chose different lengths of time for apnea testing. The Harvard criteria (1968), 3 minutes; University of Minnesota (1971), 4 minutes; National Institute of Neurological Diseases and Stroke (1977), 15 minutes; Minnesota Medical Association (1978), 3 minutes; President's Commission (1981), 10 minutes; AAN (1995), 8 minutes; and AAN (2010), 8–10 minutes. This variation is, at least in part, a function of how certain the various criteria set writers wanted to be.

Some of this variation may represent different understandings of scientific knowledge, but more may be at stake. The influence of normative judgments on the apparently scientific criteria sets is most clearly revealed in the choice of the time period over which tests should be repeated. Despite guidelines for over twenty years and the willingness to revise the guidelines as new evidence is discovered, the current data show that there is wide variability in determination of death in both pediatrics and adults.[19]

Consider the fact that different criteria sets propose repeating tests over different time periods: Harvard, 24 hours; Minnesota Medical Association, 12 hours; National Institute of Neurological Diseases and Stroke, 6 hours; President's Commission, 6 to 24 hours; and the most recent set, which proposes no clear time period for repeat tests. Part of the difference is the result of increasing scientific knowledge that has accumulated over the years. As more experience is gained, greater certainty is plausible and the time period for repetition can be reduced. Part of the difference, however, is a function of attitudes about how the possibility of error should be handled.

Two types of errors are possible: Someone might falsely diagnose the death of the brain or might erroneously conclude the brain is alive when it is dead.. Falsely diagnosing the death of the brain would mean labeling someone as having a brain without function when, in fact, functions remained. That seems like a serious error. Nevertheless, every diagnosis and prognosis has some possibility of error. The National Institute of Neurological Diseases and Stroke report said, "Rarely (1 percent of cases) the original reviewer diagnosed ECS [electro-cerebral silence] and the review panel considered that biological activity was present. This 99 percent accuracy seems adequate for basic criteria." In other words, the members of the group were willing to adopt criteria that called some people dead when they actually retained brain function 1 percent of the time based on a review panel's judgment. They thought that error was tolerable.

It is reported anecdotally that patients pronounced dead by traditional cardiac criteria are pronounced erroneously as much as 5 percent of the time. When one realizes that the patients falsely pronounced are nevertheless very near death, some would consider the errors not necessarily critical.

People also worry about the other type of error one might make: falsely labeling someone as living when they are, in fact, dead. In the case of death based on brain criteria, one sometimes worries that patients with loss of all functions of the brain might be for a time considered still alive when they are not.

Choosing the length of time to repeat the tests is, in part, related to which type of error is of greater concern. If one wanted absolute certainty that brain function would never return, one could insist on repeating tests endlessly, thereby never judging too quickly. Picking the length of time for repeat tests is not only a function of advancement in scientific knowledge; it is also an evaluative judgment about the relative concern about the two types of error. The more one is concerned about falsely pronouncing death, the longer one will want to repeat tests. The more one is concerned about calling people alive when they are dead, the shorter the time period for repeating the tests. Choosing the time period must be based on balancing these two types of errors.

It may be that something as technical as choosing the gain on the machinery used for the EEG raises similar fact/value issues. The higher the gain, the less likely one is to miss small electrical potentials. One must make value-based choices about how small a potential is too small to worry about. For example, some neurologists have suggested that small electrical potentials may come off real brain tissues (not be artifact or electrical potentials off of other body tissues), but be only cellular level activity. If one believes that only supercellular brain activity counts as a sign of life, then one would be inclined to ignore mere cellular activity and therefore attempt to exclude electrical potentials so low that they only indicate cellular activity.

Problems with the Whole-Brain Definition: The Alternatives

The simple equation of brain death with "irreversible coma" by the Harvard committee should give us pause. Was it really this integrating capacity the committee members had in mind? If so, why did they substitute the term *irreversible coma*? There is another way to put the problem with a whole-brain definition of death. Can it really be true that some mere brain-stem reflex—the gag reflex, for example—can make the difference between being alive and being dead? The current whole-brain view holds that, if one minor function survives, then the individual is alive, but without it, the individual is deceased. Can this view, taken literally, be defensible?

Several alternatives have been proposed to the whole-brain view. Depending on how we understand "integrating capacity," three other positions deserve special consideration. These are referred to as brain-stem death, somatic death, and higher-brain death. The latter two are the subjects of the next two chapters, but first a word about so-called brain-stem death.

The British discussion of the definition of death focuses on "brain-stem death" rather than the death of the whole brain. It is difficult to establish how important this distinction is. The attention given to the brain stem can be attributed largely to two influential British contributors to the discussion, Bryan Jennett and especially Christopher Pallis.[20] As Pallis puts it: "I conceive of human death as a state in which there is irreversible loss of the capacity for consciousness combined with irreversible loss of the capacity to breathe (and hence to maintain a heartbeat). Alone, neither would be sufficient. Both are essentially brain-stem functions (predominantly represented, incidentally, at different ends of the brain stem)."[21]

Thus, Pallis concludes that "the necessary and sufficient component of brain death is death of the brain stem."[22] Conversely, most American commentators have resisted the brain-stem formulation, insisting that all functions of the entire brain (including the brain stem) must be destroyed for death to occur. For example, the US President's Council on Bioethics in 2008 specifically said that brain-stem criteria are not sufficient for the declaration of brain death because, although a dead brain stem will nearly always indicate a dead higher brain, this would not be so in the case of a primary lesion of the brain stem.[23]

If the brain stem is destroyed, arousal may not be possible, but it seems plausible that the information of consciousness may still be stored in the higher-brain centers. It is at least theoretically possible that some functions related to mentation—dreaming, for example—may be possible. Those who insist that death should be pronounced only if all functions of the brain are lost have been reluctant to accept death pronouncement based solely on brain-stem destruction.

Two problems with the Pallis notion of brain-stem death arise. First, as we have noted, it is theoretically possible that brain tissue above the brain stem, particularly the cerebrum, may still be alive and retain information considered important. Second, if defenders of brain-stem death are concerned only about consciousness and respiration, they have no reason to test for other brain-stem functions, such as the many reflexes mediated though this portion of the brain. Although the presence of the gag reflex or the eye blink reflex was sufficient for a defender of the Harvard criteria or any advocate of the Uniform Determination of Death Act to consider someone still alive, Pallis would not find such brain-stem-mediated nerve circuits intrinsically important.

In spite of clinical and conceptual differences between the whole-brain and brain-stem formulations, there is considerable agreement that the practical differences are minimal. Both the Americans and the British will pronounce death based on the irreversible loss of neurological functions, but consider someone alive who retains brain activity, including activity regulating respiration. The other two alternatives to the whole-brain concept of death, somatic and higher-brain concepts of death, differ substantially. They are the subjects of the next two chapters.

Notes

1. Harvard Medical School, "A definition of irreversible coma: Report of the Ad Hoc Committee of the Harvard Medical School to Examine the Definition of Brain Death," *JAMA* 1968;205: 337–40.

2. Jonas H, "Philosophical reflections on human experimentation," *Daedalus* 1969;98 (2): 219–47.

3. Institute of Society, Ethics and the Life Sciences, Task Force on Death and Dying, "Refinements in criteria for the determination of death," *JAMA* 1972;221: 48–53.

4. President's Commission for the Study of Ethical Problems in Medicine and Biomedical and Behavioral Research, *Defining death: Medical, legal and ethical issues in the definition of death* (Washington, DC: US Government Printing Office, 1981), 32–35.

5. Ibid., 33.

6. Bernat JL, Culver CM, and Gert B, "On the definition and criterion of death," *Annals of Internal Medicine* 1981;94: 389–94.

7. President's Commission for the Study of Ethical Problems in Medicine and Biomedical and Behavioral Research, *Defining death*, 2.

8. "Report of the Medical Consultants on the Diagnosis of Death to the President's Commission for the Study of Ethical Problems in Medicine and Biomedical and Behavioral Research"; President's Commission for the Study of Ethical Problems in Medicine and Biomedical and Behavioral Research, *Defining death*, 165; Flowers WM, Patel BR, "Persistence of cerebral blood flow after brain death," *Southern Medical Journal* 2000;93: 364–70.

9. Harvard Medical School, "Definition," 337–38.

10. Mohandas A, Chou SN, "Brain death: A clinical and pathological study," *Journal of Neurosurgery* 1971;35: 211–18.

11. Walker AE, et al., "An appraisal of the criteria of cerebral death: A summary statement," *JAMA* 1977;237: 982–86.

12. Cranford RE, "Minnesota Medical Association criteria: Brain death—concept and criteria, part I," *Minnesota Medicine* 1978;61: 561–63.

13. "Report of the Medical Consultants," 159–66.

14. Quality Standards Subcommittee of the American Academy of Neurology, "Practice parameters for determining brain death in adults: Summary statement," *Neurology* 1995;45: 1012–14.

15. The President's Commission does, however, list severe illnesses and metabolic abnormalities (i.e., hepatic encephalopathy, hyperosmolar coma, and preterminal uremia) as confounding conditions to be excluded.

16. Academy of Medical Royal Colleges, *A Code of Practice for the Diagnosis and Confirmation of Brain Death* (Portsmouth, UK: PPG, 2008).

17. Wijdicks EFM, et al., "Evidence-based guideline update: Determining brain death in adults," *Neurology* 2010;74: 1911–18.

18. Nakagawa T, Ashwal S, Mathur M, Mysore M, and Committee for Determination of Brain Death in Infants and Children, "Guidelines for the determination of brain death in infants and children: An update of the 1987 task force recommendations—executive summary," *Annals of Neurology* 2012;71: 573–85.

19. On pediatrics, see Mejia RE, Pollack MM, "Variability in brain death determination practices in children," *JAMA* 1995;274: 550–53; Mathur M, Petersen L, Stadtler M, et al., "Variability in pediatric brain death determination and documentation in southern California," *Pediatrics* 2008;121: 988–93; on adults, see Greer DM, Varelas PN, Haque S, Wijdicks E, "Variability of brain death determination guidelines in leading US neurologic institutions," *Neurology* 2008;70: 284–89.

20. Jennett B, "The donor doctor's dilemma: Observations on the recognition and management of brain death," *Journal of Medical Ethics* 1975;1: 63–66; Pallis C, "ABC of brain stem death: Reappraising death," *British Medical Journal* 1982;285: 1409–12; Pallis C, "ABC of brain stem death: From brain death to brain stem death," *British Medical Journal* 1982;285: 1487–90; Pallis C, "ABC of brain stem death: The argument about the EEG, *British Medical Journal* 1983;286: 284–87.

21. Pallis, 1982, "ABC of brain stem death: Reappraising, p. 1410.

22. Ibid., 1409. Almost identical views have been expressed by the Academy of Medical Royal Colleges. See Academy of Medical Royal Colleges, *A code of practice for the diagnosis of brain stem death* (London: UK Department of Health, 1998); Academy of Medical Royal Colleges, *Code of practice.*

23. US President's Council on Bioethics, *Controversies in the determination of death: A white paper by the President's Council on Bioethics* (Washington, DC: US President's Council on Bioethics, 2008), 32.

Chapter 5

The Circulatory, or Somatic, Concept of Death

One of the two major sets of alternatives to the whole-brain definition of death is a more traditional definition holding that death is somehow related to the irreversible loss of the flowing of essential bodily fluids—blood and breath. The standard American legal definition of death, based on the Uniform Determination of Death Act, includes two ways in which death can be determined: the direct measurement of the loss of all functions of the entire brain, or the irreversible loss of circulatory and respiratory function. The fact that death can be determined based on the loss of circulatory and respiratory function has caused great confusion and has recently been the subject of increased attention.

A persistent minority of Americans and others has continued to insist that death is only properly understood as the irreversible loss of circulatory and respiratory function. Some come to this conclusion based on religious belief. Orthodox Jews, for example, relate life to breath and often deny that someone who has irreversibly lost brain function is dead if respiratory and circulatory function remain. A number of sophisticated philosophers and physicians have also continued to hold this view.[1] Although precise numbers are difficult to determine, it seems likely that about 10 percent of the US population insists on some version of a circulatory definition of death.[2]

In December 2013 a twelve-year-old girl, Jahi McMath, suffered severe bleeding after throat surgery at an Oakland hospital. The loss of blood led to the permanent loss of brain functions as measured by standard tests, a fact confirmed by three sets of physicians, including one from a court-ordered independent expert neurologist. The hospital staff proposed to follow the standard practice of declaring her dead based on brain function loss, but her mother, Nailah Winkfield, disagreed. Although apparently she first disagreed that brain function was lost, eventually she took the position that, even if brain function had been lost, she was not dead as long as circulation and respiration remained (even if the respiration was the result of ventilatory support).[3] Although her position was a minority one, it should be apparent that there is no scientific basis for refuting it. She simply believes that her daughter should be treated as alive as long as she continues to respire and circulate blood.

The court finally permitted the hospital staff to declare Jahi dead in accordance with California law. It went on, however, to face the additional question of whether the staff could stop ventilatory and other support. The court finally arranged for her to be released to the medical examiner while still on a ventilator. The medical examiner then released the body to her mother, thus permitting the mother to transfer her to an undisclosed facility that was willing to provide medical support for her legally dead body, which the mother insisted should be considered still alive. As of this writing (September 2014), no final disposition has been reported.

It is technically possible in some instances to maintain a body with a dead brain for months or even years. In chapter 8 we take up the question of whether the law should permit those who have an objection to the standard law basing death on brain criteria to opt for the traditional circulatory definition. We shall also take up the question of who should bear responsibility for the costs involved.

Two Measurements of Death

This second basis for determining death—by measuring circulatory and respiratory function loss—introduces considerable ambiguity. It sounds like the traditional concept of death, which has variously been referred to as "cardiac," "circulatory," or "respiratory." At its worst, the inclusion in the law of both neurological and respirocirculatory means of pronouncing death has sometimes been understood as offering two different meanings of death, with the puzzling possibility that one could be simultaneously dead and alive— dead by one meaning, and alive by the other. For example, someone like Jahi McMath with irreversible loss of all functions of the brain, but with circulation and respiration retained mechanically, could be dead by brain criteria but alive by circulatory criteria.

Circulation as an Indicator of Brain-Based Death

More careful commentators have held that there can be only one meaning of death for the human being, although there could be two different methods of determining that death has occurred. The proponents of this single-meaning interpretation who accept some version of the brain-based concept of death, such as that in the Uniform Determination of Death Act, have generally held that humans should be deemed dead when all brain functions are irreversibly lost, but that there are two alternative ways of measuring that state. They claim that, typically, it is sufficient to establish loss of circulatory and respiratory function. They note it is a biological fact that, in the normal case, absence of circulation and respiration inevitably means the brain has been destroyed.

We need to be aware, however, that in special circumstances, it is possible that the brain function has not been destroyed when circulation has been lost irreversibly. In the first seconds, perhaps minutes, after circulation has been lost, some brain functions may still be possible. Thus, though circulation loss is usually an indirect indicator of brain status, there may be exceptional circumstances when it is not.

If people look at circulation and respiration to determine whether brain function has been lost, they are merely using these measurements as a shortcut to establish the death of the brain tissue. Some, such as Alex Capron and others, claim we have always meant by death the loss of bodily integrating capacity under the central control of the brain and that establishing irreversible loss of circulation and respiration has simply been a traditional and simple way of documenting the loss of that integrating capacity.[4]

Circulation Loss as Intrinsically Important

Others doubt that death has been understood throughout history as the loss of bodily integrating capacity. They hold that, traditionally, human death has meant something like the irreversible loss of circulation and respiration—fluid flow. Apparently, Jahi McMath's mother, when she is willing to acknowledge that her daughter's brain function is permanently lost, holds this view that circulation and respiration are intrinsically important if she continues to claim her daughter is alive, even though she acknowledges that brain function has been irreversibly lost.

The Meaning of Death Changed in the Late Twentieth Century

Among those who think that the loss of circulation and respiration was the traditional understanding of the concept of death, two views are possible about what death has come to mean. Some hold that in the late twentieth century, the majority of us changed to a bodily integrating, neurological view. They still might rely on fluid flow loss as an indicator that someone has died, but not because circulation and respiration are intrinsically important. Rather, they would now look to fluid flow, much as Capron and others would, as a sign of loss of integrating capacity. If fluid flow has been lost in such a way that brain integrating capacity is destroyed—that is, brain tissues have ceased to function—then the loss of capacity to breathe and circulate blood is an indirect sign that death—that is, loss of brain function—has occurred.

Those who hold that loss of neurological integrating capacity has always been what we meant by death, and also those who hold that this has recently become the dominant view, would logically hold that the loss of circulation is a measure of death (i.e., irreversible loss of brain-mediated bodily integrating capacity) only when circulation has been lost long enough for brain tissue to be destroyed. A few seconds of absence of cardiac activity would not count as death because brain-based integrating capacity would not have been lost irreversibly. The critical empirical question for someone using cardiac arrest as an indirect measure of brain status would be, "How long can the brain go without blood flow and still recover at least some of its integrating functions?" There are cases of loss of circulation for at least 2 to 3 minutes, which, if circulation is restored, are compatible with some level of brain function. To be sure, such trauma to the brain might leave the individual with irreversible damage—perhaps to the level of an irreversible coma or permanent vegetative state—but not the complete loss of brain integrating capacity. For someone who looks at circulation loss as an indicator of irreversible loss of all functions of the entire brain, the critical question is how long a period of documented circulation loss is compatible with restoration of some integrative brain function. The answer is apparently at least several minutes.

The Meaning of Death Remains the Irreversible Loss of Fluid Flow

Still others (like Jahi McMath's mother), however, have clung to something like the fluid flow concept as intrinsically important to classifying humans as alive. They have held that people are alive as long as the capacity for fluid flow remains (even if it can be established that brain function is irreversibly lost). We can refer to this as the circulatory, or somatic, conception of death—the view that the presence of circulation is intrinsically important, regardless of brain status (we shall see why it is called somatic). Although data are difficult to come by, perhaps about 10 percent of Americans have stubbornly remained committed to this circulatory concept of death.[5] Under it, someone with circulating blood is considered alive, even if only because respiration was maintained by a ventilator or other means of artificial respiration. The individual is alive even if there is clear evidence of the irreversible loss of all functions of the entire brain.

For one who holds this view, a different empirical question is critical: "How long can an individual endure loss of circulation and still have that circulation restored (even if brain function is not reestablished and therefore the brain's integrative activity is gone forever)?"

In cases of potential organ procurement following death based on circulatory criteria, somewhat different questions are thus at stake for those who see the circulation as an indirect indicator of brain-function loss and those who see it as intrinsically important. Protocols for the donation of organs following circulatory death (typically abbreviated DCD, for "donation after circulatory death") need to establish that death has occurred before organ procurement. Typically, they involve pronouncement of death after a sufficient period of cardiac arrest so that circulation cannot be reestablished. As we have seen, it is critical whether this reversibility is physiologically impossible or merely legally and morally impossible (because someone has refused life support).

DCD and Evidence of Death

DCD protocols typically rely on mere legal irreversibility (sometimes now called permanent loss of function). The two different understandings of the role of circulation in establishing that death has occurred turn out to require two different criteria for establishing permanent loss, and therefore death.

Time until Brain Function Is Lost

For those who view circulation loss as only indirect evidence of the loss of brain function, the critical question, as we have seen, is how long circulation must be lost to cause the irreversible loss of brain function. It turns out that very little attention has been devoted to this question. Clearly, the brain can go for a few minutes without circulation and still have at least some functions survive. Exactly how long is an empirical question that needs more attention. Anyone using loss of circulation as indirect evidence of the loss of brain function should be interested in this question.

Time until the Heart Cannot Restart Itself (Autoresuscitate)

For those who view circulation loss as intrinsically important, the critical question is how long circulation must be lost before it cannot (or will not) be reestablished. In the context of a decision not to attempt resuscitation, this view that circulation is intrinsically important implies that circulation loss must be long enough so that autoresuscitation is not possible, that is, long enough so that the heart function will not restart spontaneously.

Extensive literature exists trying to answer this question. The early DCD protocol at the University of Pittsburgh used a 120-second period of asystole before concluding that a heart would not autoresuscitate.[6] The more conservative Institute of Medicine Committee on Organ Procurement and Transplant Policy called for 5 minutes.[7] Others, even more conservative, have insisted on as long as 10 minutes. These would be the times that one would have to wait before declaring death based on circulatory criteria, assuming that the basis for pronouncing death was the intrinsic importance of circulation and the legal impossibility of a reversal occurring in the face of a valid refusal of life support. Logically, the possibility of autoresuscitation is important only if circulation per se is intrinsically important, not if we are using circulation as indirect evidence of brain status. It is quite possible that brain tissue could be destroyed from anoxia before (or after) autoresuscitation became impossible.

Circulatory Death and Organ Procurement

The concept of death based on circulatory criteria is important not only for those who believe that some people with dead brains may not be dead people but also for those who are interested in procuring organs from some people who do not meet the tests for the irreversible loss of brain function. Because the criteria sets for establishing the loss of brain function generally require the repeating of tests for periods of 6 to 24 hours, many people who are pronounced dead relying on traditional circulatory criteria do not qualify to be organ donors based on brain function loss. That has led many to consider procuring organs from those pronounced dead based on circulatory criteria.

Two Kinds of Cases

Two groups of patients are considered feasible sources of organs following irreversible loss of circulation. The first group includes heart attack and accident victims who are brought to hospitals for emergency treatment. They suffer cardiac arrest before or after their arrival, and the attempted resuscitations fail. These people are eventually pronounced dead based on the irreversible loss of circulatory function. These have come to be referred to as "unplanned" cases; that is, cases where the stoppage of circulation was not planned.

The second group involves patients under care for critical illnesses who decide to exercise their right to refuse further life support. When that support is withdrawn, they will die. Because that was the expected outcome, these have been referred to as "planned" circulatory deaths. Some patients offer to become organ donors before the withdrawal of treatment. It is clearly illegal to take organs from dying persons until they are declared dead; no organ procurement organization in the United States would do so. However, the University of Pittsburgh Medical Center, initially, and now many centers have developed protocols whereby such volunteers could be taken to the operating room preceding the withdrawal of life support with the intention that as soon as the heart stops and death is pronounced, organs will be procured. Although the unplanned and planned groups raise somewhat different moral and policy issues, they are often considered together, as they are here.

It is striking that the death of the brain has become so ingrained as the "real" definition of death for organ procurement purposes that some, especially in Germany, have come to doubt that people who suffer irreversible cardiac arrest are really dead. Nevertheless, American law states that death can be based on irreversible cessation of either heart or brain function.

Issues in Procuring Organs from Patients Considered Dead by Circulatory Criteria

In spite of the doubters, there is a substantial consensus among those who approve of any allograft organ transplantation that, once proper permissions have been obtained, there is nothing ethically controversial about procuring organs from dead people and that it makes no difference in principle whether the death is measured by brain criteria or circulatory criteria. Individuals are just as dead either way. (Hence we plead that we not refer to individuals as "brain dead" or "heart dead." They should be thought of simply as "dead.")

The procurement of organs from asystolic patients who are dead—whether they are dead as a result of trauma, myocardial infarction, or a decision to forgo life support—appears at first not to present overwhelming problems. Nevertheless, three issues potentially add complexity to this apparently easily-won consensus: respecting the integrity of members of the procurement team, determining that the source of the organs is really dead, and establishing whether there has been a valid consent not only for donation but also for the steps necessary to prepare the body for donation.

The Rights and Welfare of the Caregivers

For reasons that are not entirely clear, some members of the health care team may be deeply troubled by procuring organs from recently deceased patients who are declared dead using circulatory criteria. They may be traumatized by discontinuance of resuscitation efforts or termination of life support, the perfusion of the body, and the removal of organs from a still-warm body in which, in some cases, a heart has beat only minutes previously. Some may have become so convinced that death should really be based on irreversible brain function loss that they are not satisfied that someone is dead when the death is measured using circulatory criteria. This appears especially to be a problem in Germany, but it can occur anywhere.

The emergency and operating room staff members will normally play only a preliminary role, assisting the patient and family in deciding to cease life support, participating in perfusion in the case of trauma and cardiac arrest patients, and preparing the body to be taken to the operating room in the case of patients with advance directives forgoing treatment. Even if there is a careful separation of the procurement team from other caregivers, the problems for professional staffs are potentially serious. Health care teams are normally militantly committed to attempting to prolong life, but they will be aware that, in the case of unplanned arrests, others are standing by with very different objectives in mind and, in the case of planned arrests, that the purposeful cessation of treatment followed by organ procurement is being contemplated. Procurement team members will need to understand that they are dealing with a truly dead body for which proper organ donation has occurred. This will be particularly true in the moments preceding perfusion, when patients will feel warm and manifest some signs often taken to be signs of life.

Compassion for nurses and other professionals on the team requires careful preparation and ample opportunity for those who have reservations to withdraw from the perfusion and procurement processes. This may be particularly troublesome for emergency room staff members who may not be intimately involved with organ procurement on a daily basis. With care and compassion, these problems can probably be avoided.

The Organ Source Must Really Be Dead

A more difficult problem raised by procuring organs from those pronounced dead by circulatory criteria may turn out to be establishing exactly when they are dead. Common wisdom used to suggest that, though it was more difficult to measure death based on brain criteria, measuring death based on heart or circulation loss was straightforward. Now it appears that exactly the opposite may be the case.

The asystolic heart can surely be used as a measure of the death of the individual after prolonged asystole, but there are important reasons why death should be pronounced (and organs procured) as quickly as possible. The Pittsburgh protocol in its original form called for death pronouncement after 2 minutes of asystole. It was claimed that at this point autoresuscitation was impossible, but it cannot be denied that cardioversion could be accomplished mechanically at this point. As we have seen, it is debatable whether a heart's stoppage should be considered "irreversible" if it could be restarted, but will not be because a decision has been made not to do so and, in fact, in the case of a valid treatment-refusing advance directive, it would actually be illegal to attempt resuscitation. This is what we have referred to as the difference between physiological and legal irreversibility, and what others have referred to as the difference between irreversible and permanent loss of function.

Even more perplexing is whether an individual should be considered dead during the period when a heart could be restarted by people with expert skills and sophisticated equipment if those people and equipment are not available. The concept of irreversibility has suddenly become much more complex. Moreover, depending on the exact meaning of irreversibility, the brain tissue is not necessarily dead at the point when the heart is determined to be stopped irreversibily. This raises the problem that in Pittsburgh, a patient could after 2 minutes be called dead while his brain continued to be living, a problem that is addressed below. If the concept of death actually refers to the state in which the body no longer functions as an integrated whole and that functioning as an integrated whole requires activity of the brain, then the exact moment of irreversible circulation loss is not precisely when integrated functioning of the body as a whole is lost.

The significance of these subtle distinctions is not necessarily great in cases where the patient or surrogate has made an advance decision not to resuscitate, but in patients suffering unexpected cardiac arrest this could raise serious problems. The initial working presumption of the trauma team must be that resuscitation should be pursued. Longer periods of asystole would be necessary to establish irreversibility, and, therefore, there may be longer periods of warm ischemic time. This means that, ethically, there must be a sharp separation of responsibility between the organ procurement team and the resuscitation team. This could mean that a longer period of asystole will be necessary in order to establish that the heart has really ceased function irreversibly (and has done so long enough to cause irreversible brain function loss, if that is the understanding of what it means to be dead). If the resuscitation team has been trying unsuccessfully for a long time to resuscitate, the heart may be asystolic for much more than 2 minutes. Having organ procurement on the agenda creates an incentive to cut resuscitation time because more lengthy attempts could diminish the value of organs. Regardless, according to current law, if the heart is really dead (however "dead" is defined), the dead donor rule will be satisfied (or will be satisfied as soon as enough time has passed for brain destruction to occur). Because the organs can survive as much as 30 minutes of warm ischemia, shifting to a longer period of asystole, say 5 minutes, probably need not pose an insurmountable problem.

A more serious question lurks beneath the surface, however. Although there is a clear recognition in statutory definitions of death that death may be pronounced based on the irreversible loss of either circulatory or brain activity, the possibility of organ procurement based on death pronouncement following short periods of asystole poses a new challenge. Especially if periods as brief as 2 minutes of asystole are used for pronouncing death (based on the irreversible loss of circulatory function), it seems likely that the brain tissue is really not dead at this moment. In fact, much of the literature advocating such death pronouncements really does not even present firm evidence that the patient is unconscious. The vision of pronouncing a patient dead after only two minutes of asystole (while brain tissue still lives) starkly poses the question of whether someone really ought to be considered dead if the brain tissue is still alive. The asystolic organ source may force the participants in the definition-of-death debate to reconsider whether someone can really be pronounced dead based on the loss of circulatory function alone.

It had previously been assumed that if irreversible cardiac arrest had occurred, then all brain functions would necessarily have ceased. That turns out to be not quite true. If brains can function even briefly after irreversible circulatory arrest can be determined to have occurred, then society must reassess whether it should continue to accept a policy according to which death can occur when either circulatory or brain function is lost. This challenges society to reexamine whether it really wants to treat people as dead when brain function exists. Of course, in routine cases of prolonged circulatory arrest, we could continue to pronounce death without measuring brain function. Surely all brain function has been destroyed with prolonged circulation stoppage. But in planned arrest, we may want to insist that enough time pass following circulatory arrest not only to foreclose resuscitation but also to assure the irreversible loss of brain function.

The reasonable conclusion seems to be that, quite to our surprise, the emergence of donation after circulatory death has challenged our established definition of death that states simply that death may be pronounced when there is irreversible loss of either brain or circulatory function. From the point of view of those who hold the now-mainstream view that death is the irreversible loss of all functions of the entire brain, this received position should be amended to make clear that, if circulatory function loss is used as an indicator of death, it must be only because it is an accurate predictor that brain function has been irreversibly lost, not because the loss of heart function per se is significant. It is becoming more and more clear, at least to those who advocate brain-based death pronouncement, that it is the brain's function that is critical, not the beating heart. Thus, if we can interpret irreversibility to mean "will not start again" rather than "cannot be started again," we still must use irreversible circulatory function loss to pronounce death only when the loss accurately measures the irreversible loss of brain function. Two minutes of asystole does not do this. Some longer time does. The neurologists need to tell us exactly how long the heart function must be stopped in order to say safely that the brain will never function again. Five minutes of asystole appears to be a much safer time period than 2 minutes. Perhaps even a longer time is necessary.

Conversely, for the minority who have persistently held, or have reverted to, the view that death means irreversible loss of bodily integrative functions independent of the brain—those who opt for Shewmon's view (see below) or the view of the minority of the US President's Council on Bioethics—then it really is irreversibility of circulation that is critical, whatever the state of the brain at that point.

The Organs Must Really Be Donated

Another truly difficult problem in procuring organs from the asystolic trauma or heart attack victim is what can be done, legally and ethically, with the deceased before obtaining appropriate permission from the next of kin. Proposed protocols for such procurement call for minimizing warm ischemia time. This means femoral cannulation and perfusion or extracorporeal membrane oxygenation (ECMO) as soon as possible after death is pronounced. The procuring surgeon would often desire to perfuse before the relatives have been contacted, or at least before they have given permission for organ procurement. The most critical legal and ethical question thus becomes whether perfusion can precede permission for procurement. Generally, it is feasible to obtain permission before actual organ procurement, but often not before perfusion. Here, two potential policy concerns deserve attention.

HUMAN RESEARCH REGULATIONS

First, at least during the early phase, such efforts at organ procurement following cannulation and perfusion might be conceptualized as research on human subjects. The Regional Organ Bank of Illinois, which made an early attempt at procurement after what is now called death based on measurement of circulatory loss, conceptualized its work as an experiment subject to institutional review board review and approval.[8] Federal regulations require that all institutions having multiuse assurances for conducting research on human subjects based on local institutional review board approval must secure the informed consent of the subjects or the subjects' surrogates.[9] Normally, this consent must be obtained before initiating the investigational interventions. This would appear to require consent preceding perfusion or another effort to preserve organs, not simply before procuring organs.

It is true that federal regulations provide for limited exceptions to the consent requirement. However, exceptions are permitted only when getting the consent would make the investigation impossible. It might be argued that, if procuring organs from asystolic patients is investigational, the perfusion should be exempt from the consent requirement on this basis. In order to qualify for an exemption under federal regulation, however, four conditions must be met: the risk must be no more than minimal, the patient (or surrogate) must be debriefed afterward, the rights and welfare of subjects must be preserved, and the situation must be such that the research could not practically be carried out any other way.[10]

However, one of the rights of human subjects of research is the right to give an informed consent before participating. Thus we are left with the odd situation that one can waive consent only when rights are protected, but one right is the right to consent. If giving consent is a right, then no waiver of the federal consent requirement would ever be acceptable for any research. In fact, even if the use of such techniques as perfusion or ECMO is not thought to be experimental, consent for treatment is still required and, by law, consent for the use of the body to begin the process of procuring organs is required, even if the patient is considered deceased.

Even if this argument does not succeed, a waiver would appear not to be acceptable in the case of research on organ procurement from patients declared dead based on circulatory loss. Waivers are permitted only when the study could not otherwise be conducted. In fact, a consent requirement would not make it impossible to procure organs from those pronounced dead by circulatory criteria, although it would make it more difficult and might delay the project. It is the nature of an investigation that only a modest number of consents would need to be obtained successfully. Even if most heart attack and trauma victims would not have surrogates reachable in time, some will arrive with valid organ donation cards and others will arrive with relatives who have the legal authority to consent to the perfusion and other preliminary organ-preserving interventions as well as organ procurement. The Baby Fae experimental baboon heart experience at Loma Linda University (discussed in greater detail in chapter 14) shows that with perseverance, some families can be reached and that some of those who are reached would give permission.

Having argued that the waiver provision in the federal human subjects regulations does not provide an out for the advocate of interventions to preserve the donation option following death pronouncement based on circulatory criteria, there is, at the level of law, another response. The federal regulations technically do not apply to body parts or materials from deceased individuals.[11] That would appear to provide a legal out. However, it does not seem to provide an ethical one. Ethically, the consent requirement is designed to show respect for the individual. The duty to show that respect does not cease at death—as is seen by our expectation that economic wills should be respected as well as the traditional requirement in organ procurement that organs not be taken from known objectors. Thus, even if the technical requirements of the human subjects research regulations may not restrict perfusion before consent and other interventions for the purposes of preserving organs, the underlying ethical concerns might do so.

The Uniform Anatomical Gift Act

The second locus of potential problems is the legal and ethical requirements that specifically address organ procurement. Under the Uniform Anatomical Gift Act, all US states require that consent be obtained—from the patient or next of kin—before procuring organs.[12] Various people have offered a number of arguments for not violating the dead body, arguments that we examined in chapter 3. For example, some argue that even after death, the integrity of the human body must be respected. Some say the body does not belong to the society but to the individual, who has the authority, while still alive, to refrain from cooperating.

After death, responsibility for the body reverts to the next of kin. There are important social reasons why we should continue to show respect for the individual by honoring his or her wishes about the body's treatment after death occurs. For religious or secular reasons, individuals may object to the state assuming control over the body to serve its purposes. Even more plausible is objection to procurement personnel—who are, after all, merely individual private citizens—claiming the right to perfuse the body for the potential benefit of strangers.

We know that some significant minority, perhaps a quarter of the population if we go by refusals to donate when asked, objects to donating organs.[13] Most of these individuals probably also object to perfusion. Some religious traditions, such as Judaism, have a strong prohibition on mutilation of the corpse, at least if it is not done to preserve another identifiable life. Therefore, the perfusion itself will offend some people. If a deceased patient possesses a valid donor card or has otherwise registered intent to donate, there is no problem. With next-of-kin permission, there is none either (assuming the deceased has not registered an objection). But absent such consent or permission, there is a potential problem.

Some people might mistakenly claim that inserting a catheter before consent preserves the family's option to donate until informed consent can be exercised, and therefore is more respectful of the patient's autonomy or informed consent. This claim, however, shows a misunderstanding of the notions of autonomy and consent.

Autonomy generates a liberty right—a right to be left alone. It is on the basis of this liberty right that both patients and potential organ donors must be asked before their bodies are violated with medical interventions. Autonomy in no way gives one the right to be a subject of a medical procedure, either an experiment or an organ procurement. In fact, even if organs are donated, the procurement organization has the legal and ethical right to refuse to procure them. The only relevance of autonomy to perfusion is that any perfusion preceding consent violates the individual's autonomy rights. This is true not only for the significant minority of the population that would refuse to consent to donation if asked but also of the group that would consent if asked, but that would object to invasion of the body without being asked.

Ways Around Absence of Explicit Consent

There are three possible ways around the problem of the absence of explicit consent. We consider deferred consent, presumed consent, and conscription without consent.

Deferred Consent

First, some have suggested turning to a "deferred consent," that is, getting the consent for both the perfusion and the organ procurement from the next of kin after the perfusion has taken place. Bruce Miller and others have shown, however, that deferred consent is no consent at all. Even if one agrees to proceed, there is no way that one can claim justification for the perfusion based on such deferred consent.[14] Debriefing and even getting approval after the perfusion process does not constitute a consent for the perfusion. Some will refuse to give approval after the fact. Even if permission is obtained after the fact, such approval does not equal consent. Consent must exist at the time of the intervention if it is to serve as the basis for justifying the perfusion.

Presumed Consent

Second, one may attempt to justify perfusing on the grounds of a concept of "presumed consent." But there is terrible confusion over the meaning of presumed consent. Many people mistakenly confuse presumed consent with policies authorizing organ procurement without any consent. Thus, as we explain in chapter 10, people mistakenly say that many European countries have presumed consent laws for organ procurement when in fact none do. What they have are laws authorizing procurement without consent, a policy that is consistently rejected by the more autonomy-loving, individualistic American society. Even if the law contains an "opting-out" provision, whereby one can execute a document recording objection to procurement, it is not possible to presume that everyone who has not executed such a provision in fact would want to have their organs used. Many people do not respond, either because they are not aware of the legal provisions or simply do not express their refusals in writing. There is no basis for presuming the consent of those who have not opted out; and, in fact, the European laws do not claim to be based on a presumption of consent.

There would be nothing wrong with presuming consent, provided there were an empirical basis for supporting the presumption. Thus, as we suggest in chapter 10, it raises no problems to presume consent for emergency treatment of the trauma victim in the emergency room—because it is clear that almost everyone would, in fact, consent not only to treatment but also to a policy that presumes the consent.[15]

Presently, however, there is no basis for such a presumption of consent to the perfusion. We need data, probably hospital-specific data, showing the willingness of an adequate percentage of patients to agree to the presumption of consent for perfusion.[16] Probably data showing with 95 percent certainty that such a presumption is correct should be considered adequate. There is no definitive argument for a specific percentage, but we would, in effect, be predicting that the specific patient would have consented (or would have agreed to perfusion without consent). If we are wrong in that prediction, we would be illegally proceeding without consent. We would be violating the rights of the deceased. Short of such a basis for presuming consent, it is hard to see how presumed consent can provide a basis for perfusing.

Even if one could establish that, say, 75 percent of a particular hospital's asystolic patients would have favored perfusion without consent, that would not be sufficient to justify perfusing the other 25 percent in the absence of a formal, publicly debated policy authorizing invasion of the dead body without consent. The two groups—those who would approve of perfusion without explicit consent, and those who would not—are not symmetrical regarding their rights. Each member of the group who would object to perfusion can be said to have a right violated—the right not to have one's body invaded without consent. Conversely, no members of the group who would approve perfusion would have any right violated if the perfusion were omitted.

Rights normally have reciprocal obligations. In fact, generally, one is not a bearer of a right if no one has a reciprocal obligation. But no one is obligated to perfuse and procure organs. This is true even if explicit consent has been given; and it is even more obviously true if no consent has been given. Anyone who feels strongly that it would be a good thing to have his or her body perfused and organs procured has the right to make an explicit donation, including an authorization to perfuse. In this case, perfusion can take place without any additional consent. But absent a documented prior consent, no one has the right to violate the body—and surely no one has a duty to do so.

Conscription without Consent

There is only one other way to justify perfusion before explicit consent has been given. That is to change public policy to accept perfusion without consent. Efforts have been made to change US policy for procuring organs to one of routine salvaging without consent, such as many European countries have adopted. They represent very different cultures, however. Although the United States has consistently rejected routine salvaging laws—even those with opting-out clauses—we have not yet had a public debate on perfusion without consent. As long as a significant number of people object to organ procurement, there is reason to assume that they would also object to laws permitting perfusion without consent; but a proposal to the state legislatures to authorize perfusion preceding consent could be attempted. One jurisdiction, the District of Columbia, has actually passed such an exemption.[17]

It is conceivable that in other jurisdictions, enough people who object to procurement without consent would have less objection to perfusion before consent, provided there was a statutory authorization. Plausibly, this might be the view of some members of the group who would donate but who have never documented their willingness to do so. Still, with about a quarter of the population objecting to organ procurement under the best of circumstances, and others objecting in principle to bodily invasions without consent, it seems unlikely that such a law would be adopted in most jurisdictions. We believe that it would not be wise to violate a person's autonomy by perfusing without consent and without statutory authorization.

There are limited examples of legal authorizations to invade a human body without consent, even in cases where we have reason to believe that the individual would have objected. Military conscription is one example. Such conscription is usually presumed to authorize invasions, even medical invasions, without consent.[18] The policy decision that troops in Desert Storm could be given experimental vaccines without their consent also illustrates a national policy of legal authorization to treat without consent.

Also, laws providing limited authorization for an autopsy without consent provide an analogy.[19] Controversy exists over whether the law permits taking corneas and tissues during an autopsy. To the extent that the law permits such removal without consent, this would be another precedent for public policies providing legal authorization for procurement without consent. What is critical here is that whenever persons are conscripted into service to others without their consent, specific statutory or judicial law must provide the justification.

Our conclusion is that there is no problem with perfusing and procuring organs from asystolic patients who have in the past authorized donation—even without next-of-kin permission. The advanced consent for medical use of the body for transplants includes consent to the procedures necessary to procure the organs, including the perfusion. There is also no problem with procurement based on next-of-kin permission before perfusion. However, absent such explicit consent or permission, one must either presume consent—a presumption that has not yet been validated—or adopt a public policy authorizing perfusion without consent.

Moving to Explicit Authorization

If deferred and presumed consent for perfusion before having received permission to procure organs is unacceptable and no explicit conscription without consent has been authorized, there is only one other way to justify perfusion of a dead body before consent or to justify any of a number of treatments of still-living persons for the purpose of preserving organs. This is to gain explicit, specific consent. We propose that such permission to perfuse following death be part of every organ donation and that permission to treat a still-living body for the purpose of preserving organs both be incorporated into model advance directives.

Advance directives have long been advocated as a device for patients to express their desires about terminal treatment. These usually have been used as treatment-refusing advance directives. Recently, we have discovered that they pose a potential problem for organ procurement. It seems reasonable that most people who execute treatment-refusing advance directives also support procurement of their usable organs after their deaths. They fail to realize that a refusal of any life-prolonging treatment would also rule out the use of ventilators, blood pressure regulators, and other treatments that would be useful for the short term to preserve organs but have the side effect of extending life. Recently, some clinicians who have gained respect for the patient's instructions in an advance directive have taken them literally and have refused to provide even short-term intervention to preserve organs if the side effect will be to possibly extend the patient's life.

The obvious solution is that all who write an advance directive should consider including specific language that addresses the issue of organ donation. With this in mind, one of us (RMV) has drafted the following wording for his advance directive, where after referring to the decision to forgo life-supporting intervention, the following sentence is added: *"In making such a decision, the decision maker should take into account my desire to preserve organs and tissues for procurement."*

Does Planned Donation Unethically Hasten Death?

The type of organ procurement that follows the withdrawal of life support and a planned death raises an additional ethical question. Certain drugs—anticoagulants, such as heparin, and vasodilators, such as pheltolamine—can be given in the hours before the withdrawal of life support for the purpose of improving the preservation of the organs.[20] Some of these drugs may actually in rare occasions shorten the life of the dying organ donor. But others could lengthen the time it takes for death to occur.

This has led to considerable controversy, particularly in Cleveland, where a case led to an exposé on the CBS television program *60 Minutes*. Critics of a Cleveland Clinic protocol for procuring organs following death based on circulatory criteria proclaimed that the administration of particular medications had actively shortened the donor's life and was therefore unethical and illegal. Some have doubted that the drugs involved actually do shorten the patient's life; but even if the life is not shortened, the drugs' administration is not for the donor's benefit and has therefore been criticized.

Of course, if drugs are administered to the donor before death for the purpose of preserving organs for transplant, the donor (or surrogate) would need to be informed of this intervention and consent to it (perhaps as part of an advance directive). But assuming that such consent is obtained, would the practice be objectionable?

Even some very conservative physicians and theorists have argued that, even if death is hastened, it is not the intention of the physician to hasten death—it is a side effect. Traditional medical ethics has always found such side effects morally tolerable, provided that they are not the direct intention of the actor and that the risk of the side effect is undertaken for proportionally good reasons. The death, in effect, becomes an "indirect" or "double" effect, one that has always been recognized as morally acceptable—even in conservative Catholic moral theology, in secular philosophy, by the American Medical Association, and in American law.[21] Conversely, such interventions may have the unintended consequence of prolonging the dying patient's life or even stabilizing the patient at a point short of death. These possibilities need to be explored with the patient or surrogate, and the fact that they are used to preserve organs rather than for patient benefit needs to be explained. They can be used only with appropriate consent. Physicians who subscribe to the pure, unmodified form of the Hippocratic Oath believe that they are justified in their actions only on the basis that they are for the benefit of the patient. That ultra-individualistic ethic is, however, widely rejected among contemporary physicians. They support research for the benefit of society, responsible cost containment, and public health efforts—all of which are undertaken for the benefit of other parties than the patient. Most relevant, they generally support the procurement of kidneys from living donors and do so not for the benefit of the donor. Whether physicians accept such procedures for the benefit of others, certainly most laypeople do. In fact, the entire organ procurement endeavor is precisely for the benefit of others, never for the benefit of the donor (unless the live-donor cases are considered beneficial to the donor—a claim we will examine in chapter 12). Hence, the mere fact that the drugs are given for the benefit of the potential organ recipient does not make the administration unethical, provided that donor consent is obtained.

The real controversy is over the possibility that these drugs would shorten the donor's life. Of course, some object to all cases of the withdrawal of life support. Many right-to-life advocates do, and so do some Orthodox Jews. They will, no doubt, also disapprove of giving the drugs that hasten death in order to preserve organs. The real issue is whether, among those who have come to accept the legitimacy of withdrawing of life support and the procuring of organs from such a planned demise, administering a drug that hastens death is also acceptable.

This may look to the untrained observer like a case of converting a forgoing of life support into an active killing. Because intended, active killings are generally considered unethical and are illegal, the implication is that administering the drugs that might shorten life potentially converts the planned DCD protocol into a homicide, a very inauspicious development for the physician who administers the drug. In fact, the Institute of Medicine panel that studied what are now called DCD protocols was divided and quite confused about the use of such medications.[22] The report's authors seemed to believe that if the drug administration actively causes death, then such administration is automatically unethical and illegal.

More careful examination, however, makes clear that the moral and legal analysis is more complex. This may be yet another case that can be analyzed under the "doctrine of double effect." The general formulation of this doctrine is that such harmful side effects are morally tolerable, provided that four conditions are met: (1) The intention behind the action must be to produce the good effect, and not the evil one; (2) the evil must not be the means of achieving the good effect; (3) the action, itself, cannot be intrinsically evil; and (4) the good effect must be proportional to the evil one.[23] One key to this doctrine is that its adherents believe an unintended evil can be tolerable even if one can foresee that it will occur.

Not everyone accepts the doctrine of double effect. Some consider it too conservative—claiming, for example, that if the good consequences exceed the evil ones, that should be sufficient to justify the action. Those who hold this more liberal view might even believe that the direct, active killing of the terminally ill with their consent in order to obtain organs would be justified.[24] This liberal interpretation has been widely rejected, however.

Likewise, some reject the doctrine of double effect, claiming that it is too liberal. They say that if intentionally producing a death is morally wrong, then one that is foreseen should also be wrong, even if it is not the actor's intention to produce the death. They claim that the mere lack of intention in the mind of the actor cannot make the action moral, provided that the evil is foreseen. Nevertheless, this doctrine is widely accepted as a middle position, one that tolerates some foreseen deaths while simultaneously affirming that it is always wrong to intend death.

This doctrine has led some opponents of abortion to the conclusion that it would be acceptable to remove a cancerous uterus even if the patient happened to be pregnant (and therefore that a fetal death would result). If the patient and the surgeon can honestly say that their intention is to remove the cancer and not to cause the fetal death, then the death can be tolerated. Likewise, the doctrine has led to the conclusion that it could be acceptable to administer pain-relieving drugs if necessary to relieve a patient's pain, even if the known side effect was respiratory depression that could contribute to hastening the patient's death. These views are now widely accepted, even by Catholic moral theologians who consider it unethical in all cases to directly intend hastening of death.[25]

The application of the doctrine in the narcotic pain-relieving cases is important for the question of administering drugs to patients who could potentially be declared dead based on circulatory criteria. If the intention is not to hasten the death of the donor but to preserve the organs in order to provide benefit to a recipient, then the doctrine of double effect can potentially apply. It seems obvious that if the drug is given, the purpose is not to hasten the patient's death. It is not the quicker death that preserves the organs. If the physicians injected potassium for the purpose of producing a quick cardiac arrest, that would be a different story—a directly intended causing of death. We can assume, however, that the purpose of administering the heparin or phentolamine is not to get the donor dead more quickly. Hence, the practice seems to meet the criterion that the hastening of the death is not directly intended. Moreover, it is not the hastening of death that is the means to the good intended end. The drug has a mechanism of action that is independent of the death of the donor. Thus the second criterion of the doctrine is satisfied.

Surely, the administration of the drug is not intrinsically evil. The third criterion is easily satisfied. This leaves the question of whether the good achieved—providing higher-quality organs for transplant, potentially for several patients, and perhaps saving one or more lives—is proportional to the harm done. One might argue that hastening a death is a tragedy (although the hastening is only a matter of minutes), but we must realize that the case only arises for a patient who has decided that his or her prognosis is so bleak that it is appropriate to withdraw life support, even though doing so will inevitably lead to a rapid death. If we can accept the negative effect of the inevitable death of the patient, surely, the fact that this death will occur a few minutes earlier is a minimal harm—if it is considered a harm at all.

The result seems to be clear: The harm to the donor is minimal, and the benefit to several other critically ill human beings could be enormous. As long as the death is not intended, any holder of the doctrine of double effect should have no moral objection to the practice of administering medications in order to preserve organs, even if the unintended side effect may be the hastening of the donor's death.

If this is our conclusion in the case where the drug is administered to preserve organs in the planned deaths based on circulatory criteria, then it is obvious that administering any drugs that have a less dramatic impact on the demise of the donor will also be acceptable. The act of choosing to become a donor is a noble one. Many such donors will realize that, as long as the decision to withdraw life support is reached independently from the organ donation decision, there is nothing morally objectionable. In fact, many would conclude that the benefit to others is a legitimate part of the patient's decision to withdraw support. If such a donor has reached the decision to withdraw life support on his or her own and is adequately informed about the use of drugs to help preserve organs, it seems that many in this position would also consent to the use of the drugs. If they do, and if the burdens sustained are minimal or nonexistent, then the practice of administering the drugs with the consent of the recipient seems morally defensible—in fact, it seems morally the right choice.

The DCD Protocols

The significance of these distinctions may be seen in three developments involving DCD protocols that implicitly rely on different interpretations of what it means to be dead by circulatory or cardiac criteria. Let us briefly consider each development.

The Infant Heart Transplant Cases

A controversial protocol at the University of Colorado was designed to procure hearts for transplant from newborn infants with conditions incompatible with life. Often referred to as the Boucek protocol (after the head of the team that developed the protocol), the protocol identified infants whose parents had made independent, valid decisions to forgo life support.[26] The investigators withdrew life support, waited for circulatory arrest, and then waited further for a period chosen to establish the impossibility of autoresuscitation. For the first case, they waited 3 minutes; for the second and third cases, they waited only 75 seconds. Death was pronounced, the hearts were procured, and then they were transplanted. The investigators found that the hearts could be restarted and function successfully.

Several problems arose that are relevant to the concept of death. First, it should be clear that waiting enough time to rule out autoresuscitation is plausible only if the legal and moral impossibility of restoration of circulation is intrinsically important. It does not establish that circulation could not be restored with intervention. (In fact, the restoration of heart function following transplant implies that it could be restored.)

There were more problems. No consensus, peer-reviewed criteria existed for establishing the waiting time to rule out autoresuscitation in newborns. Hence, even the 3-minute wait time, which is arguably within the range of the standard of practice for adults, cannot be assumed for children.[27] Even if the 3-minute time were defensible, moving to 75 seconds of asystole was without precedent.

Moreover, we have seen that many people would rely on evidence of a lack of circulation as indirect evidence that the brain has irreversibly lost its capacity to function. Even if the 3-minute or 75-second waiting time was somehow found to be sufficient to rule out autoresuscitation, it surely is not sufficient time to presume that brain function was lost. If one is relying on the irreversible loss of circulation as indirect evidence of brain function loss, this would certainly be an error in this case. Surely, brain function was not irreversibly lost in 75 seconds, and plausibly the capacity for brain function was not lost in 3 minutes. These cases raise the question of what precisely is meant by cessation of circulatory function. The investigators made clear that the heart function was restored (albeit in another infant who received the transplant). Some of us raised the question of whether it can be said that cardiac function ceased irreversibly if the plain evidence was that heart function was restored.[28]

The members of the Boucek team defended their action by claiming that the restoration of heart function was irrelevant because death was pronounced based on establishing the irreversible loss of circulatory function. The infants pronounced dead never had their circulation restored and therefore were dead by circulatory criteria. Even if we assume that irreversibility is based on the legal impossibility of restarting circulation in infants with a valid decision to withdraw life support, it is clear that a more precise articulation is required of what it means for circulation to cease. The authors of the early legal definitions of death, such as the Uniform Determination of Death Act, never faced the question of whether loss of circulation followed by restoration of heart function so that it maintains circulation in another body would still count as irreversible loss of circulation.

   This raises a complex question: The choice of the time period for waiting after asystole before death is pronounced is based on the supposed belief that autoresuscitation would be impossible after either 180 or 75 seconds. This belief, if empirically supported, would be grounds for claiming death, provided that circulation was independent not only of the fact that the heart function would be restored but also of the question of whether brain tissue was still alive. Conversely, if irreversible circulation loss is merely a basis for determining the status of the brain, there is no reason to assume that the infants pronounced dead after 180 or 75 seconds of asystole had irreversibly lost all functions of their brains. Quite to the contrary, there is strong reason to believe that the brain tissue is not dead and in fact retains the capacity to perform certain functions after 75 seconds and possibly after even 180 seconds. This is especially true for infants, whose brains are more resilient than those of adults. Pronouncing death in the Boucek cases requires the controversial assumption that death can be pronounced when circulation has irreversibly ceased (not counting the heart circulating blood in another body), regardless of the fact that the infants' brains undoubtedly retain a capacity to perform at least some functions. If death by circulatory criteria is based merely on the claim that circulation loss is indirect evidence of brain status, the Boucek infants could not be considered deceased at the time death was pronounced. The protocol requires that circulation loss is intrinsically the determiner of death, that the continued function of the heart to provide circulation outside the body can be ignored, that as little as 75 seconds of asystole is sufficient to claim the impossibility of autoresuscitation (without a peer-reviewed consensus), and that this time period can be used for newborns in addition to adults.

The New York City DCD Protocol

Although Boucek and his colleagues were making claims implying that they viewed circulation as intrinsically the sign of life (and its loss, death), another protocol was emerging that was designed to attempt to obtain organs from heart attack victims who were the subjects of unsuccessful rescue attempts by emergency responders. Those behind this protocol seemed to defend their work by assuming that circulation did not matter as long as heart function had ceased. A report from the New York City UDCDD [Unplanned Donation after Circulatory Determination of Death] Study Group seems to rely on assumptions that contradict the Boucek group.

   The NYC UDCDD group was attempting to develop a social consensus about pronouncing the death of heart attack victims for whom resuscitation was unsuccessful.[29] After the failed resuscitation and death pronouncement based on cardiocirculatory arrest by the rescue squad, a second team would be standing by, whose members would intervene to provide maximal effort to preserve organs (other than the heart) so that transport to a hospital could take place in such a way that the organs could be procured. This second team, in order to maximize organ preservation, would offer cardiac massage and ECMO. This would, in effect, restore circulation, which raises the question of whether the heart attack victim had actually experienced irreversible loss of circulation. Their defense was that as long as the heartbeat was not restored, the reestablishment of circulation did not matter.

This seems to be an obvious contradiction to the reasoning of the Boucek team. Boucek's group said that reestablishing a heartbeat did not matter because the circulation was critical; the New York group said that reestablishing circulation did not matter, because the heart was critical. Now, for the first time, we need to know precisely what it is about the circulatory system that would permit us to pronounce death. Is it the irreversible loss of circulation (as Boucek's group claims) or the irreversible loss of a heartbeat (as the New York group claims)?

The Michigan ECMO Project

The story gets even more complicated, however. A group at the University of Michigan has experimented with ECMO for many important uses in medicine. This group undertook the application of ECMO technology for the purpose of preserving organs for transplant.[30] They were aware, however, that a reestablishment of circulation would raise questions about whether their patients were dead. In order to avoid reanimation, they devised an ingenious plan of inserting catheters in the carotid arteries with balloons that could be inflated so that the ECMO would restore circulation to the body but not to the head. Hence, the brain would be allowed to deteriorate without the supply of oxygen that would otherwise come from the ECMO. They defended their approach by claiming that, because the restoration of circulation did not reanimate the brain, the recipients of the ECMO were still dead. Obviously, this defense works only if one is viewing absence of circulation as evidence of brain status. The recipients of the ECMO would be dead if, and only if, circulation was indirect evidence of brain status, not if circulation to the body were intrinsically important.

Both those who believe that circulation is intrinsically important and those who believe that it is important as indirect evidence for the loss of the body's integrating capacity have referred to this basis for pronouncing death as "circulatory death." In the past decade a new understanding of death pronouncement based on circulation loss has emerged. It views circulation loss not as evidence of brain function loss but rather as the loss of the body's capacity to perform integrated functions independent of the brain. This position, articulated best by Alan Shewmon, deserves careful attention.

Shewmon's Somatic Concept

The most influential advocate for something resembling the circulatory concept of death is the neurologist Alan Shewmon. He has accepted the concept of death as the irreversible loss of bodily integrating capacity, but he notes that "most somatically integrative functions of the body are not brain-mediated."[31] He claims that substantial capacity for such integration continues to be possible, even in the absence of brain function. He points out that a body with a completely destroyed brain can be maintained (albeit with considerable medical support) and that with maintenance of ventilatory support and proper nutrition and hydration, many systemic, complex integrative functions remain possible. He cites homeostasis, elimination, energy balance, maintenance of body temperature, wound healing, fighting of infections, development of febrile response, cardiovascular and hormonal stress responses, successful gestation of a fetus, sexual maturation of a child, and proportional growth as capacities that have all been maintained in a so-called brain-dead body.[32] He has persuasively argued that, if somatic integrating capacities are what are critical for determining whether a human body is dead or alive, then it is clear that the mere death of the brain cannot be taken as human death.

Thus, Shewmon has put forward a somatic concept of death that identifies a wide range of integrative body functions, not merely circulation and respiration. Nevertheless, he associates his position with the traditional respiratory and circulatory definition, noting that "both *circulation* and *respiration* (in the technical, biochemical sense linked to energy generation) are presupposed as means to many, if not all, of the above functions" (italics in the original).[33] Therefore, there is a close compatibility between his somatic concept of death and the views of those who adhere to the more traditional circulatory and respiratory definitions, at least those who hold that we have looked to circulation and respiration in pronouncing death because these functions have been considered intrinsically important (and not mere indirect indicators of brain status).

The result has been that, over the past decade, there has arisen more doubt about the whole-brain-based definition of death than was anticipated in the last decades of the twentieth century. Now not only those who traditionally thought circulation and respiration were an intrinsic sign of life, but also those who adopt the more sophisticated somatic integrative concept, are unwilling to accept the whole-brain basis for pronouncing the death of humans, including some who would nevertheless accept procuring of life-prolonging organs from certain persons before their deaths, that is, those who have come to reject the dead donor rule.[34] Those who hold this view still represent a small minority in the United States and most other Western countries. The view, however, has gained more credibility lately, as seen by the seriousness with which it was taken by the US President's Council on Bioethics.

The Two Definitions of the US President's Council on Bioethics

The US President's Council on Bioethics has identified two different definitions of death. One of these definitions—referred to as "position one"—rejects a neurologically based definition and closely follows Shewmon's work. Position one was adopted by two of the council's eighteen members (Alfonso Gomez-Lobo and council chair Edmund D. Pellegrino)—closely mirroring the estimated 10 percent of the US population that has never accepted neurological definitions.[35]

Having been challenged by Shewmon's persuasive claim that many bodily integrative functions exist outside the brain and that they remain possible even after the death of the brain, the majority of the President's Council has nevertheless adopted a brain-oriented definition of death, which is referred to as "position two." It has identified more or less the same group as dead as was singled out by the view that assumed the brain was responsible for bodily integrative functions, but now offered a new conceptual foundation. The majority have claimed that a more compelling view of a body functioning as a whole requires "the work of self-preservation, achieved through the organism's need driven commerce with the surrounding world."[36] This interaction with the surrounding world requires the functioning of the brain, and thus the council's majority view provides a new basis for the defense of the neurological standard—what we have referred to as the whole-brain basis for pronouncing death.

This new level of complexity in defining death and differentiating the various roles that circulation might play in death pronouncement has created a much more complicated and confusing set of issues for death pronouncement in relation to organ procurement. This is particularly true for the organ procurement that can be associated with death pronouncement based on circulatory or somatic death.

Although the circulatory or somatic view has gained some status in the past few years in its conflict with the whole-brain view, the more neurologically oriented definition of death that insists on the irreversible loss of all functions of the entire brain has also met competition from another, more liberal view: the higher-brain view. It is to this third major definition that we now turn.

Notes

1. Miller FG, Truog RD, *Death, dying, and organ transplantation* (New York: Oxford University Press, 2012); Lamb D, *Death, brain death and ethics* (Albany: State University of New York Press, 1985); Shewmon, DA, "The brain and somatic integration: Insights into the standard biological rationale for equating 'brain death' with death," *Journal of Medicine and Philosophy* 2001;26: 457–78.

2. See Siminoff LA, Burant C, Youngner SJ, "Death and organ procurement: Public beliefs and attitudes," *Kennedy Institute of Ethics Journal* 2004;14: 217–34.

3. This case description is based on the work of Wells J, "Mother of brain-dead Jahi McMath defends ventilator decision," *Los Angeles Times*, Feb. 24, 2014, http://articles.latimes.com/2014/feb/24/local/la-me-ln-mother-jahi-mcmath-defends-decision-20140224; Onishijan N, "A brain is dead, a heart beats on," *New York Times*, Jan. 3, 2014, www.nytimes.com/2014/01/04/us/a-brain-is-dead-a-heart-beats-on.html?_r = 1; Veatch RM, "Let parents decide if teen is dead," Jan. 2, 2014, www.cnn.com/2014/01/02/opinion/veatch-defining-death/.

4. Capron AM, Kass LR, "A statutory definition of the standards for determining human death: An appraisal and a proposal," *University of Pennsylvania Law Review* 1972;121: 114. See also President's Commission for the Study of Ethical Problems in Medicine and Biomedical and Behavioral Research, *Defining death: Medical, legal and ethical issues in the definition of death* (Washington DC: US Government Printing Office, 1981), 40–41. Capron was executive director of the Commission.

5. Siminoff, Burant, Youngner, "Death."

6. "University of Pittsburgh Medical Center Policy and Procedure Manual," *Kennedy Institute of Ethics Journal* 1993;3: A-1–15.

7. Institute of Medicine, Committee on Organ Procurement and Transplantation Policy, *Organ procurement and transplantation: Assessing current policies and the potential impact of the DHHS final rule* (Washington, DC: National Academy Press, 1999).

8. "Non-heartbeating donor procurement attempted," *UNOS Update* 1992;8 (6): 15.

9. US Department of Health and Human Services, "Federal policy for the protection of human subjects; notices and rules," *Federal Register*, June 18, 1991;46: 28001–32.

10. Ibid., 28017.

11. Ibid., 20813.

12. For both the text of the act and comment, see Sadler, AM, Sadler BL, Stason EB, "The Uniform Anatomical Gift Act: A model for reform," *JAMA* 1968;206: 2501–6.

13. The data from the 1990s indicated about half were willing to donate; Gallup Organization, *The American public's attitudes toward organ donation and transplantation, conducted for the Partnership for*

Organ Donation (Boston: Partnership for Organ Donation, 1993). More recently (based on data for 2009–12) authorization rates have ranged from about 54 percent to 83 percent, depending on the ethnicity of the patient and family. "Summary of analyses for authorization rate by OPO and ethnicity," www.organdonationalliance.org/wp-content/uploads/2013/11/data-summary-info-unos-oct-2013.pdf.

14. Miller BL, "Philosophical, ethical, and legal aspects of resuscitation medicine, I: Deferred consent and justification of resuscitation research," *Critical Care Medicine* 1988;16: 1059–62.

15. Meyers DW, *The human body and the law*, 2nd ed. (Stanford, CA: Stanford University Press, 1990), 128–29; *Canterbury v. Spence* 488 Fed. 2d. 772, 778; *Stafford v. Louisiana State University* (1984, LA App.) 448 So. 2d. 852.

16. Examples using this methodology are Faden RR, Becker C, Lewis C, et al., "Disclosure of information to patients in medical care," *Medical Care* 1981;19: 718–33, and Winer R, Veatch RM, Sidel VW, Spivack M, "Informed consent: The use of lay surrogates to determine how much information should be transmitted," in *The patient as partner: A theory of human-experimentation ethics*, ed. Veatch RM (Bloomington: Indiana University Press, 1987), 153–68.

17. District of Columbia Code, Annotated Title 2, Chapter 15, "Anatomical Gifts." DC Code '2-1509.1 (1998).

18. Deardorff SE, "Informed consent, termination of medical treatment, and the federal tort claims act—a new proposal for the military health care system." *Military Law Review* 1987 Jan;115: 68, 74.

19. Chayet, NL, "Consent for autopsy," *New England Journal of Medicine* 1966;274: 268–69.

20. Herdman R, Potts JT, *Non-heart-beating organ transplantation: Medical and ethical issues in procurement* (Washington, DC: National Academy Press, 1997), 39–40, 52.

21. American Medical Association (AMA), Council on Ethical and Judicial Affairs, *Code of medical ethics: Current opinions with annotations, 1998–1999 edition* (Chicago: American Medical Association, 1998), 46. Here the AMA endorses administration of pain-relieving drugs to dying patients, even though such medications may actively hasten death. The standard justification for this exception to the prohibition on active killing is that the death is not intended, i.e., the doctrine of double effect. Although the AMA endorses procurement of organs from individuals who die based on circulatory death criteria (which we now refer to as donation after circulatory death, or DCD) and supports perfusion of the deceased donor (with appropriate consent), it does not explicitly address the administration of organ-preserving drugs that might hasten death.

22. Herdman, Potts, *Non-heart-beating organ transplantation*, 52.

23. Curran CE, "Roman Catholicism," in *Encyclopedia of bioethics*, 2nd edition, ed. Reich WT (New York: Free Press, 1995), vol. 4, 2321–31; Marquis DB, "Four versions of double effect," *Journal of Medicine and Philosophy* 1991;16: 515–44; McCormick RA, Ramsey P, eds., *Doing evil to achieve good: Moral choice in conflict situations* (Chicago: Loyola University Press, 1978); Pellegrino ED, "Intending to kill and the principle of double effect," in *Ethical issues in death and dying*, 2nd edition, ed. Beauchamp TL, Veatch RM (Englewood Cliffs, NJ: Prentice Hall, 1995), 240–42.

24. E.g., see Kevorkian J, *Prescription medicide: The goodness of planned death* (Buffalo: Prometheus Books; 1991).

25. US Bishops' Committee on Doctrine, "Ethical and religious directives for Catholic health care services," *Origins* 1994;24 (27): 449, 451–62.

26. Boucek MM, Mashburn C, Dunn SM, et al., for the Denver Children's Pediatric Heart Transplant Team, "Pediatric heart transplantation after declaration of cardiocirculatory death," *New England Journal of Medicine* 2008;359: 709–14.

27. Bernat J, "The boundaries of organ donation after circulatory death," *New England Journal of Medicine* 2007;359: 669–71.

28. Veatch RM, "Donating hearts after cardiac death: Reversing the irreversible," *New England Journal of Medicine* 2008;359: 672–73.

29. Wall SP, Kaufman BJ, Gilbert AJ, et al., for the NYC UDCDD Study Group, "Derivation of the uncontrolled donation after circulatory determination of death protocol for New York City," *Transplantation Proceedings* 2011;11: 1417–26.

30. Magliocca JF, Magee, JC, Rowe SA, et al., "Extracorporeal support for organ donation after cardiac death effectively expands the donor pool," *Journal of TRAUMA Injury, Infection, and Critical Care* 2005;58 (6): 1095–1102.

31. Shewmon, "Brain," 467.

32. Ibid., 467–68.

33. Ibid., 489.

34. See, e.g., Miller, Truog, *Death.*

35. US President's Council on Bioethics, *Controversies in the determination of death: A white paper by the President's Council on Bioethics* (Washington, DC: US President's Council on Bioethics, 2008), 99, 114.

36. Ibid., 60.

Chapter 6

The Higher-Brain Concept of Death

The difficulties in developing a coherent, whole-brain-based definition of death have raised problems not only for those who identify somatic integrative functions outside the brain but also for those who question whether literally all functions of the entire brain must be lost irreversibly before neurologically based death pronouncement can occur. Shewmon, in cataloging problems with whole-brain-based notions of death, not only points to integrative functions mediated outside the brain, but also summarizes claims that have been made against the criteria sets used for brain-based death pronouncement. Several authors, starting with Halevy and Brody, have noted that some brain functions may remain in the cases of patients who meet all the criteria in the standard sets of criteria for the death of the brain.[1] In particular, Halevy and Brody observe that neurohormonal functioning, such as anterior pituitary hormone levels, have been found as have delta, theta, and alpha electroencephalographic findings as well as brain-stem-evoked potentials.[2] Thus, there exist "functions" in some brains that supposedly meet the criteria for brains that have irreversibly lost all functions.

There are two plausible responses to this paradox. The most straightforward one would be to revise the criteria to make sure that these hormonal and electrical functions are absent before death is pronounced. If the law requires all functions of the brain to be gone, then all functions ought to be tested. The other alternative is to acknowledge that, when the original proponents of brain-based death pronouncement put forward the standard that "all functions" must be lost, they really did not have in mind hormonal or electrical functions of the kind that Halevy, Brody, and others have identified. In fact, in the years since these paradoxical findings have become known, deaths based on brain function loss have continued to be pronounced using the same criteria sets that were in use prior to our awareness of this issue.

Ignoring these hormonal and electrical functions is not the only example of brain-death defenders excluding certain activities as too trivial to consider. James Bernat, the best-known defender of the whole-brain, bodily-integrating-capacity definition of death, has acknowledged that we should include only the "critical" functions, excluding certain "nests of cells" as not sufficiently important.[3] Thus, he ends up defending the "whole-brain" concept while acknowledging that some functions can be ignored.

Similarly, Pallis, in defending the brain stem concept, while suggesting that it is functionally equivalent to the whole-brain concept, identifies only consciousness and respiration as critical functions, permitting one to ignore all other brain functions, including not only the hormonal and electrical ones but also other brain stem reflexes.[4]

If one is to retain a neurologically based concept of death, it is terribly implausible to insist that all functions of the entire brain must be lost irreversibly. Every reasonable defender of brain-based death pronouncement must exclude some functions, opening up the question of just which functions should be excluded.

Henry Beecher, the Harvard committee chairman, in a 1970 lecture defending brain-based death pronouncement (what we would call the "whole-brain" view), made clear which functions he deemed essential, and he did not seem to include all the brain's functions.[5] He believed that a human is dead when there is irreversible loss of the human's "personality, his conscious life, his uniqueness, his capacity for remembering, judging, reasoning, acting, enjoying, worrying, and so on." Beecher goes on to argue: "We have proof that these and other functions reside in the brain. . . . It seems clear that when the brain no longer functions, when it is destroyed, so also is the individual destroyed; he no longer exists as a person; he is dead."

Certainly this conclusion follows from what we know about the brain, but there is a fundamental error in the argument. We have suggested that, if there is a practical problem with the more conservative heart- and lung-oriented concepts, it is that they occasionally produce false positive tests for life. Some patients with circulatory function actually have irreversibly lost all functions of the brain. If the argument is to be made for brain-oriented criteria at all, then certainly this argument must be subject to the same criticism. The functions mentioned by Beecher and summarized by the term *irreversible coma* certainly are in the brain, but clearly do not exhaust the brain's functions. Patients we would now say are in an irreversible coma, and also those who are in a permanent vegetative state (what is also referred to as "unawareness wakefulness syndrome"[6]), have purportedly irreversibly lost all the functions that Beecher enumerated but do not have dead brains. Focusing on the destruction of the whole brain may include additional nonessential functions, just as focusing on the heart and lungs did. The hormonal and electrical activities identified by Halevy and Brody, along with any other insignificant nests of cells referred to by Bernat, would surely qualify.

Which Brain Functions Are Critical?

If every reasonable defender of a neurologically based concept of death needs to exclude some brain functions, the critical question is which ones. Which brain functions are so important that their presence is a sign of life? Several candidates for functions critical to human existence have been proposed. Let us review them.

The Capacity for Rationality

Beecher's list of characteristics includes the human's ability to reason. The Latin name for our species clearly implies that reasoning capacity is somehow an essential characteristic. Could it be that it is reasoning capacity, rather than integrating capacity, that is essential? Our considered moral judgment about those members of the species who do not have any capacity for reasoning but retain consciousness is that they are still to be considered living in a very real way. They are still to have human rights, protected by both moral and positive law.

Babies lacking a language, a culture, and a capacity to reason certainly are living in a human sense, in spite of the fact that they have never executed the reasoning function. One might, of course, argue that babies have the potential for reasoning—the capacity for future reasoning. In this sense, they might be included among the category of living humans. But what of those afflicted with senile dementia, those with severe cognitive disabilities, and/or the apparently permanently psychotic? They also lack a capacity for rationality, in some cases will never have had that capacity, and in other cases will never regain it. Yet it is clear that they are still living in a meaningful sense of the term. In fact, one of the great dangers of moving to any brain-oriented concept of death is that it might place us on a slippery slope leading to the eventual exclusion of certain individuals who lack a certain minimal quality of life from the category of the human. Unless this tendency can be avoided, the dangers of movement to brain-oriented concepts may well exceed the moral right-making tendencies. Whatever may be our propensity to see rationality as the pinnacle of human functioning, it must not be the characteristic that is essential to consider humans living. We must look elsewhere.

Personhood or Personal Identity

Some contributors to the definition-of-death discussion equate the loss of personhood or loss of personal identity with death.[7] Green and Wikler, for example, claim that continuity of personal identity is essential for the existence of a person. When continuity of personal identity ends, that person no longer exists. This must surely be wrong as well. Assuming we are using the standard nonmoral definition of persons as self-aware beings, it is easy to recognize that there are human, living, nonpersons—that is, humans who lack the capacity for self-awareness—who are nevertheless alive.[8] Even if continuity of personal identity ceases, a human—the same human—still exists. Infants, the severely senile, and perhaps other humans lack self-awareness yet surely are not dead. When the advanced Alzheimer's disease patient has completely lost continuity of personal identity with his or her earlier existence, he or she continues to exist. It is not even plausible to say that he or she ceases to be the person he or she once was. Everyone would recognize that a patient who, through injury or illness, loses all continuity of personal identity—even one who could never regain that personal identity—was nevertheless the same individual. His or her spouse would still be married to him or her; his or her health insurance would still cover his or her medical costs; he or she would still be the owner of his or her property, and so forth. Any other position would produce chaos. The "new individual" in the "old person's body" would own no assets, have no family, and have no insurance coverage. Such an individual is not only not dead; he or she is still the same individual (even if philosophers might say he or she is no longer a "person" in the sense of being self-aware or having continuity of personal identity).

The Capacity to Experience

Most of the other functions mentioned in lists of essentially human characteristics—consciousness, capacity for remembering, enjoying, worrying, acting voluntarily—

characterize the human as an experiential animal. Experience is here taken in the broadest sense. Humans experience cognitively and emotionally. They cathect, comprehend, and experience through sense organs and through much more complex experiential modes. It seems clear that a human who has some vestige of consciousness, some capacity to experience in this broadest sense, could never be considered dead. To be sure, this human life may not be on the highest plane. It may be limited to a blurred vision of reality and stunted emotional experience, but it is nevertheless life of a form sufficiently human to be protected. Death behavior for such an individual is inappropriate.

Anencephalic infants are children born without functioning cerebral hemispheres, and therefore they never experience any consciousness. Although they are sometimes referred to as "brain absent," they may have a fully or partially functioning brainstem, such that they may have spontaneous respiration and therefore are living, unconscious beings by whole-brain standards, although they will never have the capacity to experience others or to have social interaction.[9]

The anencephalic infant and other humans without any capacity for consciousness raise the question of whether a being should be considered "living" if body functions such as respiration, circulation, digestion, and excretion are possible but consciousness is not. We saw in chapter 5 that the defenders of the somatic view answer in the affirmative, but most advocates for the higher-brain view would claim that, without experience—consciousness—an essential element of the being is impossible. They hold that life—for purposes of public policy—requires this capacity to experience, or something very similar.

The Capacity for Social Interaction

Although humans may be experiential, they are also social creatures. At least in the Western tradition, the human's capacity to relate to fellow humans is a fundamental characteristic—some would even say essential. Is it meaningful to speak of a living human who lacks the capacity for social interaction? We must make clear that we are not at all saying that actual social interaction must take place for a creature to be alive. We are not even saying that such interaction must have ever taken place. To say this would place the human's existence at the mercy of fellow humans. The cruel treatment of a baby who has been abandoned in a room with no human interaction should not define that baby out of existence. Presumably the capacity for social interaction nevertheless remains.

Likewise, there are cases of feral children. People have occasionally found a child that has grown up in the forest with animals. These children are called feral children. If they have no social interaction their whole childhood, they would act as animals do—they would bite, scratch, growl, and walk on all fours. They would not be able to talk, or even know that any language existed. They would drink by lapping up water, eat grass, and eat raw meat. They would not know what was considered right or wrong, and would not be able to conform to the norms of society. Similarly, children with severe autism have severely constrained capacity to experience others. It seems likely that even these extreme cases do not represent literally a complete lack of capacity for social interaction, no matter how stunted it may be. As such, we would insist on what is perhaps obvious: They are living human beings. However, if there ever were a genetic human with literally no capacity to interact socially, the question arises of whether the individual would be considered a member of the human moral community.

What, then, is the relationship between the capacity for experience and the capacity for social interaction? It is conceivable that a condition could exist that would differentiate the two capacities. But to be able to experience but not experience others would certainly be a bizarre form of existence. One of the most important experiences that humans have is social interaction. At least in the Western tradition, the human's capacity to relate to fellow humans is fundamental and integral to what we mean when we talk about what it means to be human. In fact, one could propose replacing the more traditional concepts of death (those focusing on the departure of the soul, or the irreversible cessation of fluid flow, or somatic integrating capacity) and to focus instead on the irreversible loss of the capacity for experience or social interaction, rather than the irreversible loss of integrating capacity of the body. If this is the case, the implications for the whole-brain-oriented criteria for death are great.

What emerges is what is sometimes called a "higher-brain" concept of death, one that requires only the "higher" or important brain functions to be present for one to be considered alive. The term "higher" is, of course, ambiguous and vague. It suggests that only certain brain functions are more important. These may well also be higher in anatomical location. Exactly what higher functions are critical and where those functions are located is a matter of philosophical and public policy decision.

Embodiment of Capacity

Is it simply capacity for experience and social interaction per se, or must there also be some embodiment of the capacity? Consider the bizarre and purely hypothetical case in which all of the information of the human brain were transferred to a computer hard drive, together with sufficient sensory inputs and outputs to permit some form of rudimentary experiential and social function. Would the deleting of the disk information be murder? This thought is so novel that perhaps we cannot even conceive clearly of the philosophical significance of the question. Certain worldviews influenced by the Greeks view the mind as the critical part of human existence. Liberation from the body—the flesh—is a goal. If all that is critical is mental, then presumably humans could, in theory, exist as computers.

Viewing the mind as the only essential feature of a human being, one of us has suggested, is the mistake of the "mentalists."[10] They accept that an individual could, in theory, exist completely disembodied. It seems quite possible that our concept of the essential must include some embodiment. An adult male whose mind was transferred to a little girl's body would not be the continuing existence of the adult male; it would be a chimera, a combination of two beings—something we hope would never be created. The human is, after all, something more than a sophisticated computer. At least in the Judeo-Christian tradition, the body is an essential element, not something from which humans escape in liberation. If this is the case, then the essential element is *embodied capacity for experience and social interaction*. According to this view, if either the mind or the body ceases to exist (even if the mind were to continue to exist in another body, or even if the body continued to exist without a mind), that individual would no longer exist. He or she would be dead.

We might even adopt the now-standard concept of death as the irreversible loss of the integrated functioning of the being as a whole. Only now, the "being as a whole" whose integration we have in mind is not merely somatic; it is the entire being—mind and body. The permanent collapse of the integration of the mind with the body is what might reasonably be thought of as death for all moral, social, and public policy purposes.

We opt for the general formulation that a human is dead when there is irreversible loss of embodied capacity for consciousness. This would make those who have lost all functions of the entire brain dead, of course; but it would also include those who lack consciousness, which includes the permanently comatose, the permanently vegetative, and the anencephalic infant to the extent that these groups can be identified.

Altered States of Consciousness: A Continuum

We have characterized higher-brain function to refer to consciousness, defined by William James in the 1890s to refer to awareness of self and environment.[11] Consciousness has two clinical components: (1) wakefulness, which is mediated by the ascending reticular activating system of the brain stem; and (2) awareness of self and environment, which is mediated by the cerebral cortex. A coma—an eyes-closed, pathologic state of unresponsiveness—is caused by a structural or metabolic lesion that interferes with the reticular activating system. It is usually transient.[12] A patient in a coma can progress to one of several states: (1) recover, (2) remain unresponsive, (3) progress to a locked-in state, or (4) progress to brain death. Patients who remain unresponsive are characterized as in a vegetative state, although the European Task Force on disorders of consciousness has recently proposed the more neutral term, "unresponsive wakefulness syndrome."[13] As the Multi-Society Task Force report on the permanent vegetative state (PVS) clarified the situation in 1994, those in a vegetative state (VS) have wakefulness but lack awareness: "Awareness requires wakefulness, wakefulness can be present without awareness."[14] Individuals in a VS can be aroused but are not conscious. The VS is considered permanent after three months if caused by a hypoxic-ischemic, metabolic, or congenital injury, but not until twelve months after traumatic brain injury. Some patients who remain unresponsive (or vegetative) will later progress to a minimally conscious state (MCS).

The MCS refers to individuals who have severely altered consciousness but definite behavioral evidence of conscious awareness.[15] This involves evidence that one or more of the following behaviors are observed on bedside examination: (1) simple command following, (2) intelligible verbalization, (3) recognizable verbal or gestural "yes/no" responses (without regard to accuracy), or (4) movements or emotional responses that are triggered by relevant environmental stimulae. The upper boundary of MCS is defined by the recovery of communication or functional use of objects.

To minimize errors in diagnosis and prognosis in patients with altered states of consciousness, standardized neurobehavioral rating scales have been developed. The oldest one is the Glasgow Coma Scale, originally published in 1974.[16] It lacks sensitivity to subtle changes of prognostic relevance, which has led to the development of a number of newer instruments that can distinguish between VS and MCS, with the Coma Recovery Scale–Revised (CRS-R) being the measurement of choice.[17]

The problem with the CRS-R and the other scales is that they focus on volitional behavior in patients with severe brain injury who may have fluctuating arousal levels along with impaired sensory and motor functions that can mask signs of consciousness.[18] Some studies suggest a high rate of misdiagnosis (false positives and false negatives) among disorders of consciousness. Luaute and colleagues suggest that erroneous diagnoses of MCS as PVS may reach 40 percent.[19] The natural history and long-term outcomes of MCS have not yet been adequately investigated, although the likelihood of significant functional improvement diminishes over time.[20] Luaute and colleagues found that more than 70 percent of patients in MCS emerge from MCS between one and three months after a coma's onset, and some of them recover at least partial independence in activities of daily living, but fewer achieve meaningful recovery if MCS endures from three to six months, although it is not unheard of for an individual to emerge from MCS after one year or longer.[21] As such, a time cutoff beyond which the recovery of patients in MCS cannot be expected is impossible to establish.[22] It is common experience that individuals with disorders of consciousness recover their first interaction with the environment through significant emotional stimulation, mostly provided by close relatives or caregivers.[23]

An accurate and reliable evaluation of the level and content of cognitive processing is important for the appropriate management of patients. Objective behavioral assessment of residual cognitive function can be extremely difficult because motor responses may be minimal, inconsistent, and difficult to document. This has led to the use of functional neuroimagining, which has identified some patients with consciousness who fail to show behavioral evidence of consciousness at the bedside. Two modalities that correspond with active function are [18F]-fluorodeoxyglucose positron emission tomography (FDG-PET) and functional MRI (fMRI). They work on the basis of glucose consumption by the neurons in the brain. When a person is performing or even thinking about performing a particular task, the regions of the brain that control that task increase their consumption of glucose as a source of energy. That is, glucose metabolism can be seen as a general surrogate marker for conscious experience.[24] PET involves the injection of radioactive elements that localize metabolic activity to particular areas of the brain.[25] fMRI uses strong magnetic fields to monitor the level of blood oxygenation as a marker of neural activity. fMRI is used more often than PET because of its greater availability and because it poses less risk to subjects.

To the extent that glucose metabolism is a marker for conscious experience, one would expect no metabolic activity in individuals in VS and some activity in individuals with MCS. And yet, studies have found some residual activity in some individuals in what we thought was VS.[26] In several rare cases, fMRI has demonstrated conscious awareness in patients who are assumed to be vegetative yet retain cognitive abilities that have evaded detection using standard clinical methods. Similarly, in some patients diagnosed as minimally conscious, functional neuroimaging has revealed residual cognitive capabilities that extend well beyond what is evident even from the most comprehensive behavioral assessment.[27]

Owen and colleagues reported in *Science* in 2006 a case of a woman labeled as being in VS who was able to perform two different mental imagery tasks when instructed.[28] The patient was asked to imagine playing tennis and to imagine walking through a room in her house. The fMRI results were indistinguishable from those for healthy volunteers, leading them to conclude that she was imaging those tasks.[29] Others have developed follow-up studies to convert this imagery study into a command-following paradigm, where imagining tennis would be interpreted as "yes" and walking through the house would be interpreted as "no." Monti and colleagues found that five of fifty-four patients (twenty-three in VS, and thirty-one in MCS) were able to selectively trigger motor and spatial activation on cue.[30]

The ability to accurately distinguish between MCS and PVS is very important for prognosis and appropriate treatment. It becomes even more critical for those who support higher-brain function definitions of death. Patients with PVS do not interact with their environment, but MCS patients do, such that the former may be eligible for organ donation under a higher-brain definition of death, but patients with MCS would not. Given the high degree of inaccurate diagnosis, doubt arises.

Measuring the Loss of Higher-Brain Function

If one were to propose a higher-brain function of death, the question is what criteria would be necessary and sufficient for such a declaration and what tests can determine whether the criteria have been met? Such a test will need to distinguish between individuals with permanent loss of all higher-brain function (those in coma or PVS) and those who may have some consciousness, understood as awareness of the self and the environment.

A higher-brain function conception of death must address three issues. First, researchers surmise that 30 to 40 percent of individuals classified as being in PVS are inaccurately labeled. This has important prognostic and diagnostic implications, even more so if one were to adopt a higher-brain function definition of death. Clearly, those in MCS have some consciousness and would not be dead by higher-brain function, whereas those in PVS would be. The high error rate makes one pause.

A second problem is that at the time of the multisociety task force guidelines on PVS in 1994, most patients in VS had been followed for at most one year. Today, there are more data about late recovery. Estraneo and colleagues followed fifty patients in VS for an average of twenty-six months and found that 20 percent of the sample recovered at least one sign of conscious awareness between fourteen and twenty-eight months after injury, and 24 percent emerged from MCS between nineteen and twenty-five months after injury.[31] Late recovery was more common in younger individuals with a traumatic etiology. This makes it more difficult to identify clear criteria that can be met before one who is in VS is permanently unconscious and can be classified as dead by higher-brain function.

Third, there have been recent developments with medications that have served as a "bridge" to consciousness. The first case report was described in 2000 in South Africa, where an individual who had been "semicomatose" for three years began to talk and to respond appropriately when treated with zolpidem and would revert to his semicomatose state when the medication wore off. Since then, there have been other reports of amanta-dine and the use of deep thalamic brain stimulation.[32]

Ancillary Tests

First let us consider whether the ancillary tests for whole-brain death mentioned in chapter 4 can help us identify higher-brain death.

Flat Electroencephalogram

Whereas a flat electroencephalogram (EEG) helps confirm the existence of a permanently nonfunctioning brain, the question remains whether the EEG measures whole-brain func-tion or something more limited. From the scientific evidence, the EEG apparently mea-sures simply the presence of neocortical electrical activity. If this is true, it is quite possible that some brain activity could remain in the presence of a flat electroencephalogram. Thus, though EEG activity refutes a claim of irreversible cessation of the functioning of the whole brain, the absence of EEG reading does not necessarily mean the absence of brain function. From the point of view of the higher-brain definition of death, however, could an EEG alone be a measure of death?

The problem with the EEG is that, if it measures neocortical activity, it presumably may measure any neocortical activity. Yet we have concluded that the experiential and social integrating function is the essential element in the nature of the human, the loss of which is to be called death. Once again the danger of a false positive diagnosis of living must be raised. The neocortical cells and nerve circuits responsible for the experiential and social integrating function are certainly complex. They would need to include some sensory portions of the cortex, as well as the limbic system and other areas responsible for emotion. Yet is it not theoretically possible that some cortical cells could retain via-bility and yet the person would be dead in the sense we have discussed? What, for instance, if only motor cortex cells continued to survive through some freak preservation of blood supply to a small area of the cortex or some theoretical artificial perfusion? Whether or not the EEG would be present and whether the existence of only this kind of cortical activity could be distinguished are empirical questions. At the philosophical level, how-ever, for one who sees the essence of the human to be an embodied experiential and social capacity, the presence of viable motor cells would be of no more significance than the presence of the spinal or cranial reflex arc. Thus, the concept of death being dealt with cannot be reduced without remainder to the criterion of a flat EEG. The irreversible loss of these essential functions may be compatible with the presence of some form of EEG reading. Whether empirical tests can be made to make such a distinction and whether such solely motor cell capacity could ever exist are beyond this discussion.

Blood Flow Studies

The other ancillary tests for the determination of whole-brain death do not do much better than the EEG as a means of measuring higher-brain function. Consider, for example, blood flow studies. Both computed tomography angiography (CTA) and magnetic resonance angiography (MRA) are reliable methods of measuring cerebral blood flow, and the absence of cerebral blood flow is considered an accurate marker of loss of brain function.[33] However, a person may lack upper-brain function and yet still have cerebral blood flow. A false negative result may occur, for example, if intracranial pressure is relieved by a ventricular drain that restores intracranial blood flow. CTA may also give false positives in patients with open skull defects who demonstrate minimal cerebral flood flow. An alternative to the measurement of cerebral blood flow is to measure cerebral perfusion, but these tests may also have a false negative if there is a cranial defect. These tests may be difficult to interpret.[34]

Neuroimaging

If the older ancillary tests cannot test for higher-brain death, what about the newer modalities of fMRI and FDG-PET scans? Although these modalities are useful for identifying upper-brain function, a negative fMRI does not rule out the possibility that upper-brain function exists. First, many patients in MCS have periods when they are more responsive than others. Second, some patients may have hearing or other problems that may make these tests unreliable because the patient may not receive the sensory input. Third, and most important, a negative test does not fully predict whether the patient will regain these functions in the months to come. The data about moving from VS to MCS suggest that this change can be quite slow, and there is no set time point after which recovery never occurs. This is particularly true as we learn more about techniques to bridge the arousal and awareness components of consciousness through medication or deep thalamic stimulation.

The problem of doubt returns once again—this time with doubt between the older, broader whole-brain-oriented integrating function and the more limited embodied capacity for consciousness or experiential function. As for us, the case for the concept of the human that sees experiential and social functioning as central is persuasive. The debate about the competing philosophical concepts is complex, much more complex than the original proponents of the older and more naive concept of brain death ever realized. They seemed satisfied to orient attention to brain function, failing to perceive that an irreversible coma and the death of the whole brain were not exactly the same. Moreover, they failed to perceive that neither of these might be exactly the same as the irreversible loss of experiential functions that the Harvard committee's chair indicated were crucial to being alive. Although we personally favor the more limited experiential concept, it is not clear that there exists a test or set of tests that can accurately identify those who are irreversibly unconscious and would meet the criteria for higher-brain death. However, if such tests were to be developed, we would support a law that recognizes the complexity of the debate and permits the patient or the patient's agent to choose among the plausible death concepts—a position we defend in chapter 7. Our objective in this discussion has been to push beyond the older, simpler whole-brain-oriented concept of death, which is now often used in the literature without careful definition, to achieve a more precise usage of terms. Whether humans die when they lose functions that have a primary locus in the whole brain, in a part of the brain, or in some other organs, it is a human who dies. The choice of the concept of death requires a more precise philosophical choice among these alternatives, and the use of criteria for death, in turn, depends upon these philosophical choices.

The Legal Status of Death

Because the literal whole-brain concept of death is coming under increasing criticism, it is important to understand that it remains the legal definition of death in most Western countries. Circulatory criteria for death pronouncement are incorporated into the model law in the United States, so physicians can continue to pronounce death based on loss of circulation. It remains unclear, however, whether loss of circulation is now merely an indirect measure of brain status or is itself intrinsically a sign of life. Moreover, the law states that the loss must be "irreversible," but we have seen that this term is itself ambiguous. Some insist that the loss be physiologically irreversible; but the common practice in routine death pronouncement based on circulatory criteria is that it merely be permanent. Death may be pronounced when no effort will be made to restart circulation, even though in some cases circulation surely could be resumed, at least temporarily, if resuscitative efforts were attempted.

In cases where circulation and other somatic functions are being maintained mechanically, defenders of neurological concepts of death would turn to more direct evidence of the irreversible loss of brain function. As a matter of common practice, the standard criteria for loss of all brain functions continue to be used, even though it is now increasingly clear that certain brain functions (neurohormonal and electrical) can remain when the standard criteria are met.

Unless we insist on revising the criteria for brain-based death pronouncement to measure whether these neurohormonal and electrical activities remain, we are de facto accepting neurological criteria for death that focus on less than literally all functions of the entire brain. This raises the question of the legal status of neurological concepts of death that deal with less than the whole brain—the brain stem and so-called higher-brain concepts.

No jurisdiction in the world has legalized death pronouncement if some brain functions remain. Therefore, higher-brain concepts may be important philosophically but have no legal status. It is striking that at least a large minority of people—philosophers, health professionals, and ordinary laypeople—seem to hold something like a higher-brain concept of death.[35]

Consider the study of Laura Siminoff and her colleagues published in 2004.[36] They asked citizens of Ohio to consider three well-described cases: a patient who met the criteria for death of the entire brain, a patient in an irreversible coma (who did not meet brain death criteria), and a patient in PVS. They then asked whether each should be classified as dead. Of the 1,351 who responded, 86 percent considered the first patient dead. (The remainder presumably held something like the circulatory or somatic concept of death.) However, 57 percent also considered the patient in a permanent coma to be dead—a position inconsistent with current law—and 34 percent considered the patient in PVS to be dead. Thus, in the Siminoff study, a large majority considered someone dead who had met the standard tests for losing all functions of the entire brain, but a majority also considered the comatose (but not brain-dead) patient dead, and a substantial minority considered even the PVS patient—one who was able to breathe on his or her own and went through sleep/wake cycles but was unconscious—to be dead.

Furthermore, we know that an increasing number of scholars and ordinary laypeople who would not classify any of these three patients to be dead would nevertheless endorse organ procurement from them in some cases, even though such procurement would end up killing them. That is the view of Miller and Truog.[37] It is also the view of a considerable number of respondents in the Siminoff study—67 percent of those who thought the patient meeting whole-brain death criteria was alive, 46 percent of those who thought the patient in a permanent coma was alive, and 34 percent of those who thought the patient in PVS was alive. Based on this study, a majority were willing to procure life-prolonging organs from all three of the patients, even though some who were willing to procure (431 of the total of 1,351) favored procuring believing the patient was dead; and others (305) favored procuring, even though they believed the patient was still alive.

The striking conclusion is that, at least for the citizens of Ohio in 2004, the majority were willing to procure organs from all three patients, even though only a minority would procure, believing the PVS patient was dead and that another minority would be willing to procure, believing the patient was alive, thus being willing to violate the dead donor rule. Thus only a minority believes the PVS patient is dead, and another minority is willing to procure while believing the patient is alive, even though combined they make up 55 percent of the respondents.

The confusing public policy problem is that there is no consensus on the definition of death. A large minority, perhaps even a slight majority, favors something like the higher-brain view; another large minority favors the current law, the whole-brain view and a smaller minority favors the traditional circulatory, or somatic, view. This seems to hold consistently over many years and among philosophers and theologians, health professionals, and ordinary citizens. The problem, then, is how can we develop a consistent public policy about what it means to be dead and when life-prolonging organs can be procured. This is the subject of the next chapter.

Notes

1. Halevy A, Brody B, "Brain death: Reconciling definitions, criteria, and tests," *Annals of Internal Medicine* 1993;119: 519–25. Shewmon also notes similar issues raised by Veatch RM, "The impending collapse of the whole-brain definition of death," *Hastings Center Report* 1993;23 (4): 18–24; Taylor RM, "Reexamining the definition and criteria of death," *Seminars in Neurology* 1991;28: 265–70; and Truog RD, "Is it time to abandon brain death?" *Hastings Center Report* 1997;27 (1): 29–37.

2. Halevy, Brody, "Brain death," 520–21.

3. Bernat JL, "A defense of the whole-brain concept of death," *Hastings Center Report* 1998;28 (2): 17. See also Bernat JL, "How much of the brain must die on brain death?" *Journal of Clinical Ethics* 1994;3 (1): 21–26.

4. See Pallis C, "ABC of brain stem death: Reappraising death," *British Medical Journal (Clinical Research Edition)* 1982;285 (6352):1409–12; and Pallis C, "ABC of brain stem death: From brain death to brain stem death," *British Medical Journal (Clinical Research Edition)* 1982;285 (6353):1487–90.

5. Henry Beecher, the committee's chairman, writing elsewhere: Beecher HK, "The new definition of death: Some opposing views," paper presented at Annual Meeting of American Association for the Advancement of Science, Symposium on the Meaning of Death, December 1970, 27–29.

6. Laureys S, Celesia GG, Cohadon F, et al., "European Task Force on Disorders of Consciousness: Unresponsive wakefulness syndrome—a new name for the vegetative state or apallic syndrome," *BMC Medicine* 2010;8: 68.

7. On personhood, see Lizza JP, *Persons, humanity, and the definition of death* (Baltimore: Johns Hopkins University Press, 2006); on the loss of personal identity, see Green MB, Wikler D, "Brain death and personal identity," *Philosophy and Public Affairs* 1980;9 (2): 105–33.

8. McMahan J, "The metaphysics of brain death," *Bioethics* 1995;9: 91–126.

9. Council on Ethical and Judicial Affairs of the American Medical Association, "The use of anencephalic neonates as organ donors," *JAMA* 1995;273: 1614–18.

10. Veatch RM, "The death of whole-brain death: The plague of the disaggregators, somaticists, and mentalists," *Journal of Medicine and Philosophy* 2005;30: 353–78.

11. James W, "The varieties of the religious experience, lecture III: The reality of the unseen," in *New age, new thought: William James and the varieties of religious experience*, ed. Miller LL (Denver: Brooks Divinity School; 1999), 51–54.

12. Rubin EB, Bernat JL, "Ethical aspects of disordered states of consciousness," *Neurological Clinics* 2011;29: 1055.

13. Laureys et al., "European Task Force."

14. Multi-Society Task Force on PVS, "Medical aspects of the persistent vegetative state," *New England Journal of Medicine* 1994;330: 1499–508.

15. Giacino JT, Ashwal S, Childs N, et al., "The minimally conscious state: Definition and diagnostic criteria," *Neurology* 2002;58: 349–53.

16. Teasdale G, Jennett B, "Assessment of coma and impaired consciousness," *Lancet* 1974;2: 81–84.

17. Seel RT, Sherer M, Wyte J, et al., "Assessment scales for disorders of consciousness: Evidence-based recommendations for clinical practice and research," *Archives of Physical Medicine and Rehabilitation* 2010;91: 1795–1813.

18. Owen AM, Schiff ND, Laureys S, "A new era of coma and consciousness science," *Progress in Brain Research, Volume 177*, ed. Laureys S, et al. (New York: Elsevier, 2009), chap. 28, 399–411.

19. Luaute J, Maucort-Boulch D, Tell L, et al., "Long-term outcomes of chronic minimally conscious and vegetative states," *Neurology* 2010;75: 246.

20. Giacino et al., "Minimally conscious state," 352.

21. Luaute et al., "Long-term outcomes," 250.

22. Ibid., 247.

23. Formisano R, D'Ippolito M, Risetti M, et al., "Vegetative state, minimally conscious state, akinetic mutism and Parkinsonism as a continuum of recovery from disorders of consciousness: An exploratory and preliminary study," *Functional Neurology* 2011;26 (1): 15–24.

24. Laureys C, Lemaire C, Maquet P, Phililips C, Franck G., "Cerebral metabolism during vegetative state and after recovery to consciousness," *Journal of Neurology, Neurosurgery and Psychiatry* 1999;67 (1): 121–22.

25. Fisher CE, Appelbaum PS, "Diagnosing consciousness: Neuroimaging law and the vegetative state," *Journal of Law, Medicine and Ethics* 2010;38 (2): 376.

26. Ibid., 376–77.

27. Owen et al., "New era," 408.

28. Owen AM, Coleman MR, Boly M, Davis MH, Laureys S, Pickard JD, "Detecting awareness in the vegetative state," *Science* 2006;313 (5792): 1402.

29. Ibid.

30. Monti MM, Vanhaudenhuyse A, Coleman MR, et al., "Willful modulation of brain activity in disorders of consciousness," *New England Journal of Medicine* 2010;362: 579–89.

31. Estraneo A. Moretta P, Loreto V, et al., "Late recovery after traumatic, anoxic or hemorrhagic long-lasting vegetative state," *Neurology* 2010;75: 246–52.

32. Hirschberg R, Giacino JT, "The vegetative and minimally conscious states: Diagnosis, prognosis and treatment," *Neurologic Clinics* 2011;29: 773–86.

33. Manraj KS, Heran NS, Shemie SD, "A review of ancillary tests in evaluating brain death," *Canadian Journal of Neurological Sciences* 2008;35: 409–19.

34. Wijdicks EF, "Pitfalls and slip-ups in brain death determination," *Neurological Research* 2013;35: 169–73.

35. On philosophers, see Haring B, *Medical ethics* (Notre Dame, IN: Fides, 1973), 131–36; Engelhardt HT, "Defining death: A philosophical problem for medicine and law," *American Review of Respiratory Disease* 1975;112: 587–90; Veatch RM, "The whole-brain-oriented concept of death: An outmoded philosophical formulation," *Journal of Thanatology* 1975;3: 13–30; Green, Wikler, "Brain death"; Gervais KG, *Redefining death* (New Haven, CT: Yale University Press, 1986); McMahan, "Metaphysics"; Veatch, "Impending collapse"; and Whetstine LM, "Bench-to-bedside review: When is dead really dead—on the legitimacy of using neurologic criteria to determine death," *Critical Care* 2007;11: 308, http://ccforum.com/content/11/2/208. On health professionals, see Cranford R, Smith D, "Consciousness: The most critical moral (constitutional) standard for human personhood," *American Journal of Law & Medicine* 1987;13 (2–3): 233–48; Bartlett ET, Youngner ST, "Human death and the destruction of the neocortex," in *Death: Beyond whole-brain criteria*, ed. Zaner RM (Dordrecht: Kluwer Academic Publishers, 1988), 199–215; and Machado C, "Is the concept of brain death secure?" in *Ethical dilemmas in neurology, volume 36*, ed. Zeman A, Emanuel LL (London: W. B. Saunders, 2000), 193–212.

36. Siminoff LA, Burant C, Youngner SJ, "Death and organ procurement: Public beliefs and attitudes," *Kennedy Institute of Ethics Journal* 2004;14 (3): 217–34.

37. Miller FG, Truog, RD, *Death, dying, and organ transplantation* (New York: Oxford University Press, 2012).

Chapter 7

The Conscience Clause

How Much Individual Choice Can Our Society Tolerate in Defining Death?

On the morning of March 1, 1994, a blue 1978 Chevrolet Impala pulled next to a van as it began to cross the Brooklyn Bridge. The van was carrying fifteen students from the Lubavitch Hasidic Jewish sect returning from a prayer vigil in Manhattan. As the car neared the van, a lone gunman fired at least five rounds of bullets from two separate semiautomatic weapons into the side of the van, while reportedly yelling, "Kill the Jews!" Four students were injured, two critically. One, fifteen-year-old Aaron Halberstam, was "declared brain dead, but he remained on life support."[1]

New York had, at the time, adopted a brain-oriented definition of death through judicial action and administrative regulation of the State Hospital and Planning Council and with the endorsement of the state health commissioner. It read, "Both the individual standard of heart and lung activity and the standard of total and irreversible cessation of brain function should be recognized as the legal definition of death in New York."[2] This would seem to imply that Halberstam was dead once the diagnosis of the death of his brain was confirmed. However, his parents, following Orthodox Jewish beliefs, insisted that the individual does not die when the brain dies. They would accept only a criterion based on respiratory function. The rabbis for the Halberstam family were reported to have said that Halberstam should be kept on support systems as long as his heart could beat on its own.[3] The physician, honoring the parents' wishes, refused to pronounce the death. Depending on the interpretation and individual hospital policy, this may have been legal. A sentence in the regulation requires each hospital to establish "a procedure for the reasonable accommodation of the individual's religious or moral objection to the determination as expressed by the individual, or by the next of kin or other person closest to the individual."[4]

One can hardly imagine what the result would have been if the family had placed their ventilator-dependent, brain-dead, but not-legally-pronounced-dead son in an ambulance and driven him through the Holland Tunnel to New Jersey. When they arrive in New Jersey, they are in a jurisdiction with an even more complex legal situation. New Jersey has a whole-brain-oriented criterion of death, but the law explicitly permits religious objectors to reject the use of that criterion in their own cases, thus making the patient alive until cardiac function ceases irreversibly.[5] If Halberstam had been known to hold such views, he would clearly be alive in New Jersey, assuming the law applies to minors. The law in New Jersey, however, does not explicitly permit family members to choose a circulatory or what, in chapter 5, we called a "somatic" criterion of death based on their own religious beliefs. Thus, unless his own views were known or the law were extended to permit surrogate decision making, he could not have been treated as alive.

The New York case is not the only one that has raised these complex issues surrounding religious and other dissent from the legal definition of death. In California and Florida two additional cases at about the same time pressed the issue. In California on March 27, 1994, two students whose parents live in Japan who had been shot in a senseless act of violence were declared "brain dead." According to the report, they were diagnosed as brain dead, were taken off respirators, and then were pronounced dead, even though the family was from a culture that still does not recognize brain criteria for death pronouncement.[6] They were not given any discretion to opt for a criterion of death that was preferred in their culture.

This account even suggests that the health personnel in California may have been confused. They diagnosed "brain death," which should have been enough to declare death without removing the respirators. Declaring them dead after the respirators were removed (presumably after the heart had stopped beating) implies that the ones pronouncing death did not, themselves, believe the death of the brain was the death of the individual. By contrast, we saw in the Jahi McMath case, described in chapter 5, that by 2013 a patient with confirmed irreversible loss of brain function was pronounced dead in spite of her mother's insistence that she should not be considered dead until her heart stopped. In this case, the death based on brain criteria was pronounced even though the ventilator continued to support heart function.

At about the same time as the 1990s cases, in Florida thirteen-year-old Teresa Hamilton, a severe diabetic who had been left in a coma, had been diagnosed as "brain-dead." Although Florida, like California, has a law stating that people with dead brains are dead people, the parents were insisting that she was still alive and were demanding that she be kept on what was called "life support."[7] Although the hospital was insisting that the patient was dead and its personnel wanted to stop ventilatory support on the body, they yielded to the family's wishes that her body be treated as if it were alive. Her parents pressed for a plan to send the girl home on the ventilator without pronouncing her dead. Here the family got its wishes, in spite of the Florida law.

The Present State of the Law

The New Jersey law and the New York regulation, until 1997, were unique in the world. In that year Japan adopted an even more complex law that permits brain criteria to be used to pronounce death, but only if the individual while alive has explicitly consented to both the brain-based death pronouncement and organ procurement and, then, only if the family also consents.[8] Although many countries have adopted a whole-brain-oriented definition of death, they have done so without any provision for individuals to conscientiously object for religious or other reasons.[9] Similarly, other than Japan, those countries still relying on the more traditional circulatory definition make no provision for their citizens who believe that death should be based on brain function loss. The New York regulation appears to introduce an accommodation based on family objections to a brain-oriented definition, but it actually leaves the details of the policy to individual hospitals. Because one of the requirements of each hospital's policy must be "a procedure for the reasonable accommodation of the individual's religious or moral objection to the determination as expressed by the individual, or by the next of kin or other person closest to the individual," if the hospital interpreted reasonable accommodation to include some level of individual physician discretion, a family could express dissent to one physician who is willing to accommodate, but if they happen to be dealing with another physician, that physician could refuse the request to refrain from pronouncing death.[10]

A recent report from Singapore indicated that twenty-two-year-old Swenson Tan was declared dead and his organs were procured three weeks after he lapsed into a coma following an accident in which the motorcycle on which he was riding was struck by a van. As his body was wheeled to the operating room to procure his organs, his parents and reportedly more than thirty friends and family rallied around him, protesting that they wanted him to be "kept alive."[11] Singapore's Human Organ Transplant Act allows routine organ procurement unless the individual had opted out while alive. No provision is made for next-of-kin objection.

The law in most American jurisdictions specifies that if the criteria for measuring the irreversible loss of all functions of the entire brain are met, "death shall be pronounced." In other jurisdictions, the law actually reads "death may be pronounced." This seems to imply that the physician could have the discretion much as in New York, except that the discretion is actually broader. The physician could refuse to pronounce based on his or her own personal values, economic considerations, or other factors, in addition to family wishes. Clearly, these laws seem defective if they give the physician the opportunity legally to choose whether to pronounce death based on the physician's values. The problem under consideration in this chapter is whether such discretion could be tolerated by the society if the dissent comes from the patient or the patient's next of kin.

The common wisdom has been that such discretion makes no sense. After all, being dead seems to be an objective matter to be determined by good science (or perhaps good metaphysics) rather than by individual conscientious choice. Concern is often expressed that such discretion not only makes no sense but would produce public chaos, leading to situations in which some patients are dead while medically identical patients are alive. Here, we make the case for the legitimacy of a conscientious objection to a uniform definition of death—conscientious objection that permits patients to choose while competent an alternative definition of death, provided that it is within reason and does not pose serious public health or other societal concerns. In cases where the patient has not spoken while competent (in cases of infants, children, and adults who simply have not expressed themselves), we argue that the next of kin should have this discretion within certain limits.

Concepts, Criteria, and the Role of Value Pluralism

Understanding our case for conscientious objection requires that we return to a critical point made in earlier chapters: the differences between matters of fact and matters of value in the definition-of-death debate. We argue that matters of value judgment should be open to some level of individual discretion.

The Early Fact/Value Distinction

As we have seen, early in the definition-of-death debate, commentators insisted that a basic distinction be made between two elements of the discussion. What at first appeared to be one question turned out to include at least two separate issues. First, there was a question that seemed primarily scientific: How can we measure that the brain has been irreversibly destroyed (that it has "died")? This seems like the kind of question that those skilled in neurology could answer. We have seen in chapter 4 that the neurological community, sometimes aided by others, has offered many sets of criteria, with associated tests and measures, for determining that the brain will never again be able to conduct any of its functions.[12] We have come to understand this as primarily a question for competent medical scientists.[13] (We say "primarily" because we have noted that choosing a set of criteria will involve some decisions that do not rest in science—e.g., decisions about how certain we want to be that brain function loss is irreversible.)

The second question is quite different in character. It asks whether we as a society or as individuals ought to treat an individual with a dead brain as a dead person. This question is clearly not something about which the neurological community can claim expertise. No amount of neurological study could possibly determine whether those with dead brains should be considered dead people. This is a religious, philosophical, ethical, or public policy question, not one for neurological science. When society determines that someone is dead, many social and behavioral changes occur. These are not neurological issues; they are social, normative issues about which all citizens may reasonably voice a position relying on their personal religious, philosophical, and ethical views of the world.

Democratic Pluralism and Value Variation

In a democratic, pluralistic culture, we have great insight into how to deal with religious, philosophical, and ethical controversies about which there are strongly held views and unresolvable controversy. At the level of morality, we agree to tolerate diverse opinions, and we even let a person act on those opinions, at least until their impact on the lives of others becomes intolerable. This is the position we take regarding religious dissent.

RELIGIOUS AND OTHER POSITIONS

To the extent that the disagreement is a religious or quasi-religious disagreement, toleration of pluralism seems the appropriate course. It permits people with differences to live together in harmony. And at least one major source of division over the definition of death is surely theological. The case with which this chapter opened appears not only to have been *caused* by Jewish/Muslim tensions; the moral disagreement about whether to declare Halberstam dead also has religious roots. Judaism has long been known to include persons who oppose brain criteria for death pronouncement. Not that all Jews oppose it. Rabbi Moses Tendler, a well-known moral commentator, has supported it.[14] But many Orthodox rabbinical scholars strongly oppose it, maintaining that where there is breath there is life.[15] Some Japanese, influenced by Buddhist and Shinto belief systems, see the presence of life in the whole body, not just in the brain.[16] Native Americans reportedly sometimes hold religious beliefs that oppose a brain-oriented definition of death.[17] Fundamentalist Christians, sometimes associated with the right-to-life movement, and some Catholics focusing on prolife issues, press for a consistent prolife position by opposing death pronouncement of brain-dead individuals.[18]

Conversely, mainstream Christians, both Protestant and Catholic, support a brain-oriented definition claiming that being prolife does not foreclose being clear on when life ends.[19] One Christian theological argument supporting brain-oriented definitions of death starts with the ancient Christian theological anthropology that sees the human as the integration of body and mind or spirit. When the two are irreversibly separated, then the human is gone. This view, as we have seen, places some Christian theologians in the higher-brain camp. In doing so, these theologians sometimes differentiate themselves from secular defenders of higher-brain concepts. The latter group, under the influence of Derek Parfit, stresses mentalist conceptions of the person that sometimes lead to support for a higher-brain conception that focuses exclusively on the irreversible loss of mental function without concern about the separation of mind from body.[20] By contrast, those working within Christian theology are more likely to insist on the importance of both mind and body.[21]

There are, of course, also some secular persons who support a circulatory, or somatic, definition of death. One, now dated, survey found that about a third continued to support such a definition.[22] The only plausible conclusion is that one's definition of death is heavily influenced by one's theological and metaphysical beliefs, along with one's theories of value. We have learned that in a pluralistic society, it is unrealistic to expect unanimity on such questions. Hence, a tolerance of pluralism may be the only way to resolve the public policy debate.

This conclusion seems even more inevitable when one realizes—as we have suggested—that there are not just two or three plausible definitions (whole-brain, circulatory, and higher-brain definitions); there are literally hundreds of possible variants. Some insist on irreversible loss of anatomical brain structure at the cellular level; others, only on irreversible loss of function. Some insist on the loss of cellular-level functions, whereas others insist only on irreversible loss of supercellular functions of integration of bodily function. Some might insist on the loss of all central nervous system functions, including spinal cord function (an early position of Henry Beecher, the chair of the Harvard Ad Hoc Committee), whereas others draw a line between spinal cord and brain. Among higher-brain defenders, there are countless variations on what counts as "higher": everything above the brain stem, the cerebrum, the cerebral cortex, the neocortex, the sensory cortex, and so on. Some, insisting on the loss of all brain functions, ignore electrical functions, limiting their attention to clinical functions.[23] Some are even willing to ignore functions of "nests of cells," claiming that they may be "insignificant."[24] When all the possible variants are combined, there will be a large number of positions; no group is likely to gain the support of more than a small minority of the population. The only way to have a single definition of death is for those with power to coerce others to use their preferred definition. If that single definition were the current "whole-brain" one, with a requirement that literally all functions of the brain must be gone before death is pronounced, the result could be disastrous. No one really believes that every last function of the entire brain must be irreversibly lost for a brain to be dead. That would include all electrical functions, all neurohumoral functions, and cellular functions. People's disagreement with this definition would lead to their deviating from it in practice, and this would lead to physician discretion in the absence of a workable official definition of death. Because clinicians would necessarily need to exercise discretion in deciding which functions are to be ignored, patients would be at the mercy of the discretion of the clinician who happens to be present when the question of pronouncing death arises. Even if we were willing to let some ride roughshod over others, it is very unlikely that any one position could gain majority support; in fact, it is unlikely that any single position could come close to a majority. There may be no alternative but to tolerate multiple views.

CONSTITUTIONAL ISSUES

Once the choice of a definition of death is cast in terms of theological or philosophical issues, the necessity of conscientious choice among the definitions seems more plausible. The constitutional issue of separation of church and state presses us in the direction of accepting definitions with religious groundings. Of course, the constitutional provision prohibiting the establishment of religion does not give absolute freedom of religious action. Many religious beliefs, if acted upon, could cause significant harm to others. The "harm to others" principle (or perhaps some more complex social ethical principle, e.g., the principle of justice) necessitates the state's right to limit action based on many belief systems. Snake-handling cults, religious groups that support extremes of corporal punishment for children, religious groups using hallucinogenic drugs, and sects that would practice human and animal sacrifice have all been constrained for the safety and welfare of others.

Nevertheless, the burden on the state to justify interference with religious practice is great. Defenders of the compulsory imposition of a single definition of death on a group of religious conscientious objectors to that definition would need to be supported by evidence of that group's causing significant social harm to other parties. We argue below that such harm cannot be demonstrated. Thus the New Jersey law authorizes religious objection to the state's default definition of death when there is a religious basis for objecting to the whole-brain definition. Orthodox rabbi Chaim Dovid Zwiebel casts his defense of a conscientious right of Jews to rely on a halachic concept of death (one resembling the circulatory, or somatic, definition) in terms of constitutional rights.[25] He appeals to notions of the free exercise of religion and the right of privacy or personal autonomy.

PROBLEMS LIMITING CONSCIENTIOUS OBJECTION TO RELIGIOUS OBJECTORS

A state that limits conscientious objection to religious objectors, as New Jersey has done, is likely to face potentially difficult constitutional challenges. New York's regulations, by contrast, carve out a requirement of reasonable accommodation on either religious or moral grounds. We learned from laws permitting religious conscientious objection to service in the military that restricting objection to certain types may be legally indefensible. During the Vietnam war era, some objectors had views that were clearly moral or philosophical, but they had a hard time demonstrating to others that they were religious. Especially if *religious* is defined as involving belief in a Supreme Being, many individuals whose objections seemed very similar to religious objections could not qualify. Even members of certain groups often classified as *religions* could not meet the test of belief in a Supreme Being; Buddhism, Confucianism, and Native American belief systems all look much like religions, but all fail the Supreme Being test. Gradually, the restriction of conscientious objection to religious objection was challenged and was found to be discriminatory. The concept of religious objection was gradually broadened to include many belief systems that may not, at first, appear to be overtly religious.

Some scholars who have studied the New Jersey criterion-of-death law (including some most closely involved with drafting this law) believe that its restriction of the beliefs supporting objection to the brain-oriented definition of death to those that were narrowly religious would be interpreted to also include more broadly moral objections. That, at least, is the opinion of Robert Olick, an attorney who served as the executive director of the commission that developed the New Jersey law.[26] The only reason that the New Jersey Commission on Legal and Ethical Problems in the Delivery of Health Care and the New Jersey legislature limited its provision to religious objection was political. Even during the debates before passage, some commentators were saying that objections that were not religious if religion is narrowly construed would be sustained in a legal challenge.

There are also enormous practical and moral problems with attempts to limit the New Jersey law to religion narrowly construed. At a practical level, enforcement officials would need to establish mechanisms for verifying whether an objection was truly religious. A nonpracticing Jew who had a nonreligious objection to a brain-oriented definition of death could cite his religious background, and it would be almost impossible for the state to establish whether his objection was religious. Religious objections have a clear basis for protection in the Constitution, whereas nonreligious objections, despite their logically and morally demanding the same accommodation, do not have the same level of explicit constitutional protection. Nevertheless, morally, the principle of equal respect would seem to require that if religious objections were permitted, then equally sincere and equally deeply held nonreligious philosophical objections would also be equally acceptable. If little is at stake in terms of public interest, little is lost by accepting both on equal terms.

Explicit Patient Choice, Substituted Judgment, and Best Interest

Assuming that the case is made that individuals should be able to exercise religiously or nonreligiously based conscientious choice of an alternative definition of death, should this discretion be extended to surrogate decision makers in the same manner as are terminal illness treatment refusal decisions? The New Jersey law does not explicitly permit parents or other family members to exercise choice on behalf of an incompetent patient. Conversely, the New York regulations do. They follow the pattern established for surrogate decision making in terminal illness. They permit choices "expressed by the individual, or by the next of kin or other person closest to the individual."[27] We see no reason to limit the choice to competent and formerly competent persons who have executed advance directives. Surrogates, including those legally designated by power of attorney and those with legal authority as next of kin, have decision-making authority for incompetent patients. We suggest a similar authority for deciding a definition of death. This would require substituted judgment based on what is believed to be the patient's beliefs when they are known and based on best interest judgments when they are not known. In either case an argument can be made that the surrogate should be given a reasonable range of discretion in determining what the patient would have wanted or what is in the patient's best interest.

Consider a formerly competent adult or adolescent who has never formally written a document choosing an alternative definition of death, but who has left an oral record or a lifestyle pattern that appears to the surrogate to favor an alternative definition of death, one differing from the statutory default definition. Halberstam was returning from an Orthodox Jewish prayer service when he was shot. Assuming he has not written an instruction stating a preference for a circulatory definition of death, should his parents (or other next of kin) be permitted formally to choose it for Halberstam (as, in fact, Halberstam's did, through the informal decisions in New York)? It appears that he had continued to live the religious life of his parents. There is no reason to doubt that he would choose as they did. Just as the next of kin can presently exercise substituted judgment in forgoing treatment decisions, his parents likewise should be permitted to choose on his behalf based on the values he is most likely to have held.

Some might claim that this subordinates the interests of the patient or society to the whim of the idiosyncratic beliefs of the next of kin. Below, we argue that there is little at stake for society. As for Halberstam's interests, as an unconscious individual he seems to have no explicit contemporaneous interest. If it can be said that he has any residual interests, it surely must be to have his prospective autonomy preserved. Insofar as his parents can deduce what he would have autonomously chosen if he had been able to exercise such judgment, surely they must be permitted, indeed required, to exercise that choice on his behalf.

But suppose we had no idea what Halberstam's wishes were about which definition of death should be used in his case. Or suppose he suffered his injury when he was one year old rather than fifteen or twenty-one. Clearly, in this case respecting autonomy is out of the question. The only moral alternative is to use what is considered the best concept of death. But should it be the concept of death considered best by society—perhaps some version of a whole-brain-oriented death, assuming that is the law of the state—or should it be the concept considered best by his next of kin? In the context of forgoing treatment decisions, discretion is now given to the next of kin, under the doctrine of what can be called *limited familial autonomy*.[28] Just as the individual has an autonomy-based right to choose a definition of death (or a treatment plan), so likewise families are given a range of discretion in deciding what is best for their wards. They select the schooling and religious education that so dramatically shape the system of values and beliefs of the child. They are expected to socialize the child into some value system. In a liberal pluralistic society, we do not insist that familial surrogates choose the best possible value system for their wards; we expect them to exercise discretion, drawing on their own beliefs and values. As long as the ward's interests are not jeopardized too substantially and the interests of the society are not threatened, parents and other familial surrogates should not only be permitted but should actually be expected to make a choice of a definition of death for their wards.

Limits on the Range of Discretion

Clearly, this does not mean that individuals should be able to choose literally any definition of death they please. Someone who has lost all circulatory and brain functions irreversibly, someone whose body can no longer retain cellular integrity, cannot be considered alive, no matter how strongly the individual prefers such a view. There would be serious public health concerns. Likewise, if circulatory functions and brain functions remain so that the individual is conscious, it seems clear that the individual cannot be classified as dead, no matter how strongly the individual holds such a view. (It is an open question whether such an individual should be allowed to choose to forgo life support—or even, if capable, to commit suicide—but no reasonable person would favor a public policy of permitting such a person to be labeled "dead.")

The plausible range of reasonable views includes the three major positions covered in the three previous chapters: the whole-brain, circulatory or somatic, and higher-brain views. We have suggested that the two brain-oriented views both include a substantial minority of the population, at least in Western cultures, but that a persistent minority continues to hold to the circulatory or somatic view. As we have noted, each of these includes many variants, which means that no one position commands anything like a majority of the population.

Whole-Brain versus Somatic Conceptions of Death

The New Jersey law gives the narrowest of options: between the default whole-brain-oriented definition and the single alternative of a somatic or circulatory definition. That would be a clearly acceptable choice, assuming that there are no significant societal or third-party consequences. The New Jersey plan would seem to offer a minimal range of choice.

The New York regulations are somewhat more open. They require "a procedure for the reasonable accommodation of the individual's religious or moral" views. However, all that is permitted is objection to a determination of death based on the state's preferred definition, that is, the whole-brain view. The clear implication is that the traditional somatic definition is the alternative—that is, the religiously based position of Orthodox Jews, who were the focus of the New York policy discussion. This raises the question of whether conscientious choice can be expanded to include the group of higher-brain concepts of death.

Including Higher-Brain Concepts of Death

We have suggested that more and more people are adopting the position that it is no longer plausible to hold to a literal whole-brain definition of death, in which every last function of the entire brain must be dead before death can be pronounced.[29] A case can be made that some versions of higher-brain formulations of a definition should be among the choices permitted. Under such an arrangement, a whole-brain definition might be viewed as the centrist view that would serve as the default definition, permitting those with more conservative views to opt for circulatory or somatic definitions and those with more liberal views to opt for certain higher-brain formulations. Of course, this would permit people with brain-stem function, including spontaneous respiration, to be treated as dead. Organs could be procured that otherwise would not be available (assuming the dead donor rule is retained), bodies could be used for research (assuming proper consent has been obtained), and life insurance would pay off.

If higher-brain definitions were among the plausible range of choices and surrogates were permitted to make the choice when there is no clear evidence of the patient's own preference, some might be concerned that this would give surrogates the authority to have their wards treated as dead while some brain and circulatory functions still remain. They see this as posing risks for unacceptable choices, for ending a lingering state of disability, for example. Assuming that the only cases that could be classified as dead by surrogates would be those who have lost all capacity for consciousness—that is, those who have lost all higher-brain functions—the risks to the individual classified as deceased would be minimal. We must keep in mind that surrogates are already presumed to have the authority to terminate all life support for these people. Often, this would mean that they would soon be dead by the most traditional definitions of death. This would occur within minutes, in many cases. The effect on inheritance and insurance would be trivial if they were simply called dead before stopping medical support rather than stopping before pronouncing death. Even for those vegetative or comatose patients who had sufficient lower-brain function to breathe on their own, a suspension of all medical treatment would lead to death fairly soon. Adding a higher-brain option to the range of discretion would have only a minimal effect on practical matters and would be a sign that we can show the same respect for the religious and philosophical convictions of those favoring the higher-brain position as we do now in New Jersey and New York for the holders of the circulatory position. If there are actually scores of potential definitions of death within the range from higher-brain to somatic positions, then only a relatively small minority is likely to be in agreement with the default position, whatever it may be. The wise thing to do seems to be to pick some intermediary position and then to permit people to deviate both to somewhat more liberal and somewhat more conservative positions. The choices would probably need to be limited to this range. Both public health and moral problems become severe if the scope of choice is expanded much further.

The Problem of Order: Objections to a Conscience Clause

All of this, of course, depends on the, as-yet-undefended, claim that there are no significant societal or third-party harms from permitting conscientious objection to a default definition within the range specified. The President's Commission for the Study of Ethical Problems in Medicine and Biomedical and Behavioral Research prepared an important report in 1981 reviewing the definition-of-death debate.[30] In this report the commission examined the circulatory, whole-brain, and higher-brain options. In spite of the fact that the commission's two philosophical consultants on the issue endorsed versions of a higher-brain formulation, the whole commission endorsed the whole-brain position. It gave serious consideration to the higher-brain position before rejecting it for a number of reasons, most of which can be summarized under the heading of the problems that would be created for social order.

Death as a Biological Fact

One preliminary objection that was not dwelt on by the President's Commission for the Study of Ethical Problems, but that arises in many discussions of the issue, is the claim that death is not a matter of religious or philosophical or policy choice but rather a matter of biological fact.[31] It is now generally recognized that the choice of a concept of death (as opposed to a formulation of criteria and tests) is really normative or ontological.[32] We are debating as a matter of social policy when we ought to treat someone as dead. No amount of biological research can answer this question at the conceptual level. Of course, many people could still hold that although the definition of death is a normative or ontological question, there is still only one single correct formulation. This seems to be a very plausible position, but we are not discussing the issue of whether there can only be one true definition of death; we are discussing whether society can function for public policy purposes while tolerating differences in beliefs about what the true definition is. Tolerating a Jew's or Native American's belief in a definition that is perceived by the rest of society as wrong is no different from having a society tolerate more than one belief about whether abortion or forgoing life support in the living is morally wrong. We are asking whether society can treat people as dead based on their own beliefs, rather than whether people are really dead, that is, really conform to some metaphysically correct conception of what it means to be dead, in such circumstances. It is possible to hold that there is one and only one metaphysically correct concept of death, but that, out of respect for minority views, society can treat some people who conform to this meaning of death as if they were alive.

The Possibility of Policy Chaos

One of the consistent themes in the criticism of higher-brain definitions, especially with the conscience clause, is that its adoption would lead to policy chaos. Presumably, critics have in mind the stress of health professionals, insurers, family members, and public policy processes, such as succession of the presidency. But a very similar substituted-judgment and best interest discretion is already granted surrogates regarding decisions to forgo life support on still-living patients. One would think that the potential for abuse and for chaos would be much greater in granting surrogate discretion to decide when to forgo life support. It remains to be seen what chaos would be created from conscientious objection to a default definition of death. If each of the envisioned policy problems can be addressed successfully, then we are left with a religious/philosophical/policy choice for which we should be tolerant of variation if possible and no good social reasons to reject individual discretion. Some of the rebuttal against the charge of policy chaos has already been suggested.

Potential Problems with a Conscience Clause That Includes Higher-Brain Formulations

We need to examine the purported problems that would be created by adopting a conscience clause, especially one that included a higher-brain option. We need to consider problems with the stoppage of treatment, potential abuse of the terminally ill, problems with health and life insurance, the impact on inheritance, spousal issues, the impact on organ transplants, succession to the presidency, and the effect on the presidency.

Problems with Stoppage of Treatment

One concern is that life-sustaining medical treatment would be stopped on different people with medically identical conditions at different times if conscientious choice among definitions of death is permitted. This assumes, however, that decisions to stop treatment are always linked to pronouncement of death. We now know that normally it is appropriate to consider suspension of treatments in a manner that is decoupled from the question of whether the patient is dead.[33] A large percentage of in-hospital deaths now occur as a result of a decision to stop treatment and let the patient die. Presumably any valid surrogate who was contemplating opting for a higher-brain definition of death would, if told that this option were not available, immediately contemplate choosing to forgo treatment and letting the patient die. In either case the patient would be dead within a short period of time.

The decoupling of the decision to forgo treatment from that of the pronouncement of death has led some to further decouple what we have called death behaviors, leaving agreed-upon points for various behaviors such as initiating grief, procuring organs, and terminating insurance coverage.[34] We should consider such decoupling as it was proposed in the 1970s. There are two reasons to reject it.

First, even if we further decouple death behaviors, different people with different cultural beliefs and values will still consider different times appropriate for each of the behaviors. Some will consider widowhood to begin with the loss of higher-brain function, but others only with the death of the whole brain or the cessation of circulatory and respiratory function. We would still need a conscience clause, but now we would need one for the societally defined point for each of the various death behaviors.

Second, even though some death behaviors surely may plausibly be decoupled from the declaration of death (e.g., deciding to forgo treatment), we should not underestimate the importance of having something resembling a moment of death. Socially and psychologically, we need a moment, no matter how arbitrary, when loved ones can experience a symbolic transition point, at least for a large cluster of these death behaviors. Relatives cannot send flowers one at a time as each moment arrives during a drawn-out process of death involving many different death-related behaviors. Kass won the 1970 argument about whether death was a process or an event. Although dying might be a process, death is not. There must be one defining moment of transition to which at least many of the death-related behaviors may attach.

Abuse of the Terminally Ill

For the same reasons, the risk of abuse of the terminally ill should not be a problem. There could be more concern about a family member dependent on the terminally ill person's pension opting for a somatic definition of death in order to continue receiving a pension or Social Security. Alternatively, one could be concerned that a surrogate would opt for a higher-brain definition in order to reduce hospital expenditures. These, however, seem remote possibilities.

There is also the risk of families (as surrogates) opting for a somatic definition of death when their loved ones have been declared whole-brain dead if the families know that opting for somatic death is possible. They might possibly even lie about the decedent's own wishes. In the emotional intensity of the moment, their denial that the person is dead (with denial as a normal initial psychological response to grief, strengthened by being able to see the body breathing, etc.) may lead them to demand a somatic definition not because either the decedent or even they themselves (if they were to think coolly and rationally about it) actually believe in such a definition, but as a way of (1) practically, keeping their loved one ''alive,'' and/or (2) psychologically insulating themselves from the reality of the death that has already occurred.

These abuses are all possible, but the same risks currently exist when family members or other surrogates make decisions to forgo life support. Families presently could avoid forgoing life support to continue receiving a pension or select forgoing it in order to avoid costs. They could avoid forgoing it because of their psychological need to keep their loved one alive. Falsifying the patient's wishes would be a violation of respect, but keeping a patient alive for psychological reasons already happens from time to time. Professional caregivers have means of confronting these issues and usually can bring about a satisfactory resolution. Moreover, there is no record attempting to manipulate whether a patient is classified as living having occurred in New Jersey, where the option of a somatic definition is available. If the problem did arise, the procedures currently available for review of suspected patient abuse would be available so that the surrogates could be removed from their role just as they would be now if a surrogate refused life support in a situation where the motive appeared to be the financial gain of the surrogate.

The recent case of Jahi McMath makes clear that, even if the law requires a single, brain-based definition of death, a determined family can insist that the support of bodily functions continue. If Jahi's mother had been able to insist that she was legally alive, the outcome would have been little different.

Health Insurance

There exists a potential impact on health insurance if someone chooses a definition of death that would have the effect of making someone live longer—if, for instance, a somatic definition were chosen. (If some version of a higher-brain definition were chosen, the effect would more likely be a savings in health insurance.) There is good reason to believe that the effect on health insurance would be minimal. A relatively small number of people would actively make a protreatment choice based on their preference for a somatic definition or any alternative that would require longer treatment. The small costs would probably be justified in the name of preserving respect for individual freedom on religious or philosophical matters. If the problem became significant, a health insurance policy could address the problem. Any health insurance policy must have some limits on coverage. Cosmetic surgery is usually not covered; and there are often limits on the number of days of inpatient care for psychiatric services. Many marginal procedures, including longer days of stay in the hospital, are rejected. If an insurer were worried about unfair impact on the subscriber pool if its funds were used to provide care for patients without brain function who had selected a somatic definition of death, they could simply exclude coverage for care for living patients with dead brains or offer such coverage as an additional option at an increased premium. The patient and caregivers would be left in the position in which they presently find themselves when they want a treatment not funded by insurance coverage. They could self-pay, buy supplemental insurance, rely on charity, or accept the reality that not all desired medical interventions are available to all people.

Life Insurance

The concern by life insurance companies is exactly the opposite. Insisting on a somatic definition would simply delay payment, which would be in the insurer's interest; however, selecting a higher-brain definition would make the individual dead sooner, potentially quite a bit sooner. However, most living persons with dead brains die fairly soon, either because such patients are hard to maintain or because an advance directive or surrogate opts for termination of treatment. In the case of patients who prefer a higher-brain definition of death, if they are not permitted to choose it, in all likelihood they will have advance directives forgoing life support or family surrogates will refuse that support, so these patients will die at more or less the same time that they would have if they had been permitted to choose a higher-brain definition.

Inheritance

As in the case of pensions and life insurance, some surrogate might be inclined to manipulate the timing of death to gain an inheritance more quickly. This could lead to choosing a higher-brain definition. However, as we have seen, the same surrogate already has the power to decline medical treatment, which would theoretically expose the patient to similar risks, and such cases are exceedingly rare. If a surrogate is suspected of abusing a patient by choosing an inappropriate concept of death, such a surrogate can always be challenged and removed. If one compares the risk of abuse from surrogate discretion in deciding to forgo treatment with that from deciding on a variant definition of death, surely the discretion in forgoing treatment is more controversial and more subject to abuse. Yet this has not proved to be a significant problem.

Spousal/Marital Status

Another social practice that can be affected directly by the timing of a death is the marital status of the spouse. Spouses may want to retain their status as spouses rather than become widows/widowers for various psychological and financial reasons. Or they may want to become widows/widowers so that they can get on with their lives. Conceivably, some may be ready to remarry. For example, a spouse who had been caring for a patient who was in a *permanent vegetative state* for years may have already separated psychologically from their mate even though he or she was not actually dead. This person could be ready to remarry, which could be done legally once the spouse was deceased. This problem seems quite farfetched, but it could happen. Such spouses would probably already have contemplated refusing life support and could be removed as inappropriate surrogates if it is clear that they are motivated for non-patient-centered reasons that lead to inappropriate decisions.

Organ Transplants

One significant impact of the definition of death is the availability of organs for transplant. If someone insists on a somatic or circulatory definition of death, that person would not be able to donate organs when heart function remains, even though brain function has ceased. However, anyone who selected a somatic definition of death would be unlikely to be a donor of organs if he or she were forced to be pronounced dead based on brain criteria in any case. Conversely, a person who chose to be considered dead even though lower brain function remains would be a potential organ source. Someone who wanted to have organs procured when his or her higher brain functions were irreversibly lost potentially could have his or her organs procured earlier by selecting a higher brain definition. As long as this were limited to cases where an active choice was made in favor of the higher-brain formulation, it is hard to see why there would be strong objections. With the evolution of the donation after circulatory death protocols (which we discussed in chapter 5), such persons could accomplish something similar by refusing life support to the point of death, followed by organ procurement. The outcome would be similar, except that the donor would be forced to participate in the use of a concept of death that he or she rejected and the quality of the organs might be jeopardized. As long as the cases are limited to those in which there was a valid choice for a higher-brain definition, moral or societal concern should not be raised.

Many people have pressed for a law authorizing organ procurement from living anencephalic infants.[35] The Council on Ethical and Judicial Affairs of the American Medical Associaton (AMA) temporarily endorsed such a view in 1995.[36] But it seems that the AMA council must have been muddled. If we mean by *death* nothing more than being in a condition when it is appropriate for others to engage in death-associated behaviors and we include procuring organs in the list of such behaviors, then anyone who is an appropriate candidate for procuring so-called life-prolonging organs is dead.[37] By this logic, if the AMA council really believed it was acceptable to procure organs from an anencephalic infant with remaining brain stem function, then, to be consistent, it should have claimed that such anencephalic infants are already dead (or, more accurately, have never been alive). In effect, it adopted a version of a higher-brain-oriented definition of death and, if it wanted to be consistent, it should really have claimed that it is acceptable to procure organs from anencephalic infants because they are dead (or have never been living, in the social policy sense of the term). In fact, the AMA council reversed its endorsement of anencephalic organ procurement, making its position once again consistent with a whole-brain view of the definition of death.

Succession to the Presidency

Another potential implication of choosing an alternative definition of death is that succession to the presidency or to other roles could be affected. In the United States the vice president is automatically elevated to the presidency upon the death of the president. Similar policies affect monarchies, where the successor is automatically made king. A president who chose a circulatory definition of death could thereby end his or her term of office at a different time than one who chose a whole-brain or higher-brain definition. Because, in certain circumstances, one can retain cardiac function for years, the succession of the vice president could be delayed for a long time.

Obviously, this reflects a flaw in the succession law. Under present law a permanently vegetative president is not dead and there would be no automatic succession. But as soon as the permanent vegetative state is diagnosed, there should be immediate succession regardless of whether the president is dead. One could imagine a person who is next of kin being pressured to choose a definition with an eye toward timing the succession. That could happen now in an effort to delay the succession of the governorship in New Jersey. It could happen elsewhere if discretion were permitted. But the possibility of this happening seems extremely remote. The Twenty-Fifth Amendment to the Constitution provides a mechanism for the temporary assumption of the presidency, but once a president is known to be permanently incapacitated, he or she clearly should be replaced.

The Effect on Health Professionals

A final potential problem with authorizing conscientious choice is the possible effect on the health professionals who are providing care for the patient. Nurses will be required to suffer potential emotional stress at having to continue care or cease care at a time they believe inappropriate. Physicians will face similar problems. But this is hardly a problem unique to a choice of a definition of death. Some living patients or their surrogates refuse life-supporting therapy before the nurse or physician believes it is appropriate. Yet these health professionals are simply obliged to stop according to the laws of informed consent and the right to refuse treatment. More recently, professionals have been disturbed about requests for care that the clinicians deem "futile." Patients who insisted on not being pronounced dead until their heart stopped could conceivably insist on hospital-based treatment even though their brains were dead. That is potentially the situation in New Jersey now and was temporarily the situation in California during the McMath case. But the responsibility of the health professional to deliver care deemed futile against his or her will is already a matter of considerable controversy. It will need to be resolved whether or not other states adopt the New Jersey conscience clause. The State of Texas has adopted a law permitting physicians to unilaterally stop life support on still-living terminally ill patients when certain conditions are met.[38] Most patients demanding such care are clearly not dead by any definition. The resolution could be the same for patients with dead brains as it is for terminally ill or vegetative patients, or it could be different. The law could determine, for instance, that conscious patients would have a right of access to normatively futile care (perhaps with the proviso that they have independent funding) but that permanently unconscious patients or those with dead brains would have no right of access. In any case, the impact on caregivers is not a problem unique to patients who might exercise an option for an alternative definition of death. If the concern is about the cost of additional treatment rather than the psychological effects of having to care for the patient, this is more of an insurance issue. As we have argued above, the additional cost is likely to be a minor burden on the health care system and, if it turned out to be a problem, laws could be passed requiring those who choose a somatic definition to buy supplemental insurance or a policy could be developed that makes clear that living patients with dead brains are not entitled to long-term ventilator support or other intensive care unit therapies at public expense.

Implementation of a Conscience Clause

The procedural implementation of a conscience clause would require some additional planning, but the problems would not be novel. Most are addressed in the existing Patient Self-Determination Act and required request laws (see chapter 9). The former requires the hospital staff to inquire about the existence of an advance directive upon admission to a hospital and provide assistance in executing an advance directive if the patient desires. The latter requires that the next of kin be notified of the opportunity to donate organs in suitable cases. The most plausible way to record a choice of something other than a default concept of death would be in one's advance directive. That is the kind of document that ought to be on the minds of those caring for a patient who is near death. An addition specifying a choice of an alternative concept of death would be easy; it would be crucial in the case of those who are writing an advance directive demanding that life support continue even though the brain is dead. It would be a simple clarification in the case of one asking that support be forgone when the patient is permanently unconscious. A sentence choosing a higher-brain concept of death (and perhaps donating organs at that point) would be a modest addition.

Whether the new definition-of-death laws authorizing a conscience clause should also impose a duty on health professionals to notify patients or their surrogates of alternative concepts of death is a pragmatic question that would need to be addressed. Just as Orthodox Jews presently carry the burden of notifying others of their requirements for a kosher diet and Jehovah's Witnesses carry the burden of notifying about refusal of blood transfusions, so those with alternative concepts of death would plausibly carry that burden. Something akin to the subjective standard for informed consent would apply. According to this standard, health professionals, when they negotiate a consent, are required to inform the patient of what the patient would reasonably want to know, but they are not expected to surmise all the patient's unusual views and interests. According to this approach, they would be expected to initiate discussions on alternative definitions of death only when they knew or had reason to know that the patient plausibly would have an interest in such a discussion. A clinician who knew that his or her patient was an Orthodox Jew and knew that many Orthodox Jews prefer a more traditional concept of death would have such an obligation, but would not if he or she had no reason to believe that the patient might be inclined toward an alternative concept.

Some might claim that adding a conscience clause is unnecessary because only a small group of people would favor an alternative. In fact, a not insignificant number seem to prefer a more traditional circulatory or respiratory concept of death (Jews, Native Americans, Japanese, and others who are still committed to the importance of the heart or lungs). If a higher-brain-oriented concept of death were among the options, a much larger minority would have an interest in exercising the conscience clause. In fact, there have been a number of court cases and anecdotal reports of families objecting to the use of whole-brain-based concepts. It seems reasonable to assume that these represent only a fraction of the total number of cases where patients or families would prefer either a more traditional or a more innovative concept of death.

Even if it could be shown that few people would care enough about the concept and criteria of death used to pronounce them or their loved ones dead, this is still an important issue to clarify. It is important if only the rights of a small minority are violated. It is also important as a matter of conceptual clarity and of principle. The knee-jerk revulsion with a conscience clause for alternative concepts of death probably reflects a lingering belief that deciding when someone is dead is a matter of biological fact (for which individual conscience seems irrelevant). But insisting that the choice of a concept of death be treated as a matter of philosophical and theological dispute seems to follow naturally once one realizes the true nature of the issues involved. Getting people to think why a conscience clause is appropriate for this issue has an important teaching function, as well as serving to respect the rights of minorities on deeply held religious and philosophical convictions.

Conclusion

Once one grasps that the choice of a definition of death at the conceptual level is a religious/philosophical/policy choice rather than a question of medical science, the case for granting discretion within limits in a liberal pluralistic society is a very powerful one. There seems to be no basis for imposing a unilateral normative judgment on the entire population when the members of the society are clearly divided. When one realizes that there are many variants and that no definition is likely to receive the support of a majority, pluralism appears the only answer. Having a state choose a default definition and then granting individuals a limited range of discretion within the limits of reason seems to be the only defensible option. There is no reason to limit this discretion to religiously based reasons and no reason why familial surrogates should not be empowered to use substituted judgment or best interest standards for making such choices, just as they presently do for forgoing treatment decisions that determine even more dramatically the timing of death. A default with an authorization for conscientious objection seems the humane, respectful, fair, and pragmatic solution.

Notes

1. "Man charged in shooting of Jewish students," *New York Times*, March 3, 1994.
2. "Failure of brain is legal 'death,' New York says," *New York Times*, June 19, 1987.
3. "In hospital hallways, family and friends pray for victims," *New York Times*, March 3, 1994.
4. New York Codes, Rules and Regulations, "Determination of death," title 10, section 400.16, http://w3.health.state.ny.us/dbspace/NYCRR10.nsf/56cf2e25d626f9f785256538006c3ed7/8525652c00680c3e8525652c00634c24?OpenDocument&Highlight=0,400.16.

5. New Jersey Declaration of Death Act, signed April 8, 1991; it reads, in part: "The death of an individual shall not be declared upon the basis of neurological criteria . . . of this act when the licensed physician authorized to declare death, has reason to believe, on the basis of information in the individual's available medical records, or information provided by a member of the individual's family or any other person knowledgeable about the individual's personal religious beliefs that such a declaration would violate the personal religious beliefs of the individual. In these cases death shall be declared, and the time of death fixed, solely upon the basis of cardio-respiratory criteria."

6. "Slaying suspects share a past marred by crime," *New York Times*, Apr. 1, 1994.

7. "Florida hospital seeks to end life support of comatose girl," *New York Times*, Feb. 13, 1994; "Brain-dead Florida girl will be sent home on life support," *New York Times*, Feb. 19, 1994.

8. Law Concerning Human Organ Transplants (Law No. 104 in 1997).

9. As of a decade ago, the most recent time that an international survey was conducted, Wijdicks found legal standards for organ transplantation in fifty-five of eighty countries for which he located information. To make matters more complicated, in some countries for which there was no legal standard, there existed nevertheless practice guidelines for determining brain death (implying that they may be used without further legal authorization). A total of seventy of eighty countries have such guidelines. Thus, a number of countries for which information was available (e.g., Barbados, Ecuador, Guatemala, Honduras, Egypt, Ghana, Syria, Armenia, China, Pakistan, and Vietnam) had neither law nor guidelines. In at least some of these countries, reports exist of death pronouncement based on brain criteria in spite of the absence of law or practice guidelines. See Sui WG, Yan Q, Xie SP, et al., "Successful organ donation from brain-dead donors in a Chinese organ transplantation center," *American Journal of Transplantation* 2011;11: 2247–49. Because Wijdicks was able to find no information one way or the other for more than 100 countries, it is clear that the international situation regarding brain death is quite complex and confusing. See Wijdicks EFM, "Brain death worldwide: Accepted fact but no global consensus on diagnostic criteria," *Neurology* 2002;58: 20–25.

10. New York Codes, Rules and Regulations, "Determination."

11. "Man declared brain dead after being hit by van at Hougang," SPH (Singapore Press Holdings), March 11, 2013, http://singaporeseen.stomp.com.sg/singaporeseen/this-urban-jungle/man-declared -brain-dead-after-being-hit-by-van-at-hougang.

12. Harvard Medical School, "A definition of irreversible coma: Report of the Ad Hoc Committee of the Harvard Medical School to Examine the Definition of Brain Death," *JAMA* 1968;205: 337–40; Task Force on Death and Dying, Institute of Society, Ethics, and the Life Sciences, "Refinements in criteria for the determination of death: An appraisal," *JAMA* 1972;221: 48–53; "Report of the Medical Consultants on the Diagnosis of Death to the President's Commission for the Study of Ethical Problems in Medicine and Biomedical and Behavioral Research," in *Defining death: Medical, legal and ethical issues in the definition of death*, ed. President's Commission for the Study of Ethical Problems in Medicine and Biomedical and Behavioral Research (Washington, DC: US Government Printing Office, 1981), 159–66; Cranford RE, Minnesota Medical Association criteria: Brain death—concept and criteria, part I," *Minnesota Medicine* 1978;61: 561–63; Law Reform Commission of Canada, *Criteria for the determination of death* (Ottawa: Ministry of Supply and Services, 1981); Walker, AE, et al., "An appraisal of the criteria of cerebral death: A summary statement," *JAMA* 1977;237: 982–86.

13. More recent analysis has challenged the blatant fact/value dichotomy implied in this separation of the criteria question as one for medical science and the concept question as one of religious, philo-sophical, or public policy. See Veatch RM, *Death, dying, and the biological revolution*, rev. ed. (New Haven, CT: Yale University Press, 1989), 43–44.

14. Tendler MD, "Cessation of brain function: Ethical implications in terminal care and organ transplant," in *Brain death: Interrelated medical and social issues*, ed. Korein J (New York: New York Academy of Sciences, 1978), 394–97; Veith FJ, Fein JM, Tendler MS, Veatch RM, Kleiman MA, Kalkinis G, "Brain death, I: A status report of medical and ethical considerations," *JAMA* 1977;238: 1651–55.

15. Bleich JD, "Establishing criteria of death," *Tradition* 1972;13: 90–113; Bleich JD, "Neurological criteria of death and time of death statutes," in *Jewish bioethics* (New York: Sanhedrin Press, 1979), 303–16; Rosner F, "The definition of death in Jewish law," *Tradition* 1969;10 (4): 33–39.

16. Kimura R, "Japan's dilemma with the definition of death," *Kennedy Institute of Ethics Journal* 1991;1: 123–31.

17. President's Commission for the Study of Ethical Problems in Medicine and Biomedical and Behavioral Research, *Defining death*, 41.

18. Byrne PA, O'Reilly S, Quay, PM, "Brain death: An opposing viewpoint," *JAMA* 1979;242: 1985–90.

19. For Protestants, see Hauerwas S, "Religious concepts of brain death and associated problems," in *Brain death*, ed. Korein, 329–38; Potter RB, "The paradoxical preservation of a principle," *Villanova Law Review* 1968;13: 784–92; Ramsey P, "On updating death," in *Updating life and death*, ed. Cutler DR (Boston: Beacon Press, 1969), 31–53. For Catholics, see Haring B, *Medical ethics* (Notre Dame, IN: Fides, 1973), 131–36.

20. Parfit D, *Reasons and persons* (Oxford: Clarendon Press, 1984); Green MB, Wikler, D, "Brain death and personal identity," *Phlosophy and Public Affairs* 1980;9 (2): 105–33.

21. Ramsey P, *The patient as person* (New Haven, CT: Yale University Press, 1970), xiii; Veatch, *Death*, 42.

22. Charron WC, "Death: A philosophical perspective on the legal definitions," *Washington University Law Quarterly* 1975;4: 979–1008.

23. Ashwal S, Schneider S, "Failure of electroencephalography to diagnose brain death in comatose patients," *Annals of Neurology* 1979;6: 512–17.

24. Bernat JL, "How much of the brain must die on brain death?" *Journal of Clinical Ethics* 1992;3 (1): 21–26.

25. Zwiebel CD, "Accommodating religious objections to brain death: Legal considerations," *Journal of Halacha and Contemporary Society* 17 (Spring 1989): 59ff.

26. Robert Olick, personal communication, Oct. 23, 1996; Olick RS, "Brain death, religious freedom and public policy," *Kennedy Institute of Ethics Journal* 1991;1: 275–88. Also see Goldberg CK, "Choosing life after death: Respecting religious beliefs and moral convictions in near death decisions," *Syracuse Law Review* 1984;39 (4): 427–68.

27. New York Codes, Rules and Regulations, "Determination."

28. Veatch RM, "Limits of guardian treatment refusal: A reasonableness standard," *American Journal of Law and Medicine* 1984;9 (4); 427–68.

29. Veatch RM, "The whole-brain-oriented concept of death: An outmoded philosophical formulation," *Journal of Thanatology* 1975;3: 13–30; Engelhardt HT, "Defining death: A philosophical problem for medicine and law," *American Review of Respiratory Disease* 1975;112: 587–90; Bernat, "How much of the brain must die"; Haring, *Medical ethics*, 131–36.

30. President's Commission for the Study of Ethical Problems in Medicine and Biomedical and Behavioral Research, *Defining death*.

31. For a discussion, see Gervais KG, *Redefining death* (New Haven CT: Yale University Press, 1986), 45–74; Lamb D, "Diagnosing death," *Philosophy and Public Affairs* 1978;7: 144–53; and Becker LC, "Human being: The boundaries of the concept," *Philosophy and Public Affairs* 1975;4: 334–59.

32. For normative, see Veatch, *Death*; for ontological, see Green, Wikler, "Brain death."

33. The general problem of decoupling of behavioral correlates of pronouncing death is the subject of Norman Fost's chapter: Fost N, "The unimportance of death," in *The definition of death: Contemporary controversies*, ed. Youngner SJ, Arnold RM, Schapiro R (Baltimore: Johns Hopkins University Press, 1999), 161–78.

34. Brody B, "How much of the brain must be dead?" in *Definition of death*, ed. Youngner et al., 71–82; Fost, "Unimportance."

35. Harrison MR, Meilaender G, "The anencephalic newborn as organ donor," *Hastings Center Report* 1986;16 (2): 21–23; Fletcher J, Robertson J, Harrison M, "Primates and anencephalics as sources for pediatric organ transplants," *Fetal Therapy* 1986;1 (2–3): 150–64; Walters JW, Ashwal S, "Organ prolongation in anencephalic infants: Ethical and medical issues," *Hastings Center Report* 1988;18 (5): 19–27.

36. American Medical Association, Council on Ethical and Judicial Affairs, "The use of anencephalic neonates as organ donors," *JAMA* 1995;273: 1614–18.

37. Of course, some organs (single kidneys and liver lobes) can be procured from living people. We do not insist on people being declared dead in these cases. It is considered appropriate behavior even for the living assuming that proper consents have been obtained.

38. Texas Health & Safety Code, chap. 166, subchap. A, §166.052.

Chapter 8

Crafting a New
Definition-of-Death Law

Changing current law to conform to the suggestions made in the preceding chapters is a complex endeavor, and should be done with deliberate speed—but it should be done. Three changes would be needed in the current definition of death: (1) incorporation of the higher-brain function notion, (2) incorporation of some form of the conscience clause; and (3) clarification of the concept of "irreversibility."

Incorporating the Higher-Brain Notion

Present law makes persons dead when they have lost all functions of the entire brain. It is uniformly agreed that the law should incorporate only this basic concept of death, not the precise criteria or tests needed to determine that the whole brain is dead. That is left up to the consensus of neurological experts and is likely to change as technology advances.

All that would be needed to shift to a higher-brain formulation is a change in the wording of the law to replace "all functions of the entire brain" with some relevant, more limited alternative. There are at least three options: references to higher-brain functions, cerebral functions, or consciousness. Although we could simply change the wording to state that an individual is dead when there is irreversible cessation of all higher-brain functions, that poses a serious problem. We are now suffering from the problems created by the vagueness of referring to "all functions of the entire brain." Even though referring to "all higher-brain functions" would be conceptually correct, it would be even more ambiguous. It would lack the needed specificity.

This could be given substance by referring to the irreversible loss of cerebral functions, but we have already suggested two problems with this wording. Just as we now know there are some isolated functions of the whole brain that should be discounted, so there are probably some isolated cerebral functions that most would not want to count either. For example, if, hypothetically, an isolated "nest" of cerebral motor neurons were perfused so that if stimulated the body could twitch, that would be a cerebral function, but not a significant one for determining life any more than a brain-stem reflex is. Second, in theory some really significant functions, such as consciousness, might someday be maintainable even without a cerebrum—if, for example, a computer could function as an artificial center for consciousness. The term "cerebral function" adds specificity but is not satisfactory.

The language that seems best if integration of mind and body is what is critical is the "irreversible cessation of the capacity for consciousness." This is, after all, what the defenders of the higher-brain formulations really have in mind. (If someone were to claim that some other "higher" function is critical, that alternative could simply be plugged in.) In chapter 6 we actually endorsed a concept of death related not only to consciousness but also to the capacity for social interaction. We went on, however, to suggest that we could envision no cases in which the presence of consciousness would not also permit social interactions. Likewise, we cannot envision one who possesses the capacity for social interaction without consciousness. The two, we argued, were coterminous. We are therefore content to propose a higher-brain definition of death based on the irreversible loss of the capacity for consciousness. With qualifications, we noted above about medical experts needing to make some evaluative judgments about what appear to be matters of scientific fact; we will leave the specifics of the criteria and tests for measuring the irreversible loss of the capacity for consciousness up to the consensus of neurological expertise.[1] If the community of neurological expertise claims that the irreversible loss of consciousness cannot be measured, so be it. We will have at least clarified the concept and set the stage for the day when it can be measured with sufficient accuracy

The Conscience Clause

A second significant change in the definition of death would be required to incorporate the conscience clause. It would permit individuals, when competent, to execute documents choosing alternative definitions of death that are, within reason, not threatening to the significant interests of others. Although New Jersey law permits only choosing a heart-oriented definition as an alternative to a whole-brain position, and the Japanese law permits limited options for choosing a whole-brain definition as an alternative to a circulatory definition, our proposal is to choose a default definition, perhaps a whole-brain default, and permit individuals to choose a reasonable alternative, say, a somatic or higher-brain view. Assuming some version of a whole-brain formulation—adjusted to acknowledge that minor, cellular electrical activity and probably also hormonal regulatory functions should be ignored—as a default definition, would permit choosing either somatic or higher-brain-oriented (consciousness-based) definitions as alternatives.

As we have indicated, New Jersey law presently only permits competent adults to execute such conscience clauses. This, of course, excludes the possibility of parents choosing alternative definitions for their children. We argue that, just as legal surrogates have the right to make medical treatment decisions for their wards, provided the decisions are within reason, so too should they be permitted to choose alternative definitions of death, provided the individual had never expressed a preference. Although New Jersey law tolerates only explicitly religiously based variation, we would favor variation based on any conscientiously formulated position.

As a shortcut the law could state that patients who had opted for the consciousness-based definition who had clearly irreversibly lost consciousness because of the stopping of heart and lung function could continue to be pronounced dead based on criteria measuring heart and lung function. It would have to be made clearer than in the present Uniform Determination of Death Act that this was simply an alternative means for measuring the loss of consciousness. We see no reason to continue including the alternative forms of measurement in the legal definition itself. We would simply leave those to the criteria to be articulated by the consensus of experts. As long as heart and lung function had stopped long enough to make a return of consciousness impossible, the individual could be pronounced dead based on higher-brain function loss.

Similarly, for those who rely on the default (modified whole-brain) definition, as long as heart and lung function had stopped long enough to make impossible the return of any brain function (adjusted to exclude trivial electrical and hormonal functions), the individual could be pronounced dead based on whole-brain function loss.

Clarification of the Concept of "Irreversibility"

One final change needs to be incorporated regardless of whether the higher-brain concept and the conscience clause are added to the law defining death. In chapter 3 we summarized the controversy over the notion of irreversibility that is included in the law. It has sometimes been understood to mean that the critical function—brain function, circulatory function, or higher-brain function, depending on the concept one chooses—physiologically could not be restarted. Because this implies that the physiological substrate for the function has been destroyed, this version of irreversibility is sometimes called "physiological irreversibility."

Alternatively, irreversibility has been understood to mean "will never be restarted." Sometimes the critical function could be restarted, but will not be, perhaps because needed technology or those with the requisite skills are not present or because someone has made a valid decision that resuscitation will not be attempted. For example, a patient suffering a terminal illness may have on record an advance directive refusing further resuscitation. In such a case, it would be illegal and immoral to attempt resuscitation. After one has waited long enough to rule out the restarting of function spontaneously (autoresuscitation), one could conclude that the stoppage is irreversible, in the sense that no one will try to reverse the function loss. This is sometimes called "legal irreversibility" or merely "permanent" function loss.

The original model definitions of death were typically not clear on which meaning of irreversible was intended. One might be inclined to opt for the more conservative notion of physiological irreversibility. Doing so, however, conflicts with the traditional practice of medicine. Consider an elderly patient with metastatic cancer who has an advance directive refusing life support who then suffers a cardiac arrest. Typically, a physician present, after establishing the absence of a circulatory function, will simply pronounce death. No resuscitation will be attempted, and there will be no waiting period for the body's tissues to decline to the point that the circulation could not be restored. There is simply no point in waiting. In other words, traditionally, we have measured irreversibility using the "will not be restored" definition rather than the "physiologically cannot be restored" version.

Now that the issue is clear, a model law needs to specify which meaning is intended. We recommend the traditional notion of "will not be restored"—that is, the function morally or legally cannot be restored. This is standard practice today, and it should be made explicit in the model law. We do so in the text we recommend.

A Proposed New Definition of Death for Public Policy Purposes

This leads to a proposal for a new definition of death, which would read as follows:

> There shall be three acceptable definitions of death: (1) irreversible loss of all functions of the entire brain, excluding cellular-level and hormonal regulatory functions, (2) irreversible loss of consciousness, and (3) irreversible loss of circulatory function. A determination of any of these for the purpose of pronouncing death shall be made in accordance with accepted medical standards. Definition (1) shall be the default definition according to which an individual shall be declared dead unless he or she, while competent, or a designated surrogate, legal guardian, or next of kin, as specified below, has asked that the individual be declared dead according to definition (2) or (3). "Irreversible" shall be taken to mean that a valid decision has been made not to attempt reversal, and there is an empirical basis for believing there will be no spontaneous reversal. An individual who has chosen one of these alternatives shall be declared dead according to the definition that he or she has chosen. However, no individual shall be treated as dead for public policy purposes unless he or she has sustained irreversible cessation of all consciousness and no individual shall be treated as alive for public policy purposes if he or she has irreversibly lost all circulatory and respiratory functions.

Unless an individual has, when competent, selected a definition of death to be used for his or her own death pronouncement, a designated surrogate, legal guardian, or next of kin (in that order) may do so relying on substituted judgment, insofar as information is available about the patient's own wishes. If no such information is available, the decision maker shall rely on a best-interest determination. The definition selected by the individual, legal designated surrogate, guardian, or next of kin shall serve as the definition of death for all legal purposes. If no such alternative is selected, then the default definition shall be used. Some have proposed that an additional paragraph prohibiting a physician with a conflict of interest (e.g., an interest in the organs of the deceased) from pronouncing death. We are not convinced that paragraph is needed, however.

Conclusion

It has been puzzling why what at first seemed like a rather minor debate over when a human was dead should have persisted as long as it has. Many thought the definition-of-death debate was a technical argument that would be resolved in favor of the more fashionable, scientific, and progressive brain-oriented definition as soon as the old romantics attached to the heart died off. It is now clear that something much more complex and more fundamental is at stake. We have been fighting over the question of who has moral standing as a full member of the human moral community, a matter that forces on us some of the most basic questions of human existence: the relation of mind and body, the rights of religious and philosophical minorities, and the meaning of life itself.

We are left with two options if we do not adopt the definition we propose including a conscience clause. First, we could revert to a circulatory or somatic definition of death, following the arguments of Shewmon, Miller and Truog, and the minority of the US President's Council on Bioethics.[2] We would then need to face the question of whether certain prohibitions encapsulated in the dead donor rule should be abandoned. For example, we could choose to permit organ procurement in certain limited cases before death, as endorsed by Miller and Truog, who have argued for the legitimacy of organ procurement in cases of individuals who have decided to withdraw from life support and who have also acted to donate their organs. That would, in effect, mean abandoning the dead donor rule and permitting intentional, active killing of this group of patients— killing by organ procurement. We think those drastic social policy changes are unlikely. The alternative, if we are to revert to a circulatory or somatic definition of death, is to hold to the dead donor rule and permit the procurement of life-prolonging organs only by donation after circulatory death, a substantial loss of organs, but a plausible position if one is committed to the circulatory definition of death. If that option is chosen, major social and public policy changes would be required, including amending all state and national definitions of death laws to repeal the brain-based positions. That would be a major social undertaking.

The second alternative is to opt for some version of a higher-brain definition. Individuals would be declared dead when they irreversibly lose the capacity for consciousness. A large minority of the population in Western culture appears to hold this position, but only a minority. Adopting it without a conscience clause would impose a still-controversial definition on a large number of people. We are not certain whether some version of the higher-brain-oriented definition of death will be adopted in any legal jurisdiction anytime soon, but we are convinced that the now old-fashioned whole-brain-oriented definition of death is becoming less and less plausible as we realize that no one really believes that literally all functions of the entire brain must be irreversibly lost in order for an individual to be dead. Unless there is some public consensus expressed in state or federal law conveying agreement upon exactly which brain functions are insignificant, we are all vulnerable to a slippery slope in which private practitioners choose for themselves exactly where the line should be drawn from the top of the cerebrum to the caudal end of the spinal cord. There is no principled reason to draw it exactly between the base of the brain and the top of the spine. Better that we have a principled reason for drawing it. To us, the principle is that for human life to be present—that is, for the human to be treated as a member in full standing of the human moral community—there must be integrated functioning of mind and body. This means some version of a higher-brain-oriented formulation relying on the presence of a capacity for consciousness and social interaction. At the same time, we understand that not everyone shares this view. We see no significant, unavoidable social costs in permitting people to choose, based on their beliefs and values, from among the plausible definitions—the somatic, whole-brain, and higher-brain views.

Notes

1. Even determining the criteria for measuring irreversible loss of capacity for a brain function such as consciousness involves fundamentally nonscientific value judgments. The community of neurologists, for example, would need to choose a probability level at which the prediction of irreversibility can be made. They would have to add nuanced meaning to the terms critical for the enterprise. They

would have to assume certain concepts in their work. None of these are matters about which neurologists have expertise. In theory, the lay community could disagree with the consensus of neurological experts and in such disputes over these matters the lay population would have a legitimate claim to have their preferences and assumptions used in choosing the criteria for measuring irreversible loss of consciousness. For example, if the lay population wanted greater levels of statistical significance than the community of neurological experts, there is no rational reason why the neurologists' choice of a significance level should prevail. See Veatch RM, *Death, dying, and the biological revolution*, rev. ed. (New Haven, CT: Yale University Press, 1989), 41–44; and Veatch RM, "Consensus of expertise: The role of consensus of experts in formulating public policy and estimating facts," *Journal of Medicine and Philosophy* 1991;16: 427–45.

2. Shewmon DA, "The brain and somatic integration: Insights into the standard biological rationale for equating 'brain death' with death," *Journal of Medicine and Philosophy* 2001;26 (5): 457–78; Miller FG, Truog RD, *Death, dying, and organ transplantation* (New York: Oxford University Press, 2012); US President's Council on Bioethics, *Controversies in the determination of death: A white paper by the President's Council on Bioethics* (Washington, DC: US President's Council on Bioethics, 2008).

Procuring Organs

Chapter 9

The Donation Model

We saw in chapter 1 of this book that the major religious and cultural traditions of the world do not have any clear-cut, principled objections to lifesaving organ transplants. The groundwork is in place for establishing the basic approach for a society to transfer organs from potential organ sources to others who need these organs. The focus of part II of this book is the ethics of organ procurement.

In this and the following two chapters, we first examine the general options for a basis for ethical procurement and then consider a number of specific areas of controversy. We look at three major options: donation, salvaging, and sale. We examine variations on these three as we go. Public policy could require that organs be donated by individuals or their surrogates (this is the current system in the United States and in most areas of Northern Europe). We could assume that human body parts are of no more use to the deceased and can be "salvaged" by the state to be used for medical purposes (which is the current system in most of Southern Europe, much of Asia, and parts of Central and South America). Or we could assume that human body parts belong to the individual or the family of the deceased individual in such a way that they could be sold to either the state or other individuals (this is the approach used openly in Iran and elsewhere in some extralegal transactions, and favored by some libertarians).

In the course of the exploration of these three options in this and the next two chapters, we ask whether we can presume consent of those who have not explicitly objected to donation, whether we can require hospitals or other institutions to request donation or require people to respond to such requests, and whether we can procure organs from those who are what used to be called "non-heart-beating cadavers," that is, people who have died by cardiocirculatory arrest either from accidents or intentional termination of life support. In the later chapters of part II, we also look at the ethics of procuring organs from living people, of procuring organs from HIV-positive donors and others with potentially transmittable medical problems, and of using organs from non-human animals. Finally, we look at the role of the media in organ procurement.

By 1970 much of the world was beginning to accept human-to-human (homologous) transplants as morally licit. Some pockets of resistance, reflecting deep cultural beliefs, remained in some cultures. For example, Asians, especially the Japanese, found transplants difficult to accept. In part this was because of serious doubts that the essence of a human being could be localized in the brain. In part it resulted from a 1968 attempt by a surgeon, Juro Wada, to transplant a heart, when there was widespread doubt that the surgeon had waited until the person from whom the organ was taken was really dead when the heart was procured. Native Americans were also skeptical, as were some who continued to worry about the impact of organ transplants on the abortion debate. But most people in Western culture, both secular and religious, had come to accept the exciting new technology of organ replacement. Mainstream Christianity—both Catholic and Protestant—was strongly approving. Although Judaism continued to resist a brain-oriented definition of death, some of its Talmudic scholars treated organ transplants as morally required if life-prolonging organs were procured after death, often based on death by circulatory criteria. This was more than most Christian ethicists were willing to claim. Similarly, Muslims and proponents of Eastern worldviews (Hindus, Buddhists, Confucians, and Taoists) tended to accept organ transplants, although some resistance remained.

Given the increasing acceptance of organ procurement and the enormous good that can come from transplanting these organs, the remaining issue is establishing the basis upon which the organs can be removed. As we have suggested, three major positions surfaced in the early debate. They reflect three major ethical approaches. The first of these can be called the "donation model."

The Moral Foundation of the Donation Model

The *donation model* is built on the moral notion that there is a duty to respect the bodily integrity of members of the moral community and that this obligation remains even after death. Just as there is a duty to respect the will, autonomy, and bodily integrity—the ability to decide for oneself what will happen to one's body—of a person who participates in a research project, so too is this respect required even after his or her death. We have long acknowledged the right of the individual to control the disposal of his or her assets after death. Just as there is a duty to respect the will of the individual for the disposition of assets, so we must respect his or her wishes about what will happen to his or her body.

The Duty to Respect the Deceased's Wishes

This donation model is not based primarily on concerns about consequences. True, a sophisticated utilitarian might argue that routine salvaging could produce such hostility that fewer organs would be procured using this model. Some who believe in reincarnation might, theoretically, have concerns about consequences; but as we saw in chapter 1, those who hold traditional, orthodox Christian beliefs about the resurrection of the body need have no reason to fear organ procurement. But the primary argument in favor of donation is not about avoiding harms but rather it is grounded in the ethical principle of *autonomy*.

The principle of respect for autonomy holds that others have a duty to permit individuals to live out their lives according to their own life plans—regardless of whether they have calculated the consequences so as to maximize their personal well-being. A question is sometimes raised about whether autonomy has any bearing on things after one dies. If the duty is to permit people to live out a life plan, some would ask how contravening the individual's wishes after that person's death could be a violation of autonomy. This question has generated a philosophical literature.[1] For example, a distinction is sometimes made between "experiential interests" and "critical interests."[2] Experiential interests are our normal interests in having certain experiences. These obviously cannot be fulfilled after death. Critical interests, however, are not thwarted by death. Our interest in having a particular relative receive a personal treasure, for example, can be fulfilled or blocked even after we die. Likewise, our interest in how our body is treated need not cease with death. Just as a person's objection to cremation or postmortem research binds those who survive, creating obligations that remain after a person's death, so interests in giving or refusing to give organs also can survive one's death and create obligations that remain.[3]

Suffice it to say that for our purposes, many people accept the idea that their autonomy would be violated if their wishes about the disposal of their assets are not followed after they die. So much the more would they feel that their autonomy would be violated if their wishes about the disposal of their body are not followed.

The mere fact that one will no longer be around to be aware that one's choice was violated is not really the essential issue. For one thing, if there were a general policy of disregarding people's posthumous interests, great distress would result. In the case of economic wills, if society believes that the will could be disregarded whenever more good would come if the assets were used in some other way, then all would live with the discomfort of knowing that their wishes about the future uses of their assets are not secure. More critically, we tend to feel that a wrong is committed if the individual's will is not honored, even if we believe that individuals cannot know about this when it occurs and more good would accrue if it were not honored.

A similar concern is reflected in the donation model for the use of body parts. We owe respect to the individual, limiting what we can do ethically to a person without consent. This duty of respect does not cease with the individual's death. The body is still the *mortal remains* of the individual, and his or her wishes deserve respect. Therefore, we can use the body for research, education, therapy, or transplantation only if that individual grants us permission—only if the body is made a gift to others.

This reasoning is what philosophers would call *deontological*. Derived from the Greek word for duty, the term is used to convey the idea that there are certain duties we owe to others *regardless of the consequences*. The ethical principle of respect for autonomy is one of the most profound and widely affirmed deontological aspects of Western culture. It is the foundation of the donation model. This is the model that has won the debate in the United States and in the other countries dominated by Protestant individualism, including Germany, the Netherlands, the United Kingdom, and Canada.

Surrogate Permission: The Fate of Valuable Body Parts When the Individual Has Expressed No Preference

There is one important qualification to the application of the principle of respect for autonomy as it pertains to organ donation. What should happen if there is no reason to expect that an individual has objected to donating his or her body, but this individual has left no direct evidence that the gift is intended? Can we presume that, because no objection was on record, the individual intended that his or her body be used to benefit others?

As we discuss in the next chapter, there is no reason to make such a presumption. We know that a significant minority of the American population does not want its organs used for transplants. In other cultures the percentage who would object could be even higher.

Nevertheless, even though we reject the presumption that a person who was silent about organ procurement would have wanted to donate organs, we have opened the door to donation by a surrogate—either a surrogate named by the individual while alive or, if that has not happened, the next of kin. There are several reasons to support allowing such surrogates to make this choice.

For one, the named person or nearest relative might be in the best position to know the deceased's wishes. Even if the individual has never expressed explicit wishes about organ donation, someone close to this person may be able, with varying degrees of accuracy, to deduce what the person may have wanted based on his or her knowledge of the general beliefs and values of the person. This is often called *substituted judgment*, that is, a decision based on what is known about the individual's decision making.

For another, drawing on the analogy of the economic will, we could view the body as property left at death to the family or other named parties. Just as someone who inherits assets has the right to make a gift of them to another, so it might be argued that, once the "beneficiary" receives the body, he or she then has a certain ownership interest, including the authority to make a gift of it for valid medical purposes. This explanation is controversial, however, because typically no one has a classical "property right" to a human body. At most, the literature speaks about a "quasi–property right," that is, a limited right to make certain decisions pertaining to the proper disposition of the body. Still, a quasi–property right held by the designated surrogate or next of kin could well be enough to justify a decision about organ donation.

Finally, we may view the surrogate as having some limited range of discretion in choosing how to honor the dead and dispose of the remains. The contemporary literature on the ethics of terminal care often recognizes a limited right of discretion for the surrogate decision maker, for example, in deciding in marginal cases which of two or more treatment options to pursue. This is typically limited to a choice among a reasonable set of alternatives.[4] For similar reasons the designated surrogate or next of kin might be given a limited choice about whether organs should be procured.

For some combination of these reasons, the surrogate named by the individual or, absent such naming, the next of kin is therefore given the authority to choose a mode of burial, to plan for the kind of funeral or memorial service to offer, and to make many other choices pertaining to the final rituals for the deceased.

There are, however, severe limits on the discretion of the next of kin or other surrogates. They cannot literally do anything they want with the body. As we discussed in chapter 1, they have duties as well as rights—including the duty to dispose of the remains in a respectful manner. That is why we speak of quasi–property rights over the body.[5] They are rights, but with certain duties attached that constrain the surrogate's amount of discretion.

Although infants and children generally cannot give a valid consent to donation, surrogate consent may partially address this problem. It is unlikely that a young child will have formed an opinion in advance about organ procurement; but if a minor has expressed revulsion or otherwise has objected, then the minor's opinion should be taken as a veto, even in the case of parental permission.

In the case of elderly donors, similar problems may arise. Older persons may be mentally incompetent. If they have never expressed, while competent, a willingness to donate organs, they may be in a position similar to that of minors. If so, similar reasoning should apply.

Donor Designation or First-Person Consent

The interesting case is what should happen when the wishes of the deceased conflict with those of the next of kin or another surrogate—when one party wants organs to be procured and the other does not. The ethical principle of autonomy is the basis for rights for the individual. Especially in a highly individualistic society such as that of the United States, it should be clear that the deceased's own wishes must prevail. Hence, the Uniform Anatomical Gift Act (UAGA) makes clear that an individual's refusal to agree to organ procurement takes precedence over the willingness of relatives to make the gift. The picture is slightly more complicated when the individual has made a gift and the surrogate attempts to refuse. This is now sometimes referred to as the problem of "first-person donation."

The Principles of Donor Priority over Family

In principle, a valid donation of the bodily remains made while one is alive and competent should also take precedence over the objection of the next of kin. Thus, someone with a valid donor card expressing a willingness to have organs taken for transplant should be enough to authorize organ procurement, even if the family objects.

This could pose practical problems, however. Recently, researchers reported that organs would not be procured if the family objected in 85 percent of fifty-four countries surveyed, regardless of whether the country relies on explicit consent or a law authorizing procurement without explicit consent.[6] For one, it is the family that is alive at the end. They are the ones who could sue the organ procurement organization (OPO) and the surgeons who procured the organs. The law is quite clear that the family would eventually lose such a suit, but it could make life unpleasant for the health professionals involved for awhile.

Second, procurement personnel look to the family to obtain a medical and social history in order to help rule out disease or a high-risk lifestyle that could suggest the danger of exposure to HIV or other contagious diseases. If the family objects to organ procurement, there is a good chance that it will fail to cooperate in obtaining an adequate history. There may be other ways, however, to get an adequate history, even without the help of the next of kin. If the individual dies from the irreversible stoppage of brain function following an accident, it is possible that the person was alive and lucid long enough to give an adequate medical and social history to the physicians, before dying. Perhaps the deceased was living with someone who is emotionally very close, but not the next of kin, who could supply the important history. Both law and ethics support organ procurement when the decedent has made his or her consent clear before dying, regardless of familial objection—although the organs may need to be characterized as "high risk" and require additional screening for various donor-transmittable diseases.

A good case can be made that, if the organs are otherwise suitable and an adequate medical and social history is available, the OPO has a moral duty—not merely the right—to follow the deceased's wishes and procure organs over the objection of the next of kin. Doing so may mean a confrontation with the family, but procurement is clearly supported by the law. If someone has gone out of his or her way to make a potentially lifesaving donation, that is a noble gift. Those in the transplant community, and those who are generally committed to the good that can come from organ transplants, owe it to the memory of the deceased to take on the added burden of confronting the family in order not only to honor the deceased but also to make the effort to save the lives that hang in the balance—lives the deceased was actively committed to saving. If we accept the model of donation and the moral principles upon which it is based, we will show respect for the deceased by honoring his or her wishes, including honoring any wish to refuse to participate in organ procurement, but also honoring the deceased's wish, whenever possible, to procure organs so that he or she may make a final gift of life to others. Just as a financial will cannot be overturned because of family objections, so too should a decedent's wish to donate be the final word.

The Law and Donor Priority

Over the years there have been several efforts to make clear in the law that the donor's wishes should prevail over those of the next of kin or other family members. The original UAGA of 1968, the model law upon which state laws in the United States are based, was interpreted from the beginning as giving priority to the donor's wishes. The UAGA states: "Any individual of sound mind and 18 years of age or more may give all or any part of his body for any purpose, . . . the gift to take effect upon death."[7]

The 1968 UAGA then goes on to authorize surrogate decision making, listing in order the spouse, adult son or daughter, either parent, an adult brother or sister, a guardian of the person of the decedent at the time of his or her death, or any other person authorized or under obligation to dispose of the body.[8] These surrogates, it states, may decide "when persons in prior classes are not available at the time of death, and in the absence of actual notice of contrary indications by the decedent or actual notice of opposition by a member of the same or a prior class."[9] This language seems straightforwardly to give priority to the individual from whose body the organs will be taken. And this was, in fact, the standard interpretation in the early years of the application of the act. The model law, moreover, includes the provision that "the rights of the donee created by the gift are paramount to the rights of others."[10] This is further supported by the comment added by the National Conference of Commissioners on Uniform State Laws included in its document pertaining to the act, which states that "subsection (e) recognizes and gives legal effect to the right of the individual to dispose of his own body without subsequent veto by others."[11]

In spite of the apparent clear priority of the individual donor's decision over that of the next of kin or other surrogate, it became the practice in many, if not all, OPOs to ask the family for permission to procure organs even when a valid first-person donation was available and yield to their objection if it arose. By 1983 the results of a telephone survey of organ procurement organizations conducted by the Battelle Human Affairs Research Center found that fewer than 25 percent of transplant centers would accept a written directive from a deceased person without family approval.[12] In response, the 1987 revision of the UAGA includes explicit language: "An anatomical gift that is not revoked by the donor before death is irrevocable and does not require the consent or concurrence of any person after the donor's death."[13]

In spite of this clarification and reinforcement of the priority of the donor's gift in the 1987 version, the commissioners felt obliged to revisit it again in the 2006 revision. They included an entire section on "Family Veto," reaffirming once again that "a person other than the donor is barred from making, amending, or revoking an anatomical gift of a donor's body or part if the donor made an anatomical gift of the donor's body or part."[14]

Since 2006 it has become increasingly common for OPO personnel to acknowledge the priority of donor designation over family veto. In a recent study by James Chon and colleagues, it was reported that 53 percent of the fifty-eight American OPOs always followed the donor's wishes when family disagreed, and another 45 percent did so in most cases. Only eleven of fifty-six responding OPOs would not proceed with procurement unless they had the family's consent. Although 65 percent of OPOs had encountered family objections in the past five years, most (89 percent) indicated that it occurred less than 10 percent of the time.[15] There is, of course, no legal requirement for any OPO to take a validly donated organ, but in the absence of medical contraindication or other reason to believe that that organ could not be used, there are good moral and clinical reasons why it should be taken, and increasingly it is done. Family members are diplomatically told that the gift has been made rather than asked for a reaffirmation of the gift.

Variations on the Donation Model

If donation supplied enough organs, it seems likely that everyone would be content with the donation model. The sad fact, however, is that more than a hundred thousand people are on the waiting list for organs in the United States alone. More than seven thousand people die every year for lack of an organ. Thousands more are removed from the waiting list because they become too sick to receive a transplant and presumably die thereafter. Countless others—especially those waiting for a kidney—suffer the inconvenience and medical burden while they wait.

This has led to examining many alternatives for attempting to procure more organs. The two major options—routine salvaging and markets—are the topics of the next two chapters. In the remainder of this chapter we examine strategies for increasing organ yield that remain largely within the donation model.

Routine Inquiry and Required Response

It is understandable that some are growing impatient with the donation model as reflected in the UAGA that has been in place now for more than four decades. This has led to proposals to routinize the request for organs. An early effort focused on making routine inquiry of relatives of all persons diagnosed as dead by brain criteria. Alternatively, a truly systematic and routine inquiry made to individuals while alive and competent may be more morally defensible and perhaps even more efficient.

Routine Inquiry of Next of Kin

Almost all states now have required request laws mandating that someone ask the next of kin for permission to procure organs in cases where usable organs may be obtained. In addition, at the federal level the Omnibus Reconciliation Act of 1986 requires hospitals to comply with United Network for Organ Sharing rules, including having written protocols for identifying potential donors and "assuring that families of potential donors are made aware of the option of organ and tissue donation and their option to decline."[16] Although the results are encouraging, there is a great deal that could be done to improve the process and quality of the request.

Existing routine inquiry policies are defective because they either occur at the wrong time or ask the question of the wrong person. The current routine inquiry laws ignore the dying individual and instead focus attention only on the substitute surrogate decision maker. They may pose the donation question to relatives after the patient whose organs might be procured has deteriorated to the point that he or she is beyond responding. In Western culture it is the individual himself or herself who is most responsible for choosing a life plan. That has included the right and responsibility to shape the disposal of assets after death through a legally binding will. It now also includes a first priority for the individual's own will regarding the disposal of the body and the use of body parts for medical purposes. Thus any legal requirement for routine inquiry by the next of kin about patients who are dead or are approaching that diagnosis comes too late in the process. At best, we get a substituted judgment, with family members attempting to convey what they believe would be the patient's wishes. Often what we get is the relative's personal value judgment based on the beliefs and values not of the one whose organs are under consideration but on those of the relative. Absent any wishes about the disposal of body parts expressed by the individual while competent, the next of kin has been given the discretion to donate or refuse donation; but it is hard to see why the relative's moral, religious, and philosophical position is morally relevant. At best, it is the second alternative for decision making in a liberal society.

Routine Inquiry and Required Response of Competent Persons

An alternative that received attention when donor registration was less successful was to systematize inquiries to individuals while competent to encourage them to make decisions about how they would want their bodies used upon their deaths *and then to require that they respond.*[17] Even if we maintain the donation mode of thinking about procuring organs, the argument was made that it is not too much to say that morally one ought to at least make the effort to think enough about this difficult subject to decide whether one wants to be part of the lifesaving project of organ donation, if that is feasible upon one's death. If the inquiry is presented at a time when the individual can form his or her own moral stance about organ donation and is combined with the requirement that the individual respond in some fashion (required response), the gap between those who say they would be willing to donate and those who have actually executed a written record of their donation might be reduced. The result could be an accurate record of everyone who wanted to donate, without sweeping into the process those who have some objection. Under such arrangements required requests of next of kin would be a fallback position used only when the deceased had never recorded a decision while competent to do so, either because they did not have access to the forms and the knowledge about how to execute them or because they found thinking about such matters too unpleasant.

Sometimes these inquiries to competent persons are proposed for clinical settings where the inquiry is not required legally but should be encouraged morally. Of these, many could occur in medical settings. For example, it seems reasonable that a query about one's wishes about organ procurement should become a routine part of every physician's history and physical examination. Physicians are learning that they cannot provide good and proper medical care for their patients if they do not have an idea of their patients' preferences. We are routinizing discussions of "living wills," decisions about cardiopulmonary resuscitation, and who should be one's surrogate decision maker; we should also make a discussion about organ donation a routine part of the history and physical examination. The physician whose patient fails to provide an adequate response should feel that the record is incomplete. He or she should respond with a distress similar to that expressed when the patient fails to give a clear answer to other queries in the history taking. Although the physician cannot literally demand an answer, he or she should convey that high-quality medicine requires that the record be as complete as possible. Also, queries about a willingness to donate organs should become a routine part of every hospital admission, as required by both state and federal laws.

It might be objected that this is too macabre a subject for a physical exam or hospital intake interview. It might even be seen as bad public relations, suggesting to a patient that death is a likely outcome of the encounter. But surely there are already questions posing problems of diplomacy incorporated into such sessions. Physicians ask about sexual histories; hospital intake interviews include questions about who will pay the bills. Skilled professionals learn how to pose these questions diplomatically. If these discussions occur in all routine physical exams and intake interviews, both patients and clinicians will grow accustomed to them. They will provide a good opportunity for repeated reflection and introspection.

Perhaps just as promising would be opportunities for routine inquiry outside the health care context. Routine inquiry should become a part of other social encounters, as in religious and fraternal groups. At a more formal, legal level, states could be expected to ask people about organ donation during drivers' license renewals. It would be a small additional step to require in some of these settings that the question be answered. Of course, persons would not be required to answer in the affirmative. They could even be given an opportunity to answer "I don't know" or "Undecided" to the donation question. (In that case, the surrogate decision-making provisions of the anatomical gift act would come into play.) It is critical if organ donation is part of license renewal that the motor vehicle departments' employees are well educated about organ donation so that they can respond to queries by drivers with accurate information.

Required Response in Texas

In 1991 a law went into effect in the state of Texas mandating that, when people renew their driver's licenses, they make a choice about whether to donate organs.[18] Registrants were given a choice of saying "yes" or "no" to the donation question. But there was a practical problem with the Texas law: When asked, 80 percent declined to donate, a much larger proportion of refusals than seems plausible, given what we know about the overall rates of willingness to donate.[19] Various explanations have been offered, including the lack of training and commitment of the Texas Department of Public Safety (the agency handling driving licenses) and the resistance of citizens to being forced to provide an answer.

The Texas law was repealed in 1997. A new law took effect in 2010. According to it, Department of Public Safety employees are required to ask each license applicant, "Would you like to register as an organ donor?"[20] If the applicant responds affirmatively, his or her information is added to the statewide deceased donor registry. If he or she responds negatively, no further action is taken, that is, there is no corresponding registry of declared nondonors, so declining in this setting is not a legally binding declaration of opposition to donation. (It is possible that, if the next of kin is there to hear the person decline, that could influence the next of kin's decision.) Before this change, Texas had one of the lowest donor consent rates in the country, around 2 percent of adults. By August 2010 that rate had increased to 5 percent. In 2012 Department of Public Safety employees attended training sessions specifically on organ donation, and as of January 2013 the donor rate in the state had risen to about 17 percent.[21]

An alternative would be to record both positive and negative responses, but to also provide a third alternative indicating that the registrant is undecided or otherwise does not wish to respond definitively. This would have the effect of leaving the choice to the next of kin, but still recording the objections of those who explicitly do not wish to donate, a decision that would foreclose next-of-kin involvement.

Illinois also has a mandate for choice, enacted as part of legislation that makes clear that the donor's designation is legally binding. Its donor designation through its registry has reached 53 percent.[22] California has also introduced mandated choice and has reached a registry of 34 percent of eligible adults.[23]

An Assessment of Required Response or Mandated Choice

Although some might see this type of required response or mandated choice initiative as an offensive intrusion by the state into private matters, it seems little to ask for what could have a significant lifesaving impact. All that would be asked is that one think enough about the lifesaving potential of a donation to decide one way or another, not that a particular decision be made. Our obligation to the community surely goes far enough to permit a requirement that the question be addressed.

In some settings, such as the driver's license application process, it would not be difficult to require that the question be answered. An unanswered question would be considered an incomplete application. That, after all, is what happens when other questions are not answered, such as questions about one's automobile insurance.

There are other nonmedical ways in which a routine inquiry with a required response could be arranged. One of the most practical ones would be to have an organ donation question on the income tax return. The form is completed by virtually all adults, it is updated yearly, and the data could easily be entered into a central computer at the same time as other tax data. This would mean that there would be a single national registry rather than a separate database in each state, as occurs with driver's license information. A tape of the data for just that question could be sent to the United Network for Organ Sharing or any central organ procurement agency, thus facilitating privacy protection. As long as negative answers and opportunities for expressing uncertainty were provided for, such required responses seem well within the model of affirming the primacy of the individual and the donation model. Other potentially sensitive questions, such as a willingness to make political and charitable contributions, now appear on federal and state tax forms. Although, undoubtedly, some will object, these types of nontax queries on tax forms have generally been accepted by legislatures and the general population and have been found workable. Thousands of organs, and therefore thousands of lives, hang in the balance. We know that many people are, in principle, willing to donate these organs, but they have simply never had the resolve—or the opportunity—to record their willingness to make a donation in an effective way. If we can be asked to contribute to a political party on a tax form, certainly we can be asked to record our willingness to save lives through organ donation.

Other ways to connect routine organ donation inquiries to existing computerized data banks might be possible as well. The health insurance industry maintains a centralized database of insurance records through the Medical Insurance Bureau. It could systematically include organ donation data, even classifying records lacking such data as incomplete. There is, however, already substantial suspicion among those who know of its existence that the database constitutes an unacceptable breach of confidentiality. It might not be the ideal mechanism for a required response. The census compiles a national database, which could include queries about organ donation; but that survey, even though it is national, is conducted only once a decade, and thus is not sufficiently frequent to keep an accurate and up-to-date record of individual decisions about donation. The state driving license databases and the federal income tax records seem to be the most feasible locations for this information. Of the two, the federal income tax system has the advantage of maintaining a single national database that is already computerized and is updated yearly. If we can bring ourselves to be concerned enough about a few thousand of our fellow citizens whose lives and well-being hang in the balance, the federal income tax form seems to be the ideal place to require a response to the organ donation question.

Donor Registries

The most important systematic effort to register organ donors has been led by the Donor Designation Collaborative. Launched in 2006 and operating under the name Donate Life America, it has coordinated the American national donor registration effort. Before that, states had various programs to register donors, usually through their departments of motor vehicles. Since the 1980s donation has been possible through the use of a donor card, but since 2006 the effort has been systematized; access to state registries is now available 24 hours a day, and people can enroll online or at motor vehicle departments.

As of 2012, 109,000,000 people were registered, some 45 percent of possible registrants.[24] That is up from single digits a decade earlier. Because the families of many who have not registered are willing to make donations at the time of death of a medically suitable candidate, authorization rates are now approaching 75 percent.[25]

Increasing Sophistication in Obtaining Donations

Transplant professionals at the dawn of the era of transplantation naively assumed that organ donation was a "yes" or "no" question. People either donated or did not. Early on, perhaps half of those asked, normally families of the newly deceased, agreed to donation of at least some organs or tissues.

We quickly learned, however, that the decision to donate organs was a complex, emotional, psychologically trying one and that the organ procurement community could do a great deal to influence the context of the decision. In very rough terms the combination of countless efforts has increased a typical OPO's "authorization rate" and so-called conversion rate from roughly 50 to 75 percent. The terminology itself suggests complexity. OPOs calculate an authorization rate, which is the number of successful authorizations divided by the number of potential medically suitable deaths in which a request for organs is made. They also calculate a "conversion rate" based on the number of donors from whom organs were actually obtained. (The difference is accounted for by occasional cases where the medical examiner blocks procurement after authorization is obtained, along with donors who are found unsuitable after authorization either because the donor "crashes" or there is a late discovery of medical contraindications.)

Many different variables have an impact on the authorization to procure as well as the actual conversion. There is an entire literature on social determinants of successful requests for organ donations. For example, we have learned that the request should be decoupled from the task of informing the family of the death of the patient. We also know that different people in different roles have predictably varying degrees of success. For example, procurement coordinators, with generally considerable experience and dedication, are generally more successful than critical care physicians.[26] Moreover, some people in a position to ask seem to have personalities that enable them to be more successful in gaining authorizations.

Over the years an elaborate set of strategies has emerged for increasing willingness to make a donation. For example, there is some evidence that matching the race of the person requesting the donation with the family being asked improves the donation response.[27] A "Donation Collaborative" has developed "best practice" strategies, complete with concepts like the "huddle," a team meeting of relevant personnel. Other sports metaphors have also been used, such as "scorecards." Procurement teams develop "message strategies."[28] Flags are awarded to high-performing hospitals, and considerable efforts have been made to publicize donation rates. A float encouraging organ donation appears every year in the Rose Bowl Parade. Local races, essay contests, television and radio spots, and appearances at churches, schools, and community events by OPO staff members all make donation a matter of sophisticated strategizing.[29] In addition, OPOs have in recent years modified their language from a neutral approach to families to one that has been termed the "presumptive approach," because it uses language that presumes that organ donation is the right thing to do and that when given the chance, most people will do the right thing.[30] Some have asked whether some of these efforts do not verge on manipulation and fail to encompass the moral dimensions of end-of-life care in the setting of an intensive care unit.[31] Overall, however, the minimal goal is that every potential donor of organs should be identified in a timely manner and should be approached about donation in a way that takes into account what we have learned about increasing the likelihood of a successful procurement from all who have no reasoned objection to donation.

The Limits of the Donation Model

The donation model has carried the day, at least in the United States and other countries that stress the importance of the rights of the individual. As we delineate in the next chapter, even in those countries that claim to have taken a more communitarian approach that places the interests of the community of living people over those of the individual who is deceased, the donation model has great power. Countries that authorize the procurement of useful organs without individual permission still attempt to dress their more social approach in the language of gift giving. They still talk about those from whom organs are procured as "donors." They still honor individual objections from those who explicitly refuse to let their organs be procured. And most tellingly, they still tend not to take organs when family members object.

There is only one problem with the donation model: It has not produced enough donations. As of July 2014 there were in the United States 123,116 on the waiting list for organs. A total of 28,954 organs were recovered in 2013 from 8,269 deceased donors, together with 5,989 from living donors. Almost all the living donors supplied a kidney. Liver lobes were obtained from 232 living donors, and lung lobes from 1, as well as 1 pancreas and 1 intestine. It is clear that the need is great. The disparity between the number of organs needed and procured is growing rapidly. In 2012, 6,860 Americans died while on the waiting list for an organ—up from 4,257 in 1996.[32]

Determining the number of organs that could be procured if all medically suitable patients donated their organs or had them donated on their behalf is more complicated than it seems. The number will depend on exactly which potential sources of organs are considered medically suitable, whether we include medically suitable candidates that are excluded because the medical examiner objects, how we count organs actually donated that are not recoverable (because the patient "crashes" before procurement or the medical examiner objects after consent), whether donors who die by circulatory criteria are included, and so forth. The overall result is that we are approaching 75 percent of potential donors actually authorizing procurement or having it authorized on their behalf. This is up from between 40 and 60 percent a decade ago.[33] This suggests that, assuming that the usable organs in the medically suitable donors who do not donate are comparable to those in the people who do donate, we could add about one-third to the number of usable organs procured each year if we had maximal recovery. The number of potential procurements following deaths by circulatory criteria is hard to determine.

We know that, although a substantial majority of the population would be willing to donate, only about 43 percent are registered in donor registries.[34] In many cases people who would be willing to donate simply have not done so for reasons of inertia. They simply do not know how to go about making the donation or have not taken the time and energy to do so. We also know that when family members are asked to donate organs, some refuse to do so. In some of these cases it may simply be because the family is too traumatized at the time of a loved one's death to think about the difficult subject of organ donation. Some may even regret at a later date that they failed to make the donation. The donation model is probably not the most efficient way of obtaining all the organs that people, under ideal circumstances, would be willing to give. Routine salvaging, even considering the potential backlash, is probably more efficient. Providing financial incentives or using market mechanisms, even taking into account the costs, would probably also be more efficient. These are the topics of the next two chapters.

Notes

1. Buchanan AE, Brock DW, *Deciding for others: The ethics of surrogate decision making* (Cambridge: Cambridge University Press, 1989), 128–29; Olick RS, "Deciding for incompetent patients: The nature and limits of prospective autonomy and advance directives," doctoral diss., Georgetown University, Washington, 1997; Wilkinson TM, *Ethics and the acquisition of organs* (Oxford: Oxford University Press, 2012).

2. Dworkin R, *Life's dominion: An argument about abortion, euthanasia, and individual freedom* (New York: Vintage Books, 1994), 201–4.

3. See Wilkinson TM, *Ethics and the acquisition of organs* (Oxford: Oxford University Press, 2012), 29–62, for a sophisticated discussion of posthumous harms and the moral claims of the dead.

4. Veatch RM, "Limits of guardian treatment refusal: A reasonableness standard," *American Journal of Law and Medicine* 1984;9 (4): 427–68.

5. Meyers DW, *The human body and the law* (Chicago: Aldine, 1970), 128–29.

6. Rosenbaum AM, Horvat LD, Siminoff LA, Prakash V, Beitel J, Garg AX, "The authority of next of kin in explicit and presumed consent systems for deceased organ donation: An analysis of 54 nations," *Nephrology, Dialysis, and Transplantation* 2012;27: 2533–46.

7. National Conference of Commissioners on Uniform State Laws, "Uniform Anatomical Gift Act: Drafted by the National Conference of Commissioners on Uniform State Laws and by it approved and recommended for enactment in all the states at its Annual Conference Meeting in its seventy-seventh Year, Philadelphia, July 22–31, 1968, with prefatory note and comments, approved by the American Bar Association at its meeting in Philadelphia, August 7, 1968," § 2(a), www.uniformlaws.org/shared/docs/anatomical_gift/uagapercent201968_scan.pdf. Also see Sadler AM, Sadler BL, Stason EB, "The Uniform Anatomical Gift Act," *JAMA* 1968;206: 2501–6.

8. Ibid.

9. Ibid.

10. Ibid., 7.

11. Ibid., "Comment" to § 2. This paragraph, for some unexplained reason, is omitted from the version of the document on the commissioners' website, but is included in the version published in *Uniform Laws Annotated* and is referenced by several commentators. See Blumstein J, "The case for commerce in organ transplantation," in *Politics and the human body: Assault on dignity*, ed. Elshtain JB, Clloyd JT (Nashville: Vanderbilt University Press, 1995), 176–92; Peters DA, "Protecting autonomy in organ procurement procedures: Some overlooked issues," *Milbank Quarterly* 1986;64: 241–70; and Best FL, Jr., "Transfers of bodies and body parts under the Uniform Anatomical Gift Act," *Real Property, Probate and Trust Journal* 1980;15: 806–36. It also appears in a version by the Wisconsin State Legislature in its proposed adoption of the UAGA in 1969: "Uniform Anatomical Gift Act, WI Assembly Bill 4, 1969."

12. Overcast TD, Evans RW, Bowen LE, Hoe MM, Livak CL, "Problems in the identification of potential organ donors: Misconceptions and fallacies associated with donor cards," *JAMA* 1984;251: 1559–62.

13. National Conference of Commissioners on Uniform State Laws (NCCUSL), *Uniform Anatomical Gift Act* (1987) (Chicago: NCCUSL, 1987), § 2(h).

14. National Conference of Commissioners on Uniform State Laws (NCCUSL), *Revised Uniform Anatomical Gift Act* (2006) (Chicago: NCCUSL, 2006), 29.

15. Chon WJ, Josephson MA, Gordon EJ, et al., "When the living and the deceased cannot agree on organ donation: A survey of US organ procurement organizations (OPOs)," *American Journal of Transplantation* 2014;14: 172–77.

16. Omnibus Reconciliation Act of 1986, 42 USC Sec. 1320b-8.

17. Veatch RM, *Death, dying, and the biological revolution*, rev. ed. (New Haven, CT: Yale University Press, 1989).

18. Texas General Laws 1204. See also Cotter H, "Increasing consent for organ donation: Mandated choice, individual autonomy, and informed consent," *Health Matrix* 2011;21: 618–19; and Verheijde JL, Rady MY, McGregor J, "Recovery of transplantable organs after cardiac or circulatory death: Transforming the paradigm for the ethics of organ donation," *Philosophy, Ethics, & Humanities in Medicine* 2007;2: 8, www.peh-med.com/content/pdf/1747-5341-2-8.pdf.

19. Verheijde, Rady, McGregor, "Recovery."

20. Texas General Laws, section 521.401, "Statement of gift," www.statutes.legis.state.tx.us/Docs/TN/htm/TN.521.htm#521.401.

21. George C, "Texas gains ground on registering organ donors: Organ donors turning out in force in Texas—doubling of rolls credited to law requiring DPS clerks to ask question," *Houston Chronicle*, July 27, 2010, www.chron.com/news/houston-texas/article/Texas-gains-ground-on-registering-organ-donors-1695982.php; Donate Life America, *National Donor Designation Report Card*.

22. Donate Life America, *National Donor Designation Report Card*.

23. Ibid.

24. Donate Life America, *National Donor Designation Report Card*.

25. Wynn JJ, Alexander CE, "Increasing organ donation and transplantation: The US experience over the past decade," *Transplantation International* 2011;24 (4): 324–32, esp. table 1.

26. Simpkin AL, Robertson LC, Barber VS, Young JD, "Modifiable factors influencing relatives' decision to offer organ donation: Systematic review," *British Medical Journal* 2009;338: b991; DuBay DA, Redden DT, Haque A, et al., "Do trained specialists solicit familial authorization at equal frequency, regardless of deceased donor characteristics?" *Progress in Transplantation* 2013;23 (3): 290–96.

27. Gentry D, Brown-Holbert J, Andrews C, "Racial impact: Increasing minority consent rate by altering the racial mix of an organ procurement organization," *Transplantation Proceedings* 1997;29: 3758–59; Metzger RA, Taylor GJ, McGaw LJ, Weber PG, Delmonico FL, Prottas JM, for the UNOS Research to Practice Steering Committee, "Research to practice: A national consensus conference," *Progress in Transplantation* 2005;15: 379–84; Kurz RS, Scharff DP, Terry T, Alexander S, "Factors influencing organ donation decisions by African Americans: A review of the literature," *Medical Care Research and Review* 2007;64: 475–517; Bratton C, Chavin K, Baliga P, "Racial disparities in organ donation and why," *Current Opinion in Organ Transplantation* 2011;16: 243–49.

28. Anker AE, Feeley, TH, "Asking the difficult questions: Message strategies used by organ procurement coordinators in requesting familial consent to organ donation," *Journal of Health Communication* 2011;16 (6): 643–59.

29. Joint Commission on Accreditation of Healthcare Organizations, *Health Care at the crossroads: Narrowing the organ donation gap and protecting patients* (Washington, DC: Joint Commission on Accreditation of Healthcare Organization, 2004).

30. Zink S, Wertlieb S, "A study of the presumptive approach to consent for organ donation: A new solution to an old problem," *Critical Care Nursing* 2006;26: 129–36.

31. Streat S, "Clinical review: Moral assumptions and the process of organ donation in the intensive care unit," *Critical Care* 2004;8 (5): 382–88; Rady MY, McGregor JL, Verheijde JL, "Mass media campaigns and organ donation: Managing conflicting messages and interests," *Medicine, Health Care and Philosophy* 2012;15: 229–41; Truog RD, "Consent for organ donation: Balancing conflicting ethical obligations," *New England Journal of Medicine* 2008;358: 1209–11.

32. Data from *Health Resources and Services Administration*, Organ Procurement and Transplantation Network, National Data, http://optn.transplant.hrsa.gov/latestData/step2.asp?.

33. Evans RW, Onans CE, Ascher NL, "The potential supply of organ donors: An assessment of the efficiency of organ procurement efforts in the United States," *JAMA* 1992;267: 243. This estimate is consistent with the finding of the 1993 Gallup Survey prepared for the Partnership for Organ Donation in 1993 that found that 37 percent were very likely to donate and another 32 percent somewhat likely.

34. Chon et al., "When the living and the deceased cannot agree," 176.

Chapter 10

Routine Salvaging and Presumed Consent

The donation model has dominated the theory of organ procurement in the English-speaking world, Germany, and the Netherlands. The main problem has been that it has not procured enough organs and is quite inefficient in requiring that donors actually make a documented donation decision before their death or that organ procurement organizations obtain a donation decision from the next of kin. In the earliest days of organ procurement, that was not the only model in the public policy discussion. One alternative was what was called "routine salvaging," the policy of authorizing the state to take organs from the deceased, often with the proviso (sometimes called "routine salvaging with opt-out") that people could prevent their organs from being taken after their death by recording their objection while they were alive. Sometimes this alternative is called—mistakenly, we claim below—"presumed consent." We explore routine procurement without explicit consent in this chapter. In the following chapter, we look at the third option: markets for organs and related strategies that permit organ transfer relying on financial and other incentives.

Routine Salvaging

The earliest thinking about the basis for procuring organs reflected the commonsense view that the body of the deceased—the "mortal remains"—was no longer of any use to the dead person. It was not even of any use to the surviving family. Thus a lawyer, Jesse Dukeminier, and a physician, David Sanders, proposed a model they called *routine salvaging*.[1] The idea was that no harm, in fact great good, could come from cadaver salvaging, so it was appropriate for society to routinely take any leftover viable parts without needing any formal permission.

In moral terms, this view was utilitarian. The morally right course was to be determined by estimating the total consequences of alternative courses of action and then choosing the one doing the greatest good. In this case it meant estimating the net good (the good minus any envisioned harms) that could come from simply treating useful body parts of the deceased as state property and then estimating the net good expected from alternative policies, including those that require some sort of permission be obtained to take the organs. Their conclusion was that, because no one would be harmed and some organ recipients could be given enormous benefits, the organs could simply be taken. "Salvage" without permission of the deceased or next of kin was the recommended policy.

This policy has in more recent times sometimes been called organ procurement with *presumed consent*, a concept that we explore in more detail later in this chapter.[2] Calling routine salvaging "presumed consent," we shall suggest, is a mistake—or at least an over-simplification. Thus, we shall continue to use the original, more graphic, if harsh term—routine salvaging. We do so without any implication that this approach is morally unacceptable before a review of the issues involved, noting that Dukeminier and Sanders, the original proponents of the approach, themselves used the term, obviously without implying anything negative.

The case for routine salvaging requires careful scrutiny. "Salvaging" is probably an unfortunate term, but it implies exactly what its defenders have in mind: picking over the trash and taking, without permission, what seems to have some residual value. The assumption that the human body can be used by the state without permission suggests the troublesome analogy of Nazi medical research. There, also, the presumption was made that certain humans could be used for the service of the state without permission. That is probably why Germany has been so strongly committed to the donation model.

The Nazi analogy is sometimes overused. An important difference in the case of salvaging of organs is that the humans who are being used are dead. Nevertheless, there are similarities in the reasoning. In both cases certain human bodies were considered to be outside the bounds of moral standing. Because of their lower status, they were considered accessible for others to use for their own purposes.

Even if those purposes were to turn out to be important and worthwhile, however, critics of the utilitarian approach to the use of one person's body by another consider the moral premise totally inadequate. The most obvious lesson of the Nazi experience is that one cannot use another person's body for the good of society without permission. That is the first and most critical point of the Nuremberg Code, which reads:

> The voluntary consent of the human subject is absolutely essential. This means that the person involved should have legal capacity to give consent; should be so situated as to be able to exercise free power of choice, without the intervention of any element of force, fraud, deceit, duress, overreaching, or other ulterior form of constraint or coercion; and should have sufficient knowledge and comprehension of the elements of the subject matter involved as to enable him or her to make an understanding and enlightened decision. The latter element requires that before the acceptance of an affirmative decision by the experimental subject he or she should know the nature, duration, and purpose of the experiment; the method and means by which it is to be conducted; all inconveniences and hazards reasonably to be expected; and the effects upon the health or person which may possibly come from participation in the experiment. The duty and responsibility for ascertaining the quality of the consent rests upon each individual who initiates, directs, or engages in the experiment. It is a personal duty and responsibility which may not be delegated to another with impunity.[3]

This notion of consent, which is so central to the Nuremberg approach to human subjects research, is equally critical for the second approach to organ procurement. Critics of routine salvaging have expressed similar concerns about procuring organs without explicit permission of the one from whom they are taken or, at least, a surrogate such as the next of kin. Nevertheless, as the gap between the number of people needing organs and the number of donors increases, some people—particularly in countries with less robust commitments to individualism—have developed a renewed interest in routine salvaging or procurement without explicit consent. Thus the countries of Southern Europe, Scandinavia, Asia, and South America have adopted laws that permit procurement without consent (figure 10.1).

There seems to be an unmistakable pattern: Areas of the world with more sympathy for the common good, socialism, or Catholicism tend to show up on the list. Those more individualist or Protestant tend not to. However, even the most individualistic countries, such as the United States, have endorsed some duties of their citizens to contribute to the welfare of society, imposing some such duties independent of the consent of the citizen. Thus the United States has imposed income and other taxes and has even imposed military conscription at certain periods of its history. Hence, the relation between the individual and the interests of the state is in dynamic tension, whereby even the firmest believers in individual rights and the priority of the individual over the state recognize some legitimate state interest that gives society authority over the individual and even the firmest believers in communitarian or socialist views recognize some rights of the individual.

Some involved in organ procurement have boldly embraced the salvaging model. Aaron Spital, the former medical director of the New York Organ Donor Network, in language that conjures up compulsory entry into the military, has referred to the approach as "organ conscription."[4] Most people, however, even in countries with laws authorizing procurement without explicit consent, soften the model in one way or another, adding an "opt-out" provision or referring to it as "presumed consent."

Figure 10.1 Countries Procuring Organs without Explicit Consent

Asia	France	**Scandinavia**
Singapore	Greece	Finland
	Italy	Norway
Africa	Portugal	Sweden
Tunisia	Spain	
	Costa Rica	**Central and South America**
Eastern Europe	Dominican Republic	Argentina
Croatia	(limited)	Brazil (1997–1998)
Czech Republic	Ecuador	Chile
Hungary	Panama	Colombia
Poland	Paraguay (limited)	Uruguay
Slovakia		Venezuela
Southern Europe		
Austria		
Belgium		

Note: "Limited" = case-by-case judicial approval when no next of kin is available.

An Opt-Out

One problem with routine salvaging is that some people object to having their organs procured after they die. For religious, aesthetic, or philosophical reasons, they wish to be buried whole or otherwise have their bodies remain intact. Routine salvaging would interfere with these desires. Some would insist that laws authorizing routine salvaging violate a basic right of the individual, a property right, or quasi–property right over the body that includes the authority to control what is done with the body after death. A state that routinely takes body parts without proper consent is interfering with this right.

To respond to these moral objections to routine salvaging and to decrease the practical, political problems created by those who object, some propose an "opt-out," a mechanism whereby those who object to having organs and tissues procured can register their objection and be protected from routine procurement. Various mechanisms are proposed—recording one's objection in a donor registry, carrying a donor card with a refusal to donate indicated, or otherwise documenting the fact one is opting out. This has the advantage of giving those who strongly object a way of recording their objection while still capturing the organs of those who have no principled objection to donation but simply have not had the momentum to record willingness to donate.

Libertarian Altruism and Changing the Default

The opt-out policy approach changes the "default" from nondonation to donation (or, more carefully, to the status of supplier of organs, because no act of donation need occur for organs to be procured). Such approaches have captured the attention of recent theorists dealing with "libertarian paternalism" and "libertarian altruism" in the field of behavioral economics who are addressing public policies that make use of techniques of framing and manipulation of "choice architecture" to encourage people to make good or valuable choices without infringing on their autonomy.[5]

If the goal is to structure choices so that they are better for the one doing the choosing, the policies are generally called "libertarian paternalism." Structuring retirement plan choices with regular contributions to one's 401(k) plan as the default, with the employee having to opt out rather than requiring the employee to sign up to have contributions withheld from his or her pay, would be a classic example of a libertarian paternalism. The employee is free to autonomously choose to opt out, so the claim is that the strategy is libertarian; but setting the default to produce a result that is presumed to be in the employee's long-term interest is done for paternalistic reasons—to make the employee better off.

Thaler and Sunstein specifically propose maximizing organ procurement by setting the default so that organs can be procured following death. They include an opt-out provision, insisting that the opt-out should be a minimal burden, thus preserving what they believe is the freedom of the individual to avoid having organs procured. In Thaler's words, "So long as the costs of registering as a donor or a nondonor are low, the results should be similar. But many findings of behavioral economics show that tiny disparities in such rules can make a big difference."[6] More straightforwardly, procurement policies without explicit consent are not designed to be for the benefit of the one from whom organs will be procured, but rather for the benefit of those others who will receive the organs. Hence, these policies might more appropriately be called *libertarian altruism.*[7]

Opt-Out and the Procurement Rate

Thaler illustrates his point by comparing his data on organ procurement rates in Austria, which has an opt-out system in which, according to him, 99 percent give their consent, with Germany, which has a similar culture, but an opt-in system, in which only 12 percent consent.[8]

However, the facts are actually more complex than Thaler would have us believe. First, when he says that in Austria 99 percent give their consent, what he apparently means is that only about 1 percent have recorded objections. This does not mean that anyone has actually given consent, and there is good reason to believe that, even if many, perhaps most, would consent if asked, considerably more than 1 percent would refuse. Second, when he says that in Germany only 12 percent give their consent, he apparently means that 12 percent have actually registered as donors or signed donor cards. Considerably more organs are procured, however, presumably relying on other mechanisms such as family approval in cases where the deceased has not objected. In fact, Germany has 15.3 donors of organs per 1 million population, whereas Austria procures organs (most presumably have not actually been donated by the deceased person) at a rate of 18.8 per 1 million population.[9] Thus, there appears to be a somewhat higher procurement rate in the Austrian opt-out system, but it is not nearly as dramatic a difference as Thaler would have us believe. Likewise, other countries relying on opt-out systems sometimes have high procurement rates. Spain's rate is 33.8 per 1 million population, but some other opt-out countries have rates lower than Germany's (Luxembourg, 12.0 per 1 million population; Slovak Republic, 12.1; and Cyprus, 5.7).

There is general agreement that procurement rates are multifactorial. The difference between explicit donation (opt-in) and salvaging (opt-out) is one factor that probably influences the rate. Other factors are also influential, however. These include per capita gross domestic product, health expenditure rates, religious and philosophical belief systems, the national willingness to transplant organs, and the patterns in the causes of death.[10] Scholarly studies that have attempted to use regression analyses to estimate the impact of an opt-out policy suggest that, overall, there is a modest increase in organ procurement with an opt-out system. In a study published in 2003 Johnson and Goldstein estimated, based on a regression analysis of data from seventeen European countries, a 16 percent increase in the donation rate if an opt-out system is used.[11] Abadie and Gay, in a cross-national comparative study published in 2006, estimated a 25 to 30 percent increase in organ procurement compared with countries relying on explicit consent models.[12] More recently, Horvat and colleagues have found a similar higher rate of deceased donor kidney transplants in twenty-two countries relying on routine salvaging (what they called "presumed consent") when compared with twenty-two countries with explicit consent policies.[13] They found that this relation held when controlling for per capita gross domestic product, health expenditures, and physician density.

Because the United States already has authorization and conversion rates of about 75 percent, the most that could be added would be another 25 percent. In reality, some would opt out, if an opt-out system were adopted. It is likely that some small, but undetermined, number would opt out who have currently opted in, or would have next-of-kin consent to procurement. It seems reasonable to assume that an opt-out system would add a small increase on balance to the number of organs procured from deceased, medically suitable organ sources. This increase would come from some who would have been willing to consent explicitly in advance but have never gotten around to it. It would also come from some who object in varying degrees and a significant number of people who do not care enough one way or the other to register as a donor or record an objection in an opt-out system. An opt-out system would, however, also capture organs from some people who have strong, principled objections but do not understand the mechanism of opting out or do not have the capacity to make the system work for them. Some organs would be taken from some people who have a clear objection.

Opt-Out Morality

This raises the underlying moral issue: Is it unethical to place the state in a position vis-à-vis the individual such that it can take parts of the individual's body without asking permission? What is at stake is no less than the fundamental question of the relation of the individual to the state. It is not an accident that more individual-rights-oriented, Protestant countries of northern Europe tend to favor the donation model but the countries less committed to the individual's priority to the state—the countries of Southern Europe, more socialist Scandinavia, and Asia—tend to support routine salvaging.

Adding the opt-out provision makes the philosophical underpinnings of salvaging more complex. Opt-out is surely an opening to more respect for the rights of individuals. Some may believe that there is an inherent right of the individual to object, but that it is not a strong enough right to require explicit consent. Others may be less willing to grant such a right, but rather incorporate the opt-out provision on a more practical ground of wanting to avoid the hostility to an organ procurement program that would come from someone forced to provide organs against his or her will.

One might view the opt-out choice as analogous to conscientious objection to a military draft. The overwhelming social consensus is that the state is justified in conscripting recruits into the military to serve the common good; but at the same time, the state tolerates religious objectors to war. It does so in part out of respect for the ethical concerns of those who have strong commitments to what can be considered a higher authority, and in part out of a practical need to defuse the hostility of a small group whose members would plausibly do more harm than good to the social cause. Similar reasoning may be behind the policy of including an opt-out provision in policies that would procure organs without consent.

One problem with opt-out provisions is that they may be unfair to those who are least capable of learning about and understanding the need to opt out if one does not want organs procured under a routine salvaging policy. Most likely, this would be the poorly educated, those least plugged in to mass media that would make the possibility of opting out known, and the economically poorly off. For example, those with a poor education will be less likely to be exposed to the procurement policy and understand the option of opting out. Those without automobiles and the elderly who no longer drive will be less likely to come into contact with the department of motor vehicles donor registries that could provide the mechanism for opting out. If income tax returns were to be used to document unwillingness to donate, those who do not file tax returns would be out of the loop.

Thaler and Sunstein recognize that, if the behavioral economic strategy of setting defaults is followed in a way that promotes the altruism of providing organs, at a minimum it must be easy to register dissent. One objection to opt-out policies is that it will be harder for certain groups to opt out and therefore be unfair to them.

There is also a vaguer, but pervasive, objection to opt-out policies. Some people are repulsed at the notion that the state can do something to the individual and that, if the individual does not approve, he or she must take preventive action to circumvent the state's preemptory power to intervene. At least symbolically, requiring the individual to act in order to keep his or her body parts after death may seem intrusive to those who value individual freedom.

The Morality of Salvaging

It is a provocative reality that even those countries that have adopted routine salvaging laws seem uncomfortable with the concept. They are attracted to the widely held belief that they will increase the yield of organs and will make the procurement system more efficient, thus saving more lives; but they at least want to include an opt-out provision out of respect for the concerns of the minority who have objections to the procurement of organs from the dead body.

It seems fair to say that the peoples of the world are moving on a long-term trajectory that gives more respect to the rights of the individual and is more circumspect about the use of state power to override individual choices. This is especially true when the interests of others are not jeopardized by showing such respect, but it is present even if the lives of others are at risk. It is likely that various countries with different cultures will balance the conflict between the individual and society differently, and that some will come down on the side of routine procurement without explicit consent. Even those cultures will, however, incorporate opt-outs and may continue to give families de facto veto over procurement, even if the individual has not exercised the opt-out.

Presumed Consent

Given the lingering discomfort with the salvaging model, it is important to examine the concept of *presumed consent* and the widely held linguistic convention that refers to organ procurement proposals and laws as "presumed consent" policies. Instead of going through the agony of getting actual donations, we could simply presume the consent of anyone who failed to record his or her objection to organ procurement. For many years, the idea of *presumed consent* has captured the imagination of many of those particularly hungry for organs.[14] It continues to be the dominant term to refer to policies that authorize the taking of organs without explicit consent.[15] Even if one is not categorically opposed to taking organs without consent, there is good reason to object to policies labeled "presumed consent." The term has the appearance of a desperate attempt to hold on to the model of consent and donation by using the language of consent for what is really a policy of routine salvaging, that is, taking organs without consent. It is simply dishonest to claim that we can presume that someone would consent when the empirical evidence shows that presumption would be wrong as much as half the time. It dresses salvaging in the flimsy outer garb of the consent doctrine. Instead, if one favors salvaging, it is far better to admit it openly.

In spite of the problems with the terminology, the expression *presumed consent* is so widespread that it deserves further analysis. Here is what appears to be the situation. The acute shortage of organs for transplantation has led to considerable interest in a particular type of laws that are designed to increase the number of organs procured and that are often referred to as "presumed consent" laws. Such laws are alleged in many popular and scholarly articles to exist in several European countries and Singapore, among other places. The reasoning behind recent arguments in favor of adopting a so-called presumed consent law in the United States is that if we can presume the consent of the deceased to organ procurement, there will be a substantial increase in the yield of organs.

The Difference between Presumed Consent and Salvaging

The problem with "presumed consent" is that, with a few exceptions, the existing laws never actually claim to presume consent, nor can they rightly be said to do so. They simply authorize the state's taking of the organs without explicit permission. It therefore seems wrong to call them presumed consent laws. They are, in effect, *routine salvaging* laws.[16] We believe the time has come to be more careful in distinguishing between policies of *presumed consent* and those of *routine salvaging*. Although the net outcome may be the same under either kind of policy, the underlying assumptions about the relation of the individual to society are radically different.

It is our hypothesis that those who support a societal right to procure organs without consent find it embarrassing to speak bluntly about taking organs without consent; hence, they adopt the *language* of presuming consent even when there is no *basis* for such a presumption. In doing so, they preserve the appearance of the preferred gift mode and the guise of respect for individual choice.

This desire for euphemistic language is also seen in the persistent practice of referring to persons from whom organs are taken as *donors*—even in cases, such as those involving small children, where these people could never have actually made a gift or donation. We suggest that important matters of societal relations are at stake in distinguishing between policies that allow the procurement of organs on the presumption that people would consent and those that simply take organs without consent. One form of society gives central place to the individual, holding that a person can be used by the state only with some form of consent. This has been the society of liberal Western culture, particularly the United States. It underlies the donation model and the doctrine of consent that for decades has been central not only to organ procurement but also to the practice of medicine in general.

Another form of society gives more central authority to the community or state, authorizing it to use the individual for important societal purposes even without individual consent. This form underlies routine salvaging, or the taking of organs without consent. For the purposes of this chapter, we are not pressing for one form of policy or the other. It is possible that the time has come to elevate the role of the state by adopting a routine salvaging law, at least in some societies. This seems to be the rationale behind new movements working toward enhancing communitarianism and stressing the common good in social policy.[17] It is also possible that the importance of the individual continues to require procuring organs in the gift or donation mode, whereby organs may be taken only with proper permission. The conflation of these two is, we suggest in the next sections, indeed a dangerous prospect.

The State of the Law

There is a broad tendency to claim that countries that permit routine salvaging do so on the grounds of presumed consent. In this section we show that most European countries do not use the language of presumed consent, but that it is common in Central and South America. We then explore two potential justifications for presuming consent and conclude that the arguments fail, and that taking without explicit consent would require one to hold that societal interest should take priority over the rights of the individual.

Countries with Routine Salvaging Laws

This subsection addresses countries with routine salvaging laws, with no claim of presuming consent.[18] It is striking that it is so common for commentators to refer to these laws as "presumed consent" laws. For example, according to Gerson, the French law on organ procurement adopted in 1976 is one that presumes the consent of persons who do not, during their lifetime, expressly refuse to have their organs taken upon their death.[19] However, upon examination of the law itself, one is hard-pressed to find any mention of presuming consent, overt or implicit. The law states that "an organ to be used for therapeutic or scientific purposes may be removed from the cadaver of a person who has not during his lifetime made known his refusal of such a procedure."[20] Although the law offers a provision for those willing and able to record their dissent, it is not clear why we should conclude that the rationale behind the opting-out system it establishes is based upon the presumed consent of the decedent rather than the primacy of the state. Gerson, citing a 1984 *Transplantation Proceedings* article by Cantaluppi, also attributes presumed consent laws to Austria, Belgium, the former Czechoslovakia, Finland, Italy, Norway, Spain, and Switzerland, among other countries. However, in 1984 *not one* of these laws mentioned anything about presuming consent, directly or indirectly.[21] Among the other countries that in the twenty-first century (as of August 2013) have laws authorizing organ procurement without claiming to presume consent are Austria,[22] Belgium,[23] Costa Rica,[24] the Dominican Republic,[25] France,[26] Italy,[27] Luxembourg,[28] Norway,[29] Paraguay,[30] Portugal,[31] Singapore,[32] and Spain[33]—and earlier research had also identified such laws in Cyprus,[34] Hungary,[35] Syria,[36] and the former Yugoslavia.[37] Some of these countries have been referred to in the literature as countries with presumed consent laws, yet none of them actually claims to presume consent in its legislation. (We are indebted to Thomas Gerkin for the extensive research on the laws of countries related to organ procurement.)

Laws with an Explicit Presumption of Consent

By contrast, we have located a few laws and proposed laws that do actually state a presumption of consent or its equivalent. Most of these are in countries of Central and South America, such as Ecuador and Uruguay.[38] Some have existed for many years without there being any discussion defending or criticizing the presumption of consent. For example, the Colombian law on organ procurement dated 1988 states that "there shall be a legal presumption of donation if a person during his lifetime has refrained from exercising his right to object to the removal from his body of anatomical organs or parts during his death."[39] This language is repeated in a legal decree of 2004.[40] Several other South and Central American countries—such as Argentina,[41] Chile,[42] Panama,[43] and Venezuela[44]—follow a similar pattern of using language such as "donation shall be presumed" or "the person shall be considered a donor" or "presumed to donate." In some cases the language is virtually identical in different countries, suggesting a borrowing of legislative language.

Mexico is an interesting case. It explicitly refers to the "tacit consent" of one who has not expressed his or her opposition to donation, but it permits procurement only if the actual consent of one of a list of relatives has been obtained.[45] Technically, this would impute consent to the one who is the source of the organ when all that seems to be obtained is the consent of the relative. De facto, this makes Mexico's law essentially identical to opt-in laws.

On July 2, 2013, Wales became the first English-speaking political entity to formally endorse organ procurement without explicit consent.[46] Its law, which is scheduled to take effect in 2015, specifies that organ procurement is lawful only if done with consent; but then it distinguishes between "express consent" and what it calls "deemed consent." Consent is "deemed" unless a person recorded an objection while alive, appointed someone else to handle the question of procurement upon his or her death, or has friends or family members who know of his or her objection.

In explicitly requiring (at least nominal) consent, Welsh law differs from most routine-salvage countries in Europe, which do not claim to base their laws on consent. Moreover, Wales's "deeming" of consent amounts to something like "presuming." Typically, to deem is to believe or judge something to be the case, not merely to declare it, so the rules for when consent shall be deemed would seem to reflect epistemic judgments (or presumptions) about when a person has consented rather than simply treating the person as if consent had actually be given. This seems to be a bold, if implausible, effort to clothe procurement without consent in the garb of the donation model in which consent is the foundation. Whether Wales is the first of an inevitable series of English and Germanic entities to abandon explicit consent remains to be seen.

Within the United States, at least two states have considered laws that would, if enacted, have *properly* been called presumed consent laws. In Maryland, a bill proposed on March 10, 1993, if it had not been defeated, would have allowed for the presumption of consent of those who did not opt out. It also used the language of "deeming." It read: "In the absence of specific objection by an individual expressed during that individual's lifetime, or by any of the individual's next of kin immediately following the individual's death, the individual is deemed to have consented to the donation of the individual's body or any part of the individual's body for any of the purposes specified."[47] In Pennsylvania, a subchapter titled "Presumed Anatomical Gifts," of a proposed amendment to an act, reads: "Organs and tissues may be removed, upon death, from the body of any Commonwealth resident by a physician or surgeon for transplantation or for the preparation of therapeutic substances, unless it is established that a refusal was expressed."[48] Both these proposed law changes adopted the language of presuming (or deeming) consent. This, of course, begs the question of whether consent can actually be presumed in these jurisdictions at all.

Two Justifications for Taking without Explicit Consent

If one is considering organ procurement laws that would authorize taking organs without explicit consent, two justifications might be considered. First, one might hold that the interests of others in society sometimes are so great that laws are acceptable that jeopardize the welfare of the individual and even violate some presumptive rights of the individual. Something like this stands behind income tax law and compulsory military conscription, and also lesser infringements such as driver's license requirements, laws prohibiting the practice of medicine without a license, laws requiring a prescription to buy certain potentially dangerous medications, and so forth.

The most directly analogous laws that permit society to remove organs from a dead body without the consent of the deceased or the next of kin are the medical examiners' laws authorizing an autopsy in cases where a public health risk or criminal prosecution is at stake. The societal interest is so overwhelming that the agents of society are authorized to act, even against the strong objection of the deceased or next of kin. In controversial cases, a court order might be required for the medical examiner to proceed. The consent of the deceased is considered irrelevant. If society wants to take organs in order to save lives by transplanting medically suitable ones, one might argue that the societal good justifies taking without consent in much the same way that medical examiners can conduct an autopsy without consent.

A second rationale for taking organs without explicit consent is very different. It does not rely primarily on the common good or the right of society to override individual rights. Rather, it relies on the moral concepts derived from the donation model—the right of the individual to control his or her own body and the necessity of getting the approval of the individual before the body or its parts are used for important social purposes.

Those who hold this general view may recognize that some people may be willing to agree to having their body invaded for good purposes but, for some reason, have not given that permission and are, at the critical moment, not in a position to do so (e.g., if they are already dead). To presume consent is to make an empirical claim. It is to claim that people *would consent* if asked, or, perhaps more precisely, that they would consent to a policy of taking organs without explicit permission. The reasoning behind true presumed consent laws is that it is legitimate to take organs without explicit consent because those from whom the organs are taken would have agreed if they had been asked when they were competent to respond.

This is the philosophical underpinning of the treatment for unconscious persons who need rapid intervention such as life support in an emergency room. It is widely recognized that emergency room personnel have the authority to treat such persons without waiting for them to recover to a condition in which they can give an actual consent. In these circumstances we recognize that virtually every person would want to be treated with lifesaving support and that it is acceptable to presume consent.[49] If we really doubted that a patient wanted to be treated, we would not make that presumption, but the empirical fact that virtually everyone would want to be treated justifies presuming consent.

The presumption of consent is, in effect, an empirical prediction that we can be very confident that the patients would consent if only they could. It is an open question just how confident we need to be. Especially if the patient would lose little or nothing if we did not intervene, we would want the data to be very strong before we made the claim that the patient would have consented. Otherwise, we would be violating the right not to be touched without consent of all those patients who would not in fact have consented.

Social survey evidence has, since the 1990s, made clear that if we assume people would agree to having their organs procured if they were asked, we would be wrong at least 25 percent of the time. A 1993 Gallup poll shows that only 37 percent of Americans are "very likely" to want their organs transplanted after their death, and only 32 percent are "somewhat likely." Furthermore, only about 75 percent are willing to grant formal permission for organ removal. It should also be noted that although 75 percent are *willing* to grant permission, in the 1990s only 28 percent had *actually* done so.[50] In other words, only about half the Americans who are willing to grant permission have taken the proactive steps necessary to do so, creating a large number of *false negatives*. We might expect that if America's were an opting-out system, we might also see a large number of *false positives*.

Since the 1990s the data have indicated a greater willingness to donate. The National Donor Designation Report Card for 2013 gives a national donor designation rate of 42 percent. Perhaps more relevant, the actual authorization rate reported by organ procurement organizations is in the neighborhood of 75 percent, but that includes authorizations by the next of kin.

Perhaps even more pertinent to this discussion are the relative proportions of Americans who would agree to the system of presumed consent itself, as the ethos of the presumed consent mode would seem to demand. One survey from the early 1990s, when presumed consent laws were being proposed, showed that only 38 percent of Americans agree with presumed consent, defined as a system in which doctors routinely remove organs from deceased persons unless the person indicated a wish to the contrary while alive.[51] To this day, no empirical data for the United States have ever shown majority support for presuming consent.

On the basis of even larger estimates of a willingness to donate, it is clear that there can be no ground for presuming consent. We would likely be wrong at least a quarter of the time. Claiming such a presumption is an ill-informed notion at best; it is an outright deception at worst.

Using the presumed consent doctrine as it has been developed for the justification of treatment without explicit consent as a basis for procuring organs is simply not empirically justified. It is clear that in no place in the world would there be an empirical basis for presuming that a newly dead individual would have consented to organ donation. The error rate in making this presumption would be at least 25 percent, and more in some cultures.

It is interesting to ask exactly what percentage of people would need to agree to a policy when surveyed before we can presume that individuals being treated by that policy would have consented. One's first instinct might be to assume that a majority must indicate endorsement of the policy, but that surely is wrong. It would lead to an erroneous presumption of consent almost half the time. If falsely presuming consent constitutes a violation of a right not to have one's body invaded, we cannot tolerate such a violation nearly 50 percent of the time.

One possibility is to take a figure of 95 percent approval in a survey as sufficient to presume that any one individual would have consented, if asked. That would mean that 5 percent of the time, we would have erred in presuming that the individual would have consented. (Even then, the rights of individuals would be violated 5 percent of the time.) In a society that affirms the right of the individual not to have his or her body invaded without appropriate consent, procuring organs on the basis of a presumption of consent will violate that right at least 25 percent of the time.

What is at stake, under the theory of consent, is the justification for invasion of the body. Without consent, a fundamental right would be violated, according to those who acknowledge the priority of the individual in the control of the body. It is not sufficient that a majority would not object. As in the case of emergency room treatment, support for presumption must be very strong.

Thus, even if we are justified in presuming consent for emergency room life support, there is no empirical basis for presuming consent for organ procurement. This says nothing about whether procurement without consent is justified based on a theory of what individuals owe to the common good. It does make clear that if organs are to be procured without explicit consent, the procurement cannot be based on the presumed consent concept. If we are to procure without explicit consent, we need to acknowledge that the basis for such procurement is the priority of societal interest over the rights of the individual. We need to label procurement accordingly as routine salvaging or as the conscription of organs, or with some similar term that does not imply the model of consent and donation.

What Is at Stake

What is at stake is something very fundamental: the ethics of the relation of the individual to society. A pioneer in the study of contemporary medical ethics, Paul Ramsey, introduced this issue in distinguishing between organ procurement in the modes of "giving" and "taking."[52] In liberal Western society, certain rights are attributed to the individual. Among these is the right to control what is done with one's body.

The alternative is the mode of "taking"—or what we have, following Dukeminier and Sanders, called "routine salvaging." In this model the central authority has claims over the individual without relying on the individual's consent or approval. In the donation model, the individual is prior to the state; in the alternative, the individual is subordinate. This underscores the problems associated with the casual misuse of the term "presumed consent." Many authors merely confuse presumed consent and routine salvaging, claiming that they are the same thing.[53] Others have implied that their versions of so-called presumed consent can be justified by the concept of eminent domain.[54] However, eminent domain involves the taking of private property for public use, and has no bearing on questions of consent. Clearly a system that validly presumes the consent of persons does not—cannot—rely upon notions of eminent domain.

Choosing the language of legitimating organ procurement is, in effect, choosing how we want to see the individual in relation to the state. Those who use the language of presumed consent are trying to hold on to the liberal model in which gift giving is the foundation of organ procurement. In cases where consent can validly be presumed, presumed consent seems consistent with such an orientation. However, in cases where the evidence makes clear that consent cannot be presumed, this language is simply a disguise for the less acceptable reality of the state's authority over the individual.

This in itself, of course, does not make routine salvaging wrong; it is, however, deceptive if one advocates such a relationship in the name of the more liberal mode of gift giving and consenting. Such deception is a moral affront to the members of a society that has been built upon respect for the rights of the individual.

It is worth speculating about why there is this strong propensity to use the language of presuming consent when the apparent intention is to take organs without consent. One possibility is that, at least in countries reflecting liberal political philosophy's affirmation of the rights of the individual, it is more comforting to use the language of gift giving and consent. This leaves the impression of the priority of the individual. Thus there is a strong tendency to use the language of the gift mode—to call one who supplies organs a "donor"—even in cases where the source of the organs may be a small child who never could have made an actual donation and in cases where a medical examiner rather than the individual whose organs are being taken is the one approving the procurement. The language of consent is more comfortable, and this comfortableness may be necessary to win approval for policies that de facto authorize procurement without donation. But if routine salvaging is to become public policy, it needs to be defended on its own merits rather than being disguised as a variant of the donation model.

Notes

1. Dukeminier J, Sanders D, "Organ transplantation: A proposal for routine salvaging of cadaver organs," *New England Journal of Medicine* 1968;279: 413–19.

2. Marwick C, "British ponder 'presumed consent' for organ harvesting," *JAMA* 1984;251: 1522; Caplan AL, "Organ transplants: The costs of success, an argument for presumed consent and oversight," *Hastings Center Report* 1983;13 (6): 23–32; Matas AJ, Veith FJ, "Presumed consent for organ retrieval," *Theoretical Medicine* 1984;5: 155–66; Matas AJ, Veith FJ, "Presumed consent: A more humane approach cadaver organ donation," in *Positive approaches to living with end-stage renal disease: Psychosocial and thanatological aspects*, ed. Hardy MA, Appel BG, Kierrnan JM, et al. (New York: Praeger, 1986, 37–51); Gerson WN, "Refining the law of organ donation: Lessons from the French law of presumed consent," *New York University Journal of International Law and Politics* 1987;19 (4): 1013–32; Hull AR, "Dwindling donations make presumed consent a proposal worthy of consideration," *Nephrology News & Issues* 1990;4 (10): 28–29.

3. "Nuremberg Code, 1947," in *Encyclopedia of bioethics*, revised edition, vol. 5, ed. Reich WT (New York: Free Press, 1995), 2763–64.

4. Spital A., Erin CA, "Conscription of cadaveric organs for transplantation: Let's at least talk about it," *American Journal of Kidney Diseases* 2002;39: 611–15.

5. Thaler RH., Sunstein CR, *Nudge: Improving decisions about health, wealth, and happiness* (London: Penguin Books, 2008).

6. Thaler RH, "Opting in vs. opting out," *New York Times*, Sept. 26, 2009, www.nytimes.com/2009/09/27/business/economy/27view.html?_r = 0.

7. In the case of organ procurement, some continue to refer to such policies as libertarian *paternalism.* Because any individual might be either the one from whom organs are taken or the one receiving them, it has been argued that the policy is really for the benefit of everyone and therefore is paternalistic. See Nair-Collins M, "On brain death, paternalism, and the language of 'death,'" *Kennedy Institute of Ethics Journal* 2013;23: 53–104.

8. Thaler, "Opting in vs. opting out."

9. Council of Europe, Directorate General for Health and Consumers, *Council of Europe (2007) deceased organ donors in the European Union*, http://ec.europa.eu/danmark/documents/alle_emner/sociale/081208_organ-forslag-5.pdf.

10. Rithalia A, McDaid C, Suekarran S, Myers L, Sowden A, "Impact of presumed consent for organ donation on donation rates: A systematic review," *British Medical Journal* 2009;338 (7689): 284–87.

11. Johnson E, Goldstein, D. "Medicine: Do defaults save lives?" *Science* 2003;302 (5649): 1338–39.

12. Abadie A, Gay S, "The impact of presumed consent legislation on cadaveric organ donation: A cross-country study," *Journal of Health Economics* 2006;25 (4): 599–620.

13. Horvat LD, Cuerden MS, Kim SJ, Koval JJ, Young A, Garg AX, "Informing the debate: Rates of kidney transplantation in nations with presumed consent," *Annals of Internal Medicine* 2010;153 (10): 641–49, W-214-W-216.

14. Marwick C. "British ponder 'presumed consent' for organ harvesting." *JAMA* 1984;251 (12): 1522; Caplan, "Organ transplants"; Matas, Veith, "Presumed consent for organ retrieval"; Matas AJ, Veith, FJ. 1986, "Presumed consent"; Hull, "Dwindling donations."

15. Horvat et al., "Informing the debate"; Fabre J, Murphy P, Matesanz R, "Presumed consent: A distraction in the quest for increasing rates of organ donation," *BMJ (Clinical Research Ed.)* 2010: 341c4973; Martínez-Alarcón L, Ríos A, Sánchez J, et al., "Evaluation of the law of presumed consent after brain death by Spanish journalism students," *Transplantation Proceedings* 2010;42: 3109–12; Simillis C, "Do we need to change the legislation to a system of presumed consent to address organ shortage?" *Medicine, Science, and the Law* 2010;50 (2): 84–94; Cherkassky L., "Presumed consent in organ donation: Is the duty finally upon us?" *European Journal of Health Law* 2010;17 (2): 149–64; Orentlicher D, "Presumed consent to organ donation: Its rise and fall in the United States," *Rutgers Law Review* 2009;61 (2): 295–332; Neades BL, "Presumed consent to organ donation in three European countries," *Nursing Ethics* 2009;16 (3): 267–82; Verheijde JL, Rady MY, McGregor JL, Friederich-Murray C, "Enforcement of presumed-consent policy and willingness to donate organs as identified in the European Union survey: The role of legislation in reinforcing ideology in pluralistic societies," *Health Policy* 2009;90 (1): 26–31; Rithalia et al., "Impact of presumed consent"; Pelleriaux B, Roels L, Van Deynse D, Smits J, Cornu O, Delloye C., "An analysis of critical care staff's attitudes to donation in a country with presumed-consent legislation," *Progress in Transplantation* 2008;18 (3): 173–78; Hamm D, Tizzard J, "Presumed consent for organ donation is an ethical and effective way of dealing with organ donation shortages," *British Medical Journal* 2008;336 (7638): 230.

16. Dukeminier, Sanders, "Organ transplantation."

17. Callahan D, *What kind of life: The limits of medical progress* (New York: Simon & Schuster, 1990).

18. The authors gratefully acknowledge the help of the following persons, consulted regarding foreign legislation: Francesc Abel, SJ, Edwin Bernat, Father Antonio Puca, Knut W. Ruyter, and Paul Schotsmans.

19. Gerson, "Refining the law."

20. Farfor J, "Organs for transplant: Courageous legislation," *British Medical Journal* 1977;1 (6059): 497.

21. "Austrian Law of June 1, 1982," *International Digest of Health Legislation* (hereafter, *IDHL*) 1986;37 (1): 332–33; "Belgian Law of June 13, 1986," *IDHL* 1987;38 (3):523–27; "Czechoslovakian Mandatory Directives of February 27, 1978." *IDHL* 1982;3 (3): 477–79; "Finnish Law of April 26, 1985," *IDHL* 1985;36 (4): 971–72; "Italian Law of December 2, 1975," *IDHL* 1977;28 (3): 621–27; Puca A, *Trapianto di cuore e morte cerebrale del donatore* (Turin: Edizione Camilliane, 1993), 128–33, 201–24; "Lov om tansplantasjon og avgivelse av lik m.m.," Feb. 9, 1973; "Ley de Octubre 1979," no. 30/79, art. 5.3; "Swiss Regulation of September 17, 1984," *IDHL* 1985;36 (1): 50.

22. "Bundesgesetzblatt Für Die Republik Österreich," Austria, 1982, www.ris.bka.gv.at/Dokumente/ BgblPdf/1982_273_0/1982_273_0.pdf.

23. "Justel: Législation consolidée," Belgium, 1987, www.ejustice.just.fgov.be/cgi_loi/change_lg .pl?language = fr&la = F&table_name = loi&cn = 1986061337.

24. "Detalle de leyes," Costa Rica, 1994, www.asamblea.go.cr/Centro_de_Informacion/Consultas_ SIL/Pginas/Detalle%20Leyes.aspx?Numero_Ley = 7409.

25. "Ley de Donación de Órganos y Tejidos Humanos," Dominican Republic, http://www.senado .gov.do/masterlex/MLX/docs/1C/2/11/18/1FB7.htm.

26. "Code de la santé publique: Article L1211-2," France, 2014, www.legifrance.gouv.fr/affich CodeArticle.do?idArticle = LEGIARTI000006686058&cidTexte = LEGITEXT000006072665.

27. "Disposizioni in materia di prelievi e di trapianti di organi e di tessuti," Italy, 1999, www .parlamento.it/parlam/leggi/99091l.htm. Italy's law is a less clear-cut absence of "presumed consent" than others. It mandates the creation of a medico-legal infrastructure to (1) inform the populace of this law's effects, (2) request a statement of their will concerning organ donation, and (3) inform them that failure to respond will be considered consent to donate. Though not exactly "presumed consent" per se, this seems to be at least closer conceptually to presumed consent than many other countries.

28. "Law of November 1982 regulating the removal of substances of human origin," Luxembourg, 1982, http://books.google.com/books?id = mdKmqOng268C&pg = PA256&lpg = PA256&dq = Law + of + November + 25, + 1982 + Regulating + the + Extraction + of + Substanc es + of + Human + Origin& source = bl&ots = H2ZYHl6BpJ&sig = ZAD4m YUUlcKuJGIW0stV_L7bwQ0&hl = en&sa = X&ei = r TYuUq_HKc2g4AP_y4HQAg&ved = 0CCkQ6AEwAA#v = onepage&q = Law%20of%20November %2025%2C%201982%20Regulating%20the%20Extraction%20of%20Substances%20of%20Human% 20Origin&f = false.

29. "Chapter 1: Transplantation," Norway, 1973, www.ub.uio.no/ujur/ulovdata/lov-19730209-006 -eng.pdf.

30. http://paraguay.justia.com/nacionales/leyes/ley-1246-may-19-1998/gdoc/. Accessed Mar. 30, 2014.

31. "Decreto do presidente da república no. 9/93," Portugal, 1993, http://dre.pt/pdf1sdip/1993/04/ 094A00/19611963.pdf.

32. "Human Organ Transplant Act, Chapter 131A," Singapore, 2012, http://statutes.agc.gov.sg/aol/ search/display/view.w3p≡ent = ebc9c3b4-6ca1-4ab3-811a-e018ce34e8ed;page = 0;query = DocId%3 Adb05e985-f8a0-4d61-a906-9fd39f3 b5ac9%20Depth%3A0%20ValidTime%3A19%2F08%2F2013 %20TransactionTime%3A19%2F08%2F2013%20Status%3AinforceR̃c = 0.

33. "Ley 30/1979, de 27 de octubre, sobre extracción y trasplante de órganos," Spain, 1979, www.boe.es/buscar/act.php?id = BOE-A-1979-26445.

34. "Cyprus Law of May 22, 1987," *IDHL* 1989;40 (4): 836–38.

35. "Hungarian Law of February 17, 1988," *IDHL* 1989;40 (3): 588–90.

36. "Syrian Law of December 20, 1986," *IDHL* 1987;38 (3): 530.

37. Yugoslavian Decree of October 18, 1990, *IDHL* 1992;42 (1): 46–51.

38. "Ley de trasplante de órganos y tejidos," no. 58, Ecuador, 2012, www.salud.gob.ec/wp-content/uploads/downloads/2012/09/LEYDETRASPLANTEDEORGANOSYTEJIDOS.pdf; "Ley 18.968, Donación y transplante de células, órganos y tejidos," Uruguay, 2012, http://200.40.229.134/Leyes/AccesoTextoLey.asp?Ley=18968.

39. "Colombian Law of December 20, 1988," *IDHL* 1990;41 (3): 436–37. See also the Argentinian law: "Trasplantes de órganos y materiales anatómicos Actos de disposición: Prohibiciones. Profesionales, Servicios y establecimentos, Procedimiento judicial especial (Ley 24.193, Art. 62, March 24, 1993), http://infoleg.mecon.gov.ar/infolegInternet/anexos/0-4999/591/texact.htm.

40. "Decreto 2493 de 2004, Agosto 4," Colombia, http://www.alcaldiabogota.gov.co/sisjur/normas/Norma1.jsp?i=14525.

41. "Trasplantes de organos y materiales anatomicos, Ley 24.193," Argentina, www.infoleg.gob.ar/infolegInternet/anexos/0-4999/591/norma.htm.

42. "Modifica la ley 19.451 respecto a la determinación de quiénes pueden ser considerados donantes de órganos," Chile, www.leychile.cl/Navegar?idNorma=1051662&idParte=0.

43. "General de transplantes de componentes anatomicos," Panama, www.asamblea.gob.pa/APPS/LEGISPAN/PDF_NORMAS/2010/2010/2010_572_1442.PDF.

44. "Ley sobre donación y trasplante de órganos, tejidos y células en seres humanos," Venezuela, http://200.44.118.181/sinidot/pantallas/LEY%20SOBRE%20DONACION%20 Y%20TRASPLANTE%20DE%20ORGANOS%20TEJIDOS%20Y%20CELULAS%20EN%20SERES%20HUMANOS.pdf.

45. "Ley general de salud," Mexico, 1984, www.cenatra.salud.gob.mx/descargas/contenido/normatividad/Ley_General_Salud.pdf.

46. "Human Transplantation (Wales) Bill," Wales, 2013, www.senedd.assemblywales.org/documents/s18966/Bill,%20as%20passed.pdf.

47. Maryland State Senate Bill 428, section 4-509.2.

48. General Assembly of the Commonwealth of Pennsylvania, proposed amendment to Title 20 Chapter 86, Subchapter C.

49. Appelbaum PS, Lidz CW, Meisel A, *Informed consent: Legal theory and clinical practice* (New York: Oxford University Press, 1987), 66–69.

50. Gallup Organization, Inc., "The American public's attitudes toward organ donation and transplantation," conducted for Partnership for Organ Donation, Boston, February 1993, 4, 15.

51. *Organ Donation Study*, United Network for Organ Sharing Executive Summary, Feb. 15, 1992.

52. Ramsey P, *The patient as person* (New Haven, CT: Yale University Press, 1970).

53. Silver T, "The case for a post-mortem draft and a proposed model organ draft act," *Boston University Law Review* 1988;68: 681–728; Spital A, "The shortage of organs for transplantation," *New England Journal of Medicine* 1991;325: 1243–46.

54. McNeil DR, "The constitutionality of 'presumed consent' for organ donation," *Hamline Journal of Public Law and Policy* 1989;9: 343–72; Stuart FP, Veith FJ, Cranford RE, "Brain death laws and patterns of consent to remove organs for transplantation from cadavers in the United States and 28 other countries," *Transplantation* 1981;31: 238–44.

Chapter 11

Markets for Organs

Examining the models for procuring organs, we have considered the donation model, which relies on the consent of the donor or surrogate; and the salvaging model, often mistakenly called "presumed consent," which gives the authority to the broader society to take organs from the deceased without explicit consent. But we have also long been aware of a third possibility, one that takes even more seriously the notions of an individual's rights related to ownership of the body: the model of the free market for organs, grounded in libertarian political philosophy. As it became more clear near the end of the last century that the donation model was not going to produce enough organs, strategies relying on market mechanisms began receiving more attention.[1] In the last decade serious philosophical defenses of market approaches have emerged.[2] Combined with the increasing obviousness that the donation model is not producing enough organs, the market model is stimulating a number of proposals and, indeed, experiments in public policy designed to provide financial and other incentives to stimulate organ procurement.

One good American way of making the supply of organs match the demand more closely would be to create a market for organs. Several analysts have suggested that the inertia in donation could be overcome by paying people who provide organs. According to free market principles, the price could be increased until a much greater portion of the potential is obtained. If living kidney procurement is included (and theoretically liver and lung lobes), the supply could meet the need. Any concern about the potentially enormous cost is addressed by the realization that, at least for kidneys, a transplant saves many thousands of dollars over the life of a patient compared with maintaining that person's life on dialysis.[3] Insurers currently paying for dialysis should gladly pay for the cost of purchasing kidneys and pocket the savings.

Of course, our language would probably need to change. We would then more properly speak of the *sale* of organs, not the *donation*. It is strange to see advocates of markets to buy and sell organs referring to "donation." The one from whom the organ was obtained would be a *vendor*, not a donor. Nevertheless, as we saw in the last chapter in the discussion of public policies that procure organs without consent and deceptively use the term "presumed consent," many in the transplant world have made considerable effort to maintain the language of donation—referring to gifts, "rewarded gifting," and organ donation even in the face of policies that do not involve concepts of donation and consent. Similarly, policies involving overt compensation for those supplying organs are often garbed in the language of donation.

The World's Experience with Organ Markets

The enormous value of human organs, combined with the equally enormous shortage, has led to worldwide attempts to increase the supply of organs through international trafficking. This often involves the movement of organs from those desperately needing money who have body parts that are not absolutely necessary to those who desperately need certain body parts who have enough money and are willing to use it to entice a transfer. This movement of organs is often from residents of poor countries to residents of wealthy countries. Sometimes the pattern is described as movement from countries of the South to those of the North.[4] In some cases the movement of organs has been domestic—within a country—but the economics is likely to be the same: the wealthy getting needed organs from the poor.

Basing their definition on the United Nations Office on Drugs and Crime's Protocol to Prevent, Suppress, and Punish Trafficking in Persons, Budiani-Saberi and Delmonico define organ trafficking as "the recruitment, transport, transfer, harboring or receipt of persons, by means of the threat or use of force or other forms of coercion, of abduction, of fraud, of deception, of the abuse of power, of a position of vulnerability, of the giving or receiving of payments or benefits to achieve the consent of a person having control over another person, for the purpose of exploitation by the removal of organs, tissues or cells for transplantation."[5] The United Nations has treated organ trafficking as a piece of the larger problem of human trafficking, that is, along with the international crimes of trafficking for the purposes of forced labor, prostitution, and other forms of exploitation.[6]

India and the Organ Market of Bombay

As was mentioned in chapter 1, in the earlier years of organ transplants a market for kidneys existed in India. K. C. Reddy, an Indian surgeon who procured such organs, served as a kind of broker between those who wanted to buy and those who felt compelled to sell. He seemed like a decent, respectable professional concerned about benefiting patients. He claimed that if he did not facilitate a market for organs, some other, less reputable people would (and he was probably right). He claimed he gave the poor their only chance to obtain vitally needed goods.

Buying and selling organs became illegal in India with the passage of the Transplantation of Human Organs Act in 1994.[7] This act outlaws the buying and selling of organs and allows living donation only between immediate relatives, spouses, and those united by "affection or attachment."[8] This has led to concerns that a man may marry a woman solely so that she may serve as an organ donor for him, which some see as a risk, especially in a society as patriarchal as India.[9] Concerns were also raised about the vagueness of "affection or attachment." Unrelated donor–recipient pairs justifying their donation in this way had to be approved by a state authorization committee, but these committees were accused of lacking both the infrastructure and the motivation to investigate these proposed donations. This led to the approval of several donations between Indian donors and foreign recipients, raising suspicions of organ trafficking via a legal loophole.[10] In response to these concerns, Parliament amended the act in 2008. Changes included requiring the approval of a foreign national's embassy before authorizing him or her to be either a donor or a recipient and more clearly prescribing the functioning of the authorization committee. The act was further amended in 2011, banning all transplants between unrelated Indian nationals and foreign nationals and increasing the maximum fines and jail time for violating the act's provisions.[11]

Since the passage of the Transplantation of Human Organs Act, sources estimate that the buying and selling of organs in India, while remaining widespread, has decreased, though the rate of foreign organ recipients in other countries, such as Pakistan and the Philippines, has increased at the same time.[12] A large organ-trafficking ring in the city of Gurgaon, a suburb of New Delhi, was broken up in 2008.[13] In this ring, led by physician Amit Kumar, kidneys were sold to both Indians and foreigners. The kidneys in question were obtained with varying levels of consent from the "donors." Some agreed to sell their kidneys for a price, whereas others were taken to transplant facilities under false pretenses (they were often told they were being offered a job), forcibly operated upon, and released without payment or sufficient postoperative care.[14] Authorities estimate that Kumar had been active for more than a decade and had procured organs from roughly five hundred Indians.[15]

Goyal and colleagues, writing in 2002, surveyed hundreds of kidney vendors in Chennai, a hub of paid transplantation, with fascinating results. They found that nearly all vendors gave paying off their debts as their reason for selling a kidney, that nearly half the vendors had a spouse who had also sold a kidney, that most vendors perceived their health as having declined since the operation, that most brokers and clinics paid less in exchange for kidneys than they initially promised, and that the price of a kidney had on average declined from the pre-1994 period (when the sale of organs was legal) to 2001.[16]

Pakistan

Commercial transplantation became illegal in Pakistan very recently with the Transplantation of Human Organs and Tissues Ordinance, which was issued in 2007 and ratified as law in 2010.[17] Farhat Moazam, a physician at Karachi's Sind Institute of Urology and Transplantation and a leader in the opposition to commercial transplantation, summarizes the history of organ trafficking in Pakistan thus:

> Over the first two decades of kidney transplantation in the country [the mid-1980s through the mid-2000s], family donors began to be gradually replaced by impoverished "donors" from villages "willing" to sell a kidney largely to pay off debts to landowners and cover living expenses for their families. This shift in pattern was driven by increasing numbers of private sector hospitals in the province of Punjab beginning to offer "transplant packages" to entice national and international patients who were no longer able to access similar services in Iraq (following the first Gulf war in 1990) and in India (due to the passage of the Indian Transplant Law in 1995). By the turn of the century, Pakistan had gained notoriety as the "kidney bazaar" of the world with private hospitals in major cities of Punjab running lucrative businesses worth millions of dollars using kidneys bought from the most disadvantaged in society.[18]

The shift in Pakistan from mainly familial to mainly commercial transplantation is clear: In 1991 75 percent of renal transplants were between living, related Pakistanis, whereas by 2003 80 percent were from unrelated donor/vendors and more than 50 percent of recipients were foreign nationals. Around this time, private hospitals were charging kidney recipients between $13,000 and $27,000 for "transplant packages," totaling nearly $15 million annually.[19]

In the early 2000s Pakistani and international press and policy bodies began bringing more attention to the situation of commercial transplantation and the plight of vendors. Pressure from international organizations—including the World Health Organization, the Istanbul Group against the Organ Trade, and the Sind Institute of Urology and Transplantation—led the Supreme Court in 2006 to advise the attorney general to consider legislation to curtail commercial transplantation. International pressure continued to mount from such groups as the Asian Task Force on Organ Trafficking.[20] Such guidelines were issued the following year in the form of a presidential ordinance: the Transplantation of Organs and Tissues Ordinance 2007. This ordinance criminalized the transplantation of organs from Pakistanis to foreigners, ordered the creation of a national registry and oversight body, and recommended the establishment of a deceased donor program. Following public debate and resistance from at least some members of the commercial transplant complex, including an unsuccessful suit alleging that the ordinance violated Sharia and was therefore unconstitutional, the ordinance was ratified into law by the Pakistani Assembly and Senate in 2010.[21]

The ordinance was quite effective and led to a drastic decline in the number of commercial transplantations carried out and the number of foreigners coming to Pakistan to receive organs. One transplant surgeon estimates that before the ordinance was in effect, as many as five hundred foreigners per month came to Pakistan as customer/recipients, whereas following the ordinance it was likely closer to ten. Other surgeons claimed they knew of no one continuing to transplant commercially.[22] Reports have since surfaced that commercial transplantation to foreigners may be continuing in Pakistan on a much smaller scale, primarily in the province of Punjab. These reports come mainly from physicians in other countries treating patients who have received a kidney in Pakistan.[23]

Bangladesh

According to Moniruzzaman, the organ trade is illegal but thriving in Bangladesh.[24] Moniruzzaman describes Bangladesh as an "organ bazaar" in existence for more than a decade, in spite of the fact that in 1999 the Bangladeshi Parliament passed the Organ Transplant Act, which imposes a ban on trading organs parts and also on publishing related classified advertisements.[25] It imposes imprisonment for from three to seven years and a fine of 300,000 taka (about $4,300). Still, 78 percent of the inhabitants of Bangladesh live on less than $2 a day, and the typical quoted price for a kidney is 100,000 taka ($1,400). Moniruzzaman quotes a thirty-two-year-old Bangladeshi rickshaw puller who sold one of his kidneys as saying: "When a fox catches a chicken, the little one cries. I was the chicken, and the buyer was the fox. On the day of the operation, I felt like a *kurbanir goru*, a sacrificial cow purchased for slaughtering on the day of Eid [the biggest religious celebration in the Islamic world]."[26]

China

Markets for organs in China pose a complex picture, one that is intertwined with the practice of using executed prisoners as a source of organs. In theory prisoners (or their families) have voluntarily consented to the use of their organs, although commentators in the international community have had doubts about this claim.[27] In 2006 Health Ministry officials acknowledged that most organs transplanted in China came from prisoners, claiming that this was done with consent but also admitting that government supervision was poor so that improper procurements had occurred, including some commercial exchanges.[28]

A number of reports claim that organs procured from prisoners are then sold to both Chinese nationals and foreigners. In US dollars kidneys purportedly have been sold to the Chinese for $15,000 and to foreigners for between $95,000 and $120,000. A liver reportedly commands $120,000 and a heart $140,000.[29] These fees go to the hospitals, which are government facilities.

In 2007, with the adoption of the Human Transplantation Act in China, the number of foreign transplant recipients in China is reported to have decreased by 50 percent.[30] Before these nationwide regulations went into effect, the provincial and local governments adopted various regulations, sometimes outlawing commercial sale or organs along with the use of organs from executed prisoners.[31] As in India, this decline in transplants to foreign nationals presumably led to an increase in such transplantation in the Philippines.

The first prosecution and conviction for organs trafficking did not occur until September of 2010, when seven traffickers were fined and imprisoned based on charges of operating an illegal business.[32] In 2012 the criminal code was amended to include organ trafficking as a specific crime.[33]

There is a substantial difference between what the purchaser must pay for an organ and what the seller receives. Those selling kidneys typically receive 20,000 to 30,000 yuan (about $3,200 to $5,000), whereas the price paid by the person buying such a kidney is around ten times this much, with the difference going to pay the transplant team and broker.[34] In one case a seventeen-year-old boy sold his kidney in order to buy an iPhone and an iPad. According to reports by the Chinese government's official news agency, the seller was paid 22,000 yuan ($3,450), the broker received 56,360 yuan ($8,850), the surgeon 52,000 yuan ($8,200), a hospital official 60,000 yuan ($9,450), and others assisting the broker 10,000 yuan ($1,550) and 3,000 yuan ($450).[35] The outcome in this case was particularly unfortunate, perhaps the reason the case got publicity. The seventeen-year-old suffered renal failure after the surgery. The broker, surgeon, and hospital official, along with four others, were arrested, tried, found guilty, and imprisoned for terms from one to four years. In addition, they had to pay the young man and his family compensation of more than 1.47 million yuan ($231,000).[36]

In November 2013 the Chinese government made a commitment to cease using executed prisoners' organs by mid-2014. It claimed it would then rely on a system of voluntary donations being established across the country.[37] Pilot programs of voluntary deceased donation have been tested in various provinces, and though they have met with some success, there are serious concerns as to such programs' ability to meet the need for organs in China due to low donation rates, the country's exclusive use of a circulatory definition of death, and the Chinese cultural understanding of the sanctity of the body, which causes a public reluctance to donate organs. In an attempt to mitigate this, some programs have experimented with compensating deceased donors' families, either financially or with monuments to the donor or similar compensation in the form of social honor.[38]

The Philippines

With pressures to clamp down on transplant tourism in places like India, Pakistan, and China, the Philippines emerged as a destination of choice for those seeking organs who were willing to pay. In 2004 the Philippine Medical Tourism Program was created by an executive order of the Philippine president. The program, which includes organ transplantation, generates a revenue stream and supports market forces to help develop the country's medical infrastructure.[39]

In theory, the buying of organs had been outlawed by the Anti–Trafficking in Persons Act of 2003. The prohibition, however, was without rules and regulations, so it could not be implemented effectively. It was not until 2009 that rules were finally developed.[40]

From 2002 to 2008 a government program called the Philippine Organ Donation Program compensated so-called donors. It provided those who supplied organs with 175,000 Philippine pesos (about $3,900), which is slightly more than the average annual income for a family. It also was supposed to provide ten years' free annual checkups. Fewer than 10 percent of kidney sources were included in the program, and of those who did participate, reportedly only half got the medical exams after the procurement of their kidneys that they were promised.[41]

Padilla summarizes the situation as follows: "Between 2002 and 2007, the number of unrelated donations increased by 400 percent (163–844), whereas the number of related donations increased only by 37 percent (126–73). The absolute number of transplants from deceased donors increased from 10 to 29 per year. In the same time period, the number of transplants to foreigners increased by 1200 percent (40–528), whereas the number of transplants to Filipinos increased by 89 percent (256–484). [In] 2007, 528 of the 1046 kidney transplants recorded by the Philippine Renal Disease Registry . . . were transplants to foreigners from Filipino-unrelated living donors."[42]

In April 2008 an effort was made to clamp down on the number of foreigners receiving organs from Filipinos. This was codified by the Inter-Agency Council against Organ Trafficking.[43] Before this, in theory no more than 10 percent of transplants were supposed to go to foreign recipients, but this limit was regularly exceeded.[44] By 2007 more than half of all transplant recipients in the Philippines were foreigners. In spite of the April 2008 effort, that year more than 25 percent of all transplants for the year went to foreigners. Thus, although there are efforts to restrict financial transactions involving the procurement of kidneys, especially those involving foreigners, there remains concern that the Philippines is a source of black market organ transactions.[45]

Israel

Although India, Pakistan, and the Philippines have taken their turns as major suppliers of organs from vendors who were paid, Israel has played a significant role in supporting the international organ trade as a purchaser. Israel has historically had a low rate of domestic organ procurement and transplants. This can be explained in part by Orthodox Judaism's resistance to brain death. The limited supply of domestic organs for transplants has led to significant transplant tourism, which has been facilitated by the Israeli government-supported health care system; since 1994, the system has funded international transplants by reimbursing costs. By 1996 the transplant policy of the four major health care programs had been approved by the Ministry of Health. Even if the transplant were not legal in the country where it occurred, the health care system reimbursed transplant recipients up to the amount that the transplant would have cost in Israel.[46] This led to an increase in foreign transplants, up to a peak of 155 in 2006.[47] Destinations for transplant tourism included China, Colombia, Egypt, Moldova, the Philippines, Turkey, and South Africa.[48] This situation led to both domestic and international criticism, leading to a joint anti-organ-trafficking effort between the World Health Organization and the Transplantation Society and eventually the Declaration of Istanbul condemning organ trafficking.[49]

Since 1997 a directive from the Israeli Ministry of Health has prohibited the transplanting of organs that had been paid for. Nevertheless, the buying, selling, and brokering of organs was essentially unregulated.[50] In 2008 the Israeli Knesset adopted the Organ Transplantation Law, which, in addition to supporting expanded deceased donation in various ways, ended the government's funding of transplant tourism. It provided that the health care services could cover transplants received abroad only if they conformed to laws where the transplant took place and only if they did not involve donor compensation. It also provided for criminal sanctions for organ trafficking and brokering.[51] This led to a drop of transplants outside Israel, to about thirty-five by 2011.[52] There are reports, however, that patients receiving transplants abroad can continue to receive pretransplant and posttransplant care from the Israeli health care system, thus continuing to support, indirectly, transplant tourism, including the transplanting of organs from paid vendors.[53] There are reports that, since 2008, Israel has covered expenses including some lost wages for living kidney donors. This law also gives priority to kidney donors and their families if they are in need of an organ.[54]

Moldova

Moldova is known to have played a role in organ trafficking. Recruiters are reported to have arranged for Moldovans—often poor, rural, young males—to travel to other countries, including Turkey, Ukraine, and Georgia, sometimes under the pretense of providing employment. When they reach their destination, they are persuaded to sell a kidney. Since 2000 the Moldovan government has attempted to prevent human trafficking, prosecute offenders, and protect victims.[55]

The United States

Many people have proposed markets for organs in the United States.[56] These proposals have faced serious legal and ethical challenges. The National Organ Transplant Act (NOTA) of 1984 states: "It shall be unlawful for any person to knowingly acquire, receive, or otherwise transfer any human organ for valuable consideration for use in human transplantation if the transfer affects interstate commerce."[57]

The law also clarifies what is meant by "valuable consideration": "The term 'valuable consideration' does not include the reasonable payments associated with the removal, transportation, implantation, processing, preservation, quality control, and storage of a human organ or the expenses of travel, housing, and lost wages incurred by the donor of a human organ in connection with the donation of the organ."

In 2007 NOTA was modified to explicitly permit organ-paired donation (a topic that we discuss in chapter 12).[58] The bottom line is that since the passage of NOTA in 1984, the selling of organs or paying rewards for contributing organs has been illegal.

Virginia in the 1980s

In a statement before the Subcommittee for Investigations and Oversight of the US House of Representatives' Committee on Science and Technology, which was conducting the hearings that led to NOTA, Virginia physician H. Barry Jacobs proposed to create a market for kidneys in the United States, for which he would serve as a broker, apparently in a manner comparable to Reddy in India.[59] His style was so offensive and his plan was so poorly thought out that it appears that his testimony helped seal support for NOTA, the law that prohibits a market for organs in the United States.

Pennsylvania

In spite of NOTA's apparently clear prohibition on payments for organs, in 1994 Pennsylvania passed legislation that created a program to pay an amount toward the funeral expenses of deceased donors in the state, which would be financed by an optional $1 donation made when getting or renewing one's driver's license.[60] Bill Robinson, the state representative who introduced the amendment creating this program, said that he was motivated by a desire to support and compensate donors' families, especially those with lower incomes, and that he would like the benefit eventually to increase to between $3,000 and $5,000.[61] The program was slated to start (at a rate of $300 per family, instead of the initially proposed $3,000) in the summer of 1999, but it was delayed a year and modified to apply to donors' families' food, lodging, and transportation costs instead of funeral expenses.[62] This was in response to the state Department of Health's conclusion that the funeral benefit came too close to violating NOTA's prohibition on payments for organs. In 2004 the state's Organ Donation Advisory Committee requested that the Health Department reconsider the funeral benefit, but no change was made.[63]

The program continues in this form today, with the state paying up to $300 of the food, travel, and lodging expenses of donors' families (with payment going directly to the donors rather than to the families as reimbursement). In at least one case the family of a deceased donor has received these benefits, though they occur far more often in the case of living donors, for the practical reason that the process of living donation leads to family travel and lodging expenses much more than does deceased donation. Materials on the current Web page of the program generally mention only "donors," without specifying living or deceased, though in one place it does say specifically that "family members include those persons who travel with the living donor to provide support to him/her during the transplantation process."

Thus, at least one state is willing to support donation, relying on the distinction between payment of expenses related to donation and paying directly for the organ. It has professional support. In 2003 an Ad Hoc Living Donor Committee of the United Network for Organ Sharing (UNOS) approved a resolution that supported the payment of lost wages, a proposal that has never been put into practice. While the distinction between payment for expenses versus payment for organs may be valid in the case of living donations, it is less compelling in deceased organ donation. In the case of deceased donors, payment of funeral or other expenses, which would normally be covered by the estate of the deceased, ends up with the family receiving payment that is the same as if it had been paid directly for the organs. By paying funeral or other expenses that would have been paid from the deceased's estate, the inheritance would be increased, thus resulting in greater transfer to the beneficiaries.

New Jersey and the Levy-Izhak Rosenbaum Case

In the face of the clear legal prohibition on organ trafficking in the United States, it is generally believed that the transfer of organs involving monetary payment is rare. Transplant physicians and transplant programs would have a great deal to lose if they were to violate this prohibition—potentially, they could be excluded from the transplant system. Because a transplant surgeon's colleagues have an interest in obtaining organs for their own patients and would likely know if a patient received an organ in a way that violated the UNOS allocation algorithm, manipulations of the transplant wait list for monetary payment are quite unlikely.

If there were ever a case of obtaining organs in which money played a clandestine role, it is likely to involve a living donor who is able successfully to claim an emotional relationship with the recipient when, in fact, he or she was providing the organ in exchange for a cash payment.

That is apparently what happened in a series of cases involving Levy-Izhak Rosenbaum. Rosenbaum was arrested in July 2009 as part of a large corruption investigation involving money laundering and the bribery of municipal officials. He was reported to have helped the vendors and recipients of organs concoct stories to trick hospital staffs into believing the pairs were friends or relatives. In 2011 he admitted in federal court that he had brokered three illegal kidney transplants in exchange for payments of between $120,000 and $150,000.[64] He also pleaded guilty to conspiracy to broker an illegal kidney sale. The transplants, which were reportedly all successful, took place in American hospitals. The organs came from people in Israel, who were paid between $10,000 and $25,000, and were sold to wealthy Americans, who were otherwise enduring a long wait on the American wait list. He was sentenced to two and a half years in prison and had to forfeit the $420,000 he had made brokering the transplants.

Iran

All these examples of markets for organs exist in situations where the selling of organs is illegal or at least the legal status of the sale is ambiguous. They involve black or gray markets. The obvious abuses—such as failure to screen the vendors adequately, failure to provide follow-up care, and even failure to pay the promised compensation—are sometimes attributed to the fact that there is no adequate regulation of the market, and in part to the questionable legal status of the practice. Some wonder if an aboveboard, legal market with government regulation would avoid these problems. This brings us to Iran, the only country in the world with a legal, regulated market for human kidneys.

Before 1988 Iran had the typical problem of increasing numbers of patients undergoing dialysis and limited transplantation. In 1980 this shortage led the Ministry of Health to fund travel abroad of dialysis patients to receive transplants. Between 1980 and 1985, 400 patients traveled to European countries and the United States to receive transplants at the expense of the Iranian government, mostly using living, related kidney donors. Between 1985 and 1987 two domestic kidney transplant programs were established, relying on living, related donors.[65]

The result was an expensive program of transplants outside the country, supplemented by a modest living, related donor domestic program along with a growing wait list. In 1988 efforts involving compensated living, unrelated donor renal transplantation were initiated. At first these involved individual contracts. Eventually, the government began providing a fee that, by late in the first decade of the twenty-first century, had a purchasing power somewhere in the range of $4,000 to $8,000.[66]

If that were the only payment to the vendors, a clean experiment in a market for procuring kidneys would exist, together with an allocation to recipients that did not depend on the recipient's ability to pay. The actual situation in Iran is more complex. Candidates for transplant, along with nongovernmental organizations, also provide supplemental funding, which can amount to as much as four or five times the payment by the government. Except in the poorest regions, most cases needing charity to help pay appear not to be deprived of an organ.

The details of the transactions between vendors and purchasers of organs are arranged by local organizations, with considerable variation in the practices from one region to another in the quality of the interactions between vendors and purchasers and the style and integrity of the organizations providing for the interaction.[67] Concern has been expressed about the exploitation of recipients by vendors who ask too much for an organ.[68] There is also reason to worry about the exploitation of vendors who might be offered too little. As of 2010, 70 percent of kidney transplants involved living, unrelated donors. Another 5 percent of recipients received kidneys from living, related donors; the remainder involved deceased donors.

In order to minimize transplant tourism, kidneys obtained from the living, unrelated procurement program are restricted to Iranian nationals. Non-Iranians may utilize Iranian transplant programs only if they bring their own related donors, raising questions of potential abuse if payments are made outside the purview of the Iranian government or other governments. In any case, it is estimated that fewer than 1 percent of transplantations performed in Iran are between non-Iranian pairs.

It is often claimed that Iran, by relying on its living, unrelated program, has eliminated a wait list for kidneys. This has been disputed, and an accurate picture is hard to establish, because some claim that there is limited access to the medical system or that some potential kidney recipients may be kept on dialysis rather than be listed for transplant.[69]

Ghods and Mahdavi-Mazdeh, in addition to pointing to the increase in organ supply, defend the Iranian system, claiming that it reduces the likelihood of familial coercion. They suggest that there is less pressure on relatives and spouses, especially women, to donate an organ.[70] Others have offered libertarian arguments in favor of the system, noting that the poor are better off with more choices and, in any case, also make decisions to take risks in choosing employment in exchange for monetary compensation.[71]

The Ethics of a Market for Organs

Although most of the international experience to date has focused on living persons, and in the United States, there has been at least some consideration of legalizing both living and deceased organ markets. This would require changes to the law, and thus one must first ask whether such a change would be ethical.

The Cadaver Organ Market

Some of the proposals to use markets to encourage organ availability do not rely on sales from living persons. They involve economic incentives to encourage actions to increase the supply of cadaver organs.

Various proposals have been put forward to increase cadaveric organ supply.[72] Of course, it would not work to make a payment after procurement to those who are the source of the organ. In the case of cadaver procurement, they are deceased. Some other economic incentive would need to be provided. One version would pay people to execute donor cards or to register in a state donor registry. However, this would present real problems. Because only a small portion of those who execute a donor card actually provide organs suitable for transplant, a very small fee would need to be paid to a great many people. Moreover, we would almost have to acknowledge the right of persons to withdraw consent, and it is hard to imagine a policy that could deal with such withdrawals. Presumably, the one wanting to cancel his or her donation would need to give back the incentive to cancel one's donor card. Moreover, those who really resisted donation might follow a strategy of signing up to get the incentive and then canceling if they developed a condition that would be likely to make them potential suppliers of organs. Relatives who are guardians might also try to change the consent.

A more plausible approach would be to make a payment if and when organs are procured if the donor had previously pledged to donate organs.[73] The income would go not to the deceased, but to the estate or to anyone the deceased might name. If payment were made only when an organ was actually procured (or perhaps was actually transplantable), the numbers would be much smaller and the payment could be much larger. Anyone who desired to increase the size of his or her estate for loved ones might be enticed by the payment. A similar goal could be achieved by giving a life insurance policy to anyone who signed a donor card, with the proviso that the insurance would be paid to the beneficiary only if organs were procured. At least in the case of kidney transplants, the savings from avoiding chronic dialysis would be so great that insurers might be very willing to pay a large fee to obtain organs.

All these payments would presently be illegal in the United States, but the real question is whether the law should be amended to permit them.[74] The payments could be viewed as an incentive to overcome the inertia of failing to take the steps necessary to actually commit to providing organs.

Such payments to the estates of those who had signed up to provide organs would still pose some practical problems. What should happen, for instance, if someone has signed a donor card but turns out to have marginal organs (e.g., someone at the upper limits of the acceptable age)? They, or their family, might demand the right to have their organs procured. Lawsuits for failure to procure could be envisioned. Should the same payment be made to those providing prime organs and those with less desirable ones?[75] Should the same payment be made to those who supply only kidneys and those who supply a full set of organs? What about those who supply all organs but yield only a limited number of usable ones? Should the family of someone who has ideal organs available be excluded from payment simply because no recipients for certain good organs are available?

These proposals also raise more basic ethical questions. Most Americans find the proposal for a market for organs repulsive. The arguments are complex, however. The debate often starts with the opponents claiming that life and death are too precious to be reduced to market transactions. It is believed that whether one lives or dies should not be a matter of price.

Two significantly different market arrangements have been considered. One, following the Bombay and Jacobs model, would permit those in need of organs to bargain for an available liver or heart or kidney. This would, in fact, mean that those with the greatest ability to pay would be more likely to live.

We should recognize that many other medical services are allocated by price today. Many wealthy people get a higher quality of medical services because of their ability to pay. Some of us, however, hold to the belief that, when it comes to life-and-death interventions, this ought not to be the way. The mere fact that other health services are allocated on the basis of an ability to pay does not mean that it should be this way for organs.

In the United States, however, a second way of linking organ procurement to market forces can be envisioned. We have the possibility of dissociating procurement from allocation. Relying on the market for one does not necessarily mean that we must rely on the market for the other. We could, for example, have a national organ transplant network use money as an incentive to increase the national pool of organs and still have that network allocate organs to transplant candidates without regard to payment. A national insurance plan for transplants (perhaps modeled on the Medicare funding of kidney transplants) could make organs available from the financially enhanced pool totally on the basis of medical need or predicted medical benefit. This would eliminate discrimination on the allocation side, but we would still be left with the questions about the morality of markets on the procurement side.

It is not clear that a market incentive to encourage making cadaveric organs available would be unacceptable, provided one could be identified that worked efficiently (i.e., by avoiding payments to those who would end up avoiding procurement and by not spending too much on people who were planning to give anyway).

In fact, the cadaveric organ market model may be more compatible with the donation model than many people realize. As we have seen, the donation model is built on the premise that one's body, in some important sense, belongs to oneself. We have the authority to give away body parts or refuse to make such a gift. There is a way in which we *own* our bodies. If so, selling body parts when they are no longer of any use to us but are very valuable to others is not obviously incompatible with at least some of the underlying premises of the donation model. It at least avoids the assumption that the body parts of the deceased belong to the state and can be salvaged without permission.

The Living Organ Market

Markets for living organs potentially present serious ethical problems. The stories of attempts to induce kidney procurement by offering financial incentive are rife with reports of abuses—failure to pay the promised amount; large portions of the payment by recipients going to intermediaries, hospitals, and surgeons; deception in recruiting vendors; and evidence of those enticed into selling in order to get out of debt or to improve their lot by building a home ending up as poorly off a short time after the procurement as they were before selling their organ. There are persistent reports of failures in medical follow-up, misunderstandings, and outright fraud. The evidence from Iran suggests that legalization does not necessarily eliminate these problems. A government-regulated market for vendors, with regulation to assure a fair market, adequate safety and the possession of information and with a prohibition on private payments for the allocation of organs, would pose the greatest challenge to those who have moral reservations.

There may well be cases where people would be so desperate that they would be enticed to sell a kidney or even a liver or lung lobe for a large amount of money. (There may even be some so desperate that they would sell a whole liver, lung, or heart, realizing that they would die but that their family would be spared some awful fate; but let us limit our attention, for now, to proposals to sell a single kidney.) Assuming that the vendor is an adult who is mentally competent and has been informed adequately about the risks and benefits of selling a kidney, and assuming that this person, after careful consideration, comes to the conclusion that it is better to sell the kidney and do something with the money, why should our society prohibit such sales? It cannot be that such persons have always calculated their interests incorrectly. Some people would really be better off with the money than with their second kidney (or they may be able to act more morally—taking care of loved ones in desperate need). If we are going to make such sales illegal, we need an argument that overrules the enlightened self-interest of such sellers. If we are going to do so nonpaternalistically, we need an argument that points to some feature other than the vendor's own welfare.

Some would argue that payments would be coercive, especially to the poor. The difference between incentives and coercion is a complex topic. A coercive force is one that is intended to influence another person by presenting a threat so severe that it is irresistible.[76] This immediately makes clear the fact that an offer of an enormous amount of money is not coercive, even if it is irresistible. The money is not a threat; it is an offer.

Most analyses of coercion rely on this distinction, limiting coercion to negative sanctions.[77]

Positive incentives that compel action are usually considered to be *offers* or *influences*. The analysis of these positive incentives is more complex. It is quite possible that one might respond affirmatively to a positive incentive (e.g., a cash payment) without in any way deviating from one's general life plan. Because autonomous actions are those that are in accord with one's life plan, effective positive incentives may be consistent with autonomy. For example, if someone has long thought that it would be a nice action—and one consistent with her general values—to sign a donor card but had simply never gotten around to doing it, receiving a modest incentive (either a small payment or an insurance policy of, say, $1,000, payable if organs are procured) to sign the card would not in any way violate her autonomy, even though it gets her to engage in a behavior that she had not otherwise had enough motivation to perform. Signing the card is consistent with her general beliefs and values.

Offers generally provide additional options beyond what one would otherwise have. An offer of a 10 percent bonus to change from one work shift to another adds to the range of available choices. It is hard to argue that adding an option violates autonomy. An offer of a 10 percent pay raise to go to work for a competitor likewise increases the employee's options. We normally do not think of such a competitive employment offer as immoral, even if the offer is effectively persuasive in getting someone to change jobs.

Two sorts of cases make the analysis still more complicated. These can be called the "unwelcome offer" and the "irresistible offer." An unwelcome offer is one that the recipient would rather not receive. Some offers that increase options are nevertheless ones that people would rather not receive. An offer of a new job at a 10 percent increase in wages may force many additional choices about relocation, separation from one's family, and so forth.

If the new job offer not only poses these unwelcome problems but is also an extremely good offer, it may turn out to be irresistible. A 100 percent salary increase for doing similar work may be an irresistible offer. If one prefers to relocate anyway, the irresistible offer may be very welcome and quite compatible with one's autonomy. The real issue is how to evaluate an irresistible offer that is unwelcome. Irresistibly attractive offers will force a choice on the employee. If they are nevertheless welcome offers, they are not inconsistent with autonomy; but if the offer is unwelcome, it could force one to abandon a life plan, thereby depriving one of an autonomous life. Such an individual would have more options, but would nevertheless feel constrained to abandon his or her life plan.

There is considerable dispute over whether such irresistibly attractive, unwelcome offers are ethical. Offering a large fee to persons to become live "donors" of kidneys probably fits this category, especially if the individuals are in desperate need for themselves or their families. Some will see such offers as unacceptably controlling and therefore as unethical. Others will see them as increasing options and therefore as acceptable, even though one is thereby forced to abandon a life plan. In organ procurement the fear is that financial incentives may be irresistibly attractive to those who are in desperate situations, thus forcing them to sign a "donor" card or even to become a living organ vendor.

These offers may lead to unintended consequences. One concern is that if selling organs were to become legal, then it would raise the question of whether others can demand that an individual engage in such income generation by selling organs—before declaring bankruptcy, for example. In a recent paper, Rippon argues that though "it would be better for people in poverty to sell their organs *if* given the option," it is also the case that it may "be even better for them to not have the option at all."[78] His argument is that if selling organs were legally permitted, then people in poverty might "find themselves faced with social or legal pressure to pay the bills by selling their organs," an option that does not exist where organ markets are illegal.[79]

A second unintended consequence could be that a living organ market might lead to "crowding out"—the phenomenon whereby fewer individuals would be willing to donate for free if a market existed concurrently.[80] Those who object to organ markets extrapolate from the work of Richard Titmuss, who showed how a market in blood was associated with reduced voluntary blood donations.[81] One additional variable may prove crucial. Some people who make irresistibly attractive offers of this kind may have the means to address the potential organ vendor's desperate situation using some other means. If they do, they can be seen as exploiting the desperate person's situation. So, for example, we suggest in chapter 12 that, if a transplant surgeon could have listed a recipient for a cadaver transplant but refused to do so (perhaps because his staff needed more practice with live donor procurement), thus forcing the potential recipient's spouse into accepting an irresistibly attractive offer to be a donor, that offer would be not only consistent with the spouse's life plan and irresistibly attractive but also unethical because it was exploitative. The surgeon would have forced the spouse to become a donor when he could have solved the problem in another way.

This situation reveals why proposals for markets for organs are so controversial. They are likely to involve offers of money that will have significantly different effects on people in different positions. The desperately poor may perceive the offer of money for organ donation as irresistibly attractive. But it may also be exploitative; the ones making the offer may have the resources and the responsibility to address the desperate one's problem in some other way.

For example, if Medicare were to add a financial reward for supplying cadaveric or living organs, the funds would come from the federal government. The people who were sufficiently desperate to view the offer as irresistible could face life-and-death financial crises, but the same federal government that was making the offer could have both the resources and the responsibility to provide a welfare safety net to meet these needs. Fulfilling this responsibility would remove the desperation and thus make the offer no longer irresistible.

The real issue is whether those in authority have it within their power to address the basic needs of a population, short of resorting to selling body parts. In the United States it is obvious that there are sufficient resources for a humane, safety net welfare program that should be able to provide enough resources to meet desperate needs for basic welfare without forcing people to such extremes. If those who defend markets for organs do so as a way of escaping responsibility for providing for the subsistence of a society's most needy, that is an unacceptable excuse for escaping responsibility.

However, what if we limit the positive incentives to those that are small enough to be "resistible"? As we have noted, for living donors, Pennsylvania reimburses donors for up to $300 in out-of-pocket expenses to overcome the financial barriers that may prevent live organ donation.[82] It is hard to argue that this would violate autonomy. At least for those who were already willing to donate, but simply had not developed the momentum to do so, this would be a welcome offer. But it would probably also be resistible, especially if it were modest. It probably could be crafted in such a way that it would not be seen as exploiting the desperate.

Nevertheless, monetizing organ procurement might still be perceived as unseemly. Any positive incentive will appeal more to the more desperate. Anyone who felt strongly attracted by such an incentive might well have basic needs that should be met by the government through other programs.

Payments might also be perceived as unseemly in another way. One of the great advantages of the gift-giving model is that it elevates organ donation to a level of humaneness that seems appropriate for meeting the needs of those with life-threatening medical problems. For some, financial incentives—even modest, resistible ones—change the character of organ procurement from humane gift giving among fellow members of the human community to a more commercial, businesslike transaction.

Unfair Inequality and Incentives

There is another very difficult problem with incentive payments for supplying organs. Any payment will be perceived differently by people in different financial situations. Consider the action of the UNOS Ad Hoc Committee on Living Organ Donation. It considered markets for kidneys (and conceivably even liver lobes, although the risk to the supplier of liver lobes meant that this was never seriously entertained). After some debate about proposals to amend American law to permit payment for kidneys, the committee offered the orthodox position of opposing financial markets. However, it then took up the problem that many potential family members who might be candidates to be living kidney donors faced serious financial hardship if they did. They would miss work for some weeks, be unable to carry out normal household duties, and otherwise be harmed by the act of offering to be a kidney donor to a family member or friend. It endorsed a policy of granting thirty days paid leave for state employees, a position later approved by the UNOS Board of Directors, and it supported an exploration of policies to grant reimbursement for lost income to living donors.[83]

Living kidney donation has great potential to help reduce the backlog of those waiting for deceased donor kidneys. The supply is potentially large, and higher-quality kidneys are obtained as well. Encouraging living donation is a plausible public policy until some new technology—such as an implantable artificial kidney, the use of xenografts, or generating replacement kidneys through the use of stem cells—becomes a realistic alternative.

Because the UNOS Ad Hoc Committee generally looked favorably on living kidney donation and because it understood that economic hardship, such as lost wages, was a real disincentive, it proposed that compensation for lost wages might be a policy worth pursuing. This might require a change in American law, which prohibits offering anything of valuable consideration for an organ, but the committee was sufficiently interested to begin exploring the possibility of changing the law.

It then began to encounter a problem. What would be fair compensation? Because a kidney donor will realistically miss several weeks of work and could plausibly need additional weeks to recover full capacity, the reimbursement of several weeks' wages was considered. That posed a problem, however. A highly paid business executive would need to be paid many times the compensation of an ordinary, low-income worker. In fact, the unemployed would plausibly receive nothing, and those employed as full-time, nonmonitized stay-at-home contributors to family functioning would either receive nothing or need to be paid some amount based on the hypothetical value of domestic labor. This raises questions about fairness if different people are paid widely different amounts for exactly the same contribution of a kidney. An alternative was suggested of paying six months of the average income of an American worker, but that raises a different set of problems. The business executive would receive very little in comparison with his or her normal income and would hardly have an incentive to provide a kidney. Conversely, the unemployed could find the incentive so attractive that it would once again raise questions of exploitation and irresistible offers.

The bottom line seems to be that some modest level of positive financial incentives may eventually be implemented, but it is an approach that should be tried only when all other approaches have been tried and failed. Thus, the critical question is what other compromises are available that supplement the pure donation and salvaging strategies.

Variations on the Market Model: "Rewarded Gifting"

Given what has been said above, buying organs is therefore controversial. Some see it as immoral. It is at least a violation of current American law. But the shortage of organs is real. And many people who seem, in principle, willing to donate simply have not found the momentum to do so.

Economic Rewards

Some have observed that families incur real costs when organs are donated. They propose that, even if we cannot buy organs or pay an incentive, those costs can be reimbursed. Some have gone so far as to coin the wonderfully offensive term *rewarded gifting* in attempting to salvage the donation model.[84] The implication is that organs will not be bought. Rather they will be given, in exchange for which money will be presented as a reward.

There is evidence that something like this operates in Iran. Sigrid Fry-Revere, an American lawyer-bioethicist who is the head of the Center for Ethical Solutions, has traveled to Iran to study the practice of a market there for living kidney procurement. She has noted that, although the government pays for people to supply their kidneys and recipients frequently supplement those payments with additional monetary payments, there is a tendency to continue to think of the supplying of the kidney as a "donation," whereas the payment from the recipient of the kidney is thought of as a gift in gratitude.[85]

These proposals raise subtle complications, however. In the United States all hospital costs after the death of a patient must be borne by the transplant organization. We cannot play on the fears of families that they will be billed for organ procurement, offering compensation for expenses as a strategy for stimulating them to "donate."

What, however, about paying other costs surrounding terminal care? Proposals have been made to pay the funeral costs or pay the family a "reimbursement" for travel, lodging, or meal expenses during the period of the terminal illness or time away from work.

Paying funeral expenses up to a few thousand dollars seems to be the most common proposal. But the funeral is normally paid from the deceased's estate. If funeral costs are borne by the transplant agency, the estate increases by that amount. The beneficiaries of the estate get that much more. That is almost the same as buying the organs. We say *almost* the same because new deception is involved. The participants—the family, as well as the organ procurers—may actually fool themselves into believing that they have remained in the gift-giving mode.

There is occasionally a bigger problem in paying for funeral expenses or for hospital costs. There are cases where the beneficiary of the estate—the one who will receive more if the funeral or hospital expenses are not paid from the estate—may not be the same person who makes the decision to provide the organs of the deceased. The next of kin might be the surrogate decision maker determining whether to agree to provide organs, but not the beneficiary of the patient's will. This would have the odd effect of failing to provide any incentive to supply organs while increasing the payment to the beneficiary who had nothing to do with the decision about the organs. For these reasons it might be better, or at least more straightforward, to simply pay a fee to the provider of the organs without dressing the payment up in the language of a rewarding gifting or of reimbursement for expenses.

Noneconomic Rewards

There is one way in which the concept of "rewarded gifting" might be appropriate. It is possible that nonmonetary rewards could encourage either live donation or the signing of donor cards. Community recognition of and praise for the socially noble character of the organ donor certainly seems appropriate. Even more tangible, nonmonetary rewards might be considered. Live donors, for instance, might be given some special consideration—a few bonus points—if they needed organs in the future. This plan has, in fact, been adopted. Currently, 4 points in the kidney allocation formula are awarded for those with proof that they were previously donors of a kidney, liver segment, lung segment, partial pancreas, or small bowel segment.[86] Under the new kidney allocation formula that will go into effect in 2014, those who have been prior living donors will get special priority after those who are highly sensitized, those who have a zero antigen mismatch, and minors.

Richard Schwindt and Aidan Vining have proposed one idea in the spirit of noneconomic rewards for a willingness to donate organs: a "mutual insurance pool."[87] According to their plan, an individual in the pool would receive priority for organs from other members if he or she agreed to make organs available in the event of death. Assuming that some guidelines can be developed to prevent people from joining the pool only when they anticipate needing organs, this proposal would be essentially similar to giving people bonus points if they have agreed to donate organs.

Such a program was actually created in 2002, when David Undis created LifeSharers, a nonprofit network of organ donors that gives registered organ donors preferred access to transplantable organs.[88] However, the program hit a snag. It is not clear that such priority can be achieved, because it would require UNOS or a local organ procurement organization to direct organs to a specific social group, the insurance pool. Although UNOS permits directed donations to a specific individual or hospital, it does not permit donations to a specified social group—whether this would be based on race, religion, or membership in a particular group (we discuss the concept of socially directed donation more in chapter 23). Giving special consideration to those who sign donors cards for deceased donor donation is an alternative noneconomic reward. However, its implementation could be complicated. People might not perceive the incentive to donate until they were in need of organs themselves. Giving special consideration only to those who have been donors for several years, however, might avoid the problem. Even if these two programs would not be feasible, the point is that minor, nonfinancial rewards for donors seem appropriate and should be tried more aggressively.

Notes

1. Peters DA, "Marketing organs for transplantation," *Dialysis & Transplantation* 1984;13 (1): 40–41; Peters TG, "Financial incentives in organ donation: Current issues," *Dialysis & Transplantation* 1992;21 (5): 270–73; Prottas J, "Encouraging altruism: Public attitudes and the marketing of organ donation," *Milbank Memorial Fund Quarterly/Health and Society* 1983;61 (2): 278–306; Chapman DE, "Retailing human organs under the uniform commercial code," *John Marshall Law Review* 1983;16 (2): 393–417; American Medical Association, Council on Ethical and Judicial Affairs, "Financial incentives for organ donation," *Archives of Internal Medicine* 1995;155: 581–89; Harvey J, "Paying organ donors," *Journal of Medical Ethics* 1990;16: 117–19; Barnett AH, Blair RD, Kaserman DL, "Improving organ donation: Compensation versus markets," *Inquiry* 1992;29: 372–78.

2. Taylor JS, *Stakes and kidneys : Why markets in human body parts are morally imperative* (Aldershot, UK: Ashgate, 2005); Cherry M, *Kidney for sale by owner: Human organs, transplantation, and the market* (Washington, DC: Georgetown University Press, 2005); Hippen B, "In defense of a regulated market in kidney from living donors," *Journal of Medicine and Philosophy.* 2006;30: 593–626; Wilkinson TM, *Ethics and the acquisition of organs* (Oxford: Oxford University Press, 2012).

3. According to the 2011 *Annual Report* of the United States Renal Data System, the cost of dialysis was $82,285 for Medicare patients in 2009, and the cost for supporting a transplant recipient was $29,983; United States Renal Data System, *Annual Report*, chap. 11, www.usrds.org/2011/pdf/ v2_ch011_11.pdf. The cost of a kidney transplant varies depending on many factors. Current sources estimate about $260,000, including pretransplant and posttransplant costs. See US Department of Health and Human Services, "Organ transplantation: The process," http://organdonor.gov/about/ transplantationprocess.html; and "Transplant living: Costs," www.transplantliving.org/before-the -transplant/financing-a-transplant/the-costs/.

4. Scheper-Hughes N, "The global traffic in human organs," *Current Anthropology* 2000;41 (2): 193.

5. United Nations Office on Drugs and Crime, "Human trafficking," www.unodc.org/unodc/en/ human-trafficking/what-is-human-trafficking.html?ref = menuside; Budiani-Saberi DA, Delmonico FL, "Organ trafficking and transplant tourism: A commentary on the global realities," *American Journal of Transplantation* 2008;8: 925.

6. United Nations Office of Drugs and Crime, "United Nations Convention against Transnational Organized Crime and the Protocols Thereto," adopted by the General Assembly Nov. 15, 2000, www .unodc.org/unodc/en/treaties/CTOC/index.html. See esp. "Protocol to Prevent, Suppress and Punish Trafficking in Persons," adopted by the General Assembly and entered into force, Dec. 25, 2003.

7. See Parliament of India, "Transplantation of Human Organs Act, 1994" (Act. No. 42 of 1994), http://health.bih.nic.in/Docs/THOA-1994.pdf; and Agarwal SK, Srivastava RK, Gupta S, Tripathi S, "Evolution of the Transplantation of Human Organ Act and Law in India," *Transplantation* 2012;94: 110–13, at 111.

8. Parliament of India, "Transplantation," §9.3.

9. Srinivasan S, "Health–South Asia: Hub for global organ trade," Inter Press Service, Feb. 20, 2008, www.ipsnews.net/2008/02/health-south-asia-hub-for-global-organ-trade/; Jafarey A, Thomas G, Ahmad A, Srinivasan S, "Asia's organ farms," *Indian Journal of Medical Ethics* 2007;4 (2): 52–53.

10. Srinivasan, "Health–South Asia"; Jafarey et al., "Asia's organ farms."

11. Agarwal et al., "Evolution," 112.

12. Shimazono Y, "The state of the international organ trade: A provisional picture based on integration of available information," *Bulletin of the World Health Organization* 2007;85: 957; Srinivasan, "Health–South Asia."

13. Gentleman A, "Kidney thefts shock India," *New York Times*, Jan. 30, 2008, www.nytimes.com/2008/01/30/world/asia/30kidney.html.

14. Ibid.; Ramesh R, "Indian police arrest suspected kidney snatching gang," *The Guardian*, Jan. 25, 2008, www.theguardian.com/world/2008/jan/25/india.randeepramesh.

15. Gentleman, "Kidney thefts."

16. Goyal M, Mehta RL, Schneiderman LJ, Sehgal AR, "Economic and health consequences of selling a kidney in India," *JAMA* 2002;288: 1589–93.

17. Bile KM, Qureshi JA, Rizvi SA, Naqvi SA, Usmani AQ, Lashari KA, "Human organ and tissue transplantation in Pakistan: When a regulation makes a difference," *Eastern Mediterranean Health Journal* 2010;16 (Supplement): S159–66; Moazam F, "Pakistan and kidney trade: Battles won, battles to come," *Medicine, Health Care, and Philosophy* 2013;16 (4): 925–28.

18. Moazam, "Pakistan."

19. Lahore M, "Kidney market shut as Pakistan cuts supply," *Sydney Morning Herald*, May 12, 2008, www.smh.com.au/news/national/kidney-market-shut-as-pakistan-cuts-supply/2008/05/11/12104442 44440.html; Moazam F, "Battling kidney trade in Pakistan: The struggle continues," *Bioethics Links* (Centre of Biomedical Ethics and Culture, SIUT, Pakistan) 2007;3 (1): 2.

20. The Asian Task Force on Organ Trafficking met in 2007 and 2008 and issued a report: Asian Task Force on Organ Trafficking, *Recommendations on the prohibition, prevention and elimination of organ trafficking in Asia* (Taipei: Center for Ethics, Law, and Society in Biomedicine and Technology, National Taiwan University, 2008).

21. Moazam F, "Pakistan."

22. Lahore, "Kidney market."

23. Ebrahim Z, "Organ trafficking resurfaces in Pakistan," Inter Press Service, Aug. 27, 2012, www.ipsnews.net/2012/08/organ-trafficking-resurfaces-in-pakistan/.

24. Moniruzzaman M, "'Living cadavers' in Bangladesh: Bioviolence in the human organ bazaar," *Medical Anthropology Quarterly* 2012;26 (1): 69–91.

25. Ibid., 70.

26. Ibid., 69.

27. Rothman DJ, Rose E, Awaya T, et al., "The Bellagio Task Force report on transplantation, bodily integrity, and the international traffic in organs," *Transplantation Proceedings* 1997;29: 2739–45; Bianchi S, "Death penalty: British surgeons, rights groups warn Chinese to halt organ harvesting," Inter Press Service, May 11, 2006, www.ipsnews.net/2006/05/death-penalty-british-surgeons-rights-groups-warn-chinese-to-halt-organ-harvesting/.

28. Qiu Q, Zhang F, "In organ donations, charity begins with body," *China Daily*, Nov. 16, 2006, www.chinadaily.com.cn/china/2006-11/16/content_734368.htm; Human Rights Watch, "China: Organ procurement and judicial execution in China," *Human Rights Watch–Asia* 1994;6 (9).

29. Bianchi, "Death penalty"; Boseley S, "UK transplant patients go to China for organs from executed prisoners," *The Guardian*, Apr. 19, 2006, www.theguardian.com/uk/2006/apr/20/health.china; Mufson S, "Chinese doctor tells of organ removals after executions," *Washington Post*, June 27, 2001, www.angelfire.com/co3/journal/skinned.html; "Organ sales 'thriving' in China," BBC News, Sept. 27, 2006, http://news.bbc.co.uk/2/hi/5386720.stm.

30. Budiani-Saberi, Delmonico, "Organ trafficking," 927.

31. Chunyan D, "Latest development of legal regulations of organ transplant in China," *Journal International de Bioéthique* 2008;19 (4): 61–81.

32. Tam F, "Milestone as organ traffickers jailed for first time on mainland," *South China Morning Post*, Sept. 16, 2010.

33. Li L, "New law targets organ traders," *China Daily*, Feb. 28, 2011, www.chinadaily.com.cn/cndy/2011-02/28/content_12085094.htm.

34. Blum J, Zhuang P, "Police bust black market kidney ring in Wuhan," *South China Morning Post*, Aug. 21, 2013; Zhuang P, "16 charged over sale of 51 human kidneys," *South China Morning Post*, March 1, 2012; Zhuang P, "Illegal organ trade thrives," *South China Morning Post*, March 27, 2012.

35. Zhuang, "Illegal organ trade"; Xinhuanet, "Seven imprisoned in C China kidney trading case," Nov. 29, 2012, http://news.xinhuanet.com/english/china/2012-11/29/c_132008001.htm.

36. Xinhuanet, "Seven imprisoned"; Zhuang, "Illegal organ trade."

37. Hui L, Blanchard B, "China to end use of prisoners' organs for transplants in mid-2014," Reuters, Nov. 2, 2013, www.reuters.com/article/2013/11/02/us-china-organs-idUSBRE9A011N20131102.

38. Xiaoliang W, Qiang F, "Financial compensation for deceased organ donation in China," *Journal of Medical Ethics* 2013;39: 378–79; Li L, "Pro-life: China acts to address legal barriers and conduct awareness campaigns to boost organ donation," *Beijing Review*, Apr. 16, 2012, www.bjreview.com.cn/nation/txt/2012-04/16/content_446617.htm; Xumin S, Mingchang Z, "Body and organ donation in Wuhan, China," *Lancet* 2010;376: 1033–34.

39. Department of Tourism of the Republic of the Philippines, "Medical tourism portal," www.tourism.gov.ph/Pages/MedicalTourismPortal.aspx; Olarte AM, "And now, hospitals as tourist spots," *i Report* (Philippine Center for Investigative Journalism), Sept. 2006, http://pcij.org/stories/and-now-hospitals-as-tourist-spots; Turner L, "Commercial organ transplantation in the Philippines," *Cambridge Quarterly of Healthcare Ethics* 2009;18: 192–96.

40. Padilla BS, "Regulated compensation for kidney donors in the Philippines," *Current Opinion in Organ Transplantation* 2009;14 (2): 120–23; Torres T, "Philippines say no to organ trafficking," *Philippine Daily Inquirer*, June 24, 2009, http://globalnation.inquirer.net/news/breakingnews/view/20090624-212208/Philippines-says-no-to-organ-trafficking.

41. Padilla, "Regulated compensation," 121.

42. Ibid., 121.

43. Inter-Agency Council against Trafficking, "Rules and regulations implementing section 4(g) of Republic Act No. 9208, otherwise known as the Anti–Trafficking in Persons Act of 2003, in relation to section 3(a) of the same act, on the trafficking of persons for the purpose of removal or sale of organs," 2009, www.transplant-observatory.org/SiteCollectionDocuments/wprlegethphl6.pdf.

44. Conde CH, "Philippines bans kidney transplants for foreigners," *New York Times*, Apr. 30, 2008, www.nytimes.com/2008/04/30/world/asia/30phils.html.

45. "Philippines tries to reduce sales of kidneys for transplant," *Voice of America (VOA) News*, Oct. 27, 2009, www.voanews.com/content/a-13-2007-03-19-voa16-66771412/564304.html.

46. For the cost in Israel, ibid., 93–94; for foreign transplants, ibid., 86–87.

47. Lavee J, Ashkenazi T, Stoler A, Cohen J, Beyar R, "Preliminary marked increase in the national organ donation rate in Israel following implementation of a new organ transplantation law," *American Journal of Transplantation* 2013;13: 780–85.

48. Efrat A, "The rise and decline of Israel's participation in the global organ trade: Causes and lessons," *Crime, Law and Social Change* 2013;60: 81–105; Finkel M, "Complications," *New York Times Magazine*, May 27, 2001, 26–33 ff; Greenberg O, "The global organ trade: A case in point," *Cambridge Quarterly of Healthcare Ethics* 2013;22: 238–45; Padilla B, Danovitch GM, Lavee J, "Impact of legal measures prevent transplant tourism: The interrelated experience of the Philippines and Israel," *Medicine, Health Care, and Philosophy* 2013;16: 915–19.

49. Ronen M, "How much is a kidney worth?" *Yedioth Ahronoth*, Feb. 3, 2000; Finkel, "Complications"; International Summit on Transplant Tourism and Organ Trafficking, *The Declaration of Istanbul on Organ Trafficking and Transplant Tourism*, *Kidney International* 2008;74 (7): 854–59.

50. Efrat, "Rise and decline," 87.

51. Ibid., 94–95.

52. Padilla et al., "Impact," 783.

53. Greenberg, "Global organ trade," 241–42.

54. "Encouraging Organ Donation: The Israeli Method," July 2014, http://us3.campaign-archive2 .com/?u = 865d4e1d343803cca3cdd0158&id = ee820fa629&e = fdfa9044d3.

55. Lundin S, "Organ economy: Organ trafficking in Moldova and Israel," *Public Understanding of Science* 2012;21: 226–41; Office of the Special Representative and Coordinator for Combating Trafficking in Human Beings, Organization for Security and Cooperation in Europe, *Trafficking in human beings for the purpose of organ removal in the OSCE region: Analysis and findings*. Vienna: Organization for Security and Cooperation in Europe, 2013; Scheper-Hughes N, "Parts unknown: Undercover ethnography of the organs-trafficking underworld," *Ethnography* 2004;5: 29–73; Social, Health and Family Affairs Committee, Parliamentary Assembly of the Council of Europe, *Trafficking in organs in Europe*, Doc. 9822, Strasbourg: PACE, 2003.

56. Peters, "Marketing organs," 40–41; Cohen LR, "Increasing the supply of transplant organs: The virtues of a futures market," *George Washington Law Review* 1989;58: 1–51; Hansmann H, "The economics and ethics of markets for human organs," *Journal of Health Politics, Policy, and Law* 1989;14: 57–85; Peters TG, "Life or death: The issue of payment in cadaveric organ donation," *JAMA* 1991;265: 1302–5; Peters, "Financial incentives"; Cherry, *Kidney for sale*; Hippen, "In defense of a regulated market."

57. US Public Law 98-507, Oct. 19, 1984, *National Organ Transplant Act (NOTA)* 98 Stat. 2339.

58. US Public Law 110–144, 110th Congress, "An Act to amend the National Organ Transplant Act to provide that criminal penalties do not apply to human organ paired donation, and for other purposes," www.gpo.gov/fdsys/pkg/PLAW-110publ144/pdf/PLAW-110publ144.pdf.

59. Jacobs HB, "Statement before the Subcommittee for Investigations and Oversight of the Committee on Science and Technology," in *Procurement and allocation of human organs for transplantation: Hearings before the Subcommittee on Investigations and Oversight of the Committee on Science and Technology, US House of Representatives, 98th Congress, Nov. 7 and 9, 1983* (Washington, DC: US Government Printing Office, 1984), 259.

60. Pennsylvania Department of Health, "Organ donation incidental expenses family benefit plan," www.portal.state.pa.us/portal/server.pt/community/organ_donation_awareness/18861/ organ_donation_incidental_expenses_family_benefit_plan/557829.

61. Snowbeck C, "Program offers funds for funeral arrangements of organ donors," *Pittsburgh Post-Gazette*, Apr. 19, 1999.

62. Snowbeck C, "Organ donor funeral aid scrapped: Health department fears conflict with federal law," *Pittsburgh Post-Gazette*, Feb. 1, 2002.

63. Scolforo M, "State reconsiders paying funeral costs for organ donors," *Pittsburgh Post-Gazette*, Feb. 1, 2004.

64. "Guilty plea to kidney-selling charges," *New York Times*, Oct. 27, 2011, www.nytimes.com/2011/ 10/28/nyregion/guilty-plea-to-kidney-selling-charges.html?_r = 0; Evans E, "'Black market' cash-for

-kidneys trader Rosenbaum gets 2-1/2 years in prison," http://usnews.nbcnews.com/_news/2012/07/12/12695621-black-market-cash-for-kidneys-trader-rosenbaum-gets-2-12-years-in-prison.

65. Ghods AJ, Savaj S, "Iranian model of paid and regulated living-unrelated kidney donation," *Clinical Journal of the American Society of Nephrology (CJASN)* 2006;1: 1136–45.

66. For the best extended, English-language account of the Iranian program, see Fry-Revere S, *The kidney sellers: A journey of discovery in Iran* (Durham, NC: Carolina Academic Press, 2014). Also see Ghods, Savaj, "Iranian model"; Bagheri A, "Compensated kidney donation: An ethical review of the Iranian model," *Kennedy Institute of Ethics Journal* 2006;16: 269–82; Delmonico FL, "The alternative Iranian model of living renal transplantation," *Kidney International* 2012;82: 625–26; Ghods AJ, "Ethical issues and living unrelated donor kidney transplantation," *Iranian Journal of Kidney Diseases* 2009;3: 183–91; Ghods AJ, Mahdavi M, "Organ transplantation in Iran," *Saudi Journal of Kidney Diseases and Transplantation* 2007;18: 648–55; Griffin A, "Kidneys on demand," *British Medical Journal* 2007;334: 502–5; Heidary Rouchi A, Mahdavi-Mazdeh M, Zamyadi M, "Compensated living kidney donation in Iran: Donor's attitude and short-term follow-up," *Iranian Journal of Kidney Diseases* 2009;3: 34–39; Larijani B, Zahedi F, Ghafouri-Fard S, "Rewarded gift for living renal donors," *Transplantation Proceedings* 2004;36: 2539–42; Mahdavi-Mazdeh M, "The Iranian model of living renal transplantation," *Kidney International* 2012;82: 627–34; Nourbala MH, Einollahi B, Kardavani B, et al., "The cost of kidney transplantation in Iran," *Transplantation Proceedings* 2007;39: 927–29. Some people, including some in Iran, persist in referring to those who supply kidneys as "donors." The term used by Fry-Revere of "sellers," or the term "vendors," seems more appropriate; but, as Fry-Revere points out, some of those supplying kidneys really think of the transaction as a gift, even though they end up being compensated, suggesting an explanation for why the term "donor" persists.

67. Mahdavi-Mazdeh, "Iranian model"; Fry-Revere, *Kidney sellers*.

68. Mahdavi-Mazdeh, "Iranian model."

69. Ghods, Savaj, "Iranian model."

70. Ghods, Mahdavi, "Organ transplantation."

71. Mahdavi-Mazdeh, "Iranian model."

72. United Network for Organ Sharing, Ethics Committee, Payment Subcommittee, "Financial incentives for organ donation," June 1993, http://optn.transplant.hrsa.gov/resources/bioethics.asp?index = 4; American Medical Association, Council on Ethical and Judicial Affairs, "Financial incentives for organ procurement: Ethical aspects of future contracts for cadaveric donors," *Archives of Internal Medicine* 1995;155: 581–89; Peters, "Financial incentives."

73. See, e.g., Dossetor JB, Manickkavel V, "Commercialization: The buying and selling of kidneys," in *Ethical problems in dialysis and transplantation*, ed. Kjellstrand CM, Dossetor JB (Boston: Kluwer Academic Publishers, 1992), 61–71.

74. US Public Law 98-507, Oct. 19, 1984, *National Organ Transplant Act (NOTA)* 98 Stat. 2339.

75. This term suggests that the butcher shop metaphor would be quite precise for markets in human flesh.

76. Faden R, Beauchamp TL, in collaboration with King NNP, *A history and theory of informed consent* (New York: Oxford University Press, 1986), 339–40.

77. See, e.g., Nozick R, "Coercion," in *Philosophy, science and method: Essays in honor of Ernest Nagel*, ed. Morgenbesser S, Suppes P, White M (New York: St. Martin's Press, 1969), 440–72.

78. Rippon S, "Imposing options on people in poverty: The harm of a live donor organ market," *Journal of Medical Ethics* 2014;40: 145.

79. Ibid., 148.

80. See, e.g., Rothman SM, Rothman DJ, "The hidden cost of organ sale," *American Journal of Transplantation* 2006;6: 1524–28; and Malmqvist E, "Are bans on kidney sales unjustifiably paternalistic?" *Bioethics* 2014;28: 110–18.

81. Titmuss RM, *The gift relationship: From human blood to social policy* (London: George Allen and Unwin, 1970). Ben Hippen argues that permitting kidney sales in Iran has increased supply; but again, the data are difficult to confirm. See Hippen BE, *Organ sales and moral travails: Lessons from the living kidney vendor program in Iran*, Cato Policy Analysis 614, March 2008, www.cato.org/publications/ policy-analysis/organ-sales-moral-travails-lessons-living-kidney-vendor-program-iran.

82. For cadaveric organs, one could imagine a host of "resistible" offers; one could imagine a small incentive to stimulate people to sign the line on the driver's license indicating a willingness to provide organs, e.g., a $3 reduction in the driving license fee if the donor line were signed—either for or against donation, or even a policy of paying the estate of the deceased $1,000 if any organs were procured that could be used by the organ procurement organization. At least the latter has been tried in Pennsylvania.

83. OPTN/UNOS Ad Hoc Living Donor Committee, "Interim Report," July 21, 2003, Chicago.

84. For uses of the term, see Daar AS, "Rewarded gifting," *Transplantation Proceedings* 1992;24: 2207–11; Dossetor JB, "Rewarded gifting: Is it ever ethically acceptable?" *Transplantation Proceedings* 1992;24: 2092–94; Wesley AJ, "Pro: Rewarded gifting should be tried" *Transplantation & Immunology Letter* 1992;8 (1): 4, 6; Murray TH, "The moral repugnance of rewarded gifting," *Transplantation & Immunology Letter* 1992;8 (1): 5, 7; Kahan BD, "Rewarded gifting—pro and con: Bringing the arguments into focus," *Transplantation & Immunology Letter* 1992;8 (1): 3.

85. Fry-Revere, *Kidney sellers*, 98ff.

86. OPTN Policies, 8.4.F, http://optn.transplant.hrsa.gov/ContentDocuments/OPTN_Policies.pdf.

87. Schwindt R, Vining A, "Proposal for a mutual insurance pool for transplant organs," *Journal of Health Politics, Policy and Law* 1998;23: 725–41.

88. See the website for LifeSharers, www.lifesharers.org/.

Chapter 12

Live-Donor Transplants

The Living Donor

Transplants are generally premised on the dead donor rule. The general rule, which we have described in chapter 3 in part I, is that the source of organs must be dead before organs are procured.[1] One clear exception to the dead donor rule is the more traditional situation when a living, related donor offers tissue or solid organs in a way that is not life-threatening. Provided there is adequately informed consent, these living donations are morally acceptable. This includes solid tissue—such as blood, bone marrow, and sperm—as well as the donation of solid organs and organ parts, provided the donor can be expected to survive with the parts that remain.[2] This type of situation has included the transplanting of a single kidney, a lobe of the liver, lungs, and even pancreatic tissue.[3] The dominant organ of concern, however, is the kidney, and thus we deal primarily with the kidney in this review of the ethics of live donation of organs. In this chapter we first describe the range of living donor transplants (some of which are quite innovative) and then explore the ethical issues raised.

The first successful living kidney transplants occurred between identical twins in 1954. That they were identical twins was critical, given that there were no effective immunosuppression drugs. Living donation would not grow in popularity until the development of immunosuppression. Initially, transplants only occurred between genetic relatives—both because of greater rejection with greater histo-incompatibility as seen between non-genetically related individuals and also because of suspicions about donor motivation. As immunosuppression improved, there was greater willingness to accept spouses and then friends. Finally, some transplant programs even began to consider purely altruistic live donors of kidneys to strangers when the donors had no expectation of any reward beyond the satisfaction of helping another human being in need. Because we do not want to imply that those who donate to family members and friends are not also in some sense "altruistic," these donors to strangers are now often called "nondirected donors" or "Good Samaritan" donors.

Aaron Spital has documented the evolving attitudes of US transplant centers' willingness to accept spouses, friends, and strangers as living donors. In 1987 he found that 76 percent of programs would consider spouses as potential donors, 48 percent were willing to accept friends, and fewer than 10 percent were willing to accept strangers.[4] By 1993 these proportions had increased to 88 percent, 63 percent, and 15 percent respectively for spouses, friends, and strangers; and by 1999 more than 90 percent of programs were willing to accept friends as living donors and almost 40 percent were willing to accept strangers.[5] The general public is even more accepting. A telephone survey in 2001 found that more than 90 percent of respondents believed donation by close friends is acceptable, and 80 percent felt the same about strangers. Most (76 percent) claimed they would be willing to donate to a close friend.[6] Several factors contributed to this greater willingness to accept emotionally related donors: (1) an increasing gap between the number of deceased donors and wait list candidates, (2) improved results reported in the literature, and (3) ethical support for accepting such donors in the literature.[7]

Expanding Living Donors: Paired Live-Donor Exchanges and Variants

Some living donors are unable to donate to an emotionally related candidate. Typically, this would involve ABO incompatibilities, but could also occur for other reasons (e.g., positive T-cell cross-matches or size incompatibilities). One solution is the use of powerful desensitization strategies whereby the potential recipient undergoes pre-transplant treatment to be able to tolerate a prospective donor's organ. Some centers are achieving excellent results.[8] An alternative proposed by one of us, in 1997, in cooperation with colleagues at the University of Chicago, examined the ethics of permitting an exchange between two donor–recipient pairs, a concept that had been proposed by Rapaport more than a decade earlier, and had been put into practice by Park and colleagues in South Korea in the early 1990s.[9] The results would be transplants to genetically and emotionally unrelated individuals, but the motivation of the donor would be to serve the interests of his or her intended recipient, who could be either genetically or emotionally related. We refer to this type of live-donor exchange as "living-donor paired exchanges."

Balanced Pairs

The simplest, least controversial exchange would be between two pairs (typically, with each pair being members of a family or friends, one of whom needs a kidney and the other of whom is willing to donate). One family involves a donor of blood type A (hereafter referred to as an A-donor) and a recipient of blood type B (hereafter referred to as a B-recipient). This represents a blood incompatibility, so there can be no direct donation. However, if there is another pair in another family involving a B-donor and an A-recipient, an exchange can take place. The A-donor could give a kidney to the A-recipient—typically, a stranger. In exchange, the B-donor could give a kidney to the B-recipient. The main problem that we envisioned at the time was practical: In order to avoid the possibility that one of the donors would change his or her mind, it is good to do the two procurements simultaneously, preferably in the same hospital to avoid having to transport the kidneys. However, finding a donor–recipient pair of blood type A-B respectively and another of blood type B-A respectively at the same institution that have a negative cross-match turned out to be more difficult than we had initially envisioned. Although we imagined that all four procedures (the two procurements and the two implantations) would be done at one institution, it soon became clear that larger pools of donors and recipients were needed than were available at a single institution, and thus regional programs developed.[10] Today, the National Kidney Registry is a private organization set up to help arrange such paired exchanges. The United Network for Organ Sharing (UNOS) also has established a registry of donors and recipients willing to participate in a paired exchange.

Once the ethics of performing living paired exchanges was outlined in the medical literature, transplant personnel began to consider variations on the theme. The first was to move from two-paired living donor paired exchanges to multiparty living donor exchanges.[11] For example, three pairs of donors and recipients might be able, in rare circumstances, to have a three-way exchange. For example, if an A-donor wanted to donate to a sibling of blood type O, the A-organ could be placed in someone of blood type A who had a family member of blood type AB who was willing to donate. That AB-organ could then be placed into an AB-recipient who had a family member of blood type O who was willing to donate but could not directly donate because of a cross-match problem. The O-organ could be implanted into the original O-recipient, assuming there was no cross-match issue. Three organs would thereby be procured and transplanted, even though none of these donors could have donated directly to their own family member needing an organ. This is fairly straightforward ethically, but would require a very rare set of circumstances for all three candidates and their family-member donors to be ready at the same time.

Unbalanced Pairs

A second idea was to promote paired exchanges even if one pair could donate directly (compatible pair) but the other pair could not (incompatible pair). Because one of the pairs could have exchanged directly while the other pair could not, these exchanges are called "unbalanced" exchanges.

For example, we know that O-donors are universal donors. Imagine that donor number 1 has blood type O and was planning to donate to his sister (recipient number 1) of blood type A. This donation could take place directly (and typically does). However, in the next examination room was donor number 2, who has blood type A and who wanted to donate to his brother (recipient number 2) of blood type O. This cannot occur because someone with A-blood cannot donate to someone with O-blood. Although donor number 2 cannot donate to his sibling (recipient number 2), he could donate to the first recipient. Donor number 1 could donate to either recipient. If donor number 1 and recipient number 1 agree to the exchange, then both recipients can receive a kidney; otherwise, only recipient number 1 would receive a kidney. Donor number 1 could be motivated either to get a healthier kidney for his or her recipient (e.g., if donor number 2 were much younger) or to be able to help two individuals in need of a kidney.[12] The problem—as explored by one of us with Steve Woodle, a transplant surgeon now at the University of Cincinnati—was how to offer the option without being coercive.[13] We discuss this problem later in the chapter.

Chains

Another variant is the move from paired exchanges to chains involving three or more donations in which the catalyst is a nondirected donor. The last recipient is a candidate from the wait list who need not have a paired donor.[14] The longest chain to date involved thirty donors and thirty kidneys and was described in the *New York Times*.[15] It was cata-lyzed by a nondirected donor, procured asynchronously, involved one compatible pair, and was ended by giving the last paired kidney to a candidate on the wait list who did not have a prospective living donor. Although there are concerns that donors in asynchronous chains may renege once their intended recipient receives a kidney, this has been relatively uncommon in the National Kidney Registry's experience to date.[16]

List-Paired Exchanges

An additional live-donor plan is closely related to the original paired living donor exchanges already described. A donor who is incompatible with a desired recipient (e.g., a spouse or relative) might donate an organ to the deceased donor wait list in exchange for priority on the deceased donor wait list for the donor's chosen recipient. This is known as a "list-paired exchange." Once the donor had had a kidney removed, it would be allocated to a candidate on the deceased donor wait list according to normal allocation rules. In exchange, the person designated by the donor would be elevated to the top of the deceased donor wait list to receive the first compatible organ.

Intuitively, this may appear to mean that everyone on the deceased donor kidney wait list would be as well off or better off than they were before. (They might be considered slightly better off because one person would have been removed from the wait list, improving the situation of every person waiting who was positioned below the person removed.) However, this ignores the fact that the wait list actually consists of multiple wait lists—one for each blood type. The most likely donor–recipient pair willing to partic-ipate in a list-paired exchange would be a living donor of non-O blood type (A,B, or AB) who would be donating to a recipient of blood type O. This would mean, for example, that a candidate on the blood type A wait list would benefit, but the paired recipient would now go to the head of the blood type O wait list (hereafter referred to as the O–wait list). Wait list candidates of blood types O have longer average waiting times (particularly compared to candidates of blood types A and AB), and allowing paired recipients of blood type O to move to the head of the wait list will only extend the wait time of the other O–wait list candidates. As such, though the overall candidate pool benefits, there are identifiable groups whose members will be made worse off (again, because the most likely reason to participate is donor–recipient pair with blood type non-O and O respectively, the O–wait list candidates are the most likely to be pushed down on their wait list).[17] In contrast, when a list-paired exchange is used for an ABO-identical donor–recipient pair who cannot donate directly due to sensitization, then the paired recipient merely takes the place of this other candidate who was already near the top of the list, avoiding the problem of crossing wait lists and potentially harming candidates who are already on the longer wait lists.

The Ethics of Live Donation: Two Approaches

There are two major ethical approaches to living donor cases. One focuses on benefits and harms to the recipient and the organ source, what we have referred to as consequen-tialist or utilitarian ethics. The other focuses on autonomy and whether donation is truly voluntary, what we have described as a more deontological approach.

Benefits and Harms

In the early 1990s the UNOS Ethics Committee endorsed living donor transplants, including those involving genetically unrelated individuals.[18] It began this discussion deeply divided. The transplant surgeons were very concerned about risks to donors. These include physical risks. For kidneys, that issue would be essentially the same whether the donor was genetically related, unrelated, or involved in a paired exchange. The main difference is that the benefit to the recipient could be somewhat less with a donor who is not genetically related because of somewhat lower graft survival rates. With advances in immunosuppression, that difference is shrinking.[19] The rejection risk for the nongenetically related donor today is less than what it was for the genetically related donor of the 1970s or 1980s. The risks also include psychological risk to the donor if the graft is rejected or if the recipient dies.

Conversely, the nonclinicians focused on harms to the potential donors if they were not permitted to donate: the devastating sense of loss and the anger at the system that will not let an individual save his or her spouse or other family member. The consequences to the potential donor could be devastating.

The risks and benefits of paired exchanges and their variants to donors and recipients are almost the same as those of direct donation to a genetically unrelated relative or friend. The only differences would involve the timing of the transplant and possibly, when the recipients are in two different hospitals, the need for the donor to have his or her organ procured in an institution that is not the one he or she might otherwise have chosen. (Paired exchanges involving two different hospitals must involve either the transport of the procured organs or the movement of either donors or recipients to the second hospital. Although traditionally this process involved the movement of people, there has been a trend to the movement of organs, even when they are in separate cities.[20])

In such a situation, a true utilitarian would consider net utility, all things considered.[21] There appears to be a clear expected benefit to the recipient or recipients. Arguably, there would be a net benefit to the organ sources as well. In the end, the UNOS Ethics Committee chose to accept living donations, including emotionally related donors.[22] In 2007 Congress passed the Charlie Norwood Act, which affirmed that swaps between donor–recipient pairs were legal; and in 2008 UNOS approved a pilot program for kidney paired exchanges.[23]

Nonconsequentialist Ethics

Those who consider moral factors other than consequences focus on the rights and responsibilities of the parties involved. They hold that ethics is not exclusively a matter of benefiting the patient and protecting the patient from harm. The old Hippocratic ethics was grounded in the benefits and harms approach.[24] It was pure paternalism. But that consequence-based ethic could theoretically justify procuring organs from living sources without consent—in cases where a physician believed the patient would be harmed more by refusing to donate. A more social ethical approach would also consider the benefits and harms to the other parties involved, including the recipient, which could easily make procurement from living organ sources acceptable and even mandatory—theoretically, the surgeon would be expected to procure organs for such transplants even without the organ source's consent. Those who insist that there is more to ethics than maximizing good consequences will consider the other factors as morally crucial.

Competent Adults

Ethics is, according to this second view, a matter of rights and responsibilities, not merely benefits and harms. This is the approach of Immanuel Kant and the rights-oriented tradition of liberal political philosophy. In exploring how nonconsequentialists handle the rights and responsibilities of living organ procurement, let us focus first on competent adults.

THE AUTONOMY-BASED RIGHT TO CONSENT TO DONATION

Does a consenting adult have a right to make decisions about his or her own body; for example, does such a person have a right to refuse medical treatment? In a liberal society the answer is surely "yes." This is the ethical basis for decisions of people to refuse life-sustaining medical treatment. The right is usually understood to be only a liberty-right, that is, a right to refuse to be touched without one's permission. It has not normally been understood to entail an entitlement right, that is, a right of access to a medical procedure and the means to obtain that procedure. Hence, traditionally, a person would have the right to consent only in cases where a provider is willing to cooperate. This is the basis for participation in research involving human subjects. It is also the ethical basis for living, genetically related donations. And it could be the basis for living, non–genetically related donations from relatives, friends, and even strangers as well as paired exchanges and donations to the cadaver pool. If potential donors are substantially autonomous agents, they have the right to either give or refuse consent to medical procedures that are consistent with their freely chosen life plans. At least until very recently, it has not been suggested that one has a right to be a donor if a surgeon is not willing to cooperate; but assuming a willing surgeon, a source of funding, and the like, the willing donor's consent is the basis for legitimating the donation.

OPPOSITION TO AUTONOMY AS THE BASIS FOR LIVE DONATION: TWO COUNTERARGUMENTS

Concern about preserving an "out" for the donor. One objection to grounding the ethics of live donation in the autonomy of the substantially competent adult is that consent requires that the parties be adequately informed and that providing such information may put pressure on the potential donor to provide the organ. In response, some transplant surgeons have cooperated in creating "outs" for family members who really would rather not donate but perceive that a straightforward refusal will damage their relation with the potential recipient. Surgeons have been known to provide a "medical excuse."

This plan to mislead the recipient, of course, is an equivocation at best and an outright lie at its worst. It is a statement intended to mislead the recipient into believing that a physiological reason exists why the organ donation cannot take place when, in fact, the reason is rooted in the will of the donor. Kantians and other nonconsequentialists who consider lying and equivocation prima facie ethically wrong will find reason to criticize such practices.

Today, the idea of providing a medical excuse is rejected on the grounds that providing medical misinformation is both ethically wrong and potentially dangerous. But the need to give a potential donor an "out" persists. The solution is one that a Kantian can accept. It is based on the right to privacy. It rejects the idea that the recipient has the right to health information about the prospective donor. Rather, today, the attitude among transplant providers is that the donor is a patient and has a right to privacy and confidentiality. As such, all that the prospective candidate has a right to know is whether the donor can donate. Whether the donor is rejected due to ABO-incompatibility or because the donor is scared or feels coerced, the transplant team's answer to the recipient should be the same: The donor is not a viable candidate—and the team should offer no additional explanation.[25]

However, how to maintain an opt-out is more complicated in an era when donors who are rejected for ABO-incompatibility can now participate in a paired exchange or chain that allows a potential donor to donate to any number of strangers, with at least one of whom he is ABO-compatible and nonsensitized. Although potential recipients may be suspicious of their family member who states, "I am told I am not a viable candidate," the potential recipient has no right to additional information from the team.

Irresistibly attractive offers. A second problem with grounding the ethics of live donation in autonomy and consent is that some would consider the offer to be an organ donor for a spouse or close friend "irresistibly attractive"—that is, it is impossible to reject, an "offer one cannot refuse." The availability of paired exchanges and chains simply increases the potential problem, because familial donors will have less excuse for failing to donate. If the offer to donate were considered irresistibly attractive, so the argument goes, it would no longer permit an autonomous choice by the potential donor.

The problem of irresistibly attractive offers was encountered in chapter 11 when we were considering markets for organs and whether money payments for organs would be coercive for the poor, who might be forced to sell their organs to meet desperate needs for income. There, we saw that *coercion* may not technically be the correct term. The most careful definitions of coercion include the requirement that coercion involve a "threat" rather than an "offer" and that the threat be irresistible and intentional.[26] Moreover, coercion must be distinguished from pressure or manipulation. The core issue, for our purposes, is whether the offer, whatever it is called, renders the decision maker substantially nonautonomous.

Autonomous actions are actions that one chooses based on one's own life plan— according to one's own beliefs and values. Just as accepting money payments for an organ may be consistent with one's life plan, so might deciding to become a live donor. Choosing to make a modest sacrifice of one's own health for the benefit of one's spouse or family member is plausibly consistent with one's life plan. Likewise, making such an offer to a close friend can be consistent with one's own life plan. Even making such an offer to a stranger might be consistent with the life plans of some competent adults. Offers cannot violate one's autonomy simply by being terribly attractive.

But this does not mean that all offers that are attractive are ethical. We saw in chapter 11 that we also need to consider whether the offer is "unwelcome" and "exploitative."

Whether an irresistibly attractive offer is ethical will depend on the mindset of the potential donor as well as on the state of the person making the offer. In this case the offer to a relative to become a candidate for live donation may or may not be welcome. A spouse, for example, may truly be eager to do "anything" to save a husband or wife and not be concerned that the offer is made, but other relatives may find the offer quite unwelcome even if that relative perceives there is no way to resist.

With regard to whether the offer to become a live donor is exploitative, usually this will not be the case. Normally, the health professional presenting the live donor option will discuss the alternatives of dialysis and deceased donor donation and not try to take advantage of the potential donor's desire to help the recipient. However, given the widening gap between candidates and deceased donors, the waiting time is more than five years in certain parts of the country, and transplant professionals are becoming more assertive in encouraging candidates to seek out living donors.

What would be unethical, however, would be a scenario where transplant surgeons offer living donation to a friend or relative of someone in kidney failure, but only after they have withheld an available deceased donor organ. If a surgeon were to withhold a deceased donor organ in order to gain practice in procuring from live donors, that would of course be unethical. It would force the family member to become a live donor. But assuming that the living donation is being considered because the surgeon has nothing else to offer (short of a long and perhaps fruitless time on a wait list), then the mere fact that the offer seems powerfully attractive to the potential donor cannot by itself make the offer immoral, any more than offering painful cardiac surgery to a critically ill heart patient would be considered unethical because it was so attractive an offer compared with the available alternatives. When there are no plausible alternatives to transplanting from a living donor, then there is nothing unethical about making overpoweringly attractive offers to potential donors.

The problem of perceived pressure to donate is just as great for living, genetically related relatives as for non–genetically related ones. In fact, by this analysis, strangers are the least likely to be pressured into consenting. The focus on respect for autonomy provides an argument for accepting volunteers who are strangers, at least for bone marrow and, arguably, for kidneys as well. What might be thought of as the "coerciveness" of an offer to donate is merely an offer that is terribly attractive given some relatives' commitment to their loved ones' survival. It is not unethical because it "coerces" the "donor" and therefore violates the donor's autonomy—unless it exploits the commitment to the recipient to force the donor's behavior when other options were available that were not fairly presented. The coercion felt by potential donors may be increased with the new options of paired exchanges and chains, which remove some of the medical reasons that would have previously excluded a living donor.

Incompetent Organ Sources

Although this analysis heretofore seems to provide moral support for adults who autonomously choose to donate organs (regardless of the degree of kinship), it says nothing about the use of small children, infants, or the mentally incompetent as organ sources.

THE ANALOGY TO HUMAN SUBJECTS RESEARCH

The problems of organ procurement are in many ways like those of conducting research on human subjects. In both human subjects research and organ procurement, human beings are being "used" for the benefit of other humans. If we accept the model of gift giving, we commit to the position that humans must offer their bodies or organs rather than having them taken for public purposes. This was the position taken earlier in this book, and it is generally the position of the American transplant program as well as the human subjects research enterprise. However, unless some provision is made for surrogate decisions to authorize the use of bodies or body parts from incompetents, the implication is that they could never be procured from infants, children, or others who have never been competent. Using one human as a means to benefit another, whether in human subjects research or transplantation, requires consent; and incompetent persons cannot give consent. Hence, in both human subjects research and organ procurement, we must face the issue of surrogate consent for the use of incompetents for a purpose that is primarily for the benefit of another.

There is somewhat more ambiguity about the requirement for access to a cadaver in human subjects research. Most interpretations hold that the federal human subjects research regulations apply only to research on living humans.[27] Nevertheless, many hold that the principle of respect for persons requires some form of consent for research on tissues of the deceased. We generally accept a limited authority of parents to give that permission to do research on deceased minors and, under even more rigid conditions, on living minors. Even if the human subjects regulations do not apply to the deceased, the clear meaning of the Uniform Anatomical Gift Act is that consent or permission is required for *all* uses of the dead body, whether for transplant, education, therapy, or research.

We generally recognize that the parent or guardian of a living minor can give permission for research on the minor. Not all medical ethical commentators accept this approach.[28] However, this is the dominant view,[29] as well as the view expressed in both medical ethical codes and federal regulations.[30]Research that is not connected with therapy that promises benefit for a child or other incompetent person is permitted with surrogate permission, provided certain conditions are met, including the requirement that the risk to the incompetent person is strictly limited. Of course, in the case of a deceased incompetent, it is hard to imagine what risk there would be in organ procurement. Respect for the body would certainly be required, but normally surrogate permission should be sufficient to permit such research. Likewise, it should be sufficient for organ procurement.

"DONATION" FROM INCOMPETENT PERSONS

On the procurement side of transplants, we have stressed that infants and young children can never be "donors." They cannot give consent to have their organs used for a transplant. The younger ones cannot even comprehend the idea of transplantation. For this reason, we continue (as we have done throughout this book) to avoid calling any minors donors. As with mentally incompetent adults, we use the more noncommittal term "organ source."

We begin with the basic premise that children and other incompetent persons are part of moral communities. As such, they are the bearers of rights. However, they also have a very limited responsibility to contribute to the community. For instance, as a society we acknowledge the legitimacy of involving them in minimal risk research.[31] We impose the condition of parental consent in order to protect against abuse; but with proper consent and other standards, a *minimal* imposition of social service on incompetents is morally tolerable, perhaps even essential to nurturing a responsible citizen.

Probably, children have a greater obligation to their family members than they do to participate in minimal risk medical research, so marginally more risk may be acceptable. Several court cases in the United States have supported this conclusion regarding procuring organs for transplant from living, incompetent siblings. The more philosophical question is on what basis such approval might be given. Three arguments have been put forward in favor of procurement from certain minors, and these arguments mainly hold for adult incompetent persons as well.

The first argument is the argument from benefit to the incompetent person supplying the organ. The first legal case presented below developed the notion that it can actually be in the interests of the donor to donate a kidney—even when the organ source cannot consent for himself or herself. Although the potential organ source was an adult, his mental retardation rendered him like a child in all relevant respects. By contrast, the second case suggests some moral limits on the use of this argument.

Strunk v. Strunk. A Kentuckian named Tommy Strunk, a twenty-eight-year-old married employee of the Penn State Railroad and a part-time student, was suffering from chronic glomerulus nephritis.[32] His dialysis treatments were reaching the point at which they could not continue much longer. He needed a transplant. His mother, father, and a number of collateral relatives were tested and found incompatible. His brother, Jerry, however, was found "highly acceptable." The problem was that Jerry was a twenty-seven-year-old who was committed to the Frankfort State Hospital, a state institution for the "feebleminded." He had an IQ of approximately thirty-five and was further handicapped by a speech defect, making it difficult for him to communicate. The mother of the two men petitioned the court for authority to proceed with the transplant by procuring a kidney from Jerry to be transplanted to his brother.

Although Jerry was not a minor, he was described as having a mental age of six years. The court concluded that it was actually in Jerry's interest that his brother receive his kidney. Jerry was described as "greatly dependent upon Tommy, emotionally and psychologically, and . . . his well-being would be jeopardized more severely by the loss of his brother than by the removal of a kidney."[33]

The moral logic was identical to that of a parent offering permission or "proxy consent" for a therapeutic treatment for their child. The transplant was obviously therapeutic for Tommy, the recipient. But the court took the view that the transplant was also "therapeutic" for Jerry. It offered him the benefit of increasing the chances of his brother's survival and the capacity to provide support for Jerry. If that was true, then this was not a case of using the incompetent sibling solely for the benefit of the mentally healthy brother. It was a case of acting so as to benefit the incompetent one.

In re Richardson. Although the court accepted this "patient-benefit" argument in the *Strunk* case, it seems clear that it would not apply in all cases of obtaining organs from children or other incompetent organ sources. A second case suggests an interesting contrast. Four years later a case was heard in the Louisiana courts involving a similar set of circumstances.[34] Thirty-two-year-old Beverly Jean Richardson was in need of a kidney transplant. She had only months to live. (The reasons are unclear why dialysis would not have been successful in bridging until a cadaver organ could be obtained.) The most acceptable organ source was her brother, seventeen-year-old Roy. He, however, was, in addition to being a minor, also severely retarded, having a mental age described as that of a three- or four-year-old.

Richardson's parents relied on the *Strunk* case, attempting to argue that it was in Roy's interest to provide a kidney for his older sister. But the court did not accept this argument, concluding that "such an event is not only highly speculative, but in view of all of the facts, highly unlikely."[35] The reasons are not spelled out, but reports about the case suggest that the sister was not close to the institutionalized young man. The fact that he had been institutionalized suggests that he was not likely to be dependent on his sister. Moreover, the court observed that Roy's condition gave him a short life expectancy. The facts of this case failed to support the claim that it would have been in Roy's interest to be the source of an organ for his sister, taking into account the medical risks and discomfort of the organ procurement surgery.

The second argument is the argument from the duty of incompetents to others. Some have observed that it is a bit of a stretch to defend procurements of organs from incompetents solely on the grounds of benefit to the source of the organ, but that this may be an unnecessary standard in any case. In the sphere of human subjects research, many now reject the standard that experimental treatments may be undertaken for incompetents only when it is in their interest to do so. Under the most rigorous standards that legitimate research only when it is for the benefit of the subject, even risk-free research could not be permitted when it does not promise some benefit to the subject.[36] Surely, the welfare of children and other incompetents is a very high priority; but, it is argued, even children are part of larger social communities and have some limited obligations to be altruistic.[37] In the case of research, risk-free research seems justifiable, provided that other obvious conditions are met: that the research could not be carried out on competents who consent, that parents give their permission, and that older minors who are able give their assent are preferred over younger minors.

If risk-free research is permissible, it must be because even incompetent minors owe something to the communities of which they are a part. This suggests the second kind of argument that has been brought forward to support the procuring of organs and tissues from minors and other incompetents—a social debt that each of us owes to society. This debt to the community might even justify research with minor risks—such as a needle stick or wearing of electronic monitoring equipment to measure heart rate. For these kinds of reasons, federal regulations permit children to participate in research that has only minimal risks, and even greater than minimal risks under certain special circumstances.[38]

If such bonds of community permit imposing minor risks on children who cannot consent merely to benefit strangers, it might be plausible for somewhat more serious risks to be imposed on children to benefit other members of their immediate families. In families in dire straits from poverty or natural disaster, we assume that the parent's duty to do whatever is beneficial for the child is attenuated by the critical limits placed on the family. Although parents are expected to make extreme sacrifices for the welfare of their children in such circumstances, they are not expected to make a total sacrifice. They must pay at least some attention to their own needs (if for no other reason than that it is in the child's interest that the parent remain capable of providing continuing care). It is even more obvious that the parents may compromise one child's interest for the benefit of their other children.[39] Even in more ordinary circumstances, we might expect parents to require children to make some modest contribution to others—as part of the child's socialization into the role of responsible moral citizen. Thus children may be expected to contribute a portion of an allowance to a charity or religious organization. They may be required to compromise their own interests as part of the process of learning altruism. Many would consider that children have some limited form of a duty to make personal compromises in order to benefit others, especially those in greater need or those who are part of the child's family. Being part of a family requires some form of limited duty to others, even for minors who cannot be said to be substantially autonomous and capable of choosing to be altruistic. It is this reasoning that has been offered to support organ and tissue procurement from children and other incompetents.

It is not clear exactly what the limits should be on imposing such family-serving risks. Surely, the risks should not be as great as we would permit a competent adult to accept. Procuring a pint of badly needed blood from an older child to be transfused into a needy sibling when no other source was available seems well within the limits we are talking about. A hospital ethics committee on which one of us (RMV) served used this argument years ago to justify a bone marrow procurement from a living nine-month-old infant sibling who was the only feasible source of marrow for a brother suffering from leukemia. The infant would be at risk of needing a blood transfusion if she were a bone marrow source. We were concerned about possible hepatitis or HIV transmission to the infant along with the pain. After much deliberation, we came to think that the risk was justified. The procurement proceeded without adverse consequences. A decade later, the American Academy of Pediatrics (AAP) has acknowledged this to be a morally acceptable risk to the healthy donor child, even a child who is too young to understand what is happening.[40] Today, parents may even conceive a child, often through in vitro fertilization and preimplantation genetic diagnosis, in order to create a human leukocyte antigen–identical sibling, known as a "savior sibling," who can provide bone marrow or stem cells to an ill older sibling.

Procuring a kidney is a step beyond procuring bone marrow. The kidney will not regenerate, and the surgery is much more substantial. It seems reasonable that the presumption should be against such procurements unless there is no other alternative, there is a reasonable likelihood of success, and the parents can make the case that the child is an integral part of the family unit. Only if such requirements are met, procuring a kidney for transplant to a family member who has no other source for an organ and who can no longer be maintained on dialysis, may possibly be within the limits of what we can impose on a child or an incompetent person.

One of us (LFR) was instrumental in developing the AAP policy that permits minors to serve as living donors without judicial review if done according to strict criteria, including a role for a living donor advocate to work with the potential donor child.[41]

Although the AAP document permits donations by minors, it was not meant to liberalize the practice but rather to restrict it. And though reasonable people may differ on whether ever permitting such contributions from nonconsenting minors goes too far, forty-eight cases of kidney donation and fifteen cases of liver donation by minors have been documented in the UNOS database since 1988.[42]

Probably the kidney is as far as donation by minors can go ethically. Liver and lung lobe procurement, even from consenting adults, raises serious problems due to the greater risks of the surgery to remove it.[43] It is surely more than we should ask of minors and other incompetents. If we ask the question "What does one human being owe to others?" we will frame the question properly. Competent potential donors can then have considerable leeway to decide to donate, providing that any organs donated are not considered life-prolonging. From incompetent patients, we should be severely limited in what we can expect. Surely we do not expect incompetents to provide organs whenever the benefits to others will be greater than the harm expected for the one who is the source of the organs. But some modest contribution may be morally tolerable. From the nonconsequentialist perspective, it is not the risk and benefit that is critical; it is what we have a right to expect.

The third argument is the argument from the wide discretion that parents have in fulfilling their duties to their child. The basis for this third argument to support the participation of children and other incompetent persons as organ sources is found in two additional cases involving minors.

Nathan v. Farinelli was one of twenty-two cases in which the Supreme Judicial Court of Massachusetts issued decrees authorizing transplant operations between 1957 and 1974.[44] (Of note, the Court never rejected a request.) Although in most cases the court justified its decree on the grounds that the procurement of the organ served the best interest of the organ source, in this case the court stated that it was not its duty to decide what was in the "prospective donor's best interest," but only to determine whether the parents took all the risks and benefits into consideration. The court found that the parents had fulfilled their duty and that the parents' decision should be binding.

The second case was *Hart v. Brown*, in which the parents petitioned to allow a child of seven years and ten months to serve as the source of a kidney for her identical twin sister.[45] The defendants were the physicians who refused to perform the operation and the hospital that refused to allow the use of its facilities "unless the court declares that the parents and/or guardians ad litem of the minors have the right to give their consent to the operation upon the minor twins." The court relied heavily on *Bonner v. Moran*, which involved skin grafting from a fifteen-year-old boy to his cousin at a time when such a procedure was still experimental and the procedure was not being done for the benefit of the donor.[46] The court held that the consent of the parent was necessary. It also referred to *Strunk v. Strunk*, in which the court authorized the parent to give her consent because it would serve the incompetent brother's best interest.[47]

In both *Bonner* and *Strunk* the courts were focusing on the right of parents to consent to their child's participation. In *Strunk* the parent was held to a "best interest" standard; but in *Bonner* the parent was not. Based on these cases, the court in *Hart v. Brown* found that "natural parents of a minor have the right to give their consent," although it did hold that their consent should be "reviewed by a community representation which includes a court of equity."

Even in *Hart v. Brown*, however, the need for court oversight was waning, as the court itself noted that the procedure was becoming standard of care. Today, court intervention is no longer sought, although the AAP recommends a living donor advocate for the child who is the source of the organ to ensure that the child's interests are being adequately considered.[48] That is, parental consent is necessary, but there must be some standards to which they are held, or at least some limits to their discretion.

As we saw above, when the justification for allowing minors and other incompetents to serve as organ sources was based on their duty to others, it was felt that bone marrow and kidney was as far as one could go. Likewise, when we think of what is the limit to parental discretion, one of us (LFR) has argued for the same limitations.[49] From a nonconsequentalist perspective, it is what parents have a right to authorize in the private realm of the family to promote family intimacy and integrity.

In the end, consideration of both the limited duties of incompetent persons to society (or, more narrowly, to one's family) and the right of parents to decide what activities are appropriate for their children are relevant moral considerations. Imposing the requirement of parental consent is a strategy for assuring that not too great a burden is imposed on children and incompetent persons. Beyond that, however, our society gives parents a limited authority to decide what is best for their children and the extent to which their children should contribute to others, even if doing so is not necessarily in their medical best interest. Thus we rely on parental discretion, but we also impose limits on the parental decision.

The Assent of Older Minors

The human subjects regulations pertaining to children impose an additional requirement. In the case of older children, they must be asked to "assent" to participation. *Assent* differs from *consent* in that it does not require that the person have the capacity to comprehend and make a reasoned choice, but only requires an affirmative acceptance of another's decision on his or her behalf. In research not involving therapy, in addition to obtaining parental permission, the investigator must ask older children for their assent.[50] If they decline, the children cannot participate. The same reasoning might be applied to tissue and organ procurement from older children.

The Limits of Parental Autonomy

Both the justifications that as members of the human moral community even incompetents owe certain minimal obligations to serve others and the need to respect broad parental discretion in how they raise their children must be examined to determine the limits of a minor's participation as a living donor. The ethical permissibility of exposing them to some degree of physical risk to benefit others seems particularly true when the others are members of the same family and the risks to the incompetent are minimal, such as in the procurement of blood or bone marrow. It would not support minors serving as solid living organ donors except in very rare circumstances, given the degree of risks that they pose. Despite our moral concerns, however, as we have noted, the UNOS database documents several dozen kidney and liver donations by minors, and there are additional cases reported in the literature.[51] There is also a case report of a thirteen-year-old donating a small bowel to an identical twin.[52]

A valid exception to the rule that prohibits minors from acting as living solid organ donors is the minor who serves as a domino donor. A domino transplant occurs when an organ recipient serves as a living donor.[53] For example, a minor with cystic fibrosis may undergo a heart-lung transplant because of end-stage pulmonary disease, and the removed heart may be "healthy" enough to be used for a solitary heart transplant. In that case, the recipient may simultaneously serve as a donor. In such cases, the procurement of the organ poses no additional medical risk to the donor and the use of organs ought to be permissible on the basis of normal standards of parental consent.

In 2000 the Live Donor Consensus Panel enumerated four criteria to justify the participation of minors as live solid organ donors: (1) Donor and recipient are both highly likely to benefit, (2) the surgical risk for the donor is extremely low, (3) all other deceased and living donor options have been exhausted, and (4) the minor freely assents to donate without coercion (established by an independent advocacy team). Although no lower age limit was stated, it was clear that the minor should have the ability to give an informed assent. The AAP adopted these criteria, suggested a lower limit of eleven years, and added a fifth criterion, that the emotional and psychological risks to the donor are minimized. The AAP adopted similar requirements for a child to serve as a bone marrow donor, including the need for an independent living donor advocate, although it was willing to allow for bone marrow donation at all ages and sometimes without assent, on the grounds that the risks were much more limited. In fact, it is fair to say that the focus of the AAP and the Live Donor Consensus Panel was to permit parental permission on the grounds that parents have the authority to expose their children to low-risk activities even if it is not in the child's medical best interest on the grounds of minimal obligations, as opposed to attempting to justify activities on the grounds of promoting some organ source benefit. However, to ensure that the risks are minimal for the particular child, the AAP requires a living donor advocate for all living donations by minors, and additional consultation with psychiatric or developmental pediatrics for minors with cognitive disabilities. In both bone marrow and living tissue donations by minors, the AAP also limited the minor to intrafamilial donations to ensure that minors are donors of last resort. The AAP was not willing to modify any conditions for identical twins because even though such a donation provides greater benefit to the recipient (who will not need immunosuppression), and by extension, to the family, the risks to the donor are unchanged. This again supports the position that the moral justification for allowing parents to authorize their child's participation is based on a minimal obligation owed to all family members and not on donor benefit.

Exchanges and Chains

The ethics of live donor exchanges add only modest complications to the analysis. However, several variations on the theme must also be examined.

Balanced Exchanges

A paired exchange leads to organ transplants to genetically unrelated individuals, so the risks and benefits are comparable to those of living, emotionally related donation. We have seen that this is increasingly considered acceptable. The motivation of the donors is certainly understandable. It is precisely the same as donating directly to one's relative.

The timing of paired exchanges poses some additional problems. For either technical or practical reasons, the ideal time for transplant for the two recipients and two donors may not be the same. However, if one donor contributes a kidney to the other donor's intended recipient prior to the time of the second nephrectomy, some guarantee would need to be in place that the second donor would not change his or her mind. However, it is hard to imagine how such a compulsory, uncancellable pledge to donate would be ethical or legal. This will probably mean that the pair of transplants would need to occur simultaneously, even if the timing is not ideal for some of the parties. In the original protocol, one of us (LFR) and colleagues recommended that both donor–recipient pairs have their surgeries simultaneously, such that both donors would have the option to renege up until the time of surgery.

Paired exchanges could involve kidney patients of the same surgeon. If so, and if the organs are procured simultaneously, presumably one of the transplant recipients would need to accept someone other than his or her chosen surgeon. If different surgeons are involved, this problem would be avoided. If they are at different institutions, then either the donors or the recipients will need to travel to another hospital (or the organs would need to be transported). The trend has been to transport the organ rather than the individual. This does raise questions if different hospitals have different standards or different levels of quality, factors that presumably should be disclosed to all—creating a complicated situation for all involved, but one that presumably can be overcome. Given that paired kidney donation raises few new risks, those who accept direct living kidney donation will probably accept paired kidney exchanges.

Unbalanced Exchanges

The move from paired exchanges between two incompatible pairs to an unbalanced exchange—which involves one compatible and one incompatible pair—may seem at first to raise no new issues. Those who support unbalanced transplants focus on donor autonomy and the right of a living donor to donate an organ to his or her loved one or to a stranger in exchange for another kidney for his or her intended recipient. They note that the risks to the donor are unchanged, although they concede that it is not clear if giving a kidney directly to a loved one versus swapping one's own kidney to get a kidney for a loved one has the same emotional benefit. Although there may be no choice when the swap involves two incompatible pairs, the compatible donor–recipient pair in an unbalanced exchange does have a choice. What impact this has on donor benefit is not known; it is also not clear whether the recipient who is willing to consent to a direct donation from a family member will always consent to getting a kidney through a swap. A recipient may be concerned about disease transmission for himself or herself, and may also be concerned about asking a loved one to donate to a stranger.

Those who believe that such donations should not be offered focus on the process of asking a potential donor compatible with his or her loved one to consider donating to a stranger and getting a different (i.e., similar or better-quality) kidney in return. The concern is how to ensure that the donor who could donate directly is participating voluntarily in an exchange. When this was first proposed, one of us (LFR) and colleagues were concerned that it would be an "irresistible offer" if made by the transplant team—how could one say no to the requesting team? It would require the donor to say, "I want to be selfish and donate directly to my emotional recipient." The donor may find the offer irresistible in that to refuse to help two people when it costs the same as helping one person seems selfish, even though the prospective donor may have preferred not to have been given the opportunity. This becomes a particularly difficult situation if the other donor–recipient pair has already been identified.

How can this offer be done ethically? One way to avoid an irresistible offer is to offer all options upfront. Roodnat and colleagues describe a process in the Netherlands where all potential living donors attend a pretransplantation meeting in which alternative living donation options are described.[54] Of 1,046 donors evaluated, 492 donated directly. Fifty-one nondirected donors were evaluated, 37 of whom donated. Of the 503 who were ineligible to provide a direct donation, 52 participated either in exchange or chain programs, and 7 were pending at the time of publication.[55] To the extent that all options are mentioned upfront, some compatible donor–recipient pairs may elect to participate in chains. We believe it is ethically appropriate to inform donor–recipient pairs of the possibility of alternative live donor transplant strategies at the time when they initiate their evaluations in order to empower them to consider the potential benefit of chain or exchange participation for the recipient of the pair and for other recipients, even if they subsequently learn that they are compatible. But offering this possibility to donor–recipient pairs after they have been found to be compatible may mean offering them something that they wish they had not been offered.

Chains

A major ethical issue that arises in the move from paired exchanges to chains is the inability to perform these chains simultaneously. Although this concern led to the initial recommendation that all procedures should be done simultaneously, the National Kidney Registry's data show that chain donors rarely renege.

A second problem with chains is that typically the chain will start with a nondirected donor who would otherwise donate directly to the wait list, but now will be given the opportunity to begin a chain and help many more people. The utilitarians rejoice, as will most nondirected donors, who will find the ability to benefit five or ten people better than benefiting one life. Those who value fairness, however, may express concern, because chains consist of candidates who have potential living donors and are better off than those on the wait list who do not have a potential alternate source. One solution for this problem is that chains end, and so the last recipient of a chain does not need to have a paired living donor and thus he or she can be a candidate without a potential living donor.

Those who focus on fairness may also express concern, particularly when the nondirected donor is of blood type O. If chains and exchanges were not permissible, then the nondirected donor would have given to an O–wait list candidate; but now the nondirected donor will give to a recipient whose donor can continue the chain, and this recipient may be of any blood type. The concern is familiar: Because O-candidates can only receive from O-donors, the O-candidates are worse off, and directing nondirected donors of blood type O to donate to an individual of any blood type who can catalyze a chain makes those on the O–wait list worse off. Because candidates on the O–wait list already have one of the most difficult times getting an organ, the chain will make things even worse for one of the worst-off groups on the list.[56]

List-Paired Exchanges

Placing the live donor's organ in the deceased donor organ pool in exchange for first priority for a suitable organ for one's desired recipient is, in many ways, a much more efficient plan. It avoids the problems of arranging simultaneous donations in paired exchanges. It is even more convenient than chains that may occur over weeks or months and may end prematurely because a donor either becomes ineligible or reneges. Most important, it would make live donation available in many more cases. The donor–recipient pair would not be restricted to the rare instances when a suitable cross-exchange can be arranged. For example, if blood type is the basis for the donor/recipient incompatibility, no paired exchanges would ever involve donors of blood type O. However, the donor in each case could donate to the deceased donor wait list. In virtually all cases, someone on the wait list would be able to use the organ.

This raises a new set of ethical issues, however. As mentioned above, though list-paired exchanges increase the number of transplants performed, candidates on the wait list of blood type O would be made worse off if most donors are of non-O blood types and their recipients are of blood type O. One of us (LFR), in cooperation with a colleague, predicted that this would happen in 2000.[57] Region 1 obtained a variance from UNOS to be allowed to perform list-paired exchanges. Of their first seventeen list-paired exchanges, only one living donor was of blood type O (trying to donate to a positive cross-matched recipient of blood type O), but all seventeen recipients of kidneys from the wait list were of blood type O.[58]

One of us (RMV) raised the question, what if candidates on the O–wait list agreed to these harms? The idea was that inequalities that do not benefit the worst off can be ethical if the least well off consent to waive the requirements of Rawlsian justice. To answer this question, the other author (LFR) and colleagues sought to determine the attitudes of candidates regarding paired exchanges and their variants. We interviewed approximately a hundred dialysis patients. What we found is that approximately half the patients of blood type O supported list-paired exchanges, even though they understood that these would place them at an even greater disadvantage. Surprisingly, we also found that approximately half the patients of blood types A, B, and AB rejected list-paired exchanges as being unfair to those of blood type O. Interestingly, those who did not know their blood type (those who could be said to be behind the Rawlsian veil of ignorance) were most supportive of list-paired exchanges.[59] But the bottom line was that approximately half those who are worst off were not willing to be harmed even incrementally more, thereby negating the argument that such inequalities could be acceptable if those who are worst off voluntarily waived the requirements of Rawlsian justice.

One of us (RMV) then suggested a compromise. Non-O living donors might be allowed to contribute to the wait list and have their paired recipient receive an O-organ in exchange, but a limit could be imposed on the number of such exchanges. When this occurs, the persons of blood type O on the wait list will be passed over when the deceased donor's O-organ is diverted to the recipient paired with the living non-O donor. One can calculate the predicted additional waiting time this will produce until another O-organ becomes available. For example, in one organ procurement organization, an O-organ became available on average every three days. This means that every O-blood-type candidate on the wait list above the recipient paired with the living donor will wait, on average, an additional three days for a transplant. (Those below the recipient paired with the living donor will be unaffected by the exchange.) By setting a limit on the number of exchanges, one can control the predicted additional wait time. Setting a limit of ten exchanges at any one time would, for example, mean that the O-candidates would wait, on average, thirty additional days, which may seem like a tolerable compromise. Some adjustments might have to be made to deal with highly sensitized people on the wait list, but this approach suggests a basis for a limited list-paired exchange with control of the extent of the unfairness to O-candidates.

The compromise, however, did not work in practice; and in theory it may not be consistent with egalitarian justice, a key component of a fair allocation system. Despite the variance that permitted the Region 1 organ procurement organization to do any number of list-paired exchanges, the transplant team conceded that the O–waiting time on the deceased donor wait list had increased by several months due to the priority given to list-paired recipients, even though only a handful were waiting at any given time. As such, they elected to limit the number of such donations and list-exchange recipients to three at any time to keep the extra wait low.[60] One of us (LFR) also argued against the compromise on the grounds that egalitarian justice would prohibit this type of exchange because it harms those candidates of blood type O who do not have a living donor and are therefore one of the worst-off groups.[61]

The Right of Persons to Become Donors

There is one final problem worth addressing. If competent persons may donate organs to family, friends, and perhaps even strangers as an act of charity without violating any moral principles and incompetents may have a very limited altruism imposed upon them for the welfare of the family, then do people have a *right* to become living donors of organs, even if transplant surgeons object?

When expressed in terms of a "right," we are referring presumably to free choices made by competent individuals, not to decisions by some family members to procure organs from other, incompetent members. Suppose that a parent of a child who is severely ill with kidney or liver failure is aware that he or she could be the one last hope for saving the child's life. If this person chooses to donate an organ, does the transplant surgeon have a moral duty to cooperate and perform the transplant, even if the surgeon has reservations (e.g., believing the risk to the donor is too great or the chance of success too small)?

Or consider another case of which we are aware. A woman without children wanted to donate a liver lobe (admittedly a risky procedure) to her husband, who had primary liver cancer. His only chance to survive was a liver transplant, and his tumor was on the margin of being so large that he would not qualify for a liver from the list of deceased donor organs. His chance of surviving with a transplant was estimated to be 5 to 10 percent. Because of his poor prognosis, he was not listed for a deceased donor liver. However, the woman loved her husband and wanted him to survive. Moreover, he was the sole source of their support. If left widowed, she would have no obvious means of generating income. She felt compelled out of love and perhaps self-interest to do what she could to help him survive. Does she have a right to become a liver lobe donor, and if so, do surgeons have a moral duty to cooperate?

We raise this as a moral issue, not a legal one. We assume that, at least for now, no surgeon will be forced by law to perform this type of surgery against his or her will. But under what conditions could a potential organ donor make a moral demand that his or her organs be procured?

The Futile Care Analogy

This question closely parallels the debate in the United States and elsewhere over so-called futile care.[62] People are increasingly demanding the right to life-prolonging treatment even in cases where the clinician believes the procedures will do no good. The interesting cases are those where the intervention (with ventilator or medication) might temporarily prolong the life of a permanently comatose, vegetative, or inevitably dying patient. Increasingly, clinicians are refusing to perform these procedures. And patients or their surrogates are going to court to obtain an order to be treated.

The American courts have uniformly recognized that when certain conditions are met, a right of access to care will be supported that generates an obligation for hospitals and individual clinicians.[63] We are speaking only of interventions that can be expected to prolong life and that are not burdensome, at least in the case of an incompetent recipient. The physician must be competent to provide the care, and an ongoing patient–physician relationship must exist. When all these conditions are met, the courts have generally ordered treatment.

This creates interesting questions for transplants. If we are inclined to recognize the right of people with minority views to preserve their own lives or the lives of loved ones by court-ordered continuation of life support, would a willing potential donor of organs have a similar right to have his or her organ procured and transplanted even if the clinician objected?

For now, the working presumption is that there is no such right. Granting a right to have one's organs procured could be supported by secular liberal ethics, as well as Jewish and Christian moral theology. However, it would violate the Hippocratic ethic that the physician's intervention must be for the benefit of the individual who is treated. It would also violate the Hippocratic ethic that specifies it is the physician's judgment about benefit that is decisive. Recent shifts in American law and ethics have now largely abandoned the idea that it is the physician's judgment of benefit and harm that is decisive. The *Quinlan* opinion clearly rejected the professional standard in favor of judgments by the patient or the valid surrogate. Of course, there would need to be limits on the risk to the donor and the recipient, and there would need to be some reasonable probability of success. But even then, whether a court would mandate living donor surgery over the conscientious objection of a surgeon is not clear-cut. Regardless of whether a court would intervene, would a parent or a spouse have some sort of moral right to have a kidney or a liver lobe procured in order to attempt to benefit greatly or even save the life or a loved one?

Limits to the Rights of Donors

It has obviously been considered unacceptable to transplant nonrenewable life-prolonging organs such as a heart or liver or lungs from a living donor. This remains the current conclusion for practical purposes, although some theorists, particularly libertarian theorists, debate whether this prohibition should be absolute. To our knowledge, no individual has attempted to petition the court to be allowed to be a living heart donor. The closest case of which we are aware is a man who petitioned to be allowed to donate his second (and only remaining) kidney to his daughter, who had been the recipient of his first donation. Although the procedure would not have killed the donor, it would have left him in need of renal replacement therapy for the rest of his life. The surgeon refused, the institutional ethics committee affirmed his right to refuse, and the procedure was not performed. A few months later, a paternal uncle served as a living donor for the man's daughter.[64]

Moral theorists, however, have considered variants that are even more controversial.[65] First, at least in theory, one might be able to find two persons, each of whom needed an organ part that could be procured without ending the life of the donor (e.g., a kidney, liver lobe, lung lobe, or pancreas portion). If the two persons needed different organs or organ parts, they could theoretically each serve as the other's donor. Of course, this approach would raise complicated technical questions: whether the organ parts procured would be sufficiently healthy if they came from a person in serious organ failure from another organ; and whether the parties could survive surgery at two sites simultaneously. Certainly, such persons would be highly motivated and would be able to understand the burdens from both the donor's and recipient's points of view.

A more controversial proposal would be to identify a group of persons, each of whom was in organ failure for a single organ but whose other organs remained healthy. These might involve persons needing a liver, lung, heart, pancreas, and so forth. (Presumably, considering what is contemplated, kidney recipients would not be interested.) This small group, after being educated about the fact that they would all be dying soon without replacement organs, could be asked whether they wished to volunteer for a lottery in which the loser would be anesthetized and have all his or her usable organs removed for the benefit of the others in the lottery. This would involve living, nonrelated donation that would actively cause the death of the lottery loser.

One can see that, if people were facing rapid certain death without such an arrangement, the lottery could be perceived, from the perspective of all parties before they know who the loser in the lottery was, as being in the rational interests of all involved. Conversely, this would be a clear violation of the dead donor rule. The surgeon procuring the organs would be guilty of an illegal act—a murder. The fact that the murder was humane, rational, and consented to by the parties would not exonerate the murderer under current law.

Almost everyone would probably find such life-ending organ donation by lottery morally repulsive. What is striking is that such an approach seems clearly to be in the self-interest of those who would play the lottery, and all but one would clearly come out better while the loser would be little worse off. The opposition to legalizing such an approach must rest on the core ethical premise of the dead donor rule: There is something morally wrong with actively and intentionally killing another human being, at least one who is innocent and wants to live. Unless we are willing to create a critical exception to the dead donor rule, such survival lotteries will need to remain illegal.

A lottery in which living persons would agree that one should die to save the rest would be a frontal assault on the dead donor rule. However, what if there were a variant on the lottery proposal that would be consistent with the dead donor rule? Imagine that lottery were to take place in a state like Oregon where assisted suicide is currently legal. This lottery could probably already take place if the proposal were modified so that the loser chose physician-assisted suicide and the organs were procured after his or her death. Now the opposition would need to argue that the use of physician-assisted suicide is only acceptable in autonomous adults who have a poor quality of life and believe that they are better off dead—and thus is not to be used when the candidate loses a lottery that, if he had won it, would have led to his consent for a desperately needed organ. The lottery is an irresistible offer at best; murder at worst.

These and other variants have not only been proposed by moral theorists. Jack Kevorkian, the American physician promoting assisted suicide, proposed procuring life-prolonging organs preceding a physician-assisted death.[66] Similarly, one could consider, for example, a person dying from a condition from which an unaffected organ could be salvaged. One of us (RMV) once corresponded with a death row inmate who wanted to be executed in such a way that his organs could be procured.[67] Surgeons, however, will overwhelmingly refuse to cooperate in such lethal organ procurements, even if the quality of their consent is impeccable and the potential donors are inevitably going to die soon (from disease, physician-assisted suicide, forgoing of life support, or execution), regardless of organ procurement, on the grounds that as moral agents, they cannot be forced to kill.[68] Even if a surgeon could be found, that would still not be sufficient; the proponent of such a plan would need to convince multiple surgeons, multiple surgical teams, and multiple institutions to participate in the procurement and allocation of each organ. Suffice it to say, it would require a sea change in many transplant professionals, one that does not appear to be on the horizon.

Conclusion

The ethics of procuring organs from living donors poses no moral questions that are truly new. In one way or another, we have faced them before for transplants, medical research, and other areas of medical ethics.

We now know that the old Hippocratic Oath is inadequate for twentieth-century medicine. It violates the autonomy of the patient, would prohibit most medical research, and would make all living donor organ transplants extremely difficult. However, if we turn to the more appropriate ethic of rights and responsibilities rather than merely benefits and harms, an ethic that recognizes social responsibilities and social relationships within moral communities while guarding against simple utilitarianism, then the procurement of organs from living people becomes more defensible.

Notes

1. Robertson JA, "Relaxing the death standard for organ donation in pediatric situations," in *Organ substitution technology: Ethical, legal, and public policy issues*, ed. Mathieu D (Boulder, CO: Westview Press, 1988), 69–76; Fost N, "Organs from anencephalic infants: An idea whose time has not yet come," *Hastings Center Report* 1988;18 (5): 5–10; Arnold RM, Youngner SJ, "The dead donor rule: Should we stretch it, bend it, or abandon it?" *Kennedy Institute of Ethics Journal* 1993;3 (2): 263–78.

2. Of course, the adequately informed consent of the donor is still required. There is considerable hand-wringing about whether family members or others contemplating donation of lifesaving organs can really make a rational choice to give their consent. Some people report that, when learning of a loved one's need of an organ, the decision is immediate—without the benefit of an adequate information session upon which to make the choice. Sometimes such decisions are thought to lack freedom. For an example, see Majeske RA, Parker LS, Frader JE, "In search of an ethical framework for consideration of decisions live donation," in *Organ and tissue donation: Ethical, legal, and policy issues*, ed. Spielman B (Carbondale: Southern Illinois University Press, 1996), 89–101. In fact, some offers in such cases may be irresistibly attractive. This may lead to instantaneous decision, but that need not imply that the decision is not "adequately" informed. Some offers are so obviously compatible with one's basic commitments and life plan that very little if any information is needed. Such poorly informed decisions may nonetheless be autonomous and consistent with one's life plan. These donors, of course, should be worked up psychologically, but the ethics of consent seems rather straightforward. We discuss these issues later in the chapter.

The risk of mortality from a kidney donation is small, but real. It is estimated to be about 0.03 percent; Allen RDM, Lynch SV, Strong RW, "The living organ donor," in *Organ and tissue donation for transplantation*, ed. Chapman JR, Deierhoi M, Wight C (New York: Oxford University Press, 1997), 165. There is also concern about long-term risks of the donor developing renal failure leading to a need for the second kidney. Until recently, the transplant community held the position that the risk of end stage renal disease in living donors was the same as the risk in the general population. See, for example, Ibrahim HN, Foley R, Tan L, Rogers T, Bailey RF, Guo H, et al., "Long-term consequences of kidney donation," *New England Journal of Medicine* 2009;360: 459–69. However, two recent articles suggest that living donors may be at a small increased risk. See, for example, Mjøen G, Hallan S, Hartmann A, Foss A, Midtwedt K, Oven O et al., "Long-term risks for kidney donors," *Kidney International* 2014;86: 162–167; and Muzaale AD, Massie AB, Wang MC, Montgomery RA, McBride MA, Wainright JL, Segev DL, "Risk of end-stage renal disease following live kidney donation," *JAMA* 2014;311: 579–86.

3. Barr ML, Belghiti J, Villamil FG, et al., "A report of the Vancouver Forum on the care of the live organ donor: Lung, liver, pancreas, and intestine data and medical guidelines," *Transplantation* 2006;81: 1373–85; Pruett TL, Tibell A, Alabdulkareem A, et al., "The ethics statement of the Vancouver Forum on the live lung, liver, pancreas, and intestine donor," *Transplantation* 2006;81 (1): 1386–87; Ethics Committee of the Transplantation Society, "The Consensus Statement of the Amsterdam Forum on the Care of the Live Kidney Donor," *Transplantation* 2004;79: 491–92.

4. Spital A, "Unconventional living kidney donors; attitudes and use among transplant centers," *Transplantation* 1989;48: 243–48.

5. Spital A, "Unrelated living kidney donors: An update of attitudes and use among US transplant centers," *Transplantation* 1994;57: 1722–26; Spital A, "Evolution of attitudes at US transplant centers toward kidney donation by friends and altruistic strangers," *Transplantation* 2000;69: 1728–31.

6. Spital A, "Public attitudes toward kidney donation by friends and altruistic strangers in the United States," *Transplantation* 2001;71: 1061–64.

7. Terasaki PI, Cecka JM, Gjertson DW, Cho YW, "Spousal and other living renal donor transplants," *Clinical Transplantation* 1997: 269–84; Murray TH, "Gifts of the body and the needs of strangers," *Hastings Center Report* 1987;17 (2): 30–38; Levey AS, Hou S, Bush HL Jr., "Sounding board: Kidney transplantation from unrelated living donors," *New England Journal of Medicine* 1986;314: 914–16; Evans M, "Organ donations should not be restricted to relatives," *Journal of Medical Ethics* 1989;15: 17–20; Matas AJ, Garvey CA, Jacobs CL, Kahn JP, "Nondirected donation of kidneys from living donors," *New England Journal of Medicine* 2000;343: 433–36.

8. Becker LE, Susal C, Morath C, "Kidney transplantation across HLA and ABO antibody barriers," *Current Opinion in Organ Transplantation* 2013;18: 445–54.

9. Rapaport FT, "Living donor kidney transplantation," *Transplantation Proceedings* 1987;19: 169; Rapaport FT, "The case for a living, emotionally related international kidney donor exchange registry," *Transplantation Proceedings* 1986;18(Suppl. 2): 5–9. Park K, "Emotionally related donation and donor swapping," *Transplantation Proceedings* 1998;30 (7): 3117; Park K, Moon JI, Kim SI, Kim YS, "Exchange donor program in kidney transplantation," *Transplantation* 1999;67: 336–38.

10. Woodle ES, Goldfarb D, Aeder M, et al., "Establishment of a nationalized, multiregional paired donation network," *Clinical Transplantation* 2005: 247–58; Hanto RL, Reitsma W, Delmonico FL, "The development of a successful multiregional kidney paired donation program," *Transplantation* 2008;86: 1744–48.

11. "Doctors perform 3-way kidney swap," ABC News, Aug 4, 2003, http://abcnews.go.com/GMA/story?id=124899&page=1; Duke A, "5-way kidney swap offers hope for unmatched donors," CNN Health, April 3, 2011, http://www.cnn.com/2011/HEALTH/04/03/california.kidney.swap/index.html.

12. Veatch RM, "Organ exchanges: Fairness to the O-blood group," *American Journal of Transplantation* 2006;6: 1–2; Ratner LE, Rana A, Ranter ER, et al., "The altruistic unbalanced paired kidney exchange: Proof of concept and survey of potential donor and recipient attitudes," *Transplantation* 2010;89: 15–22.

13. Ross LF, Woodle ES, "Ethical issues in increasing living kidney donations by expanding kidney paired exchange," *Transplantation* 2000;69: 1539–43.

14. See Gentry SE, Segev DL, Montgomery RA, "A comparison of populations served by kidney paired donation and list-paired donation," *American Journal of Transplantation* 2005;5: 1914–21.

15. Sack K, "60 lives, 30 kidneys, all linked," *New York Times*, Feb. 19, 2012.

16. Veale J, Hil G, "The National Kidney Registry: 175 transplants in one year," *Clinical Transplantation* 2011: 255–78.

17. In the past decade kidney wait list candidates of blood type B now have a longer wait time than kidney candidates of blood type O. One could argue to prohibit all ABO-incompatible wait list pairs unless it involves a kidney donor of blood type B because this way the B-wait list candidates (who are the worst off) will be helped.

18. Burdick JF, Turcotte JG, Veatch RM, "Principles of organ and tissue allocation and donation by living donors," *Transplantation Proceedings* 24 (1992): 2226–37.

19. Terasaki PI., Cecka JM, Gjertson DW, Takemoto S, "High survival rates of kidney transplants from spousal and living unrelated donors," *New England Journal of Medicine* 1995;333: 333–36.

20. Segev DL, Veale JL, Berger JC, et al., "Transporting live donor kidneys for kidney paired donation: Initial national results," *American Journal of Transplantation* 2011;11: 356–60.

21. Spital A, "Living kidney donation: Still worth the risk," *Transplantation Proceedings* 1988;20: 1051–58.

22. Burdick, Turcotte, Veatch, "Principles."

23. HR 710, 110th Congress, Charlie W. Norwood Living Organ Donation Act (2007), www.govtrack.us/congress/bills/110/hr710; Victorian B, "National Kidney Paired Donation Program: OPTN/UNOS approves components for pilot," *Nephrology Times* 2008;1 (8): 17.

24. Veatch RM, *A theory of medical ethics* (New York: Basic Books, 1981).

25. Ross LF, "What the medical excuse teaches us about the donor as patient," *American Journal of Transplantation* 2010;10: 731–36.

26. Faden R, Beauchamp TL, in collaboration with King NNP, *A history and theory of informed consent* (New York: Oxford University Press, 1986), 337–73.

27. US Department of Health and Human Services, "Federal policy for the protection of human subjects," *Code of Federal Regulations* 45, part 46, rev. June 18, 1991, repr. March 15, 1994.

28. Ramsey P, "Consent as a canon of loyalty with special reference to children in medical investigations," in *The Patient as person*, by Ramsey P (New Haven CT: Yale University Press, 1970), 1–58.

29. Earlier ethicists supporting the morality of children's participation in research include McCormick RA, "Proxy consent in the experimentation situation," *Perspectives in Biology and Medicine* 1974;18: 2–20; Ackerman TF, "Fooling ourselves with child autonomy and assent in nontherapeutic clinical research," *Clinical Research* 1979;27: 345–48; and Bartholome WG, "Parents, children, and the moral benefits of research," *Hastings Center Report* 1976;6 (6): 44–45. There are a number of more recent full-length manuscripts on the topic as well as edited collections. See, e.g., Ross LF, *Children in medical research: Access versus protection* (Oxford: Clarendon Press, 2006); and Wender D, *The ethics of pediatric research* (New York: Oxford University Press, 2010); Kodish E, ed., *Ethics and research with children: A case-based approach* (New York: Oxford University Press, 2005); Grodin MA, Glantz LH, *Children as research subjects: Science, ethics, and law* (New York: Oxford University Press, 1994); Field MD, Berman RE, for Institute of Medicine, Committee on Clinical Research Involving Children, *The ethical conduct of clinical research involving children* (Washington, DC: National Academies Press, 2004). All support the morality of the participation of children in some research, including research that does not offer the prospect of direct benefit.

30. World Medical Association, "Declaration of Helsinki—1989," in *Encyclopedia of bioethics*, rev. edition, vol. 5, ed. Reich WT (New York: Free Press, 1995), 2765–67; US Department of Health and Human Services, "Additional protections for children involved as subjects in research: Final rule," 45 CFR 46, *Federal Register: Rules and Regulations* 48 (no. 46, March 8, 1983): 9814–20.

31. National Commission for the Protection of Human Subjects of Biomedical and Behavioral Research, *Research involving children: Report and recommendations* (Washington, DC: US Government Printing Office, 1977).

32. *Strunk v. Strunk*, KY, 445 SW2d 145 (1969).

33. Ibid., 146.

34. In re Richardson, LA App., 284 So.2d 185 (1973).

35. Ibid., 187.

36. Ramsey, "Consent."

37. McCormick, "Proxy consent."

38. US Department of Health and Human Services, "Additional protections."

39. Ross LF, *Children, families, and healthcare decision-making* (Oxford: Clarendon Press, 1998).

40. American Academy of Pediatrics, Committee on Bioethics, "Policy statement: Children as hematopoietic stem cell donors," *Pediatrics* 2010;125: 392–404.

41. Ross LF, Thistlethwaite JR, Jr, and American Academy of Pediatrics Committee on Bioethics, "Policy statement: Minors as living solid organ donors," *Pediatrics* 2008;122: 454–61.

42. US Department of Health and Human Services Organ Procurement and Transplantation Network, "Data: View data reports—national data," http://optn.transplant.hrsa.gov/latestData/step2.asp?.

43. Shaw LR, Miller JD, Slutsky AS, et al., "Ethics of lung transplantation with live donors," *Lancet* 1991;338: 678–81; Kramer MR, Sprung CI, "Living related donation in lung transplantation: Ethical considerations," *Archives of Internal Medicine* 1995;155: 1734–38.

44. *Nathan v. Farinelli* (Eq. no 74-87 [Mass, July 3, 1974]); Baron CH, Botsford M, Cole GF, "Live organ and tissue transplants from minor donors in Massachusetts," *Boston University Law Review* 1975 (55): 159–93.

45. *Hart v. Brown* (29 Conn Supp 368) 1972.

46. *Bonner v. Moran* 126 F.2d 121 (1941).

47. *Strunk v. Strunk*, KY, 445 SW2d 145 (1969)

48. Ross, Thistlethwaite, and American Academy of Pediatrics, "Policy statement."

49. Ross, *Children.*

50. US Department of Health and Human Services, "Additional protections," 9819.

51. US Department of Health and Human Services Organ Procurement and Transplantation Network, "Data"; Delmonico FL, Harmon WE, "The use of a minor as a live kidney donor," *American Journal of Transplantation* 2002;2: 333–36.

52. Berney T, Genton L, Buhler LH, et al., "Identical 13-year-old twins have donated small bowel: Five-year follow-up after pediatric living related small bowel transplantation between two monozygotic twins," *Transplantation Proceedings* 2004;36 (2):316–18.

53. Lowell JA, Smith CR, Brennan DC, et al., "The domino transplant: Transplant recipients as organ donors," *Transplantation* 2000;69: 372–76.

54. Roodnat JI, Kal-van Gestel JA, Zuidema W, et al., "Successful expansion of the living donor pool by alternative living donation programs," *American Journal of Transplantation* 2009;9: 2150–56.

55. Ibid.

56. In recent years, B-candidates have an even longer wait than O-candidates, due in part to the fact that blacks disproportionately have blood type B and blacks make up more candidates and are less likely to have a living donor. Thus, it is no longer the case that O-candidates are the worst off. But they still have a much longer wait than those of blood type A or AB.

57. Ross, Woodle, "Ethical issues."

58. Delmonico FL, Morrissey PE, Kipkowitz GS, et al., "Donor kidney exchanges," *American Journal of Transplantation* 2004;4: 1628–34.

59. Ackerman PD, Thistlethwaite JR Jr, Ross LF, "Attitudes of minority patients with end-stage renal disease regarding ABO-incompatible list-paired exchanges," *American Journal of Transplantation* 2006;6: 83–88.

60. Delmonico FL, Morrissey PE, Lipkowitz GS, et al., "Donor kidney exchanges," *American Journal of Transplantation* 2004;4: 1628–34.

61. Ross LF, Zenios S, "Practical and ethical challenges to paired exchange programs," *American Journal of Transplantation* 2004;4: 1553–54. See also Ross LF, "The ethical limits in expanding living donor transplantation," *Kennedy Institute of Ethics Journal* 2006;16: 151–72.

62. Veatch RM, Spicer CM, "Medically futile care: The role of the physician in setting limits," *American Journal of Law & Medicine* 1992;18: 15–36.

63. *In the Matter of Baby K*, 832 F.Supp. 1022 (ED VA 1993); *Administrator of Estate of Rideout, et al. v. Hershey Medical Center, Dauphin County Report*, 1995, 472–98; *Velez v. Bethune et al.* 466 SE 2d 627 (GA App. 1995); *In re Jane Doe, a minor, civil Action File No. D-93064*, Superior Court of Fulton County, State of Georgia, October 1991. (Cf. a newspaper article by Gina Kolata reporting a case that may have been decided to the contrary, but for which there is no published opinion). See Kolata G., "Court ruling limits rights of patients; care deemed futile may be withheld," *New York Times*, Apr. 22, 1995.

64. Ross LF, "Donating a second kidney: A tale of family and ethics," *Seminars in Dialysis* 2000;13: 201–3.

65. Some of these arrangements are discussed by Harris J, "The survival lottery," *Philosophy* 1975;50(191): 81–87; and Kamm FM, *Morality, mortality, volume I: Death and whom to save from it* (New York: Oxford University Press, 1993), 226–28.

66. Kevorkian J., *Prescription medicide: The goodness of planned death* (Buffalo: Prometheus Books, 1991), 33 passim.

67. The correspondence is published in Vedau HA, "A condemned man's last wish: Organ donation & a 'meaningful' death," *Hastings Center Report* 1979;9 (1): 16–17.

68. Ross, "Donating a second kidney."

Chapter 13

High-Risk Donors

A *variety of factors* can make organs procured for transplant less suitable in the eyes of transplant surgeons and potential recipients. Some organs are medically marginal due to donor age, some because they were damaged during the procurement process, others because of too long a warm ischemic time, and still others because they come from patients with diseases that could be transmitted to the recipient. Some of these diseases are so troublesome that they clearly rule out the organs for anything but research. Metastatic cancer is an example.

In the mid-1980s, the first cases of human immunodeficiency virus (HIV) transmission from deceased kidney donors to their recipients were documented in France and Austria.[1] Later that decade, the first documented cases of HIV transmission occurred between living donors and their recipients in the United States.[2] This led to changes in practice regarding the timing of HIV testing and to the identification of risk factors that would qualify an individual as a "high risk" donor.

Under an amendment to the National Organ Transplantation Act in 1988, the recovery and transplantation of HIV-positive donor organs were prohibited.[3] Though this may have seemed reasonable in the 1980s and 1990s, when so much about HIV was not known and treatments were not available, it overlooked the possibility that some people, including some who were already HIV-infected, could be at death's door and might consent to an organ from such a donor. For years, however, there has been great interest in overturning the law, and this position was buttressed by successful case reports from South Africa regarding transplanting HIV-positive organs into HIV-positive recipients.[4] In November 2013 legislation was passed that made it legal to procure and transplant HIV-positive organs into HIV-positive recipients.[5]

HIV is only one of a number of infections that are transmissible through solid organ transplantation. Donors can transmit a wide range of viral infections, from cytomegalovirus and Epstein-Barr virus to HIV, hepatitis B virus (HBV), and hepatitis C virus (HCV).[6] Cancers have also unwittingly been transmitted from donors to recipients. In November 2004 the Organ Procurement and Transplantation Network (OPTN) enacted Policy 4.6, which requires reporting by a transplant center of a confirmed or suspected donor-derived disease transmission to the organ procurement organization (OPO), which must then report the transmission to the OPTN. In 2005 only seven reports were made, but this increased to sixty and ninety-seven in 2006 and 2007, respectively.[7]

214

The 1994 guidelines for preventing disease transmission were focused exclusively on HIV.[8] These guidelines were not updated until 2013, when the Public Health Service issued new guidelines that address not only HIV but also HBV and HCV.[9]

In this chapter we argue that recipients should be informed about the risk of donor-derived disease transmission from living and deceased organ sources and that these organs should be used if the candidates consent. We also argue that even HIV-negative candidates should be allowed to consent for HIV-positive organs, particularly for vital organs.

The Types of High-Risk Organs

Donors can transmit infections and cancers. Not all infections are the same in degree of infectivity, severity, and impact on quality of life, and not all cancers are the same in likelihood of metastasis. Different practices and policies should hold, then, depending on a number of factors. We first consider HIV and hepatitis and then turn to other viruses and cancer.

HIV and Hepatitis

The most problematic type of high-risk organ is the one from a donor at risk for viral infection. HIV and hepatitis are of particular concern.

Cases of Transmission

On November 13, 2007, the *New York Times* reported that four transplant recipients had contracted HIV and HCV from a deceased organ donor.[10] This was the first known documented case of HIV transmission from an organ donor to a recipient since 1987, and the first reported case of cotransmission of HIV and HCV. The donor had tested negative for HIV and HCV antibodies, although both infections were later confirmed by nucleic acid testing (NAT) in the stored donor sera.[11] This was followed by a report of HIV transmission from a living donor in New York City in 2009.[12]

HBV and HCV are common causes of cirrhosis and hepatocellular carcinoma and a frequent indication for liver transplantation.[13] Both can also be transmitted during an organ transplant from donor to recipient. When the donor is known or suspected to be infected with HBV, a judgment is made about whether the risk is worth it. Although intentionally risking transmission is very troublesome to clinicians, patients may consider the risk worth it, especially if the alternative is certain, rapid death. Moreover, there is a high prevalence of naturally occurring immunity to hepatitis B, so immune recipients might be located. Pretransplant vaccination and the use of posttransplant immunoprophylaxis against HBV can also significantly reduce donor transmission, although the risk is not zero.[14]

There is also evidence that HCV is transmitted via transplantation. The viral therapies against HCV were traditionally not as effective as those against HBV and were poorly tolerated, but newer oral therapy cocktails have recently been found to be quite effective and may change this.[15] Virtually all individuals who receive an HCV-positive organ become infected with HCV, with variable degree of expression, and what impact the new antiviral cocktails will have on expression remain to be seen. The current practice is to only use HCV-positive organs in HCV-positive recipients. Practice is also organ specific. Only HCV-positive kidneys are used routinely, and they are only transplanted into HCV-positive kidney candidates. The acceptance of an HCV-positive donor kidney reduces time and therefore morbidity on the wait list, but it also causes a slightly greater chance of needing a liver transplant due to chronic HCV infection.[16] HCV-positive candidates are eligible for both HCV-positive and HCV-negative kidneys, and the results are not equivalent. The data show that HCV-positive candidates who receive an HCV-positive kidney have a 2 percent lower survival rate at three years than an HCV-positive candidate who receives an HCV-negative kidney.

For other organs the use of an HCV-positive donor graft also has worse outcomes. A study by Gasink and colleagues published in 2006 showed overall worse outcomes for heart transplant recipients who received a heart from an HCV-positive donor, whether or not the recipient was HCV-positive.[17] There is a broad consensus not to utilize HCV-positive heart donors, except for the critically ill who are not expected to survive without a transplant.[18] In liver transplants, HCV-positive donor grafts can be transplanted into HCV-positive recipients with virtual 100 percent recurrence of HCV infection.[19] Virtually all HCV-negative donor grafts implanted into HCV-positive recipients will become infected with HCV over time. There are few studies that have examined the impact of HCV transmission through transplantation on posttransplant outcomes and the clinical course of a donor-derived infection versus a recurrence.[20] Again, the impact and effectiveness of the new antiviral cocktails remains to be seen.

Mandatory Screening

Currently, all potential organ donors, both living and deceased, must be tested for HIV, HBV, and HCV using a screening test that is licensed by the US Food and Drug Administration.[21] Although all donors must be tested for antibodies to HIV, anti-HBc and HBsAg, and anti-HCV and HCV NAT, the guidelines propose additional testing when risk factors are identified by history. Risk factors include high-risk sexual activity, injecting drug users, incarceration in the preceding twelve months, people newly diagnosed with certain sexually transmitted infections because of possible coinfection, and people who have been on hemodialysis in the preceding twelve months because of its associated risk of contracting HCV.[22]

History Taking

Living donors and family members of deceased donors must be informed that a detailed history of the potential donor is necessary to determine whether the potential donor is in a "high risk" group for certain donor-transmittable infections and cancers and that this history must be communicated to any transplanting center. The person consenting to procurement should be informed that a screen will be performed for "for medical acceptability for organ donation and that such tests may be the basis for not using the organ in transplantation." There should be a consent to the screening as well as the organ procurement. The persons giving the consent must be informed that screening includes testing for HIV, HBV, and HCV, and what a positive and negative test mean. They must be made aware that a positive test may lead to not using the organ, even if already procured. They must be informed that they will be told if any of the screening tests come back positive and what this may mean for them. Living donors must also be informed that repeat testing may be necessary, depending on their risk-taking history.

PROBLEMS ARISING FROM SCREENING WITHOUT EXPLICIT CONSENT OF THE NEXT OF KIN

In a still-living patient, detecting HIV, HBV, or HCV can have medical, social, and psychological implications. Although it is important that people know their status given the myriad of treatments that now exist, it is not a good thing for patients to be screened without understanding that the testing is going on.

Disclosure that a potential deceased donor was HIV positive or is infected with HBV or HCV can have implications for third-parties. Spouses or close relatives learning unexpectedly that their loved one was positive can leave them in a difficult and psychologically stressful position. They may be forced unexpectedly to confront the possibility that they themselves may have been exposed. The next of kin or any other party with authority to consent to organ procurement must be told upfront that testing for HIV, HBV, and HCV is to be performed, and the procurement team must reach an explicit understanding with that person about what will be done with the results. The only possible exception might be screening persons who have already recorded their consent to be organ donors—by signing a donor card, by registering in a first-person donor consent registry, or by agreeing to donation after circulatory death through a planned treatment stoppage, as discussed in chapter 5.

THE EMERGENCY EXCEPTION TO SCREENING FOR HIV, HBV, AND HCV

The United Network for Organ Sharing (UNOS) permits one exception to the screening requirement. In the case of nonrenal organs, when there is an "extreme medical emergency" in the eyes of the staff of the procuring OPO and the recipient institution, an organ may be used without screening, provided that the consent of the recipient or next of kin is obtained.[23]

Donors with High-Risk Lifestyles

The purpose of insistence on obtaining an adequate medical and social history is to rule out potential donors who do not test positive but may nevertheless be infected with the virus. This can occur if the exposure is so recent that antibodies have not formed. Screening has improved and current NAT reduces the "window period"—during which a donor tests negative but is actually positive and can transmit infection. Although UNOS only requires the use of NAT testing for HCV, HIV NAT, or HIV antigens, there are additional tests that can be used when a risk factor is identified or suspected.[24]

Disclosure to Recipients

Halpern and colleagues found that standards for the disclosure of HIV and hepatitis risk and consent were informal and nonstandardized at the time when the cotransmission of

HIV and HCV from a single deceased donor occurred.[25] In August 2008 UNOS implemented a policy that required surgeons to obtain special informed consent before transplanting a high-risk donor's organs, although it does not require that the transplant center inform the candidate who may receive the organ which activity—for example, whether intravenous drug usage or high-risk sexual activity—places the donor at high risk. This is true for both living and deceased donors. A living donor may decide that he or she does not want the intended recipient to know of his or her high-risk activities. In that situation, the donor should be excluded and the candidate should be informed that "the donor was not suitable," without any additional information regarding what made the donor not suitable.[26]

Although positive donors are not eligible to donate to negative recipients, both HIV-positive as well as hepatitis-positive donors are now permitted to donate to positive recipients, and there is a greater willingness within the transplant community to accept such organs. However, first and foremost, a diagnosis of HIV, HBV, or HCV in a donor belongs to the donor, and if the recipient is negative, the donor is not permitted to donate. In these cases, the recipient should only be informed that the donor is not eligible to donate—it is up to the donor if he or she wants to share the reason.

Although information about donor infections or risks of infections with HIV, HBV, or HCV belongs to the donor, the transplant community generally takes the position that, if the donor wants to donate, then the recipient has the right to this information. This reflects a double standard in that donors do not have the right to specific information about the health of the recipient. Rather, the OPTN guidelines (Policy 12.2h) state: "The donor must be informed that any transplant candidate might have risk factors for increased morbidity or mortality that are not disclosed to the potential donor"; that is, a recipient has the right to know whether the donor has a disease such as HCV, but the donor does not have the right to know this about the recipient.[27] One can argue that this unilateral standard makes sense because it is only the donor who can infect the recipient. However, donors may believe that to give a proper consent, they have the right to know the likelihood of patient and graft survival, which may be affected by a recipient's health problems. For example, HCV is a major cause of liver failure. Living donors may want to know if their intended recipient's liver failure was caused by HCV because HCV is known to recur in virtually all liver transplants and is the main cause of graft loss.[28]

Organ Sources without Medical or Social Histories Available

Although a potential donor or organ source for whom no history can be obtained because no relative knows the information or the relatives are uncooperative may have been excluded from the procurement process in years gone by, today these individuals would be viewed as high-risk donors and described to organ procurement agencies as such. They should undergo the additional testing that is recommended for high-risk donors, but organs would still be procured if appropriate consent exists (e.g., permission from a first-person consent registry).

Other Diseases

Although transplant teams focus on avoiding the procurement and allocation of organs with HIV, HBV, and HCV, other viral infections and also cancers are transmissible. Given the absolute shortage of organs, policies must balance known and potential risks with known and potential benefits.

Human T-Lymphotropic Virus Type 1/2 (HTLV-1/2) Antibody

In the 1990s UNOS policies had provisions for screening and excluding persons infected with the HTLV-1 virus. Exceptions were again permitted for an "extreme medical emergency."[29] Although endemic in certain parts of the world (Japan, the Caribbean, and Sub-Saharan Africa), it is of low frequency in the United States and Europe.[30] Most individuals infected with HTLV-1 remain asymptomatic throughout their life, although it can present as adult T-cell leukemia/lymphoma and HTLV-1 associated myelopathy. There is also an HTLV-2 virus, but its pathogenicity in humans remains uncertain, although cases of neurological disease, inflammatory arthritis, and lymphocytic leukemia have been reported.[31] In 2001 the first cases of HTLV-1 infection acquired through organ transplantation from one asymptomatic carrier were reported in Europe.[32] At least three cases of transmission were reported in the United States as of 2009.[33]

Assays for the detection of HTLV-1/2 have been available since the middle of the 1980s. Early assays were poor at detecting HTLV-2, but new assays developed in the 1990s detected both HTLV-1 and -2, with additional testing needed to distinguish between the two.[34] In the United States an enzyme-linked immunoabsorbent assay was used to screen organ donors until the end of 2009, when Abbott Pharmaceuticals stopped making the assay.[35] The test was sensitive but lacked significant specificity, and therefore its positive predictive value was low in the United States, where seroprevalence is low.[36] Its use was further complicated by the need for confirmatory testing, and none of these tests were approved by the US Food and Drug Administration.[37] Given the low prevalence, high false positive rate, and lack of an approved confirmatory test, the OPTN/UNOS Ad Hoc Disease Transmission Advisory Committee in 2010 "opined that elimination of pretransplant HTLV-1/2 screening was a reasonable option."[38]

Other Viral Illnesses

So far we have focused on HIV, hepatitis, and HTLV-1/2, but there are other viruses, specifically the herpes virus family, that are far more ubiquitous. Herpes virus includes cytomegalovirus (CMV), herpes simplex viruses (1 and 2), Epstein-Barr virus, varicella-zoster virus, and the emerging pathogens human herpes virus (6, 7, and 8).[39]

In the case of CMV the exclusion of positive organs would significantly decrease the supply. Between 40 and 80 percent of donors of kidneys are seropositive.[40] Although some transplant programs, at least historically, reserved CMV-negative organs for negative recipients with a decrease in morbidity and mortality and graft loss from primary infection, current practice is not to have separate wait lists, but rather to provide prophylactic antiviral regimens and immunoglobulins.[41] The policy of separate wait lists raised serious equity questions for two reasons. First, all candidates, both those who are CMV positive and those who are CMV negative, do better with a CMV-negative organ, and so reserving CMV-negative organs for CMV-negative recipients gives them an unfair advantage. Second, fewer recipients are negative than donors, such that the CMV-negative candidates get to jump the queue for a better organ—an organ that would be better, however, in virtually all candidates and not just in those who are CMV negative.[42]

Today, guidelines for the management of expected donor-derived infections from CMV are well established and are frequently incorporated into routine posttransplant care at most transplant centers.[43] If a donor is suspected of or known to be CMV positive, antivirals are usually begun in the immediate or very early posttransplantation period and are continued for a finite period of time (e.g., three to six months). Despite this, there is a high rate of late-onset disease.[44] Factors for recipients developing late-onset CMV even after posttransplant prophylaxis include CMV-negative recipient status, a shorter course of prophylaxis, higher levels of immunosuppression, and allograft rejection.[45] An alternative to prophylactic treatment is preemptive therapy, in which treatment is begun once viral replication reaches a certain assay threshold. This requires extensive monitoring, which is not always feasible but has the advantages of lower rates of late CMV, more selective drug targeting, decreased drug cost, and avoiding associated toxicities.[46] In all transplants with a CMV-positive donor, a decision will need to be made about whether the risk of CMV infection is tolerable as a side effect of obtaining the usable organ.

Case reports about the transmission of other viruses during transplantation include rabies, West Nile Virus, and the virus-causing Creutzfeldt-Jakob disease—all of which had deleterious outcomes and go back to the need for thorough history taking and testing of the donor when found to be high risk. In addition to viral transmission, there are case reports of donor-derived transmission of bacteria, fungal parasites, syphilis, tuberculosis, and yeast infections.[47]

Cancer

To be absolutely safe, one could argue that any history of cancer should be an absolute contraindication to donation. Donor origin cancer (DOC) in transplant recipients may be transmitted with the graft (donor-transmitted cancer, DTC) or develop subsequently from the graft (donor-derived cancer, DDC).[48] Although historically all individuals with a past medical history of cancer were excluded from donation, with the exception of low-grade skin cancers and primary brain tumors that have not been subjected to any surgical manipulation, there has been some acceptance of donors who have been cancer free for over five years.[49] The risk of procuring organs from donors with a history of cancer is that even an apparently cancer-free organ can harbor microscopic cancer cells, which can then metastasize. There are case reports of various donor origin cancers, including death from metastatic, donor-derived ovarian cancer in a male recipient.[50]

The risk of donor origin cancer transmission is low. In the United States over a thirty-three-month period (April 1994–December 1996), UNOS reported 14,705 deceased donors, of which 257 had a past history of cancer. A total of 650 organs (397 kidneys, 178 livers, and 75 hearts) were transplanted from these 257 donors. Twenty-eight recipients of organs from donors with a past history of cancer developed posttransplantation tumors (the 28 DOC were 18 skin, 2 posttransplant lymphoproliferative disease, and 8 solid cancers). During a mean follow-up of 45 months (range, 30–61 months), no recipients developed a later onset cancer from the donor.[51] In a more recent study of UNOS data,

Ison and Nalesnik analyze 146 reports of malignancies in donors with 20 confirmed transmissions.[52] Likewise, in the United Kingdom, between January 1, 2001, and December 31, 2010, from a group of 14,986 donors, 18 recipients developed a donor-originated cancer, although none of the donors was known to have cancer at the time of donation.[53]

Living donors have also transmitted cancer. The first reported case was the transmission of breast cancer from a donor wife to recipient husband; but lung, lymphoma, and renal cell carcinoma transmission have also been reported.[54]

Keeping in mind that many people on the wait list end up dying for want of an organ and that some cancers can be determined to be unlikely to have metastasized, it seems that some potential transplant recipients who are nearing death from their organ failure would rationally be willing to accept an organ from someone with a malignancy that appears not to have spread. More critically, we can raise questions about whether it would ever be in the interests of someone on the wait list for an organ to accept a transplant procured from someone known to have cancer. Surely, a surgeon should be troubled with the thought that his or her actions might be the cause of a cancer in a transplant recipient. Conversely, those surgeons should also realize that, without the transplant, their patient will die needlessly. It is hard to imagine an argument supporting a categorical prohibition on an organ transplant from organ donors with cancer. Necessity seems to have won, as the transplant community has reluctantly realized that it will need to accept some donations from sources with a past history and even some with active cancer (e.g., low-grade glioblastoma multiforme).[55] Even melanoma, which was previously seen as an absolute contraindication, has undergone reevaluation. Despite a case report of donor transmission of malignant melanoma in a lung transplant recipient thirty-two years after curative resection,[56] Dr. James Guarrera, surgical director of adult liver transplantation at New York–Presbyterian Hospital / Columbia University Medical Center, was quoted in the *New York Times* in June 2012, stating that "many centers, including our own, have used donors with a history of earlier-stage melanoma which had no signs of recurrence for many years."[57]

Should Transplant Patients Receive High-Risk Organs?

Having identified several kinds of high-risk organs, we need to ask whether they should ever be transplanted into patients who need organs. We consider, first, those in need of organs who themselves are virus positive. Then we consider the even more controversial case of the virus-negative recipient. Finally, we examine the resistance of surgeons to transplanting high-risk organs.

Virus-Positive Recipients and Transplant

Attitudes about donors and recipients infected with HIV or hepatitis are evolving. Although HIV-positive patients were initially excluded from the transplant wait list, data from the 1990s showed that they did quite well, and they are now listed for all solid organs.[58] Likewise, today candidates with HBV and HCV are wait-listed for organs because they are expected to benefit from a transplant, even though HCV liver candidates have a 100 percent risk of HCV recurrence in the transplanted liver, which may eventually cause graft failure unless the newer antivirals can prevent it.

Historically, organs from high-risk candidates and those from whom no history can be obtained were discarded. Today, these organs are used, although in general they are only given to candidates who are also positive. A strong case can be made to procure, offer, and transplant both vital and nonvital organs from virally infected donors and from those donors who are at high risk but for whom no history can be obtained. Of course, the potential recipients should be informed that these are "high-risk organs," that is, organs for which we cannot establish a "clean" history, or even that they are known to be infected organs. Some patients might decline, but others might accept. At least for those who are at the end stage of their organ-specific disease that makes them a candidate for a transplant, they might prefer such a risk to the alternative of certain death.

If a case can be made that HIV-positive recipients should have the right to accept organs from HIV-positive donors, a case can also be made that an HIV-positive candidate has the right to refuse a low-risk organ in order to leave it for a lower-risk candidate. Although that kind of altruism seems to be beyond the call of duty, it would be hard to criticize someone who made such a choice. However, there is no guarantee that the next person on the list is HIV negative or that the candidate who passes up the organ will be offered another organ.

HIV-Negative Recipients in Desperation

This suggests an even more controversial proposal: If it is reasonable for HIV-positive persons to accept organs for which HIV cannot be ruled out, and maybe even for organs from persons known to be positive, is there ever a case where it would be rational for an HIV-negative person to accept an organ known to be HIV positive? If death is the only alternative for someone who cannot obtain a negative organ, we do not see why someone would decline. There is no firm evidence on the incidence of transmission in such a situation. The risk surely should be presumed to be high. But the risk of dying without a transplant may also be very high. Given the fact that people with HIV are now living with medication cocktails for many years symptom free, we can imagine some people preferring this risk to a certain, rapid death.

Why Do Surgeons Fear High-Risk Organs?

The fear of transmitting HIV through organ transplantation has had a significant impact on physicians' practice. Lauren Kucirka and colleagues surveyed transplant surgeons regarding high-risk donors following the 2007 national headlines describing the first case of HIV transmission in more than fifteen years.[59] Almost one-third of the surgeons stated that the case report changed their practice with a decreased use of high-risk donors, increased emphasis on informed consent, and increased use of NAT testing (which is an expensive, labor-intensive test that can identify more recent HIV infection than antibody testing but is also known to have a higher rate of false positive results).[60] However, in 2013 the HIV Organ Policy Equity (HOPE) Act was passed, which repealed the proscription from using known HIV-positive organs for transplant into HIV-positive recipients.[61]

Whether this will change attitudes of using high-risk organs in HIV-positive as well as HIV-negative recipients remains to be seen.

Are Surgeons Afraid of Infection?

Surgeons and other health professionals are traditionally committed to benefiting patients and protecting them from harm. This could lead them to resist the transplantation of high-risk organs. Implanting an infected organ sounds terrible. No one would like the possibility of performing a successful, lifesaving transplant only to see the patient die of an infection introduced from the surgery. This concern, however, seems implausible in cases where the patient has a high probability of dying without a transplant.

Surgeons may also be concerned that they themselves will be infected from handling virus-positive organs. Their self-interest may incline them to avoid risk to themselves from participating in such transplants. This seems like an implausible explanation of resistance to transplanting organs at a risk for HIV or other viral infections, because health professionals are routinely at risk for HIV and other infectious diseases. They put themselves in harm's way when they handle HIV-positive tissue and organs. The procuring team is particularly exposed to contaminated blood and fluids. They understand the necessary precautions. They regularly provide treatment for HIV-positive patients. Many health professionals are remarkably dedicated in their service during epidemics. They have a generally good record of maintaining their presence in the face of infectious disease. And they show dedication in caring for infected patients, even at significant personal risk.

Physician Fear of Iatrogenic Death

Despite the risk to personal safety, most surgeons routinely operate on HIV-positive patients outside the context of transplant. Why then do many physicians resist transplantation of positive organs? Part of the explanation may be fear of iatrogenic disease and death. Physicians do not want to be the cause of a patient's death, even if risking exposure would be the rational thing for a patient to do. We see this in surgeons who militantly oppose letting so-called do-not-resuscitate orders remain in effect in the operating room.[62] Even though a patient may have very carefully thought out reasons why resuscitation should not be attempted, surgeons may flatly refuse to perform surgery on a patient who will not suspend his or her do-not-resuscitate decision, even though that patient understands that resuscitation in the operating room may be easier and more successful than when it is performed elsewhere.

The real issue seems to be that physicians, especially surgeons, simply do not want to be the direct cause of the patient's death. This may also stand behind many physicians' insistence on a distinction between omitting and withdrawing life support. Although almost all theorists, lawyers, and policymakers insist that there is no valid distinction between the two, many clinicians still feel a powerful emotional resistance to actively withdraw support, even when the patient insists upon it.[63]

In the case of transplanting HIV-positive organs, the issue is the physician's role in the causal chain. Philosophers recognize both actions and omissions as potentially leading to causal responsibility. If a physician were to refuse to implant an HIV-positive organ for which the patient had consented because it might lead to the patient's death, the surgeon would become responsible for the patient's dying for lack of an organ, just as he or she would be if the death were to result from implanting an infected organ. The surgeon, indeed, enters the causal chain by implanting the organ, but he or she can also enter that causal chain by refusing the patient's request for the surgery.

Many physicians concerned about medical ethics are quick to point out that a professional is not required to treat a patient simply because the patient demands it. In fact, the right of the physician to refuse to treat is by no means absolute. As we saw in the previous chapter, several legal cases have been brought to the courts where patients demand so-called futile treatment, that is, treatment that will only extend life temporarily and at a burden that many feel is unacceptable. These cases raise the issue of whether a physician can refuse to deliver temporary life-prolonging treatment on the grounds that the benefits are not worth it. In general these cases are decided in the patient's favor—even though the benefits may be very minimal and very brief.[64]

The dilemma for a surgeon with the opportunity to implant an HIV-positive organ should be seen as more like that of an anesthesiologist than it is like a physician who withdraws life support at the patient's request. The anesthesiologist knows every time anesthesia is administered that there is some finite risk of an unintended adverse reaction that could kill the patient. The lethal effect is not expected; surely it is not intended, but it is foreseen that occasionally such accidents happen. But this does not lead the anesthesiologist to refrain from practicing his or her art. It would, in fact, be immoral to refuse to anesthetize merely because we foresee that occasionally a bad event, even death, may be actively caused by the action. So, likewise, implanting an HIV-positive organ (or a high-risk one) may be the only rational thing for a surgeon to do. The policy of refusing to procure all organs from this class of donors forecloses the possibility of this lifesaving surgery in patients, some of whom may already be HIV positive and quite able to understand and take the risk.

It is hard to predict whether a surgeon would be required by a court to implant an HIV-positive organ in a patient who was dying and demanded the transplant. Certainly, the expected benefit to the patient is greater than in the more classical "futile care" cases. But the complexity of the procedure is also greater. Perhaps the eventual conclusion of a court would be on the side of the surgeon refusing to operate.

Although the law may not require a physician to treat in these cases, it is hard to see on what ethical grounds the refusal would rest. The surgeon surely cannot claim that his or her personal risk is too great. Surgeons routinely perform surgery on HIV-positive patients. He or she cannot even claim the operation would be futile (in the sense of being doomed to fail to achieve the objective sought). In some cases, the benefit measured in expected days of survival will surely be much greater with the HIV-positive transplant than without it. The moral imperative for a licensed health care professional to use his or her professional skill to significantly increase the life expectancy of an ongoing patient is powerful. Even if the law would not require such surgery, ethics surely does.

A Proposal for a Policy Change

People are dying today for want of organs. Some of them are already infected with HIV, HBV, or HCV, and they understand enough about the risks of exacerbating the infection to be able to choose between a good chance at living with an infected organ or dying without one. Others are not infected but are willing to take the risk rather than die for lack of an organ.

HIV-, HBV-, and HCV-Positive Organs

We propose that all patients be asked when they are placed on the wait list for an organ whether they would be willing to accept an otherwise medically suitable HIV-positive, HBV-positive, or HCV-positive organ or an organ from a source at high risk for HIV, HBV, or HCV. They should be further told that, if such an organ is not in their interest at the present time, they would have the opportunity at any time to add their name to the group of those willing to accept such an organ. They would, of course, also be permitted to withdraw their name at any time, just as they have the opportunity to consent to receiving other nonideal organs (e.g., older organs, organs procured after donation after circulatory death).

For any patient willing to receive such an organ, a discussion with his or her surgeon should then take place, including information about whether the surgeon is willing to implant such an organ if it were to become available. Although we have argued that surgeons who are committed to doing what is best for their patients should feel themselves under moral pressure to agree to do the surgery, we would not force any unwilling surgeon to engage in the surgery against his or her will. If the surgeon declined to agree to the potential of doing the surgery with an infected or high-risk organ, that should be a stimulus for the physician and patient to explore, whether or not they have a mutually acceptable agreement. The patient would, of course, be free to change surgeons, seeking one willing to pursue what is in the patient's interest if the original surgeon declined to do so.

If such information were part of the database for patients on the wait list, we could then make a rational judgment about the probability of an organ from a positive or high-risk donor being used if it were procured. We would then expect all OPOs to facilitate organ procurement of such organs unless they could establish that there was little likelihood of anyone using the organ at the time the procurement decision had to be made.

We realize that it is often impossible to run the program to establish whether there is a suitable, willing recipient before the organs would need to be procured. From the wait list supplemented by data on patient willingness to accept positive and high-risk organs, however, the probability of the organ being used could be calculated. As long as the probability of being used was similar to that of other organs that are procured, then it ought to be retrieved.

Other High-Risk Organs

We cannot discuss in detail the policy issues of transplanting all kinds of high-risk organs. The concept we are advocating, however, should be clear. Whenever an organ is known to be infected or perceived to be a high-risk organ, it should be offered to patients on the wait list. The reasonable way to do this, when feasible, is to ask the transplant candidate in advance whether he or she would be willing to accept such an organ. This policy has been followed for what has been termed "expanded criteria donors" (ECD), including donors over the age of sixty or those over fifty with at least one complicating condition, such as hypertension, high serum creatinine, low glomerular filtration rates, or obesity. It is also used for organs from those who died from a cerebrovascular accidents. In the newly adopted kidney allocation formula, donors will no longer be classified as ECD, but a similar approach could be used for transplanting organs from donors with high kidney-donor-profile-index (KDPI) scores; and in fact, the new allocation model will require that transplant teams get affirmative consent from candidates that they are willing to accept a kidney with a KDPI greater than 85 percent, analogous to the ECD policy of asking patients in advance whether they would be willing to accept an ECD. Then, when such a kidney becomes available, the computer match run could be generated, limiting the recipients to those who had agreed to accept such organs.

We are proposing that a similar approach based on recipient choice be used for other kinds of high-risk organs, including those from donors with cancer and infections. Thus, for example, we would normally reject organs from potential donors with a history of cancer, but if the potential recipient's condition is critical, organs from patients with a cancer history may make sense, especially if the tumor appears not to have metastasized and the tumor is not in the organ being transplanted. When possible, the patient's willingness to accept such an organ should be established in advance. In unusual situations, such as an emergency where a patient's medical status has recently changed, ad hoc decisions about the use of high-risk organs will need to be made. Hence, consider the case of Sarah Murnaghan, who made the news in June 2013. Sarah needed a lung transplant because of cystic fibrosis and successfully challenged the policy that placed her at low priority for adult deceased donor lungs. When her first set of adult lungs was rejected, an ad hoc decision had to be made to transplant a second set of lungs from a patient with pneumonia, a choice the surgeons would rather have avoided, but, when the only alternative was certain death, the use of such lungs seems more plausible. In this case, the gamble paid off, and Sarah was discharged several weeks later.

In general, high-risk organs will need to be used in certain cases when the alternative is less attractive. Whenever possible, the patient on the wait list should be asked in advance, and a record of the patient's consent or refusal of consent should be entered into the database. In emergencies and in cases where the patient is unlikely to get another organ in a timely manner, transplanting the high-risk organ may be reasonable, provided the patient or surrogate consents.

Notes

1. Prompt CA, Reis MM, Grillo FM, et al., "Transmission of aids virus at renal transplantation," *Lancet* 1985;2: 672; L'Age-Shehr J, Schwarz A, Offermann G, "Human immunodeficiency virus transmission by organ donation: Outcome in cornea and kidney recipients," *Transplantation* 1987;44: 21–24.

2. Kumar P, Pearson JE, Martin DH, et al., "Transmission of human immunodeficiency virus by transplantation of a renal allograft, with development of the acquired immunodeficiency syndrome," *Annals of Internal Medicine* 1987;106: 244–45; Quarto M, Germinario C, Fontana A, Barbuti S, "HIV transmission through kidney transplantation from a living related donor," *New England Journal of Medicine* 1989;320: 1754.

3. National Organ Transplantation Act (NOTA), 42 USC 273 et seq.

4. Muller E, Kahn D, Mendelson M, "Renal transplantation between HIV-positive donors and recipients," *New England Journal of Medicine* 2010;362 (24): 2336–37; Muller E, Barday Z, Mendelson M, Kahn D, "Renal transplantation between HIV-positive donors and recipients justified," *South African Medical Journal* 2012;102 (6): 497–98.

5. HR 698, S.330: HIV Organ Policy Equity (HOPE) Act, introduced Feb. 14, 2013, and signed by the president Nov. 21, 2013, www.govtrack.us/congress/bills/113/hr698.

6. Morris MI, Fischer SA, Ison MG, "Infections transmitted by transplantation," *Infectious Disease Clinics of North America* 2010;24: 497–514.

7. Ison MG, Hager J, Blumberg E, et al., "Donor-derived disease transmission events in the United States: Data reviewed by the OPTN/UNOS Disease Transmission Advisory Committee," *American Journal of Transplantation* 2009;9: 1929–35.

8. Rogers MF, Simonds RJ, Lawton KE, Moseley RR, Jones WK, "Guidelines for preventing transmission of human immunodeficiency virus through transplantation of human tissue and organs," *Morbidity and Mortality Weekly Report (MMWR) Recommendations and Report* 1994;43 (RR-8): 1–17.

9. Seem DL, Lee I, Umscheid CA, Kuehnert MJ, "PHS guideline for reducing human immunodeficiency virus, hepatitis B virus and hepatitis C virus transmission through organ transplantation," *Public Health Reports* 2013;128 (4): 247–343.

10. Grady D, "Four transplant recipients contract HIV," *New York Times*, Nov. 13, 2007, www .nytimes.com/2007/11/13/health/13cnd-organ.html?_r = 0.

11. Ahn J, Cohen SM, "Transmission of human immunodeficiency and hepatitis C virus through liver transplantation," *Liver Transplantation* 2008;14: 1603–8.

12. "HIV transmitted from a living organ donor—New York City, 2009," *Morbidity and Mortality Weekly Report (MMWR)* 2011;60 (10): 297–301.

13. Crespo G, Marino Z, Navasa M, Forns X, "Virus hepatitis in liver transplantation," *Gastroenterology* 2012;142: 1373–83.

14. Ibid.; Singer AL, Kucirka LM, Namuyinga R, Hanraha C, Subramanian AK, Segev DL, "The high-risk donor: Viral infections in solid organ transplantation," *Current Opinion in Organ Transplantation* 2008;13: 400–404.

15. Terrault N, "Liver transplantation in the setting of chronic HCV," *Best Practice and Research Clinical Gastroenterology* 2012;26: 531–48; Kowdley KV, Lawitz E, Poordad F, et al., "Phase 2b trial of interferon-free therapy for hepatitis C virus genotype 1," *New England Journal of Medicine* 2014;370: 222–32; Sulkowski MS, Gardiner DF, Rodriguez-Torres M, et al., "Daclatasvir plus sofosbuvir for previously treated or untreated chronic HCV infection," *New England Journal of Medicine* 2014;370: 211–21.

16. Carbone M, Mutimer D, Neuberger J, "Hepatitis C virus and nonliver solid organ transplantation," *Transplantation* 2013;95: 779–86; Kucirka LM, Peters TG, Segev DL, "Impact of donor hepatitis C virus infection status on death and need for liver transplant in hepatitis C virus-positive kidney transplant recipients," *American Journal of Kidney Diseases* 2012;60 (1): 112–20.

17. Gasink LB, Blumberg EA, Localio AR, Desai SS, Israni AK, Lautenbach E, "Hepatitis C virus seropositivity in organ donors and survival in heart transplant recipients," *JAMA* 2006;296: 1843–50.

18. Qamar AA, Rubin RH, "Poorer outcomes for recipients of heart allografts from HCV-positive donors: Opening the silos," *JAMA* 2006;296: 1900–1901.

19. Abdala E, Azevedo LS, Campos SV, et al., "Use of hepatitis C–positive donors in transplantation," *Clinics* (São Paulo) 2012;67 (5): 517–19.

20. Singer AL, Kucirka LM, Namuyinga R, Hanraha C, Subramanian AK, Segev DL, "The high-risk donor: Viral infections in solid organ transplantation," *Current Opinion in Organ Transplantation* 2008;13: 400–404.

21. Seem et al., "PHS guideline," 252, figures 4 and 5.

22. Ibid., 251.

23. UNOS, "Policy 2.2.3.4," http://optn.transplant.hrsa.gov/PoliciesandBylaws2/policies/pdfs/policy_2.pdf.

24. Seem et al., "PHS guideline."

25. Halpern SD, Shaked A, Hasz RD, Caplan AL, "Informing candidates for solid-organ transplantation about donor risk factors," *New England Journal of Medicine* 2008;358: 2832–36.

26. Ross LF, "What the medical excuse teaches us about the potential living donor as patient," *American Journal of Transplantation* 2010;10: 731–36.

27. OPTN, "Policy 12.0: Living donor," http://optn.transplant.hrsa.gov/PoliciesandBylaws2/policies/pdfs/policy_172.pdf.

28. Crespo G, Marino Z, Navasa M, Forns X, "Viral hepatitis in liver transplantation," *Gastroenterology* 2012;142: 1373–83.

29. Rosner F, "Artificial and baboon heart implantation: The Jewish view," *Archives of Internal Medicine* 1985;145: 1330.

30. Armstrong MJ, Corbett C, Rowe AI, Taylor GP, Neuberger JM, "HTLV-1 in solid-organ transplantation: Current challenges and future management strategies," *Transplantation* 2012;94: 1075–84; Andersson S, Thorstensson R, Godoy Ramirez K, et al., "Comparative evaluation of 14 immunoassays for detection of antibodies to the human T lymphotropic virus types I and II using panels of sera from Sweden and West Africa," *Transfusion* 1999;39: 845–51.

31. Roucoux DF, Murphy EL, "The epidemiology and disease outcomes of human T-lymphotropic virus type II," *AIDS Review* 2004;6 (3): 144–54. Also see Andersson et al., "Comparative evaluation."

32. Toro C, Benito R, Aguilera A, et al., "Infection with human T-lymphotropic virus type I in organ transplant donors and recipients in Spain," *Journal of Medical Virology* 2005;76 (2): 268–70.

33. Ison MG, Nalesnik MA, "An update on donor-derived disease transmission in organ transplantation," *American Journal of Transplantation* 2011;11: 123–1130.

34. Andersson et al., "Comparative evaluation."

35. Kaul DR, Taranto S, Alexander C, et al., "Donor screening for human T-cell lymphotrophic virus 1/2: Changing paradigms for changing testing capacity," *American Journal of Transplantation* 2010;10: 207–13.

36. Ibid.

37. Ibid., 208.

38. Ibid.

39. Slifkin M, Doron S, Snydman DR, "Viral prophylaxis in organ transplant patients," *Drugs* 2004;53: 2763–92.

40. Ho M, "Epidemiology of cytomegalovirus infection," *Reviews of Infectious Diseases* 1990;12 (suppl 7): S701–10.

41. Ackerman JR, LeFor WM, Weinstein S, et al., cited by Natov SN, Pereira BJG, "Transmission of disease by organ transplantation," in *Organ and tissue donation for transplantation*, ed. Chapman, JR, Deierhoi M, Celia W (New York: Oxford University Press, 1997), 125.

42. Kuo H-T, Ye X, Sampaio M, Reddy P, Bunnapradist S, "Cytomegalovirus serostatus pairing and deceased donor kidney transplant outcomes in adult recipients with antiviral prophylaxis," *Transplantation* 2010;90: 1091–98.

43. Kotton CN, Kumar D, Caliendo AM, et al., "International consensus guidelines on the management of cytomegalovirus in solid organ transplantation," *Transplantation* 2010;89: 779. See also Kotton CN, Kumar D, Caliendo AM, et al., "Updated international consensus guidelines on the management of cytomegalovirus in solid-organ transplantation," *Transplantation* 2013;96: 333–60.

44. Harvala H, Stewart C, Muller K, et al., "High risk of cytomegalovirus infection following solid organ transplantation despite prophylactic therapy," *Journal of Medical Virology* 2013;85 (5): 893–98.

45. Kotton et al., "Updated international consensus," 341.

46. Ibid.

47. Natov SN, Pereira BJG, "Transmission of disease by organ transplantation," in *Organ and tissue donation*, ed. Chapman, Deierhoi, Celia, 120–51; Gottesdieneer KM, "Transplanted infections: Donor-to-host transmission with the allograft," *Annals of Internal Medicine* 1989;110: 1001–16; Schwarz A, Hoffman F, L'age-Stehr J, Tegzess AM, Offermann G, "Human immunodeficiency virus transmission by organ donation: Outcome in cornea and kidney recipient," *Transplantation* 1987;44: 21–24; Eastlund T, "Infectious disease transmission through cell, tissue, and organ transplantation: Reducing the risk through donor selection," *Cell Transplantation* 1995;4 (5): 455–77; Morris, Fischer, Ison, "Infections."

48. Desai R, Collett D, Watson CJ, Johnson P, Evans T, Neuberger J, "Cancer transmission from organ donors: Unavoidable but low risk," *Transplantation* 2012;94: 1200–1207.

49. Kauffman HM, McBride MA, Delmonico FL, "First report of the United Network for Organ Sharing Transplant Tumor Registry: Donors with a history of cancer," *Transplantation* 2000;70: 1747–51.

50. Bellati F, Napoletano C, Nuti M, Benedetti Panici P, "Death from metastatic donor-derived ovarian cancer in a male kidney transplant recipient," *American Journal of Transplantation* 2009;9: 1253.

51. Kauffman, McBride, Delmonico, "First report."

52. Ison MG, Nalesnik MA, "An update on donor-derived disease transmission in organ transplantation," *American Journal of Transplantation* 2011;11: 1123–30.

53. Desai et al., "Cancer transmission."

54. Kauffman HM, McBride MA, Cherikh WS, Spain PC, Marks WH, Roza AM, "Transplant tumor registry: Donor-related malignancies," *Transplantation* 2002;74: 358–62.

55. Chapman JR, Webster AC, Wong G, "Cancer in the transplant recipient," *Cold Spring Harbor Perspectives in Medicine* 2013;3: a015677. See also Watson CJ, Roberts R, Wright KA, et al., "How safe is it to transplant organs from deceased donors with primary intracranial malignancy? An analysis of UK Registry data," *American Journal of Transplantation* 2010;10: 1437–44.

56. Bajaj NS, Watt C, Hadjiliadis, D, et al., "Donor transmission of malignant melanoma in a lung transplant recipient 32 years after curative resection," *Transplant International* 2010;23: e26–e31.

57. "Ray CC interviewing Guarrera JV: Donation details," *New York Times*, June 11, 2012.

58. Kuo PC, Stock PG, "Transplantation in the HIV + patient," *American Journal of Transplantation* 2001;1: 13–17.

59. Kucirka LM, Ross RL, Subramanian AK, Montgomery RA, Segev D, "Provider response to a rare but highly publicized transmission of HIV through solid organ transplantation," *Archives of Surgery* 2011;146: 41–45.

60. Ibid.

61. HOPE Act, as cited above.

62. Cohen PJ, Cohen CB, "Do-not-resuscitate orders in the operating room," *New England Journal of Medicine* 1991;325: 1879–82; Smith AL, "DNR in the OR," *Clinical Ethics Report* 1994;8 (4): 1–8; Reeder JM, "Do-not-resuscitate orders in the operating room," *AORN Journal* 1993;57 (4): 947–51; Micco G, Cohen NH, "Do-not-resuscitate orders in the operating room: The birth of a policy," *Cambridge Quarterly on Healthcare Ethics* 1995;4: 103–10; American College of Surgeons, "Statement on advance directives by patients: 'Do not resuscitate' in the operating room," *Bulletin of the American College of Surgeons* 1994;79 (9): 29.

63. President's Commission for the Study of Ethical Problems in Medicine and Biomedical and Behavioral Research, *Deciding to forgo life-sustaining treatment: Ethical, medical, and legal issues in treatment decisions* (Washington, DC: US Government Printing Office, 1983).

64. Veatch RM, Spicer CM, "Medically futile care: The role of the physician in setting limits," *American Journal of Law & Medicine* 1992;18 (1&2): 15–36; for the most famous court case, see *In the*

Matter of Baby K, 832 F. Supp. 1022 (ED VA 1993). Other cases include *In Re The Conservatorship of Helga Wanglie*, State of Minnesota, District Court, Probate Court Division, County of Hennepin, Fourth Judicial District, June 28, 1991; *Rideout, Administrator of Estate of Rideout, et al. v. Hershey Medical Center*, Dauphin County Report, 1995, 472–98; and *Velez v. Bethune et al.*, 466 SE 2d 627 (GA App. 1995). Also see Kolata G, "Withholding care from patients: Boston case asks who decides," *New York Times*, Apr. 3, 1995; and Veatch RM, "So-called futile care: The experience of the United States," in *Medical futility: A cross-national study*, ed. Bagheri, A (London: Imperial College Press, 2013), 9–13.

Chapter 14

Xenotransplants

Using Organs from Animals

Baby Fae was born October 12, 1984. She was born with hypoplastic left heart syndrome, a condition in which the left atrium and ventricle are seriously underdeveloped.

The baby was transferred from a community hospital to Loma Linda University Medical Center, a medical facility associated with the Seventh-Day Adventist Church and its medical school. The mother was told that the baby's condition is usually fatal within the first week of life. A Norwood procedure, a palliative two-stage surgical procedure was explained to them. They were told that the procedure was generally unsuccessful. The mother left the hospital with the baby.

Four days later the pediatrician called the mother informing them of the possibility of a xenograft cardiac transplant, that is, a transplant of an organ taken from a nonhuman animal. The mother, accompanied by the grandmother and a friend, met with Dr. Leonard Bailey, a surgeon at Loma Linda who had been developing a proposal for experimental xenografts. He reviewed the Norwood procedure and explained to them that a human heart transplant was unlikely because size-matched and histocompatible infant human hearts only rarely become available.

The mother consented to the xenograft transplant after reviewing and signing a form that summarized the procedure.

Initially the transplant appeared to be successful, but then the baby's condition worsened, and she died November 15th. There was considerable dispute over the cause of death. There were initial reports that the tissues did not show evidence of cellular graft rejection. A report that the death was related to a blood-type mismatch was disputed.

Following the death and enormous publicity, there was widespread criticism. The problems raised included claims that animal-to-human transplant was intrinsically unethical as a violation of divine orders of creation, concern that the family was inadequately informed, the suggestion that this was an abuse of a baby in a procedure that was more for the purpose of advancing knowledge than serving the baby's interests, and the claim that it was an unethical use of scarce resources.

A National Institutes of Health (NIH) team visited the site and prepared a report reviewing these charges. The report praised the candidness of Loma Linda personnel and acknowledged that internal reviews of the protocol had taken place by an ad hoc committee in the department of surgery as well as a neonatal cardiac transplantation committee, the hospital ethics committee, the executive committee of the medical staff, and the advisory committee to the Loma Linda vice president for medical affairs in addition to the institutional review board required to review all human subjects research. The review team was critical of some shortcomings in the consent procedure: the expected benefits were thought to be overstated, it failed to discuss the possibility of searching for a human heart, and it failed to explain the institution's compensation policy. The controversy surrounding the case and lingering moral doubts about the wisdom of xenografts have led to a voluntary moratorium on such procedures in the United States.[1]

Transplanting of organs from one species to another conjures up images filled with ethical controversy. When the source or recipient species is a human being, that controversy is particularly acute. Because xenotransplants into humans are medical procedures, the ordinary, traditional ethical requirements must of course be met. There must be an adequately informed consent and protection of confidentiality. There must be adequate review, especially of any procedures that are experimental. Any discussion of the ethics of xenotransplantation must be premised on the expectation that all these standard requirements of medical ethics will be fulfilled.

Assuming that adequately informed consent is obtained and that the decision by the prospective patient or surrogate is not clearly contrary to the patient's interests, what are the special ethical problems of transplantation between humans and other species? Although many more xenotransplants have been performed from human to animal species than the other way around, here we focus primarily on those cases where the nonhuman species is the source of the cells or the organ. (As we have suggested in the case of infants, children, and the mentally retarded, it is not acceptable to refer to the nonhuman as a "donor." Clearly, the animal did not decide to engage in an act of gift giving the way some humans do when they are appropriately called donors.) We begin with a history of xenotransplantation. We then address five special ethical problems raised by xenotransplantation: (1) the natural law problem, (2) the animal rights problem, (3) the problem of nontherapeutic interventions, (4) the problem of scarce resources, and (5) the virus issue.

The History of Xenotransplantation

Baby Fae's case was not the first attempt at animal-to-human xenotransplantation. There were a flurry of such procedures in the early part of the twentieth century, and in the 1960s with attempts at kidneys, livers, and hearts from chimpanzees, baboons, pigs, and lambs into humans.[2] Although Reemtsma had one successful xenotransplantation using a chimpanzee kidney that survived for nine months in a twenty-three-year-old woman, most xenotransplanted kidneys lasted only days to weeks, and the hearts and livers had even shorter success rates, often ending with hyperacute graft reactions.[3]

Despite the negative publicity surrounding the death of Baby Fae, research on xenotransplantation persists, in part because the gap between human organ supply and patient demand grows. However, new concerns have also been raised. One concern is that viral infections are "being transmitted from nonhuman primates, as exemplified by the HIV pandemic."[4] This concern led to a decision in May 1999 by the US Department of Health and Human Services (HHS) to halt the use of nonhuman primate tissues for transplantation, because there was insufficient information to assess the risks posed by these procedures. Many other Western countries have also placed a moratorium on these procedures. In 2004 the World Health Organization (WHO) promulgated World Health Assembly Resolution WHA57.18, which urged member states to "allow xenotransplantation only when effective national regulatory control and surveillance mechanisms overseen by National Health Authorities are in place."[5] And yet, such clinical trials have been performed, both before and after the passage of the WHO resolution. Sgroi and colleagues collected information from January 1994 to September 2009 and identified a total of twenty-nine human applications of xenotransplantation, including seven that were currently ongoing. The treatments were performed in twelve different countries, nine of them having no regulation on xenotransplantation.[6]

Pigs are an alternate potential source for xenotransplantation, and they have been used for decades for structural tissues, such as pig heart valves and tissues for ligament reconstruction and even intestinal submucosa for bladder repair. These procedures involve removing the pig cells from the tissues, which are then repopulated by human recipient cells.[7] By contrast, current attempts at porcine xenotransplantation seek "to provide viable pig organs and cells that will continue to function after clinical transplantation" to treat many conditions, including organ failure (with hearts, livers, and kidneys), diabetes (using porcine islet cells), neurodegenerative diseases (using neuronal cells), and blindness (with corneas).[8]

The shift to porcine transplants, however, also raises infection concerns. In 1997 Patience and colleagues showed that porcine endogenous retroviruses (PERVs) could infect human cells in culture.[9] According to the International Xenotransplantation Society, this led to a reduction in research support in this area and to widespread public concern about moving xenotransplantation into clinical trials.[10] In addition to PERVs, other infectious risks from pigs include porcine hepatitis E, circoviruses, and herpesviruses.[11]

A second problem with the use of porcine organs is that all nonprimates possess a cell surface antigen containing the epitope known as Galalpha1-3Balbeta1-4GlcNAc-R (alpha-Gal), to which all humans have complement-fixing antibodies that cause immediate rejection of the animal cells when transplanted into humans.[12] This has led to a number of strategies to overcome xenorejection, including genetic modification of animal cell donors.

Human allotransplantation is not limited to solid organs but also involves cells and tissues. Human islet cell allotransplantation has had some success, but it is limited both by the relatively small number of donors and the need for several pancreati for each recipient.[13] Likewise, research on porcine islet cell xenotransplantation has been ongoing for more than two decades. Between 1990 and 1993 ten adults with type 1 diabetes were transplanted with pig fetal islets, injected either intraportally ($n = 8$) or under the kidney capsule ($n = 2$). No clinical benefits were observed, although porcine C-peptide was measured for 200 to 400 days in some of the recipients.[14]

In 2002 Valdes-Gonzalez and colleagues claimed to have cured one of twelve children with type 1 diabetes and reduced the insulin requirements in five others after transplantation of porcine islet cells encapsulated in hollow fibers with porcine Sertoli cells (cells found in the testes), which are assumed to have immunomodulating properties.[15] This study was criticized by the international community because it was performed in Mexico, outside internationally recognized regulatory conditions, and used techniques that had not been proven to be effective in animal studies before being attempted in humans.[16] It was also criticized for choosing children as the first subjects of a first-in-human research study.[17] Despite these criticisms, the researchers published long-term data in 2010 that found no evidence of PERVs during a 4.6- to 8-year follow-up.[18]

Elliott, on behalf of Living Cell Technologies, describes a clinical trial of porcine islet cell transplantation in New Zealand that is being performed under strict national regulatory oversight by the New Zealand Department of Health.[19] The study enrolled eight adult patients with long-standing proven type 1 diabetes with hypoglycemic unawareness.[20] Preliminary results in 2011 show a modest reduction in insulin requirement and a reduction of unaware hypoglycemia and total hypoglycemia scores. Elliott and colleagues note that "evidence of xenosis in the xenotransplant recipients [has] been diligently sought but not found," which they credit to the credential of the source herd used.[21]

An alternative to animal-derived organs and sources will be regenerated human cells, tissue, or organs that will restore or establish normal function. The evolving field of "Regenerative Medicine," as it is known, may include "the use of soluble molecules, gene therapy, stem cell transplantation, tissue engineering and the reprogramming of cell and tissue types."[22] In the case of islet cells, two different regenerative approaches that are showing promise are (1) the development and implementation of microencapsulation technology, in which the porcine cells are enveloped and therefore isolated from the recipient such that the recipient's immune system is not aware of their existence and does not try to destroy them; and (2) the development of a porcine pancreas extracellular matrix "to serve as a scaffold that approximates the biochemical, spatial and vascular relationships of the native extracellular matrix," which is then decellularized and repopulated with human stem cells.[23]

Special Ethical Problems Raised by Xenotransplantation

Although all transfers of body parts from one party to another raise ethical issues, when the transfer is from animal sources to humans, there are five special ethical problems: (1) the natural law problem, (2) the animal rights problem, (3) the problem of nontherapeutic interventions, (4) the problem of scarce resources, and (5) the virus issue. This section examines these problems.

The Natural Law Problem

The first problem that is unique to xenotransplantation is whether the intermixing of biological material from different species somehow violates fundamental morality in and of itself. We have seen that this question was raised in Baby Fae's case. Especially when we transplant vitally important and emotionally significant organs such as hearts, are we tampering with nature in a way that goes beyond what humans are supposed to do? Are we, to use religious language, violating God's plan for creation? This question was initially raised when concern was expressed about the transplantation of organs from one human to another. There is, likewise, an initial feeling of shock if not repulsion by many people when they think of baboon organs replacing those of humans.

Some have maintained that the human is unique, not in any way in continuity with other species. Anyone who holds this view might be uncomfortable with xenotransplantation from animal to human. It is therefore important to realize that there are no principled objections from the major religious traditions to the transferring of material from one species to another, even if it involves humans. The Catholic theologian Richard McCormick, a member of the NIH panel reviewing the Loma Linda cardiac xenograft transplant, raises the issue and refers to the "special concern" about cross-species grafts.[24] He focuses primarily on the more practical psychological problems of xenografts—how people will be viewed by others and themselves—and not on any violation of the natural law that would be involved. Although it is a special problem, it is not "insuperable."

Orthodox Jews go even further in affirming the fundamental morality of cross-species transplants. Fred Rosner, one of this country's leading authorities on medical ethics in Judaism (who happens also to be a physician), has examined the problem of cross-species transfer. He concludes that "the preservation of human life is of infinite and supreme value."[25] Provided the rules for the respectful treatment of animals are followed and the standards governing human experimentation are met, and a human being stands a chance of benefiting from the procedure, then it is permissible in Jewish thought to use an animal's organ to save a human life.

Although the movement of essential organs from one species to another at first appears shocking, it involves no more of a violation of any natural law than does the movement of an organ from one human to another, as long as the animal is treated respectfully. This issue needs further exploring.

The Animal Rights Problem

The qualifier that the animal must be treated respectfully suggests a second possible problem with xenografts. Assuming that the therapeutic use of xenografts occurs primarily to humans from other species, some may argue that this is an abuse of animals. In fact, this issue also arose in Baby Fae's case.

The animal rights movement is increasingly powerful and has raised objections to xenografts. Anyone who has fundamental objection to the use of animals for any human ends would logically object to interspecies transplants for the purpose of benefiting humans.

Tom Regan, a professor of philosophy committed to the animal rights perspective, refers to the baboon as "the other victim."[26] Charging anthropocentrism, he argues that animals are experiencing subjects who command respect. They cannot be viewed solely as means for the support of other living beings.

Regan's view is being taken increasingly seriously, and at least it has been a force sufficient to overcome patterns of abusive brutality and unnecessary slaughter of animals for research purposes. The broader question of animal rights clearly cannot be resolved within the explicit context of xenografts. It does seem clear, however, that if there is ever a case for using an animal for the benefit of humans, it would be when the sacrifice of one animal will offer the possibility of saving an identifiable human life. The case for xenograft use of animals is, for example, much stronger than the case for any general use of animals in research laboratories, for food, or for sport. Jews, for example, will object to animal experimentation solely to satisfy human curiosity.[27] They and many others, however, find that at least some uses of animals are acceptable. Animals are thus viewed as morally distinct from humans, with their own moral claims.[28]

There is another dimension to the animal rights concern. It is apparently still a minority of the population that objects in principle to animal research. Yet the reduction of animals to instruments of human welfare could take on an added perspective if xenografts were to become acceptable. Clearly, one of the major problems of human to human transplantation is inadequate tissue compatibility. If it can be established that animals such as primates can be sources of badly needed organs for human transplantation and that their immune systems are similar to those of humans, then there would be a greatly increased incentive to breed large numbers of primates so that eventually there could be a "grocery store" approach, with primates available on the shelf to provide virtually all the thousands of tissue-type combinations that might be needed by humans. Revulsion against this image of thousands of primates bred specifically for their organs may increase the possibility that people will join the camp of those who object to using animals, especially sensate animals, for human ends.

The Problem of Nontherapeutic Interventions

The third major objection to xenografts that has emerged, especially in conjunction with the Baby Fae procedure, is the concern that Baby Fae was, in effect, the unconsenting subject of an experiment on a human being that had no therapeutic justification. It is now common to distinguish between interventions that are justified for their therapeutic intent (even if they are novel or experimental procedures) and interventions that are solely for research purposes. This distinction was once referred to as the difference between therapeutic and nontherapeutic research. And though this language has been criticized, the underlying distinction remains valid between those interventions justified by considerations of the potential welfare of the patient and those justified by the potential value of the knowledge to be gained.[29]

A number of critics have questioned Baby Fae's xenograft on the grounds that it constituted a nontherapeutic intervention—that it was really done just to see what could be learned, with no hope of benefit for the baby.[30] If that were true, it would be a valid criticism. It is widely recognized that novel procedures, especially nontherapeutic ones, should first be tested on consenting adults when possible. And such procedures are justified for testing on nonconsenting subjects only when the risks are very minor.

There is room for controversy, however, over whether Baby Fae had a realistic chance to benefit. Some have argued that Baby Fae could not consent to the experiment. The parental permission to operate has also been questioned. There is some public doubt that the parents had adequate information about the alternatives. The review by the Office for the Protection from Research Risks—now the Office of Human Research—casts some doubt on the adequacy in this case. In any case, we assume that adequate consent based on the duty to communicate what parent(s) would reasonably want to know would be a minimal necessary condition for ethically acceptable surgery.

Some have gone on to argue that even if the parents did have adequate information, they did not have the right to volunteer their child for a procedure so experimental that it could be said that it was undertaken for the knowledge to be gained rather than for the patient's benefit. We are increasingly coming to the conclusion that parents, in making medical decisions for their wards, must attempt to approximate the ward's interests. A parental decision that the xenograft best served their child's interests does not strike us as totally unreasonable. We are increasingly coming to the conclusion that society should not insist that the parents have made the most reasonable choice. According to this view, their choice should simply be tolerated, provided that it is a choice within the realm of reason.[31] Although the most reasonable parental decision might have been against the surgery on the grounds that it did not serve the baby's interests, we are not persuaded that the parental decision was so unreasonable that it should have been overridden.

Considering the alternatives available to Baby Fae, it is hard to fault parents who opt for a chance of success, no matter how slim. A principle is emerging in the contemporary debate about parental and guardian decision making that helps to justify a parental choice for a xenograft—assuming that the parents are adequately informed and not pressured into a decision, beyond the natural pressures caused by the critical illness of their daughter.

Today it is increasingly recognized that the decision about whether a child will benefit from a novel procedure should first be made by his or her parents. Parents will differ in such judgments, but if the parents were to conclude that the xenograft was more in their daughter's interest than any available alternative, normally their judgment should not be challenged. It should be reviewed and overturned only in those cases where the parental judgment was so unreasonable that it would constitute child abuse.[32] It would need to be beyond the limits of reason.[33] We do not see how anyone could conclude that the parents who opted for a xenograft heart transplant for their dying daughter when their options were so constrained were beyond reason when they judged it to be not only potentially beneficial but also the best option available to them. Assuming that their consent was adequately informed and voluntary, such parental choice strikes us as well within reason. Thus even if we agree that it would be wrong to conduct xenograft experiments on non-consenting patients who did not stand to benefit, it would not follow that they should never be tried on those patients who could benefit, according to their own judgment, if they are competent, or according to the reasonable judgment of their guardians, if they are not.[34]

Resource Allocation

This brings us to a fourth controversy surrounding the ethics of xenotransplantation. It has been argued that even if xenotransplantation does not violate any law of nature, does not violate any rights of animals, and does not necessarily constitute nontherapeutic interventions on nonconsenting subjects, it still consumes significant resources that would be better spent elsewhere. Xenotransplantation, according to this argument, surely constitutes an exotic technological innovation with a low probability of short-term payoffs. The critics ask whether our resources would not better be spent on more basic interventions in preventive care and more simple treatments.

A number of people have suggested that even if the animal rights issues and consent problems were to be solved, it would be unethical to spend hundreds of thousands of dollars on exotic, high-technology care when others in our society are doing without the basics of preventive care, maternal and child health services, and other essential medical assistance. This argument—which is usually offered against experimental transplant surgery, such as Baby Fae's—deserves further attention.

Resource arguments rest fundamentally on a cost/benefit reasoning that is insensitive to basic questions of social justice and, therefore, is incompatible with the Judeo-Christian tradition. The observation that appears to drive the critics of expensive, high-technology medical interventions is that more good could be done if the resources currently invested in the Baby Faes of the world were instead spent on primary care. But even assuming that this is true, it does not follow that care should be so diverted. The hidden moral premise is that net utility in the aggregate should be maximized as a matter of social policy, even when aggregating utility masks any consideration of the distribution of benefits and harms. Although that may be good act utilitarianism, it violates both the moral insights of the Judeo-Christian tradition and sound, secular theories of justice.

This argument takes us into the center of the ethics of distributive justice. It hinges in large part on how one ought to evaluate benefits. Two basic strategies are available for assessing how resources ought to be distributed. The first, the approach dominating much contemporary health planning and public health, emphasizes the maximization of the aggregate net welfare that will come from an investment in health care. It is the strategy that leads to the methods of cost/benefit and cost-effectiveness analysis, two devices that are really nothing more than sophisticated strategies for adding up the benefits and harms of alternative courses of action. The underlying philosophical premise is that of utilitarianism—doing the greatest good for the greatest number.

Under such an ethic of distribution, xenografts are quite frankly going to be difficult to justify. It is the approach that leads to invitations to imagine how many immunizations against measles could be provided for the cost of one organ transplant. Conceivably, even on these grounds, xenografts would come out ahead in the calculation. The short-term benefits are admittedly not very large, but if there were a success, the reward would be great. Moreover, in the long term, countless lives might be saved, not only from hearts but also from other organ transplants. It is nevertheless quite difficult to imagine that spending equal resources on xenografts and preventive medicine would lead to greater net benefits in the aggregate from the xenografts.

There is a second way of assessing the ethics of distribution, however. This second alternative is emphasized in part III of this book, where we deal with the allocation of organs. Some people argue that it is a mistake to look only at the net aggregate benefit from alternative courses of action. They say that, instead, one should focus on the special needs of special groups. The least well off among us, according to this second strategy, have special priorities. According to John Rawls, the basic institutions of society should be organized so that the interests of the groups that are least well off are served.[35] This suggests that policies should be developed to devote significant resources to the least well off, even if the payoff for society as a whole is not efficiently maximized.

Others, who consider themselves egalitarians, reach a similar conclusion, arguing that resources should be organized so as to provide for greater equality. One of us (RMV) has examined this question in depth.[36] If we understand it correctly, much of the Judeo-Christian tradition holds to this theory of distribution, a theme we develop further in chapter 17. The important thing to note here is that resources get skewed toward the least well off rather than toward approaches that simply produce great aggregate societal benefit.

Although the application of this egalitarian principle of justice to health care is complex, a case can be made that this principle requires that, whenever possible, an individual should be given an opportunity for health care equal to that of any other individual. This probably means that there are enough resources for both primary prevention and high technology. If a choice must be made, however, the resources should go to the least well off. According to egalitarian justice, primary care would get priority only if those who did not get it would be worse off than those needing, but not receiving, the high-technology interventions.

What does all this mean for xenotransplantation? Where do those who might receive xenograft transplants stand in relation to others in society? Are they among the least well off? At first, it would appear that anyone who is sick enough that a xenograft is likely to be of benefit is in very bad shape, plausibly among the least well off in society. We are convinced that this is true for some, but not all, possible xenograft recipients.

The critical question is whether we should evaluate how well off people are at one moment in time or over their lifetimes. Some older persons are admittedly very sick at the moment, but they may well have had long, productive, enjoyable lives. If this over-a-lifetime perspective is adopted, then some persons who have completed their life cycles could be said to have very low claims on societal medical resources, even though they will not live long without treatment. Conversely, the very young who are critically ill would appear from the over-a-lifetime perspective to be very poorly off indeed. They are in danger of dying without having had the benefits of many years of life. This perspective would place Baby Fae at or near the top of the list in terms of how poorly off she is. She and similarly ill infants could easily be considered the worst off in society.[37] (These issues are explored further in chapter 20.)

This suggests that even if xenografts are not terribly efficient in improving societal health statistics—that is, mortality and morbidity rates—there are claims of justice from certain among our number for significant investments in resources. If a xenograft is, according to the parental judgment, likely to offer some chance of benefit for an infant who is surely among the least well off in society, and if we are members of a society that responds to the needs of the neediest, then a xenograft for that infant is going to have a high-priority claim of justice. And it will have this claim even if the payoff is not very great and even if other critically ill patients—those who have had long, happy lives—do not have such a priority claim. Thus even if consenting adults ought to be first from the standpoint of a theory of informed consent, it may be that infants whose needs are great instead deserve the highest priority.

The Virus Issue

The fifth issue is viral infection. In the case of human-to-human transplants, the risks to the transplant recipient—risks of being exposed to HIV, cytomegalovirus, cancer, and other diseases, along with rejection risks and graft–versus–host disease—could be evaluated and accepted or rejected by the recipient. The same is true for any theoretical risk to which the xenotransplant recipient will be exposed from endogenous viruses from other species. As Fishman and colleagues explain, the "term 'xenosis' (also 'direct zoonosis' or 'xenozoonosis') was coined to reflect both the unique epidemiology of infection of source animals used for xenotransplantation and experience with immunocompromised patients that indicates that novel pathogens may emerge as a cause of infection, including organisms not normally associated with human disease."[38] These pathogens pose a risk to the recipient, to his or her intimate contacts, to his or her health care professionals, and even to the broader community. This may be the most difficult issue to surmount.

The Science of Cross-Species Virus Transmission

Concern about the small, but real, risk that viruses could be transmitted from primate animals to humans receiving organs and then from the human organ recipient to other humans was the basis for the May 1999 decision by HHS to halt nonhuman primate xenotransplantation. With the history of the HIV virus having moved from nonhuman animals to humans still vivid in our consciousness, even a small risk raises great concern. Particularly in an immunosuppressed patient, viral recombination could pose a potential threat.[39]

Some of the concerns about the use of primates as organ sources have been mitigated by the development of the transgenic pig as a potential source.[40] Pigs are easily bred, are already mass-produced for human consumption, and offer an anatomical and physiological fit that is encouraging for human transplants. However, the discovery that PERVs could infect human cells in vitro has caused much consternation.[41]

The Precautionary Principle

The contemporary xenograft infection risk policy is based on "the precautionary principle," which first emerged in German environmental policy in the 1970s and subsequently became incorporated into many multinational treaties and declarations.[42] Today various versions of the principle are in use; an early, classic formulation is Article 15 of the 1992 Rio Declaration on Environment and Development: "In order to protect the environment, the precautionary approach shall be widely applied by States according to their capabilities. Where there are threats of serious or irreversible damage, lack of full scientific certainty shall not be used as a reason for postponing cost-effective measures to prevent environmental degradation."[43] An alternative formulation is found in the Wingspread Statement of 1998: "When an activity raises threats of harm to human health or the environment, precautionary measures should be taken, even if some cause-and-effect relationships are not fully established scientifically. In this context, the proponent of an activity, rather than the public, should bear the burden of proof."[44]

The precautionary principle has its advocates, who argue that it is common sense to "proceed with caution"; and it has its opponents, who fear that it will stifle innovation, or who oppose it on more theoretical grounds.[45] Some argue that the precautionary principle is no more than a risk/benefit calculation, whereas others argue that it includes qualitative risks that are often ignored in classic risk/benefit calculations because the risks are not quantifiable.

The field of tissue transplantation (illustrated by blood transfusion) adopted the precautionary principle in response to the "perceived failure to appropriately address issues of scientific uncertainty in the transfusion transmission of hepatitis C and HIV."[46] Not all believe that this has been beneficial. Wilson notes that "the adoption of the principle to address theoretical risks has resulted in highly risk adverse policy which has both enhanced the safety of the blood supply but also contributed to rising costs." He also notes that its application can also create risks to health by reducing the donor supply.[47]

Marc Germain, Smaranda Ghibu, and Gilles Delage, conversely, argue that the precautionary principle was effective in the case study of the potential threat of variant Creutzfeldt–Jakob disease (vCJD) to transfusion safety at the turn of the twenty-first century.[48] Because it was thought (although not yet known) that vCJD could be transmitted by blood transfusions, risk mitigation strategies for transfusion were employed. One such strategy was to limit donations from people who traveled to areas in which the agent was known to exist. Germain and colleagues describe the policy of "geographical deferrals" applied to the vCJD threat as "an unadulterated application of the precautionary principle."[49] They also note that it "is also one of the few instances where the same basic precautions were widely applied by the transfusion community across the developed world."[50] They distinguish the use of the precautionary principle from a zero-risk paradigm, which would have prohibited all donors who had traveled to areas where mad cow disease existed. Rather, "the policy was a compromise between the purely theoretical risks of a full-blown vCJD crisis vs. the real risks and costs associated with donor deferrals. In other words, the principle of proportionality itself dictated that our precautions should not aim for zero risk."[51] As the authors note, "eventually, vCJD was shown to be transmissible by transfusion, a fact that could be seen to vindicate the precautions that were taken. However, the overall vCJD threat to transfusion now appears to be extremely small. In fact, there is no indication that geographical deferrals ever prevented a single case of transfusion-transmitted vCJD."[52]

The proposal to use the precautionary principle in xenotransplantation can also be traced to the turn of the twenty-first century.[53] The determination that PERVs could infect human cells in vitro challenged the safety of porcine xenotransplantation, both for the recipient of a transplant and possibly for the people who have contact with that patient. This led to arguments in support of invoking the precautionary principle.[54]

More than a decade later, however, the data consistently fail to show any risk from porcine organ or tissue transplanted into humans.[55] Nevertheless, in 2012 Fishman and colleagues published a WHO consultation on xenotransplantation-associated infectious risk in which they employed the precautionary principle approach, and they concluded that there was a need (1) to develop "surveillance programs to detect known infectious agents and, potentially, previously unknown or unexpected pathogens"; and (2) to deploy appropriate procedures and assays to identify xenogeneic infection, even though the risk is generally thought to be low because it is irresponsible to wait until a risk is confirmed.[56] The main problem with this approach is that it does not provide a risk level except zero, at which point the precautionary principle becomes overly burdensome relative to the potential benefits that such research could provide.

Consent and Withdrawal Issues

In 2004 an HHS Secretary's Advisory Committee on Xenotransplantation was formed and published several reports. A 2004 draft report, titled "Informed Consent in Clinical Research Involving Xenotransplantation," examined the special challenges pertaining to informed consent in xenotransplant research, including (1) public health risks, such as the transmission of infectious agents in pig-to-human xenotransplantation, and how these risks should be monitored and managed; (2) the need to inform intimate contacts, health care professionals, and the general public about issues relating to xenotransplantation; and (3) informing third parties, such as the intimate contacts of research participants as well as the public at large, about the risks associated with xenotransplantation. In addition to the usual descriptions of risks, benefits, and alternatives, the committee stated that the consent process for early clinical trials in xenotransplantation should also include relevant results from animal studies and early human studies. A unique consent issue would be a discussion of the public health responsibilities of the recipients of xenotransplantation products. These responsibilities are quite broad ranging—from the need for lifelong follow-up; to the collection, testing, and archiving of biological samples to behavioral modifications (including the use of barrier methods in all sexual activities); to the lifelong need to inform intimate contacts and future health care providers of the xoonotic infection risk and to decline to donate blood and other body fluids and tissues.[57] The committee argued that consent must include "the prospective participant's understanding and agreement to comply with public safety measures (including lifelong monitoring, temporary isolation if indicated, and autopsy)."[58]

The problem with this committee's recommendation for lifelong monitoring is that it ignores the fact that a central component of ethical research participation is the subject's right to withdraw at any time. This principle is found in the Nuremberg Principles, as well as the Declaration of Helsinki and the US Code of Federal Regulations regarding human subjects protections. This would hold even if the xenotransplant failed and/or the xenograft were removed.

Many agree with the committee's requirements for lifelong monitoring and the need for the recipient to waive his or her right to withdraw. Spillman and Sade propose that xenotransplant candidates must make a Ulysses-type contract (like that employed in clinical psychiatric treatment), whereby the patient, though competent, consents to a treatment plan that proscribes withdrawal when the patient loses decisional capacity.[59] Azofra and Casabona argue that in xenotransplantation clinical trials, "the need of complying with a specific surveillance plan arguably outweighs the individual's right to withdraw."[60] They view the surveillance from a public health perspective, which can intrude on individual autonomy if the public's well-being is at risk.

We acknowledge the need for careful follow-up with xenograft recipients and how this clashes with the right that all research participants have to withdraw from research. We maintain that xenograft recipients must have the right to withdraw from research, even if they may be required to provide samples from time to time to ensure that they do not pose a pandemic risk. However, the limits on their curtailment of movement and their obligation to undergo monitoring must be minimized. The research protocol should enumerate the ideal frequency of data collection that xenograft recipients will be asked to undergo, but it should also enumerate those samples that will be mandatorily collected based on a possible public health threat, a number that would clearly decrease over time as the safety of xenografts is reaffirmed. A data safety monitoring board should prospectively be in place to provide opportunities for the xenograft recipient, the research team, and the public health authorities to renegotiate the frequency of such monitoring as data continue to accumulate about the safety of the intervention. However, a zero-risk policy is both too intrusive and not practical, given that some viral risk may exist that we cannot currently identify because we do not have the tests to identify them or the knowledge to realize that they are pathogens.

Our proposal, then, concedes that the subject will not have full autonomy to completely withdraw because of the potential public health threat that he or she poses, which justifies mandatory participation. But he or she will not be required to undergo the extensive data observation that researchers might otherwise plan.

The Ethics of Third-Party Risks

The risk of xenotic infections is not limited to the xenograft recipient. There is a possibility that other human beings will also be exposed (just as they are with HIV). This means that when the recipient of a xenograft consents to the xenotic infection risk, he or she is in effect consenting to some risks to other parties.

This, of course, poses serious ethical problems. It would seem fair that those other parties who are put at risk should need to agree in some way to that risk. Close relatives, such as spouses, may be among those most at risk, and they are theoretically capable of being educated about the risk and consenting to it. However, some of those at risk will inevitably be children and others incapable of both making autonomous choices and consenting. Also, direct consent to the risk is not feasible for distant relatives, friends, and strangers. The real question, then, is whether potential transplant recipients who are willing to take their own personal risks of viral infection in order to get an organ have a right to take these risks without securing any explicit approval from the other exposed parties. This is essentially a problem of what economists would call the "externalities" of such decisions—risks that the decision maker may not take into account in making his or her choice.

The concern, however, is not just for viral transmission between intimate contacts but also the possibility that a xenotransplant recipient could start a worldwide pandemic. This was discussed in a consensus statement by the International Xenotransplantation Association: "Indeed, the SARS and H1N1 influenza experiences have taught us that infections travel at a high speed and may spread at a global level in a matter of weeks. . . . In light of such observations, all reasonable precautions must be taken to manage the potential infectious danger related to xenotransplantation procedures and to prepare the global public health community to respond to any infection in a coordinated manner to contain the spread."[61]

Given this serious concern, the recommendations propose to monitor third parties who have intimate contact with the xenograft recipient: a spouse or other family member, and the primary caregivers. The threat of xoonotic transmission from xenograft transplant recipient to intimate contacts has led to guidelines for the screening of intimate contacts (including pets) for viral illnesses at various points after a xenotransplant. Indirectly, then, the intimate third parties also become research subjects, which raises the question of whether their consent must be obtained. It is also not clear how long the risks may be present, nor how long these third parties will need to be subject to screening. However, because blood and tissue samples, and also medical records, will be needed over some extended period of time, it seems obvious that they do need to consent.

What happens, then, if an intimate contact states that he or she refuses to have regular routine examinations? Should the person in organ failure be deprived of the opportunity for a xenotransplant because his or her loved ones refuse to participate?

The integral role of third parties in transplantation is not unique to xenotransplantation, but is also seen in allotransplantation. Heart transplant candidates, for example, must meet strict social criteria in order to be listed, which include living with someone who is willing to take on caregiving roles. A candidate without strong social support may be excluded from listing. A parallel, then, would be to reject potential xenograft recipients whose intimate household members refuse serial monitoring and screening or even the proposed behavioral modifications.

Part of this problem will be addressed by requiring governmental and other public agencies (e.g., HHS or UNOS) to approve the regulations or guidelines. The most restrictive standard would be that no third party be put at any risk without his or her explicit consent. That would, of course, make xenotransplant impossible. It would also make impossible most other socially worthwhile social programs—road construction, building schools, and developing a police force. A policy requiring explicit, individual consent is not plausible.

A possible alternate approach would be to endorse xenografts only if it can be shown that the benefits from the xenograft can be expected to exceed the harms—including the harms to third parties. This would be the utilitarian justification. There are two problems with this criterion, however. First, the quantification of both expected benefits and harms is almost impossible. The problem is not just the usual one of having to quantify uncertainties and subjective goods and harms; it is also that the potential benefits and harms are both almost unlimited. On one hand, if xenografts from a commonly available animal such as a pig become successful, thousands—and eventually millions—of additional life-years could be the result. On the other hand, if the worst fears were to be realized, another HIV-scale pandemic or worse could result.

The real issue is whether it is morally defensible to assess the aggregate benefits and risks. This process would involve relying on potentially large benefits to the xenograft's recipient to offset the risks to society, which may not be fair to members of society who are exposed largely to harms without their consent. Another approach would be to base the decision on the principle of justice, focusing on the needs or interests of the worst-off persons. As we have seen previously in this chapter, this principle supports organizing social practices so as to benefit these worst-off people or to give them opportunities to be as well off as others, insofar as that is possible. And it would support such practices even if the effect were to be a net decrease in the amount of good in society—provided that was necessary in order to improve the lot of the worst off.

The implications of the principle of justice, though not easy to determine in the case of viral transmission risk via xenotransplants, may turn out to be easier to estimate than if the principle of utility were the criterion. People so ill that they are candidates for a transplant are surely not well off. Those on wait lists who are so ill that they are willing to volunteer to be pioneers in an experiment to transplant organs from pigs or other nonhuman animals are probably particularly poorly off. They would be members of the kind of group that would have a special claim grounded in the principle of justice, a claim for society to adopt social practices that are designed to benefit them, even if the interests of others in society are in conflict.

But even very sick people in organ failure would not be helped if they were to contract a serious viral disease from a pig. That risk, however, is one that people desperate for an organ transplant might rationally be willing to take. Thus, assuming that they are reasonably well informed and rational about their decision to take the chance on a xenograft, their choice to undergo the procedure would be understandable and, for egalitarians, justified.

Still, someone approaching this issue from the perspective of the principle of justice would need to ask whether others in society have interests that must be taken into account. Surely they do, and it would be decent for potential xenograft experimenters to take these interests into account. But how ought society to take them into account in deciding policy about whether to permit volunteers to receive experimental xenografts when we do not know the risk of virus transmission?

The justice theorist, at least one who interprets justice as requiring organizing practices to serve the interests of the worst off among us, will ask whether it is possible that the others at risk from the introduction of the virus into the human species could plausibly end up even worse off than the transplant candidate. And any such even-worse-off bystanders would have a legitimate claim to block the xenograft experiment.

Although it cannot be denied that someone who became infected via human-to-human transmission of the hypothetical virus from a xenograft recipient could be even worse off, it is important to note how unlikely that would be, for three main reasons. First, the xenograft recipient would be in double jeopardy. He or she would be very poorly off from organ failure—organ failure so severe that the individual is willing to risk an experimental xenograft. Second, if it should turn out that some virus was indeed a danger to humans, that recipient would also be a victim of the virus. If we are trying to identify who is the worst off, the person with severe organ failure combined with the serious viral infection is surely worse off than the one contending only with the virus. There is more to consider. The dose of the virus received by the transplant recipient is quite likely to be larger than one passed on to other humans through blood, body fluids, or another mode of transmission. If the seriousness of the risk is dose-dependent, the transplant recipient is statistically in a worse position.

Third and finally, there is a technical problem in how we calculate how poorly off people are. If the members of a large group of people each has a small chance of being exposed to a deadly disease, do we view each person statistically as being relatively well off because his or her harm is considered to be the harm of getting the disease multiplied by the probability of getting it? Or do we describe the group as being made up of many people who are well off because they will not get the disease, plus a small number who are in a very bad position because they will get it? If the former approach is used, then no one can be identified who is very poorly off, because each person is viewed as having only a small chance of getting the disease. Or if the latter approach is appropriate, then a few people are very poorly off. However, even if the latter approach is the right one, the unfortunate ones who get the viral disease are still better off than those who receive the transplant and also get the virus.

Of course, there may be some in society who are even worse off than people with the worst imaginable outcome of a virus exposure—people with amyotrophic lateral sclerosis or extreme poverty or pain, for example. According to the principle of justice, they would have prior claims. But if the virus risk issue is one of whether the risk to others in society is justified in order to benefit those needing transplants, the correct question is what can be done to benefit them, even if others who are better off are put at risk. For those who have been reasonably well informed about the risks and the alternatives and still choose to volunteer to receive the xenograft, they have a strong claim of justice to get the organ. The interests of those in society who are better off do not have the moral weight that they would in a more straightforward utilitarian analysis.

Therefore, an ethic that focuses on justice would probably be more supportive of xenografts in the face of possible viral risks than would a utilitarian one. In chapter 2 of this book, we suggested that the only considerations that legitimately compete with a principle such as justice are the other "non-consequence-maximizing" principles—veracity, fidelity, autonomy, and avoidance of killing. By contrast, beneficence and non-maleficence—maximizing the aggregate good and minimizing the aggregate evil—should come into play only when the other principles have been satisfied or when they offset each other so that beneficence and nonmaleficence are "tiebreakers."

If this is the proper approach, then the viral transmission issue would be a problem only if some getting the virus from transplant recipients were even worse off or if one of the other principles militated against permitting the exposure. For example, fidelity or promise keeping is one of these principles. If members of the public had somehow been promised that no xenografts would take place as long as there was a risk of virus transmission, the duty to keep this promise would count against the justice argument that we have presented. This seems quite unlikely, however. If the mere fear of harm to others who are actually better off than the transplant candidate is not a legitimate moral concern, then it seems that ethical support for xenografts would exist. Of course, utilitarians might reach a different conclusion, but they would need to show that the risks to the population exceeded the benefits to the transplant candidates (including all future candidates, who could eventually benefit from it having been established that animal organs were adequately safe and effective). This would be very hard for a utilitarian to show. In this case, respect for the autonomy of consenting transplant candidates would seem to support those who want to volunteer for xenografts. Thus, even a utilitarian might end up supporting policies that take prudent risks to conduct studies to see if the viral transmission problem is real.

Conclusion

Where does all this leave us? If xenotransplantation does not violate any natural law, if it is found not necessarily to violate the rights of animals, if it does not constitute research without hope of benefit for unconsenting patients, if the patient is among the least well off in society, and if the many aspects of the virus issue can be settled—if all these conditions can be met, and if the more traditional requirements of medical ethics having to do with confidentiality and consent and respect for the rights of patients can be met, then xenotransplantation will have passed the test of ethics. This is a stiff test, but one that some xenotransplantation efforts surely will be able to meet.

If so, someday the inherent shortage of human organs may be overcome. In the meantime, if our transplants are constrained by the natural limits of the supply from brain-dead and non-heart-beating deceased humans, we must face the other major challenge in the ethics of organ transplants: Who will receive this precious but scarce resource? This question of the allocation of organs is the topic of part III of this volume.

Notes

1. This summary is based on a report of the National Institutes of Health (the report of the NIH team investigating the Baby Fae transplant), *Spectrum* 16;1 (April 1985): 19–26. See also Bailey LL, Nehlsen-Cannarella SL, Concepcion W, Jolley WB, "Baboon-to-human cardiac xenotransplantation in a neonate," *JAMA* 1985;254: 3321–29.

2. American Medical Association, Council on Scientific Affairs, "Xenografts: Review of the literature and current status," *JAMA* 1985;254: 3353–57; Deschamps J-Y, Roux FA, Sai P, Gouin E, "History of xenotransplantation," *Xenotransplantation* 2005;12: 91–109.

3. Ibid.

4. Sykes M, d'Apice A, Sandrin M, "Position paper of the Ethics Committee of the International Xenotransplantation Association," *Xenotransplantation* 2003;10: 196; Michie C, "Xenotransplantation, endogenous pig retroviruses and the precautionary principle TRENDS," *Molecular Medicine* 2001;7 (2): 62.

5. Fifty-Seventh World Health Assembly, "Human organ and tissue transplantation," agenda item 12.14, May 22, 2004, www.who.int/ethics/en/A57_R18-en.pdf.

6. Sgroi A, Bühler LH, Morel P, Sykes M, Noel L, "International human xenotransplantation inventory," *Transplantation* 2010;90: 597–603.

7. Ekser B, Rigotti P, Gridelli B, Cooper DK, "Xenotransplantation of solid organs in the pig-to-primate model," *Transplant Immunology* 2009;21 (2): 87–92.

8. Ibid.

9. Patience C, Takeuchi Y, Weiss RA, "Infection of human cells by an endogenous retrovirus of pigs," *Nature Medicine* 1997;3 (3): 282–86.

10. Sykes M, Pierson RN, III, O'Connell P, et al., "Reply to 'critics slam Russian trial to test pig pancreas for diabetes,'" *Nature Medicine* 2007;13 (6): 662–63.

11. Michie, "Xenotransplantation," 62.

12. Elliott RB, on behalf of Living Cell Technologies, "Towards xenotransplantation of pig islets in the clinic," *Current Opinion in Organ Transplantation* 2011;16: 195.

13. Shapiro AM, Lakey JR, Ryan EA, et al., "Islet transplantation in seven patients with type 1 diabetes mellitus using a glucocorticoid-free immunosuppressive regimen," *New England Journal of Medicine* 2000;343: 230–38.

14. Groth CG, Korsgren O, Tibell A, et al., "Transplantation of porcine fetal pancreas to diabetic patients," *Lancet* 1994;344: 1402–4; Reinholt FP, Hultenby K, Tibell A, et al., "Survival of fetal porcine pancreatic islet tissue transplanted to a diabetic patient: Findings by ultrastructural immunocytochemistry," *Xenotransplantation* 1998;5: 222–25.

15. Dufrane D, Gianello P, "Pig islet for xenotransplantation in humans: Structural and physiological compatibility for human clinical application," *Transplantation Reviews (Orlando)* 2012;26 (3): 186, citing Valdes-Gonzalez RA, Dorantes LM, Garibay GN, et al., "Xenotransplantation of porcine neonatal islets of Langerhans and Sertoli cells: A 4-year study," *European Journal of Endocrinolology* 2005;153: 419–27.

16. Birmingham K, "Skepticism surrounds diabetes xenograft experiment," *Nature Medicine* 2002;8 (10): 1047; Sykes M, Cozzi E, "Xenotransplantation of pig islets into Mexican children: Were the fundamental ethical requirements to proceed with such a study really met?" *European Journal of Endocrinology* 2006;154: 921–22 (author reply 923).

17. Sykes, Cozzi, "Xenotransplantation."

18. Valdes-Gonzalez R, Dorantes LM, Bracho-Blanchet E, Rodríguez-Ventura A, White DJ, "No evidence of porcine endogenous retrovirus in patients with type 1 diabetes after long-term porcine islet xenotransplantation," *Journal of Medical Virology* 2010;82 (2): 331–34.

19. Elliott RB, on behalf of Living Cell Technologies, "Towards xenotransplantation of pig islets in the clinic," *Current Opinion in Organ Transplantation* 2011;16 (2): 195–200.

20. Ibid.

21. Ibid., 199.

22. Mason C, Dunnill P, "A brief definition of regenerative medicine," *Journal of Regenerative Medicine* 2008;3 (1), citing Greenwood HL, Singer PA, Downey GP, et al., "Regenerative medicine and the developing world," *PLoS Medicine* 2006;3 (9): e381.

23. Mirmalek-Sani SH, Orlando G, McQuilling JP, et al., "Porcine pancreas extracellular matrix as a platform for endocrine pancreas bioengineering," *Biomaterials* 2013;34 (22): 5488–95.

24. McCormick R, "Was there any real hope for Baby Fae?" *Hastings Center Report* 1985;15 (1): 12.

25. Rosner F, "Artificial and baboon heart implantation: The Jewish view," *Archives of Internal Medicine* 1985;145: 1330.

26. Regan T, "The other victim," *Hastings Center Report*, 1985;15 (1): 9.

27. Rosner F, "Artificial and baboon heart implantation."

28. Gorovitz S, "Will we still be 'human' if we have engineered genes and animal organs?" *Washington Post*, Dec. 9, 1984,

29. Levine RJ, *Ethics and regulation of clinical research* (Baltimore: Urban & Schwarzenberg, 1981).

30. Capron AM, "When well-meaning science goes too far," *Hastings Center Report* 1985;15 (1): 8–9; Annas G, "Baby Fae: The 'anything goes' school of human experimentation," *Hastings Center Report* 1985;15 (1): 15–17; McCormick, "Was there any real hope."

31. President's Commission for the Study of Ethical Problems in Medicine and Biomedical and Behavioral Research, *Deciding to Forgo Life-Sustaining Treatment: Ethical, Medical, and Legal Issues in Treatment Decisions* (Washington, DC: US Government Printing Office, 1983), 212; Veatch RM, "Limits of guardian treatment refusal: A reasonableness standard," *American Journal of Law and Medicine* 1984;9 (4): 427–68; Ross LF, *Children, families, and health care decision making* (Oxford: Clarendon Press, 1998).

32. Buchanan A, Brock D, *Deciding for others: The ethics of surrogate decision making* (New York: Cambridge University Press, 1989).

33. Veatch, "Limits of guardian treatment refusal."

34. However, even if one agrees that this could be seen as research that offers the prospect of direct benefit, one could still ask whether the first subjects should be children. According to the *Federal Regulations* for the protection of human subjects, research should be done first on adults who can consent for themselves before it is attempted on children. There may be times when one can justify that the research be done concurrently, but this usually requires data to show that it does not pose undue risk of harm. See Roth-Cline MD, Gerson J, Bright P, Lee CS, Nelson RM, "Ethical considerations in

conducting pediatric research," in *Pediatric Clinical Pharmacology*, ed. Seyberth HW, Rane A, Schwab M (Heidelberg: Springer, 2011), 219–44.

35. Rawls J, *A theory of justice* (Cambridge, MA: Harvard University Press, 1971).

36. Veatch RM, *The foundations of justice: Why the retarded and the rest of us have claims to equality* (New York: Oxford University Press, 1986).

37. Even if one accepts an over-a-lifetime perspective, the question remains whether Baby Fae should have been an experimental subject before there were better data to show that xenotransplantation is safe and that it held out a real possibility of clinical success. As mentioned above, the *Federal Regulations* for the protection of human subjects requires that, when possible, research be done first on adults who can consent for themselves before it is attempted on children.

38. Fishman JA, Scobie L, and Takeuchi Y, "Xenotransplantation-associated infectious risk: A WHO consultation," *Xenotransplantation* 2012;19: 72–81.

39. Brown J, Matthews AL, Sandstrom PA, Chapman LE, "Xenotransplantation and the risk of retroviral zoonosis," *Trends in Microbiology* 1998;6 (10): 411–15.

40. Bhatti FN, Schmoeckel M, Zaidi A, et al., "Three-month survival of Hdaff transgenic pig hearts transplanted into primates," *Transplantation Proceedings* 1999;31 (1–2): 958; Kozlowski T, et al., "Porcine kidney and heart transplantation in baboons undergoing a tolerance induction regimen and antibody adsorption," *Transplantation* 1999;67: 18–30.

41. Williams N, "Paving the way for British xenotransplant," *Science* 1998;281 (5378): 767; US Department of Health and Human Services, "Draft Public Health Service (PHS) guideline on infectious disease issues in xenotransplantation (August 1996)," *Federal Register* 1996;61 (185): 49920–32; Butler D, "Europe is urged to hold back on xenotransplant clinical trials," *Nature* 1999;397: 281–82; US Department of Health and Human Services, Food and Drug Administration, "Guidance for industry: Public health issues posed by the use of nonhuman private xenografts in humans (April 1999)," *Federal Register* 1999;64: 16743–44.

42. Michael B, "The precautionary principle should be used with caution—and should be applied to animal experimentation and genetic manipulation, not merely to protection of the environment," *Alternatives to Laboratory Animals* 1999;27 (1): 1.

43. United Nations, *1992 report of the United Nations Conference on Environment and Development*, Document A/CONF.151/26, vol. 1 (New York: United Nations, 1992), as cited by Steel D, "Extrapolation, uncertainty factors and the precautionary principle," *Studies in History and Philosophy of Biological and Biomedical Sciences* 2011;42: 359; Stirling A, "Risk, precaution and science: Towards a more constructive policy debate," *European Molecular Biology Organization Reports* 2007;8 (4): 309.

44. Wingspread conference participants, "Wingspread statement of the Precautionary Principle," Wingspread Conference, Racine, WI, 1998 as cited by Kumanan W, "A framework for applying the precautionary principle to transfusion safety," *Transfusion Medicine Reviews* 2011;25 (3): 178.

45. Powell R, "What's the harm? An evolutionary theoretical critique of the precautionary principle," *Kennedy Institute of Ethics Journal* 2010;20: 181–206.

46. Kumanan, "Framework," 177.

47. Ibid.

48. Germain M, Ghibu S, Delage G, "The precautionary principle in blood safety: Not quite the same as aiming for zero risk," *Transfusion Medicine Reviews* 2012;26 (2): 181–84.

49. Ibid.

50. Ibid., 181.

51. Ibid, 182.

52. Ibid.

53. Michael, "Precautionary principle," 1–5.

54. See Balls M, "The precautionary principle should be used with caution—and should be applied to animal experimentation and genetic manipulation, not merely to protection of the environment,"

Alternatives to Laboratory Animals (ATLA) 1999;27 (1): 1–5, at 1; and Michie, "Xenotransplantation," 62–63.

55. Denner J., Tonjes RR, "Infection barriers to successful xenotransplantation focusing on porcine endogenous retroviruses," *Clinical Microbiology Reviews* 2012;25 (2): 318–43.

56. Fishman, Scobie, Takeuchi, "Xenotransplantation-associated infectious risk," 72.

57. US Department of Health and Human Services, Secretary's Advisory Committee on Xenotransplantation, "Informed consent in clinical research involving xenotransplantation," draft, June 2004.

58. Ibid., vi.

59. Spillman MA, Sade RM, "Clinical trials of xenotransplantation: Waiver of the right to withdraw from a clinical trial should be required," *Journal of Law, Medicine & Ethics* 2007;35: 265–72.

60. Azofra MJ, Casabona CM, "Some ethical, social, and legal considerations of xenotransplantation," *Methods in Molecular Biology* 2012;885: 307–29.

61. Cozzi E, Tallacchini M, Flanagan EB, Pierson RN III, Sykes M, Vanderpool HY, "The International Xenotransplantation Association consensus statement on conditions for undertaking clinical trials of porcine islet products in type 1 diabetes—Chapter 1: Key ethical requirements and progress toward the definition of an international regulatory framework," *Xenotransplantation* 2009;16: 203–14.

Chapter 15

The Media's Impact on Transplants and Directed Donation

On *November 5, 1982,* eleven-month-old Jamie Fiske received a liver transplant at the University of Minnesota Hospitals. The donated liver came from a baby in Utah pronounced dead using brain criteria. Jamie had biliary atresia and had two unsuccessful operations in Massachusetts to improve bile drainage before being admitted to the University of Minnesota in September to be considered for a liver transplant. When no donor became available, her parents sent a brief statement to the wire news services and Boston newspapers, and a few stories appeared in the press. On October 28, her father, Charles Fiske, an administrator at the Boston University School of Medicine, appealed for a liver at the American Academy of Pediatrics' annual meeting in New York, urging those present "to keep your eyes and ears open for the possibility of a donor for my daughter." As reported in *JAMA*, Fiske concluded his appeal by telling "the pediatricians that her favorite toy is a stuffed musical goose that plays the song 'You Are My Sunshine, . . . Please Don't Take My Sunshine Away.'" The three major television networks publicized the story, and a week later, an organ became available.[1] Thirty years later, in November 2012, the University of Minnesota published an update stating that Jamie was the longest-surviving liver transplant candidate to date.[2]

Jamie's was not the first public appeal. In October 1981, Lauren Touhey's parents publicized her need for a liver because she suffered from hereditary tyrosinemia. The publicity brought offers from all over the United States and Canada and resulted in at least six other children receiving organ transplants, before a liver was eventually found and she had the transplant performed at the University of Pittsburgh.[3]

Although President Reagan sent well-wishes to Jamie Fiske, he took on an even greater role in July 1983 for Candi Thomas and two other children, for whom he made an appeal on his weekly radio broadcast. The following week, Reagan thanked Americans for their response, stating that more than 5,000 people in forty-seven states had called a Houston center that coordinates organ donations.[4] In April 1984, however, Reagan was criticized for his willingness to take credit in individual cases but his refusal "to support legislation that would aid thousands of transplant patients through a bill sponsored by Representative Al Gore Jr. of Tennessee."[5] The Reagan administration argued that organ procurement and allocation should be left to the private sector. Six months later, however, Reagan signed into law the National Organ Transplant Act (NOTA) of 1984.[6]

Although there are now formal organ procurement organizations (OPOs) throughout the United States and specific organ algorithms for allocating deceased donor organs coordinated by United Network for Organ Sharing (UNOS), mass media appeals continue due to the great gap in supply and demand. The intersection of the media and transplantation has been a mixed blessing. In this chapter we examine the ethical issues raised by the different roles that the media have played and continue to play in organ transplantation since the passage of NOTA and the development of national allocation algorithms: (1) direct media solicitation by individuals for a deceased donor; (2) media appeals for direct living donations; (3) patterns in media use, depending on whether the appeal is for a deceased or a living donor; (4) limits on media publicity, and (5) the use of the media by transplant programs to encourage living donations, particularly the solicitation of Good Samaritans (donors who give without an intended recipient in mind) at their centers.

Direct Media Solicitation by Individuals for a Deceased Donor

With the establishment of an organ allocation system, it would seem that the media appeals for deceased donor organs would disappear and that the media would lose interest in this human interest story. However, as the gap between demand and supply grows and candidates die on the wait list, candidates and their families look for ways to jump the queue. Hence, we continue to have cases like that of Jamie Fiske, Lauren Touhey, and Candi Thomas. In May 2004 thirty-two-year-old Todd Krampitz was diagnosed with hepatocellular cancer (HCC), and by July he was told that only a liver transplant could save his life. His liver cancer was too far advanced at that time to make him eligible for additional points that other candidates with HCC receive in order to get higher priority for a deceased donor liver transplant before the cancer grows and spreads. Afraid that he would die while waiting, his family mounted a media campaign. They purchased a billboard and developed a Web presence where they advertised his plight. Media coverage of these media attempts helped further spread the word, and in September the family of a deceased donor directed their deceased donor's liver to Krampitz.[7] He survived for only nine months. As Hopper reported in the *Houston Chronicle*, Krampitz's transplant angered many who felt he had cut the line.[8] In response Annie Moore, a spokeswoman for UNOS, stated that it was legal under the Uniform Anatomical Gift Act to donate an organ to an individual and that only "a handful" take place each year.[9] However, the public outcry led to a review of the policy and practice by both the American Medical Association (AMA) and UNOS.

The AMA's and UNOS's Positions on Soliciting Deceased Donors

The AMA Council on Ethical and Judicial Affairs prepared a report in 2006 noting that the argument in favor of public solicitation was the possible increase of the number of organs but expressing worry that public solicitation would have an impact on the equity and efficiency of the UNOS allocation algorithms.[10] Likewise, the report noted that "the OPTN/UNOS Board of Directors is on record as opposing any attempt by an individual transplant candidate (or her/his representative) to solicit a deceased donor's organ(s), if doing so would place the transplant candidate ahead of others on the wait list in a way that subverted the system's commitment to equity."[11]

In 2009 the Organ Procurement and Transplantation Network (OPTN) released a statement regarding directed deceased donation. It began by noting its legality under the Uniform Anatomical Gift Act and by most state anatomical gift laws. It also noted that at least 100 deceased donor transplants each year have occurred through directed donation and explained that it usually involves the donation of an organ to a transplant candidate related to or emotionally close to the donor or the donor's family, although sometimes it may be donated to a celebrity or stranger in response to a media report. The statement noted that many other organs from the donor are then allocated nondirectedly according to OPTN policy—meaning that the permissibility of directed deceased donor transplantation also leads to increased nondirected deceased donor organs.[12]

Individual and Social Directed Donation

The US transplant law distinguishes between a directed deceased donation to a specific person and a socially directed donation (also known as a conditional deceased donation), which is a donation to (or perhaps withheld from) a specific class. The issue was raised in the United States when a family agreed to the donation of their loved one's organs, provided the organs would only go to white recipients because their loved one had been a member of a white supremacist group.[13] Although the offer was accepted, the public outcry led to the rejection of all socially directed donations (for a more complete discussion, see chapter 23).

In the United Kingdom a similar socially directed donation was accepted in the North of England in 1998 and led to a guidance by the secretary of state for health to proscribe conditional deceased donation.[14] Whether it was meant to hold for directed deceased donation to a particular candidate is not clear. However, in April 2008 the UK media publicized the story of Rachel Leake, whose daughter, Laura Ashworth, died on April 2, two days after an asthma attack. Leake had kidney failure and could have used a kidney, but her daughter's kidneys were given to strangers on the grounds that a deceased donor's organs cannot be directed but must be allocated according to the allocation process.[15] The family was quite frustrated, especially because Ashworth had talked about serving as a living donor for her mother. Leake died a year later, in August 2009.[16] In March 2010 the National Health Service Blood and Transplant Committee issued a revised policy document that set out the circumstances whereby a request for a specific allocation of a deceased donor's organ could be considered: (1) the death of an intended living donor; and (2) an organ from a deceased donor that might benefit a close family member or friend.[17] If the regulation had been in place at the time of Ashforth's death, Leake would have been the recipient of a kidney from her daughter and might not have died from the septicemia that she fought for the last three months of her life.

Ethical Concerns about Using the Media to Obtain a Deceased Donor

In contrast with the case of Leake and her daughter, there is a broad consensus that families can direct deceased or living organs to family members and friends. This, in fact, was incorporated into the original American Uniform Anatomical Gift Act. The ethical concern arises when a deceased donor's organs are directed to a stranger who has made his or her case in the media. It is a justice issue, given that some families are more media savvy, media appealing, and politically connected, and can afford more publicity. As such, when a candidate on the deceased donor wait list "jumps the queue" due to such publicity, others claim it is unfair.

Is the claim of unfairness valid? It is, if the deceased donor would otherwise have donated to the wait list in a nondirected fashion. There are empirical data to show that media publicity has increased public awareness of the organ donor shortage.[18] If the deceased donor would not have been a donor except that his or her family was moved by the media story, then no one is hurt. However, if the decedent would have been a donor regardless, then those higher on the list have been harmed. There are only anecdotal reports to show that when a directed donation is refused by an OPO, some families agree to a nondirected donation. The solution may be to instruct OPOs to encourage families that have been moved by a story (i.e., by what is known as the power-of-the-identified-victim syndrome[19]) to understand that every person on the wait list has a story and that it is best and fairest if they donate in a nondirected fashion, but to continue to permit donations directed to specific individuals who become known to donor families through media attention while, at the same time, not tolerating donations directed to religious, racial, ethnic, or other social groups.

Another ethical concern is that solicitation diverts organs to unsuitable candidates for transplantation or to candidates who are less likely to have successful grafts. Todd Krampitz did not qualify for extra points for hepatocellular carcinoma because his cancer was too advanced. He died of a recurrent tumor less than one year after transplantation, which raised questions of whether he should have been eligible for a deceased donor's organ, even if it had been directed specifically to him.

The question of whether families of deceased donors can attach certain strings to the gift of a deceased donor's organ raises the ethical question of whether the deceased donor's kidney is a commodity that one can dispose of as one pleases or whether it is something more. Organs seem to be more than commodities, given that we do not allow "owners" to sell them. Dees and Singer suggest that it may be better to treat organs more like children (over which society has some responsibility).[20] If organs are more like children, then how they are allocated may not be solely in the domain of the decedent and his or her family. Instead, the state may have a say in the decision making, or at least may create boundaries regarding what decisions are morally permissible.

Elsewhere one of the authors (LFR) has argued that even if organs are perceived as property, transplant surgeons are moral agents who can refuse to allocate a deceased donor's organs according to the family's wishes by refusing to procure and transplant the organ.[21] Thus, though one can request to donate directedly to a particular individual, a transplant program can decide that, ethically, it will not participate. One problem with depending on the moral agency of individual physicians, however, is that it may lead to inconsistent responses—that is, some physicians or programs may decide to proceed with a directed donation, even if the reasons are distasteful. This becomes more controversial as one moves from a donation directed to an individual to a socially directed or conditional donation, where some conditions may seem more acceptable (e.g., directing a donation to candidates who are minors) than others (directing a donation to candidates who are of a certain ethnicity), which may lead some centers or OPOs to accept some conditional donations and other centers or OPOs to refuse to do so (this is further discussed in chapter 23).

The Media and Living Directed Donation

In contrast to deceased donor transplantation that focuses on impartial justice, living donation has for the most part focused on a partially autonomy-driven rationale.[22] As we saw in chapter 12 with respect to living donors, however, there have been attempts to expand living donation from genetic relatives to spouses, then to friends, and then to persons with whom one has less of a personal relationship (e.g., people at work, members of a church).

The Good Samaritan Donor

We now consider the role of the media in creating relations with people who, previously, were strangers. These donors who start as strangers are sometimes called "Good Samaritan donors" or nondirected donors. They are sometimes referred to as "altruistic" donors, but that term has been resisted because it implies that more traditional living donors are not altruistic when they donate to a relative.[23] Conversely, family donations are not purely altruistic, in that there may be a prima facie, albeit defeasible, duty to donate to a family member.[24]

The Evolution of the Good Samaritan Donor

In the early 1970s, there was a report about several Good Samaritan kidney donors, but the idea lost favor as the recipients did not fare well.[25] A quarter of a century later, improved immunosuppressants made these transplants much more likely to be successful, and in 1996, Jochem Hoyer, a German transplant surgeon, donated his kidney nondirectedly in Germany.[26] Two years later, in August 1998, Joyce Rouch donated a kidney to Christopher "Bear" Bienieck, a thirteen-year-old boy whom she did not know.[27] Rouch was a former hospice and trauma nurse who was a coordinator at the Indiana Organ Procurement Organization when she heard about the new technique of laparoscopic surgery in 1998 and decided to donate a kidney. She approached Lloyd Ratner at Johns Hopkins University. The hospital ethics committee approved the donation, and she donated in September 1999. Her story made headlines all over the world.[28] In August 1999 Minnesota began to accept "nondirected donors," and Art Matas and his colleagues published an article in the *New England Journal of Medicine* describing the first program devoted to "nondirected" living donors.[29] In the University of Minnesota program, kidneys from Good Samaritan nondirected living donors were allocated to candidates on the wait list, although they did not strictly follow the UNOS order, selecting those at their own institution (to offset time and costs of the workup). They also did not allocate strictly by the UNOS order, even within their own institution, choosing instead to only transplant those with a high likelihood of graft and patient long-term survival (e.g., patients in need of a first or second transplant and without a history of noncompliance) to maximize the utility of the gift and to gain public support.[30] In some ways, then, it is not fair to say that the living, non–emotionally related donors are completely "nondirected." Although the donors may not be choosing their recipients, the institution was doing so. The transplant team directed the organ to a candidate at their own institution who had a high likelihood of long-term graft survival, two traits that, if requested by the donor, would make the donation a conditional or socially directed donation.

Today, many so-called Good Samaritan donors are offered the option of donating nondirectedly to the list or to catalyze a kidney chain that can involve many donor–recipient pairs. In chains, the potential candidate who receives a nondirected kidney is not chosen randomly; nor is she necessarily the person at the top of the UNOS order, but rather, the candidate is an individual who has a potential living donor willing to donate to a stranger in exchange for a kidney to be obtained for her. This raises ethical concerns that the altruistic nondirected kidney donors are donating to those who are already advantaged as they have a potential living donor in contrast to many on the list who do not. Although this has been addressed by ending kidney chains with a transplant to a wait list candidate without a living donor, it still may not be fair to call these donations nondirected as they are being directed by the institutions to candidates with certain traits (either long life expectancy or those with willing paired donors). It is more accurate, then, to refer to these donors as Good Samaritan donors rather than as nondirected donors.

Soliciting for Good Samaritan Donors

Although some Good Samaritan donors are self-motivated and do not need an "identified victim" and are willing to donate nondirectly to anyone on the wait list, other Good Samaritans are motivated by an appeal by a particular person. Patients and families now seek to use the media to encourage a healthy individual to choose to become a Good Samaritan donor and to donate directly to their loved one.

One of the first solicitations for a living donor was on behalf of Camilo Sandoval Ewen, a Canadian infant born in 2001 with biliary atresia, like Jamie Fiske two decades earlier.[31] Other than the diagnosis, however, the cases were quite dissimilar. The Fiskes sought a deceased donor, whereas Camilo's parents sought media help to find a living person who was willing to donate part of his or her liver. Although Camilo was listed on the Canadian deceased donor wait list, his parents did not believe that their son could wait any longer. According to newspaper accounts, more than fifty people responded to their request for consideration as a living donor.[32] Camilo's family and the donor went to the United States for the transplant because no Canadian transplant program permitted donations between non–emotionally related individuals.[33]

Unfortunately, the case did not have a happy ending. Camilo had the liver transplant on April 7, 2001, and died within 24 hours. It turned out that the donor was known to the family and was considered a potential emotionally related donor who was in the process of being worked up in Canada, and the procedure would have been paid for by the Canadian government. However, the donor did not like how she was being treated, and so she insisted that the procedures be performed in the United States, the Canadian government refused to pay, leading to the family's appeal to raise money. The family presented their story to the media as a case where the Canadian government would not pay for a child's transplant and would leave the child to die, but a US hospital was willing to help. They raised about $200,000. When the Canadian press published the full story about how the procedure could have been done in Canada at the National Health Service's expense, financial donors were angry about being duped, and the charity group that had helped Camilo's family raise the money agreed to refund the donations.[34]

Since Camilo's case, others have sought living donors (usually for kidneys) using billboards and, in the past decade, the internet. Because Good Samaritan donors can elect to donate to a specific stranger, why should candidates not seek out their attention? The concern is that some individuals are more media savvy, more politically savvy, or cuter (who would win the media beauty contest). Thus, when the media elect to promote the needs of one patient, other patients do not get such attention, which raises questions of fairness.

Alternatively, some argue that media appeals increase community awareness, which can lead to more donations, even beyond the intended recipient. A case in point: The University of Minnesota stated that between January 2000 and July 2009, 165 children were evaluated for kidney transplants and that the families of 9 children without compatible living donors engaged the media to find willing donors. The children ranged from seven months to fourteen years of age, and their families used a variety of media; the most common media source was local television (four of the nine families), and three families used local newspapers and two used websites. One family used a church bulletin, and another used a work bulletin. Three used multiple sources. Of the nine children, four were successfully transplanted within 4.5 months and another four received deceased donor kidneys while living donor evaluations were in progress. Only one candidate could not find a match, but at the time of the publication, had two responders willing to enroll in a paired exchange. In addition, six individuals who called in response to the media campaigns became Good Samaritan donors to others on the wait list.[35] The transplant team stated that it had not encouraged the media appeals and at the time did not have a protocol to address the activity, but it has now modified its literature to include a section on "media appeals." It acknowledges the social justice issues raised by media appeals, but concludes that "the debate, as of now, is unresolved."[36]

From a social justice perspective, it may not be fair that some candidates get media attention when others do not. Conversely, if everyone had access to the media, then there would be no media interest as the stories would lose their human interest appeal. More than 120,000 individuals are currently on organ wait lists, each with a unique story. As such, one must ask, particularly in the living donor arena, whether letting some "jump the queue" benefits everyone because it leads to greater awareness and hence more donors than otherwise. That is, the media attention can encourage some who are ambivalent to donate and encourage others who are unaware about the need and opportunities for donation. And yet, when one hears about the deceitful use of the media by families like Baby Camilo's, the fear is that it can lead to a backlash.

In sum, to the extent that media coverage of candidates in need of solid organs finds donors who would not have otherwise donated, the recipient of the directed donation benefits and no one else is hurt. The only issue, then, is that the person receiving the organ gets an advantage from the media solicitation when others, equally deserving, go without. Conversely, if Good Samaritan donors could be encouraged to donate nondirect-edly to the list in response to a specific appeal, many more recipients would benefit and the equity of the UNOS allocation system would be preserved.

MatchingDonors.com

Another way to solicit living donors is by social engagement on the internet. On October 20, 2004, the first known kidney transplant to be arranged between a stranger and a candidate using a commercial company as intermediary took place at Denver's Presbyterian / Saint Luke's Medical Center after the hospital's ethics committee decided it was permissible.[37] Robert Hickey (the recipient) paid MatchingDonors.com a $295 monthly fee to advertise his need for a kidney. Robert Smitty agreed to serve as a donor. There is no fee paid to the donors at MatchingDonors.com. Although the hospital initially refused to perform the surgery, it relented after both the donor and recipient signed affidavits that no money would change hands.[38] As Art Caplan noted, the initial media attention was very positive.[39] It led to a huge increase in the number of donors signed up on the website.[40]

Again, the story did not have the happiest of endings. It turns out that Smitty had failed to pay his child support and the media attention landed him in jail. Suspicion surfaced that he had sold his kidney, a concern that was never proven or disproven.[41]

Wait list candidates at MatchingDonors.com were initially charged a monthly fee of $295 for listing, whereas donors joined for free. Accusations of unfairness led Matching-Donors to waive the fee for economic hardship.[42] As of 2008 it had arranged seventy-eight transplants at twenty hospitals, and only seven US hospitals have refused.[43]

Some of the ethical concerns raised by directed deceased donor organs apply to the directed living donors solicited on the internet. One early listing on MatchingDonor.com, for example, was a skillfully worded, emotional appeal presented in terms of grandchil-dren who wanted their grandfather to survive. It was written by the mother of the children (the daughter of the man needing a kidney). She, herself, was a health professional working in a transplant program. She clearly had knowledge and skills unavailable to many in need of a kidney.

Concerns of fairness echo here. For some, there is concern only if one assumes that the organs solicited through the internet would otherwise be available to any of the patients on the list. If not, then many on the wait list (those who would have lower priority than the successful candidate) would benefit as they would move up a notch, while those above the candidate would be neither harmed nor benefited. If these organs might have otherwise been donated nondirectedly, however, then an individual who is above the candidate on the UNOS wait list is harmed because he or she is skipped over when the organ goes to the one obtaining the organ through MatchingDonors.com.

For others, the fairness issue remains even if the organs obtained via internet solicita-tion would not otherwise be transplanted. For them, even if extra organs are obtained that would not otherwise have become available, and even if those below the one obtaining the organ actually gain an advantage while those above that person on the wait list are neither helped nor harmed, there remains a moral problem of fairness in that one person, who has no special claim to getting an organ out of turn, gets a major advantage. This problem of arrangements that give a major advantage to one person while hurting no one else (and even helping some other people a little) is the focus of chapter 23, which explores socially directed donation.

What are the other potential harms of a website like MatchingDonors.com? One concern is future exploitation of the organ recipient. One of the reasons that some programs seek to require recipient anonymity is to protect the recipient from a donor coming back years or decades later asking for some type of help, stating: "Remember that I helped you? Well now I need help." However, most donors and recipients do want to meet, and so the practice at most centers is to allow for meetings if both parties agree. To date there have been no reports of attempts at extortion by former living donors.

Another potential type of harm is institutional. Dees and Singer suggest three potential types of institutional harm: (1) if the practice undermines the whole transplant allocation system, (2) if the practice promotes the interests of some groups at the expense of others, or (3) if it leads to commodification.[44] To date, although there are theoretical grounds for worrying that MatchingDonors.com favors those with financial resources and/or those who are media savvy, there are no data to suggest that this website has undermined the organ allocation system. To address cries of inequity due to the cost of enrollment, MatchingDonors.com offers financial aid to candidates who cannot afford the fee. Finally, to date kidneys must be donated voluntarily without payment, and although it is hard to verify that there is no exchange of money from these transplants, the same can be said about transplants arranged between donors and recipients who know each other well.

Living versus Deceased Directed Media Appeals

Should the same rules apply to media appeals for both living and deceased donors' organs? Is it permissible to have different allocation processes for deceased and living donations? We already do, given that we have a national allocation for deceased organs and allow living donors to choose their family and friends, regardless of whether they are the sickest or less needy.

To the extent that one believes that deceased donor allocation should be based on principles of justice and that living donor allocation can be more partial—for example, to one's family—one may want to proscribe directed deceased donation but permit directed living donation. This would be consistent with public sentiment, in which there seems to be much greater objection to media appeals for deceased donors than for living donors because in some ways the directed deceased donor seems to have taken an organ that was otherwise a public good and allocated it to the successful media candidate. The problem with this objection is that it assumes that the decedent had planned to donate. Yet it is also possible that the decedent had left no instructions, but the members of the family are so taken by the media appeal that they move from a "no" to a "yes" when approached by the organ procurement team. In those cases, then, everyone who is wait-listed below the candidate benefits because one person is effectively removed from the wait list and those above the candidate are not harmed because there would not have been a donation. And to the extent that other organs are procured from the decedent, candidates other than the recipient of the direct donation also benefit.

Media appeals to living donors are often viewed differently given that they are a private good. One can argue that someone can give to charity or they can specify to which charity they donate. No one on the wait list can claim that they have a right to this individual's kidney. Here again, it may be that the person was an altruist and would have donated, but often strangers present to transplant programs because they hear a story on the news or know of someone, and so the personal media plea may actually be increasing the number of Good Samaritan donors.

Supporters of websites like MatchingDonors.com argue that this type of website enhances donor autonomy. No one is required to register at the site, just as no one is required to be a living donor. If an individual decides that he or she wants to donate to a stranger, he or she can choose to donate nondirectedly and allow the institution to choose their recipient; or he can look for a candidate in church bulletins and billboards; or he can choose to meet someone on line for the express purpose of donation. In an article about the oversight of OPTN/UNOS, Delmonico and Graham point out that "the OPTN cannot regulate or restrict the ways relationships are developed in our society with respect to living organ donation, nor does it seek to do so."[45]

Although donors have wide discretion on whether to donate and then to whom to donate, there are limits. First, a living donor cannot donate a vital organ like a heart or even a second kidney. In contrast, a deceased donor can set limits on what organs and tissues to donate or can agree to donate everything, including his or her hands or face. Second, a donor, whether living or deceased, cannot donate unless he or she is "healthy" enough. And even if the donor is healthy enough, a transplant surgeon can refuse to operate on a potential living donor if he or she feels that the risks are too great for that individual. Similarly a transplant surgeon can refuse to operate on a potential deceased donor if he or she feels that the organs are no longer viable (e.g., the patient died outside the 60-minute window after withdrawal of the ventilator, even if the decedent had signed a first-person authorization). Third, neither living nor deceased donors can sell their organs. Fourth, most programs will not allow a conditional directed donation for either living or deceased donors, although living donors can get around this by creating a relationship for the express purpose of finding a candidate who meets their conditional criteria. And fifth, currently it is legal to seek media attention for a deceased or living donation in the United States, although not for a deceased organ in the United Kingdom.

Limits to the Media

The interrelationship of medicine and the media is complex, and this is true for transplantation. In 1990, W. J. Brady, a Canadian journalist, stated that "transplantation, frankly is no longer a procedure which attracts the attention it did three or four years ago."[46] He also felt that the media, whether intentionally or not, had become a part of the system, but he warned the transplant community that though the media can be an ally, "that's not their prime mandate or their agenda."[47] Although the transplant community would like the media to help increase organ donation, the media gravitate to the unusual, which may explain the current interest in reporting possible examples of queue jumping and commerce.[48]

Was Brady right that the media have lost interest in transplantation? Quick and colleagues examined network television news coverage (ABC, CBS, and NBC) of organ donation from January 1990 to December 2005. Overall, they found that organ donation was the subject of 1,507 stories, which they described as "modest" interest, with the majority of the coverage described as positive.[49]

But not all the stories have been positive. When the media publicized that a nurse, Joyce Rouch, was planning in 1998 to be a non–emotionally related living donor to a teenager in Maryland whom she did not know, the world heard and it led to increases in living donations. However, when the media publicized the death of Greg Hurwitz—who had donated a liver lobe to his brother, Adam—the transplant program at Mount Sinai Hospital in New York City was temporarily suspended and the number of living liver donors dropped nationally. It has never bounced back.

Negative media portrayals have a seriously adverse impact. In an analysis of seventy-eight family discussions about organ donation, Morgan and colleagues found that the most influential information came from sensationalistic, negative media portrayals, with the myths of premature declaration of death, a black market, and corruption having the greatest influence.[50]

In the summer of 2013, transplantation seemed to make national headlines quite a lot. There was the case of Sarah Murnaghan, a young girl with cystic fibrosis whose parents used the internet and other forms of media to help challenge the UNOS lung allocation system. As a result, she received two adult double-lung transplants in June of that year. Also, there was the case of Amelia Rivera, who made the news in January 2012 when her mother said that the Children's Hospital of Philadelphia would not list her daughter for a kidney transplant because she was "mentally retarded." She did, however, receive a living kidney graft from her mother in July 2013. Anthony Stokes, a sixteen-year-old African American, was originally denied listing on the heart transplant list due to concerns of compliance, but he was eventually listed and received a transplant in August 2013.[51] All three stories challenged the equity of the transplantation process. Although they all had happy endings, what impact the negative publicity will have on deceased and living donations is still to be seen.

In additional to national news, fictional organ donation stories are featured in television shows and the movies, and these often "promote myths and fears of the organ donation process" that have a greater influence than national nonfictional news.[52]

Limiting the Publicizing of Appealing Candidates

Should there be limits on what the media reports? The decision by the media to give attention to one candidate whose story is more appealing, or whose parents are more politically savvy and therefore present their story as more appealing, leads to concerns about justice. If one candidate's story gets headline news, this person may attract a nondirected living donor, and others, perhaps equally deserving or even more deserving but who did not get media attention, will not. For example, there were approximately thirty children waiting for lungs nationally when Sarah Murnaghan was, by court order, given priority on the adult lung transplant wait list. No one—not the judge, not UNOS, and certainly not Sarah's parents—addressed the question of whether she was the most deserving child currently on the list.

Nevertheless, in the case of appeals for living donors, especially kidney donors, because this may be a kidney that would otherwise not be donated, it would seem that the candidate who uses the media successfully benefits greatly and the others are not harmed. However, whether one can prove that this same Good Samaritan would not have donated nondirectedly is difficult to know.[53] The transplant community needs to develop protocols that it should use to encourage donors enamored by an individual's story portrayed in the media to donate to the wait list rather than to the particular individual, because each candidate has a compelling story.

Limiting the Publicizing of a Family's Refusals

A second possible limit that one might want to impose is on the media's decision to publicize a family's refusal. The first such report may be a case that was adjudicated in court in 1979.[54] Robert McFall had aplastic anemia and needed a bone marrow transplant. His cousin, David Shimp, was a perfect match, but then reneged on donating. McFall went to court to force his cousin to be his stem cell donor, claiming that he would otherwise die and that if his cousin had not said he would donate, McFall would have continued his search, but it was now too late. The courts suggested that Shimp was a moral coward for reneging on a bone marrow donation but that he could not be legally coerced. The behind-the-scenes details were reported in *People* magazine.[55]

In Britain, stories about siblings refusing to donate after human leukocyte antigen compatibility was established have also made headlines. When Helen Pretty refused to donate stem cells to her brother, Simon Pretty, her brother's story was covered in several newspapers; one story was titled "I Have Been Sentenced to Death by My Sister."[56] The media had a good impact for Pretty. Although his sister was steadfast in her refusal to be a stem cell donor, his story was picked up by the international press, and many potential donors came forward. A donor was found in the United States, and Pretty received his transplant. Unfortunately, he rejected the bone marrow, and the British tabloid exclaimed, "Man Sent Home to Die," reminding the reader that his sister had refused to donate.[57]

In this case, the media helped an individual obtain a direct donation, one that might not have happened otherwise. One concern about this type of media help, however, is that there are hundreds of individuals waiting on transplant lists who do not get such coverage. But if those who sign up on international donor registries will agree to donate to another wait list candidate not covered by the media, this would be a win–win situation.

But what if the media had been successful in pressuring the sister to decide to donate? Would it be ethically permissible for a transplant program to procure the stem cells from a donor who may have felt some degree of coercion about donating? In 1998 the British tabloids helped shame a woman into donating to her sister. Angela Latham had leukemia, and her sister, Susan Squires, was found to be human leukocyte antigen–compatible, but then said she was too scared to be a stem cell donor. The media pressure eventually convinced her, and she had stem cells removed at Manchester Royal Infirmary.[58] Interestingly, the media portrayed very different stories about the end result: In one tabloid, their relationship remains rocky; but in another, they have made their peace.[59] But the case raises the ethical issue of the role of the media and how transplant programs should respond when it is clear that a donor may have been coerced to act.

The Media and Transplant Programs

As the numbers of deceased donor and living donor organs have flattened or decreased over the past few years, there has been stiff competition between transplant programs to find donors for their patients. This has led to greater acceptance of less-than-ideal deceased donor kidneys. It has also led to the acceptance of Good Samaritan donations by virtually every major transplant program (although fewer accept donor–recipient pairs that were created through internet websites).[60]

Programs also advertise their living donor transplant programs. Levinsky cites an advertisement in the *New York Times* from the University of Maryland: "Donating a kidney is a tough decision. Deciding where to go is easy."[61] His fear is that it may lead to offering donors large payments for "expenses." He concludes, "We must avoid a slippery slope on which the benefits to the transplant recipients and to the institutions that care for them come to outweigh the risks to the donors."[62] Thus, the transplant community itself will need to place limits on the appropriateness of advertising to encourage living donation, particularly by Good Samaritan donors.[63]

Is it ever ethical for physicians and hospitals to advertise to encourage living donation, particularly nondirected living donation? In a debate about the ethics of encouraging healthy adults to donate a kidney to a stranger, both Glannon and Cronin claim that the physician's responsibility is first to do no harm.[64] Both also agree that competent, healthy adults can choose to be donors. The disagreement is what role the physician should play. Glannon argues that physicians should encourage their patients to be deceased donors because it does not affect their health, but they should not encourage them to be living donors to strangers because "many patients perceive their doctors as authority figures and trust them to always act in their best interests."[65] He claims that encouraging individuals to become Good Samaritan living donors when it involves clinical risks without clinical benefit violates the trust that patients place in their physicians.

In contrast, though Cronin concedes that doctors "do not have a moral obligation to encourage stranger kidney donation," she argues that providing healthy competent adults "with adequate information about the process involved and recognizing the value of their donation is consistent with the ethos of the NHS [National Health Service], which exists for the common good."[66]

Glannon agrees that doctors should promote organ donation and transplantation, but he claims that this is a secondary duty that should not supersede their primary duty: to focus on the patient's well-being and the avoidance of preventable harm.[67] Because it seems obvious that being a living organ donor involves necessary harm to the donor—surgical wound pain and suffering, not to mention the risk of infection and the hypothetical concern about the failure of the remaining kidney—it is not clear how anyone can promote organ donation and still focus primarily on patient well-being and the avoidance of harm.

Norman Levinsky raises concerns about the conflicts of interests that are inherent in Good Samaritan donations. In a critique of the nondirected donor program at the University of Minnesota, Levinsky questions the university's policy of providing financial aid to unrelated donors (as well as to related donors).[68] Although he notes that the aid "is presumably small and is intended only to defray expenses," he worries that programs may try to compete financially for donors. His concern is validated by a perusal of the Web, where we found transplant programs and transplant advocacy programs that give tips to candidates about how to find a living donor and recommend seeking a donor both within and beyond the family. They even provide strategies to overcome barriers. For example, the University of Minnesota has a Web page for living donors that includes frequently asked questions and answers about how to pay for living expenses after a donation. The Web page states:

> ▶ If you work outside of the home, ask your employer if you qualify for any leave benefits while you're away from work. Most donors use vacation, sick leave, or short-term disability income to provide a source of income.
> ▶ Family members may help with your costs. By helping with donor expenses or household bills, they have a way to take part in the transplant experience.
> ▶ If your recipient has a fund-raising drive, some of the money may go to nonmedical expenses related to donation.
> ▶ The Transplant Center has a Living Donor Assistance Grant. This is for eligible donors who need financial help during this vital time. Ask your social worker how you can apply for these funds.[69]

The line between providing information and promoting financial incentives is thin indeed.

Conclusion

Families have turned to the mass media to encourage organ donation since the earliest days of organ transplantation, and they have done so with great success. As Kluge notes, "The identified victim syndrome is too powerful to be ignored as a public relations tool."[70] The creation of a national allocation system has partially solved this problem, but because the growth in demand outpaces the growth in supply, families continue to turn to the media to get an organ specifically for their loved one. Although directed donations may benefit all the candidates if they motivate an individual or family members who would otherwise not have donated, if the individual would have donated without the solicitation, directed donation is troublesome because it potentially takes away an organ from the person who is next on the wait list and instead gives it to a person who is more media savvy or more politically savvy but may not be in as great a need as the individual who has been bypassed. Even if the solicitation adds an organ to the system that would not otherwise have been available, some are concerned that it is unfair for those who have the resources and skills to use the media to get an advantage that they do not deserve.

Notes

1. Gunby P, "Media-abetted liver transplants raise questions of 'equity and decency,'" *JAMA* 1983;249: 1973–74, 1980–82.

2. "On this date in Minnesota history: November 5, 1982," *Minnesota Family History Research*, Nov. 5, 2012, http://pjefamilyresearch.blogspot.com/2012/11/on-this-date-in-minnesota-history_5 .html.

3. "Efforts to save a child help 6 other patients," *New York Times*, Oct. 6, 1981, www.nytimes.com/ 1981/10/06/nyregion/efforts-to-save-a-child-help-6-other-patients.html; "The Region: Liver replaced, girl, 2-1/2, improves," *New York Times*, Nov. 17, 1981, www.nytimes.com/1981/11/17/nyregion/the -region-liver-replaced-girl-2-1-2-improves.html.

4. "Six children get new livers; Reagan cites reaction to plea," *New York Times*, July 31, 1983, www.nytimes.com/1983/07/31/us/six-children-get-new-livers-reagan-cites-reaction-to-plea.html.

5. Kurtz H, "Organ transplants turn into form of patronage," *Washington Post*, Apr. 23, 1984.

6. National Organ Transplant Act (NOTA), October 19, 1984, PL 98-507.

7. Robeznieks A, "Public plea spurs new liver, and debate over technique," *American Medical News*, September 6, 2004, www.amednews.com/article/20040906/profession/309069958/4/.

8. "Hopper L. Man, who advertised on billboards for liver, dies," *Houston Chronicle*, Apr. 26, 2005, www.chron.com/news/houston-texas/article/Man-who-advertised-on-billboards-for-liver-dies-19394 75.php.

9. Robeznieks, "Public plea."

10. Council on Ethical and Judicial Affairs of the American Medical Association, "Solicitation of the Public for Directed Donation of Organs for Transplantation," CEJA Report 3-A-06, 3.

11. Ibid., citing Organ Procurement and Transplantation Network / United Network for Organ Sharing Board of Directors, "Statement regarding solicitation of deceased donation," Nov. 19, 2004, http://optn.transplant.hrsa.gov/news/newsDetail.asp?id = 374.

12. OPTN, "Information regarding deceased directed donation," May 29, 2009, http://optn .transplant.hrsa.gov/news/newsDetail.asp?id = 1254.

13. Testerman J, "Should donors say who gets organs?" *St. Petersburg Times*, Jan. 9, 1994.

14. Wilkinson TM, "Racist organ donors and saving lives," *Bioethics* 2007;21: 63–74; UK Department of Health, "An investigation into conditional organ donation: The Report of the Panel," Feb. 22, 2000, http://webarchive.nationalarchives.gov.uk/20130107105354/http://www.dh.gov.uk/ prod_consum_dh/groups/dh_digitalassets/@dh/@en/documents/digitalasset/dh_4035465.pdf.

15. Jones A, "Mother denied dead daughter's organ transplant," *The Guardian*, Apr. 11, 2008, www.theguardian.com/society/2008/apr/12/health.nhs; BBC News, "Mother denied daughter's organs," April 12, 2008, http://news.bbc.co.uk/2/hi/uk_news/england/bradford/7344205.stm.

16. Brooke C., "Mother dies a year after being denied her daughter's kidney," *Mail Online*, 23 August 2009, www.dailymail.co.uk/news/article-1208480/Mother-dies-doctors-refuse-save-life -transplant-using-daughters-kidneys.html.

17. Requested allocation of a deceased donor organ. This policy has been agreed to by all UK Health Administrations. See www.nhsbt.nhs.uk/to2020/resources/finalguidanceen.doc.

18. Hanto DW, "Ethical challenges posed by the solicitation of deceased and living organ donors," *New England Journal of Medicine* 2007;356: 1062–66.

19. Kluge EHW, "Designated organ donation: Private choice in social context," *Hastings Center Report* 1989;19 (5): 14. Kluge would not allow a directed deceased donation but supports the idea of using "media campaigns that highlight the plight of particular persons," even though the distribution would be done under national allocation syndromes.

20. The dichotomy between organs as property versus organs as something of value independent of its owners is developed by Dees RH, Singer EA, "KidneyMatch.com: The ethics of solicited organ donations," *Journal of Clinical Ethics* 2008;19 (2): 141–49.

21. Ross LF, "All donations should not be treated equally: A response to Jeffrey Kahn's commentary," *Journal of Law, Medicine and Ethics* 2002;30: 448–51.

22. Cronin AJ, Price D, "Directed organ donation: Is the donor the owner?" *Clinical Ethics* 2008;3 (3): 127–31.

23. One of us (LFR) actually argues that family donations are not purely altruistic, in that there may be a prima facie, albeit defeasible, duty to donate to a family member. See Glannon W, Ross LF, "Do genetic relationships create moral obligations in organ transplantation?" *Cambridge Quarterly of Health Care Ethics* 2002;11: 153–59.

24. Ibid.

25. Sadler HH, Davison L, Carroll C, Kountz SL, "The living, genetically unrelated, kidney donor," *Seminars in Psychiatry* 1971;3 (1): 86–101.

26. Gohh RY, Morrissey PE, Madras PN, Monaco AP, "Controversies in organ donation: The altruistic living donor," *Nephrology, Dialysis and Transplantation* 2001;16: 619–21.

27. Grady D, "The new organ donors are living strangers," *New York Times*, Sept. 20, 1999.

28. Fields-Meyer T, "Perfect stranger," *People*, Nov. 8, 1999; Milner C, "Gift of a Lifetime," *WNC Magazine*, Jan. 4, 2013, http://wncmagazine.com/feature/gift_of_a_lifetime.

29. Mates AJ, Garvey CA, Jacobs CL, Kahn JP, "No directed donation of kidneys from living donors," *New England Journal of Medicine* 2000;343: 433–36.

30. Ibid.

31. Ross LF, "Media appeals for directed altruistic living liver donations," *Perspectives in Biology and Medicine* 2002;45: 329–37.

32. Galatian, S, "Baby Camilo departs for New York," *Vancouver Sun*, March 21, 2001.

33. Ross LF, *2002*, "Media appeals," citing personal communication with Bill Barable, then director of the British Columbia Transplant Authority.

34. Ibid.

35. Verghese PS, Garvey CA, Mauer MS, Matas AJ, "Media appeals by pediatric patients for living donors and the impact on a transplant center," *Transplantation* 2011;91: 593–96.

36. Ibid., 596.

37. Davis R., "Online organ match raises ethical concerns," *USA Today*, Oct. 26, 2004.

38. Truog RD, "Are organs personal property or a societal resource?" *American Journal of Bioethics* 2005;5 (4): 14–16.

39. Caplan A, "Organs.com: New commercially brokered organ transfers raise questions," *Hastings Center Report* 2004;34 (6): 8.

40. Vallis M, "'Hero' denied his day in the sun: Ethics controversy, donor's criminal past overshadow organ donation," *National Post* (Canada), Oct. 27, 2004.

41. Ibid.

42. Caplan, "Organs.com."

43. Dees, Singer, "KidneyMatch.com."

44. Ibid.

45. Delmonico FL, Graham WK, "Direction of the Organ Procurement and Transplantation Network and the United Network for Organ Sharing regarding the oversight of live donor transplantation and solicitation for organs," *American Journal of Transplantation* 2006;6: 39.

46. Brady WJ, "The role of the media in organ donation," *Transplantation Proceedings* 1990;22 (3): 1047–49.

47. Ibid.

48. Ibid.

49. Quick BL, Kim DK, Meyer K, "A 15-year review of ABC, CBS, and NBC news, coverage of organ donation: Implications for organ donation campaigns," *Health Communication* 2009;24 (2): 137–45.

50. Morgan SE, Harrison TR, Long SD, Afifi WA, Stephenson MS, Reichert T, "Family discussions about organ donation: How the media influences opinions about organ donation decisions," *Clinical Transplantation* 2005;19: 674–82.

51. Ross LF, "President's column: Pediatric controversies in the news," *American Academy of Pediatrics Section on Bioethics Newsletter*, Fall 2013, 3–8.

52. Harrison TR, Morgan SE, Chewning LV, "The challenges of social marketing of organ donation: News and entertainment coverage of donation and transplantation," *Health Marketing Quarterly* 2008;25 (1–2): 34.

53. Aaron Spital surveyed the public and found that of those who would consider donating to a stranger, more than 90 percent would still donate, even if they could not choose the type of recipient. See Spital A, "Should people who donate a kidney to a stranger be permitted to choose their recipients? Views of the United States public," *Transplantation* 2003;76: 1252–56.

54. *McFall v. Shimp*, 10 PA D. & C. 3d 90 (July 26, 1978).

55. Neuhaus C., "A cousin's stunning refusal to donate bone marrow leaves Robert McFall facing death," *People*, Aug. 14, 1978, www.people.com/people/archive/article/0,,20071484,00.html.

56. Roberts L, "I have been sentenced to death by my sister," *Daily Mail*, March 24, 2007, www.dailymail.co.uk/news/article-444238/I-sentenced-death-sister.html.

57. Murtagh M, "To [*sic*] weeks to live; Simon sent home to die after transplant fails," *Liverpool Echo*, Aug. 4, 2007, www.thefreelibrary.com/TO + WEEKS + TO + LIVEpercent3B + Simon + sent + home + to + die + after + transplant + fails.-a0167209509.

58. Raymond C, "Sisters torn apart," *Mirror*, May 13, 1998.

59. Ibid.; Oldfield S, "A happy return to work for sister who cheated death," *Daily Mail*, March 23, 1998.

60. Friedman AL, Lopez-Soler RI, Cuffy MC, Cronin DC II, "Patient access to transplantation with an internet-identified live kidney donor: A survey of US centers," *Transplantation* 2008;85: 794–98.

61. Levinsky NG, "Organ donation by unrelated donors," *New England Journal of Medicine* 2000;343: 430–32.

62. Ibid.

63. Johns Hopkins Comprehensive Transplant Center, www.hopkinsmedicine.org/transplant/living_donors/types.html#directed; University of Maryland Medical Center, http://umm.edu/programs/transplant/services/kidney/living-donor; Barnabas Health, Renal and Pancreas Transplant Division, "Altruistic living donation," www.barnabashealth.org/services/renal/donor/altruistic.html.

64. Glannon W, "Is it unethical for doctors to encourage healthy adults to donate a kidney to a stranger? Yes," *British Medical Journal* 2011;343: d7179; Cronin AJ, "Is it unethical for doctors to encourage healthy adults to donate a kidney to a stranger? No," *British Medical Journal* 2011; 343: d7140.

65. Glannon, "Is it unethical for doctors to encourage healthy adults."

66. Cronin, "Is it unethical for doctors to encourage healthy adults."

67. Glannon, "Is it unethical for doctors to encourage healthy adults."

68. Levinsky, "Organ donation."

69. University of Minnesota, "Financial information for living donors," www.uofmmedicalcenter.org/Specialties/KidneyTransplant/Livingkidneydonorprogram/Financialinformationforlivingdonors/index.htm.

70. Kluge, "Designated organ donation."

PART III

Allocating Organs

Chapter 16

The Roles of the Clinician and the Public

The Clinician and Allocation

The allocation of organs for transplantation poses a fundamental problem for the traditional medical ethics of clinicians. Since the days of the Hippocratic Oath, clinicians have professed a commitment to the welfare of their patients. They swear to benefit the patient and protect the patient from harm. We have discovered that this traditional ethic poses problems, even for more routine medical care of patients. We now know that there is more to medical ethics than simply benefiting the patient and protecting the patient from harm. Patients have rights grounded in moral principles of autonomy, fidelity, and veracity. Perhaps the most significant moral development in the last decades of the twentieth century was the recognition that patients (at least most adult patients) were autonomous agents who could consent or refuse consent to proposed therapies. The right to refuse treatment, especially life-prolonging treatment for the terminally ill, has shaped our thinking about medical ethics.

The other major challenge to the Hippocratic, patient-benefit ethic came from recognizing a social dimension in medicine. Physicians increasingly acknowledged their obligations to society as well as to the individual patient. This has been reflected in a commitment to research medicine and to public health, and a concern for the allocation of scarce resources. Closely related has been the development of transplantation medicine. The intriguing thing about transplantation is that physicians are thrust into a set of social relations. In organ procurement from deceased donors, the physician is working not for the good of the patient from whom the organs are procured but for the good of other patients, typically patients unknown to the procuring surgeon. In organ procurement from living donors, the physician is actually placed in the awkward spot of doing harm to his or her patient for the benefit of a third party—a relative, or sometimes now even a stranger. Meanwhile, the physician who implants organs is working primarily for the good of the patient receiving the organs, much as was done traditionally, but this means that such physicians have an inherent conflict of interest, if they are expected to participate in the decision about who should receive an organ. Naturally, the physician, especially one oriented toward Hippocratic patient benefit, wants to arrange the allocation of organs so as to help his or her own patient.

271

For this reason, we soon realized that there must be a division of labor in transplantation. The health professionals working for the good of the individual patient need to be isolated from the procurement and allocation decisions. This means that a physician caring for a dying or recently deceased patient should be freed up to remain loyal to his or her patient, and isolated from organ procurement and allocation decisions. This means that a physician caring for a patient in need of an organ must be isolated from the decision about how to allocate organs. Otherwise, each physician—following the Hippocratic mandate—would arrange the allocation so as to benefit his or her own patient.

The reality, at least in the United States, is that no physician in his or her role as clinician is ever expected to allocate organs for transplantation or other scarce medical resources, such as dialysis machines, intensive care unit beds, or any other expensive or limited resource. The normal limiting factor for dialysis in the early days was the availability of machines, and more recently, it has been the funding to operate them. The US Congress has, through an amendment to the Medicare laws, categorically covered all appropriate dialysis patients. Of course, clinicians will continue to be expected to determine which patients will benefit medically from dialysis, but in the normal sense of rationing—as we were forced to allocate scarce hemodialysis machines in the 1960s—allocation need not take place. In other countries, there may be fewer machines available; but even then, we would argue, physicians in the clinical, caregiving role ought not be the ones who allocate.

For transplantation, the story is quite different. Organs are inherently scarce. It is not just a matter of money, but also of the availability of the organs themselves. The problem has become more acute because, while the need for organs continues to grow, the supply of organs has not. Even if organ availability were maximized through freedom-infringing routine salvaging of organs from the newly dead, we would still not have enough. Someone must allocate.

Yet it does not follow that clinicians are expected to do the allocating. By law in the United States organs, at least organs from deceased donors, are made available through organ procurement organizations in cooperation with the national United Network for Organ Sharing (UNOS), whose board, under legislative guidelines, sets the principles for allocation of scarce organs and creates formulas for allocating them. Local practices must conform to the UNOS policies or to authorized variances; and UNOS policies must, in turn, conform to nationally set public principles. No clinician can gain access to an organ for transplant unless he or she conforms to the decisions of the local procurement organization, UNOS, and Congress.

To take kidney allocation as an example, whenever a kidney becomes available in a local procurement organization, a nationally approved formula determines a priority list of possible recipients (a formula that has recently been revised), which is discussed in chapter 20. This formula takes into account the quality of the donor organ, an estimate of how much extra life the recipient will gain, panel-reactive antibody levels, histocompatibility, whether one has previously been a living kidney donor, whether one is a child or an adult, geographical considerations, time already spent on dialysis, and, under special circumstances, medical urgency. Whenever a kidney becomes available, a computer generates a priority list among all eligible patients awaiting a kidney transplant. The organ procurement organization (OPO) is required to offer the organ to the person scoring highest according to the allocation formula. This has the advantage of eliminating any charge of special ad hoc considerations or prejudices influencing the allocation. It also has the effect of completely removing the clinician from the allocation decision at the local level. To be sure, physicians are well represented on both the local and national boards that establish and operate the allocation formulas. Physicians, primarily transplant surgeons, make up about half the UNOS board. When other health professionals—nurses and transplant coordinators—are included, this group makes up a dominant majority of the board. Because physicians and other clinical professionals tend to have predictable and somewhat atypical ethical commitments, these commitments to particular moral perspectives may skew the allocation principles in ways that are not fully supported by the general public. For example, transplant professionals may be more committed to maximizing good outcomes than to allocating organs fairly.[1] Nevertheless, individual clinicians at the bedside do no direct allocating involving their own patients. We are convinced that this is the only morally defensible arrangement. It is the public's responsibility to make sure that the UNOS allocation formulas fairly reflect the proper moral principles. This may require readjusting the UNOS board so that it is not as heavily dominated by transplant surgeons and other health professionals. For example, the president of UNOS has always been a physician, even though a significant minority of the board has always included transplant recipients, donor family representatives, philosophers, attorneys, and representatives of community perspectives.[2] Here we would like to summarize the argument that leads to this conclusion that clinicians should not be making allocation decisions at the bedside and possibly should play a less dominant role in the policymaking process.

Allocation as a Moral Rather Than Technical Matter

In order to understand why bedside clinicians should have no role in allocating dialysis machines or transplantable organs, we need to understand why someone might be inclined to assign this life-and-death task to them. The working assumption of those who would expect clinicians to be allocators is either that allocations can be made on the basis of factual medical information about patients or that allocations should be made on the basis of the values of physicians. Our claim is that key features of allocations are not factual in the medical sense; they are necessarily evaluative, and should not be made on the basis of the personal values of physicians.

The Role of Medical Facts in Allocation

Surely medical data are relevant in deciding how to allocate scarce medical services. We should continue to expect clinicians to determine the likely outcomes of transplants in patients who are potential candidates for these services. It is certainly sound to hold that no patient should be a candidate for these procedures whose medical condition will not be affected by them. But the patient who would not be affected is not likely to want the procedures anyway. The real debate is over how to allocate in cases where more patients wanting care have medical conditions that will be affected than there are organs to meet these needs. The issue is particularly controversial when we can expect different patients to benefit to different degrees, yet all the potential recipients will benefit to some degree.

The Role of Maximizing Benefit

If we could assume that the scarce resource should automatically go to the person who would benefit the most, it might appear that clinicians would be in a good position to play a role in deciding who should get the organs. As we shall see, however, it is very implausible to allocate organs on the basis of who will get the most benefit and, even if that were the correct principle, determining what counts as a benefit is inherently controversial and independent of medical facts. One patient may have the greatest chance of survival of acute illness; another may have the greatest predicted years of survival; still another may receive the greatest relief from suffering or morbidity; and yet another may get the most satisfaction. Medical facts alone cannot tell us which of these patients will benefit the most from a transplant.

More critically, even if we knew which patient would benefit the most medically from a procedure, we cannot automatically conclude that that patient should receive the medical procedure. Social utilitarians would insist that we take into account social and other nonmedical consequences to all parties of assigning the scarce resource to a particular person—a determination about which physicians surely are not expert. They would, for example, ask not only about the benefits to the recipient of an organ but also about how much good for others providing the organ would do. Saving some lives could be thought to do more total good than saving others. People who are in responsible positions—public officials, business leaders, brilliant scientists, and so forth—will contribute more aggregate good than more ordinary citizens. In fact some transplant candidates may actually provide net disutility if they receive organs. Even if they gain benefit, it could be offset with the expected harm to others. There is, for example, a controversy over whether convicted criminals, particularly those convicted of serious, repeat offenses, should receive organs. Critics argue that, even if one takes into account the benefits to the recipient and those family members and friends who still care about the recipient, the net effect of saving the life may be negative when one considers the consequences to others.

Conversely, trying to quantify the net consequences of saving one life rather than another is an enormously controversial and value-laden task, as shown, for example, by the experience of the Admission and Policy Committee of the Seattle Artificial Kidney Center. The committee was established in 1962 to select who would get dialysis at a time when dialysis was innovative and there were an inadequate number of dialysis machines to meet demand.[3] They were asked to choose between the head of a large corporation, a poet, and the mother of three small children—to decide who would contribute most benefit to society. It was quickly noted that the people chosen for dialysis looked strangely like the members of the committee. There were even disutilities of the process of deciding which candidates would contribute most to society—paralyzing controversies over which people were most valuable. This is a controversy we will revisit below when we talk about the proper composition of the committees that design organ allocation algorithms, and again in chapter 21, when we discuss the role of status in organ allocation.

The end result of this debate was a widespread social consensus that social consequences—benefits to third parties—should be excluded from the allocation process. Some people reach that conclusion because they believe it is intrinsically wrong to give organs on this basis. They challenge the basic approach of social utilitarianism. They believe that people deserve to be treated more equally regardless of their ability to make social contributions. Others may accept social utilitarianism in principle but reach the pragmatic conclusion that allocating organs and other medical technologies on the basis of such vague and complex considerations causes more harm than good. The time spent in deciding what the long-term social consequences are of giving an organ to one person from a long list of candidates might not be worth it when one realizes how complex the calculations would be and how much discord could be generated from the feuds over the calculations.

Critics of social utilitarianism may insist that the allocation be made solely on the basis of patient-centered reasons. They would exclude all third-party effects. This is the moral principle of the Hippocratic Oath, and it seems to support the notion that physicians might be the proper allocators after all. Still, limiting allocation considerations to the effects on the potential recipient does not imply that the organ should go to the one who would benefit the most medically. Among those in the Hippocratic camp, some would emphasize considering total good in all spheres of a potential recipient's life—economic, social, educational, aesthetic, spiritual, and other benefits, as well as those measured in medical terms. This is one interpretation of the Hippocratic mandate. Making these assessments of total individual benefit would still require skills well beyond those of the bedside clinician. Others, however, would constrict the relevant considerations still further, limiting them to medical benefits, that is, the changes in morbidity and mortality expected to result from the organ graft. Deciding whether to consider medical benefits to the individual or total benefits to that recipient is, once again, a question that physicians are not in a good position to answer. In fact, we should expect that physicians might be more inclined than others to give special consideration to medical benefit. It is plausible that those who have found medicine so important that they have chosen to give their lives to the field might give special emphasis to the medical component (just as professional specialists in other areas might be biased in favor of their areas—artists emphasizing the aesthetic, clergy the spiritual, etc.). It is reasonable that specialists in any area would overemphasize their area of concern when compared with the values of the general public.

Even if we could agree that the allocation decision should be limited to expected medical benefits, that does not mean that clinicians can be considered authoritative. Certainly, they will be expert in anticipating the likely effects of a transplant, but deciding what is a medical benefit is a deceptively complicated issue. Medical benefits involve many different considerations. Some might emphasize years of expected added life, using added survival as the criterion for a medical benefit. This seems to be what is implied in the newly adopted kidney allocation formula that makes use of expected posttransplant survival rates as a basis for allocating kidneys. Others might use the predicted graft survival rates, recognizing that the person with the best predicted graft survival rate (based on, say, human leukocyte antigen–matching considerations) might not be the same person who has the longest predicted survival. In estimating the length of predicted survival, we would take into account the probability of graft survival, but also how long the person is expected to live if the graft is successful. An eighty-year-old with a zero-antigen mismatched kidney may have a shorter predicted survival rate than a twenty-year-old receiving a significantly mismatched organ.

Survival is not the only medical benefit worth considering. Some people would see the curing of disease as a legitimate goal of medicine. Some transplant recipients may still have underlying pathology, either the pathology that caused the organ failure in the first place or a concomitant disease unrelated to the organ involved. The kidney recipient may also have heart disease unrelated to the kidney problem. This heart problem may have an impact that shows up in predicted years of life following a transplant, but it may also have an impact on morbidity. Should a life expectancy of twenty years following transplant be considered the same, whether or not the survivor has incapacitating heart disease? Many would attempt to adjust the expected years of survival for the quality of the life, taking into account the presence of co-morbidities. Deciding whether to adjust years for expected quality is a controversial topic. The point here is that, if bedside clinicians were to do the allocating, they would need to decide whether to adjust life expectancy for quality and how to make the adjustment. There is a value choice to be made in deciding whether and how to make the adjustment, and physicians have no special skill making such value choices. In fact, as we have suggested, they may have unique, profession-specific inclinations, so they (or any other professional group) can be expected to make the choices atypically.

Deciding how much medical benefit will accrue from a graft is even more complex. Some people will include improved subjective sense of well-being as part of medical benefit; others will not. If two people could receive a graft with equal predicted life expectancy and equal expected medical morbidity, but one will be more "nervous" about recurring disease than the other and therefore have less of a sense of medical well-being, can we say that one person is expected to receive more medical well-being than the other, or is their expected medical benefit objectively equal? Which of these criteria would be appropriate in allocating organs? Deciding overall medical well-being will involve trade-offs among mortality, the curing of disease, relief from suffering, and the prevention of future disease. Being an expert in medicine does not give one expertise in making these trade-offs. The intellectual mistake of assuming that those who are expert on the technical aspects of a technology are also experts on the moral and other evaluative questions that one of us (RMV) long ago called *the generalization of expertise*, which is one of the primary fallacies of modern technological society.[4]

The Role of Fairness or Justice

All this discussion assumes that the goal of the decision is to use the medical resources with maximal efficiency, doing what will provide the most benefit. We have argued that physicians are not really expert in making the choices needed to determine which benefits count. But even if we were somehow to establish that physicians at the bedside were uniquely good at determining what allocation would do the most good, we need to recognize that most ethical theories deny that maximizing benefit is the proper ethic for resource allocation. Major theories of ethics insist that other considerations are morally relevant. Most important, they insist that fairness or justice be taken into account, as well as medical or social utility, in deciding what is an ethical allocation of organs.

For example, some might argue that justice requires that each candidate receive an equal chance of getting a scarce, social, lifesaving resource such as a kidney, even if not all have an equal chance of benefiting. They may insist that those who have waited the longest or those who are sickest get priority, recognizing that these patients may not be the ones who would predictably benefit the most.

We need not solve the complex ethical problem of what is the correct basis for allocating scarce resources. The point here is merely that, in principle, even perfect knowledge of the medical facts about the patients who are candidates cannot determine which patient should receive an organ or a dialysis machine. The presumption of a role for clinicians in the allocation process may be based on their expert medical knowledge of the patient, but that is an inadequate basis. The clinician is not in a good position to know anything about alternative uses of an available organ and the relative claims of candidates for receiving that organ. This perhaps suggests an important role for the clinician in providing medical data about the medical condition of the patient, histocompatibility, prognosis without treatment, and likely outcomes with treatment—but these alone cannot determine the appropriate allocation. On this basis, the clinician should provide data for those who create and run the allocation system; they should not make the allocation itself.

The Role of Clinicians' Values in Allocation

Sophisticated clinicians, especially those with knowledge of the contemporary medical ethical literature, will readily concede that all medical judgments require ethical and other value judgments and that this includes decisions about dialysis and transplants. They argue at this point that there are values inherent in the medical profession that provide the clinician with a basis for deciding.[5] They point to the traditional values of preserving life, relieving suffering, and maintaining health.

There are serious problems, however, with permitting allocations to be made on the basis of the clinician's interpretation of these traditional values of medical professionals. First, as we have seen, the medical values, in the interesting cases, lead to contradictions among themselves. The allocation that most preserves life may not be the one that best relieves suffering or promotes health. Clinicians will differ among themselves over how these conflicts should be resolved. Even if they could agree completely, it would not follow that laypeople—the ones whose lives are at stake, and the ones who created the pool of resources to be allocated—would concur in the ranking.

The problem is even more severe when one realizes that it is not at all obvious that the goal is to maximize medical values. If clinicians can disagree among themselves and can disagree collectively with the general public over the ranking of medical values, they can disagree much more dramatically over the question of how medical values would relate to social, nonmedical goods and over how pursuing the maximum good should be related ethically to other moral norms, such as promoting a just allocation.[6] Because these choices have nothing to do with medical knowledge, there is no reason why clinicians should be the ones making them. It is the general lay public that creates the money pool to support dialysis and creates the pool of cadaver organs to be allocated. They should be the ones making the moral choices relating medical to nonmedical goods and relating the pursuit of maximum benefit to maximum justice or fairness in allocation. Clinicians should remain free to give undivided loyalty to their patients. That role is incompatible with asking them to be resource allocators.

The Role of the Public in Allocation

Any discussion about who should be empowered to make health policy decisions for a scarce commodity like organs should recall the experience of the Seattle Committee in selecting dialysis candidates. It highlights the need for membership transparency because different stakeholders bring different values and biases to the table.

The Seattle Committee

The Seattle Committee consisted of seven citizens: lawyer, a minister, a banker, a housewife, an official of the state government, a labor leader, and a surgeon. At their first briefing, they were told that they would never make medical decisions; all candidates would have been cleared. In their first meetings they set up guidelines. First, they requested anonymity. Second, they drew up a list of factors that they would use to choose between candidates who met the medical criteria—age and sex, marital status and number of dependents, income, net worth, emotional stability, educational stability, education, occupation, past performance and future potential, and the names of people who could serve as references. Many of the details were described in an article in *Life* magazine written by Shana Alexander.[7]

Although the Seattle Committee was given no rules to follow, a pattern developed that promoted individuals who shared the same middle-class values as the committee itself. George Annas, in an article aptly titled "The Prostitute, the Playboy and the Poet: Rationing Schemes for Organ Transplantation," describes the generally negative reaction when the biases and selection criteria of the committee became public.[8] The *Life* article ends with one of the selected patients commenting about the fact that his life is dependent not only on the doctors and nurses and machines but also on a committee of unknown laypeople: "I guess that as long as facilities are not unlimited, somebody has to pick and choose. And then they have to go home and sleep at night. What a dreadful decision! It's like trying to play God. Frankly, I'm surprised the doctors were able to round up seven people who were willing to take the job."[9] The committee became known as "the God Squad."

Annas suggests that there are four major approaches to rationing scarce resources: the market approach, the selection committee approach, the lottery approach, and the "customary approach." He rejects the market approach on the grounds that it lacks any concern for equity—an issue we address further in chapter 17. He rejects the lottery as too inefficient. He rejects the selection committee because it uses vague, arbitrary criteria. Although one can codify the values if a pattern emerges, as it did with the Seattle Committee, such an allocation process may need a much greater diversity to ensure that all values are included, a point to which we will return. Finally, Annas examines the customary approach, which incorporates cultural norms without explicitly stating them. For example, to the extent that transplant candidates need to prove they have adequate social support for posttransplant care, the system can exclude individuals without families, such as the homeless.

Annas's concerns about the customary approach are well founded. Levenson and Olbrisch examined the psychosocial and medical criteria used by different transplant programs regarding absolute and relative contraindication to listing for hearts, livers, and kidneys. The first finding is that the criteria were strictest for cardiac programs and most lenient for kidneys. But consider two different factors: (1) intellectual disability and (2) current cigarette smoking. An IQ of less than 70 was an absolute contraindication to transplantation in 25.6 percent of heart, 10.9 percent of liver, and 2.6 percent of kidney programs, and was a relative contraindication in 59.0 percent of heart, 69.6 percent of liver, and 51.3 percent of kidney programs. This means that only 15.4 percent of cardiac, 19.6 percent of liver, and 46.1 percent of kidney programs found this criterion to be irrelevant. Cigarette smoking was an irrelevant criterion in 9 percent of heart, 63 percent of liver, and 77.3 percent of kidney transplant programs.[10]

Annas concludes his article with the recommendation that we need to have public transparent mechanisms that are fair and efficient, and that "we all need to be involved."[11] He supports an allocation process that balances equity and efficiency, and he develops criteria that are transparent, inclusive, and public—what is mandated by the 1984 National Organ Transplant Act (NOTA) and is more or less what is attempted by the UNOS Board, although he may have wanted greater public representation.

Like the Seattle Committee, the UNOS committees are all made up of volunteers. Despite the concern that physicians will have a unique perspective and that their emphasis on utility should not be put on a pedestal, the data suggest that there is more diversity within the medical community, even within the transplant community, than our previous arguments suggest. For example, numerous articles show physicians as divided about the proper weight to be given to alcoholism as a criterion for wait-listing for deceased liver transplant, a topic we discuss further in chapter 18.[12] Likewise, physicians are divided about how to balance "greatest need" with likelihood of success.[13]

But let us imagine reconstituting the UNOS committees with more members from the public. The first questions would be to determine who represents the public, and are the representatives willing to make allocation decisions? And if willing, what values would they bring to the process?

Public Perspectives

Researchers, both in the United States and abroad, have compared and contrasted physicians' attitudes regarding allocation prioritization with the attitudes of patients and of the general public. In the United Kingdom, James Neuberger and colleagues evaluated 1,000 members of the public, 200 family doctors, and 100 gastroenterologists. The study found that there was little support overall for allocating livers to those with alcoholic liver disease compared with other indications, although the public rates those with alcoholic liver disease as more deserving than the health care professionals. However, both the public and gastroenterologists thought that a person convicted of a violent crime was less deserving than the alcoholic, in contrast to the family doctors.[14]

Sears and colleagues at the University of Florida queried individuals at a state driver's license office asking about what role three psychosocial values—ability to pay, gender, and smoking history—should play in heart allocation. They found that the public did not want gender or ability to pay to influence allocation, but they were more willing to give organs to those who never smoked compared with both former smokers and current smokers.[15]

Peter Ubel and colleagues in the 1990s did a series of studies asking members of the public how they would allocate livers. He and his colleagues found that "the public places a very high value on considerations other than outcomes, particularly that of giving everyone a chance at receiving scarce resources, even if that means a significant decrease in the chance that available organs will save people's lives."[16] However, they also found that "members of the general public feel that patients who cause their own organ failure through smoking, alcohol use, or drug use should not receive equal priority for scarce transplantable organs."[17] Even when they were told that a candidate who had abused drugs in the past had the best prognosis, the respondents were less likely to want to allocate the organs to these individuals. Ubel concluded: "People's unwillingness to give scarce transplantable organs to patients with controversial behaviors cannot be explained totally on the basis of those behaviors either causing their primary organ failure or making them have worse transplant prognoses. Instead, many people believe that such patients are simply less worthy of scarce transplantable organs."[18] Thus if policies were to incorporate the raw opinions of the public, the allocation may have serious biases that may be inconsistent with the side constraint of respect for persons.

Ubel notes three recurrent themes regarding what the community wants in health care policies: (1) the public rejects policies based solely on medical utilitarianism, (2) the public places great importance on equality and need in the distribution of health care resources, and (3) the public is adverse to denying health care to groups of patients.[19] However, Ubel has also examined the challenges of incorporating public preferences into public policy: "The move from a notion that community values ought to play a role in health care decision making to the creation of health care policies that in some way reflect such values is a challenging one. No single method will adequately measure community values in a way appropriate for setting health care priorities. Consequently, multiple methods to measure community values should be employed, thereby allowing the strengths and weaknesses of the various methods to complement each other."[20]

Given the complexity of relying on the values of a "public," we point particularly to one expression of public values relevant to the allocation of organs. NOTA requires that, for the United States, organs be allocated taking into account both efficiency and equity.[21] These two principles, which we explore in chapter 17, are essentially the equivalent of the philosophical principles of utility and justice. They provide admittedly abstract guidance that is a foundation upon which allocation theory can be built when one considers the perspective of the general public.

Conclusion

Who, then, should make allocation decisions? As we mentioned above, transplant professionals make up more than half the current UNOS board. Many of the other members are living organ donors, transplant recipients, and representatives of deceased donors' families. These individuals also have vested interest in the organ procurement and allocation process and may not represent the average public citizen. Thus, to the extent that one might want allocation decisions to represent the public at large, giving voices to those with the greatest vested interest may be as problematic as giving authority to physicians.

Transplant recipients may try, even if unconsciously, to ensure that revisions to the allocation system continue to benefit people like themselves. In fact, they may be more supportive, for example, of second and third transplants than is the general public and some bioethicists, even when the data show that recipients of second and third transplants do worse.[22] Likewise, families of deceased donors may actually want to know that their recipients used this gift wisely, which may lead to a greater focus on personal responsibility for illness.

To the extent that one would want more representation of the general public, one would need to determine how much prior education the representatives would need, and there would need to be a consensus on how that education would be provided. There have been a few attempts to educate the public in "citizen juries" regarding priority setting in health care. For example, Lenaghan and colleagues held four citizens' juries that involved participant involvement for four days. They found that "given enough time and information, the public is willing and able to contribute to the debate about priority setting in health care." They concluded that "we are hopeful that this method [citizen jury] . . . may offer us a meaningful way of involving the public in decisions about priority setting in health."[23] Others have used a process of deliberative democracy or deliberative engagement to help educate the public to think and then deliberate about health priorities and various policy options.[24] Most have been on a small scale and have involved considerable time and energy on the part of the research team and the public. This would be a disincentive for frequent changes in any committee created, due to the start-up costs. Even those deliberative processes that attempted to be all-inclusive had difficulties reaching some hard-to-reach vulnerable populations.[25] Although deliberative engagement gives policymakers the opportunity to hear the voice of an educated rather than an uneducated public, it is not clear how to determine whether the educational component of these engagements is not biased, either consciously or unconsciously. Finally, there is controversy regarding what exact role the deliberations should have vis-à-vis policy.[26]

For the moment, we need not determine what the correct way is to trade off the different medical values and the correct way to balance medical and nonmedical values or how to constitute a revised UNOS committee roster. For our purposes, the question is whether individual clinicians or clinicians as a group should be empowered by the general community to choose the principles upon which allocations will be made. In the case of a formula for organ allocation, the critical question is what should be the relative weight given to medical benefit and to need or equity (efficiency and equity, in the language of NOTA). We and many others working in the field of ethical theory have our preferred answer to this question. We think fairness or equity in organ allocation should be our first priority, at least for a public system to which all in society are expected to contribute. We recognize, however, that others may give different answers. We would propose that, as a compromise, equal weight be given to each of the two considerations. This, in fact, is the answer that the UNOS Ethics Committee gave in the 1990s, when it first addressed this question directly.[27] Yet regardless of the answer, there seems to be no reason why clinicians alone should be empowered to make the choices. Although it is obviously necessary to rely on the enormous technical skills of such professionals for the data upon which specific allocation protocols will need to be based, it is a serious mistake for society to cede to those experts the responsibility for making policies such as those upon which society will allocate organs. These choices are fundamentally moral and philosophical, and they cannot be made on the basis of technical knowledge alone.

In fact, in the United States the final authority for allocation policy rests with the people. Policy is set by Congress in NOTA, and these policies are administered by the Health Resources and Services Administration, which delegates the details of carrying out policy to the Organ Procurement and Transplantation Network, which has, since 1984, been UNOS.

Notes

1. This is not to say that all transplant professionals ignore equity considerations when deliberating on allocation. In a literature review, Tong et al. show that there is broad appreciation among transplant professionals regarding the tension between equity and efficiency in organ allocation. See Tong A, Jan S, Wong G, et al., "Rationing scarce organs for transplantation: Healthcare provider perspectives on wait listing and organ allocation," *Clinical Transplantation* 2013;27: 60–71.

2. This is about to change as the UNOS Board approved a slate of nominees for open positions for the 2014–15 term. In a press release the UNOS News Bureau stated: "For the first time, neither of the two nominees for Vice President / President-Elect is a transplant surgeon, transplant physician or executive director of an organ procurement organization. James Gleason, BS, MA, is a heart transplant recipient and the husband of a donor mother; Betsy Walsh, JD, MPH, is a living kidney donor. Both have served on the OPTN/UNOS Board of Directors and on multiple committees." See OPTN Media Release, Nov. 22, 2013, http://optn.transplant.hrsa.gov/news/newsDetail.asp?id=1621. Walsh won the election and began her term as vice president on July 1, 2014. See OPTN/UNOS Board of Directors, http://optn.transplant.hrsa.gov/members/boardOfDirectors.asp.

3. Alexander S, "They decide who lives, who dies," *Life Magazine* 1962;53: 102–25.

4. Veatch RM, "Generalization of expertise: Scientific expertise and value judgments," *Hastings Center Studies* 1973;1 (2): 29–40.

5. Dyer AR, "Virtue and medicine: A physician's analysis," in *Virtue and medicine: Exploration in the character of medicine*, ed. Shelp EE (Dordrecht: D. Reidel, 1985), 223–35; Kass LR, *Toward a more natural science* (New York: Free Press, 1985); Pellegrino ED, Thomasma, DC, *For the patient's good: The restoration of beneficence in health care* (New York: Oxford University Press, 1988).

6. Frances Kamm has also observed that clinicians have a unique set of moral commitments that lead them to strive to do what is maximally beneficial for their patients. See Kamm FM, *Morality, mortality, volume I: Death and whom to save from it* (New York: Oxford University Press, 1993), 272, 293.

7. Alexander, "They decide."

8. Annas GJ, "The prostitute, the playboy and the poet: Rationing schemes for organ transplantation," *American Journal of Public Health* 1985;75 (2): 187–89.

9. Alexander, "They decide," 125.

10. Levenson JL, Olbrisch ME, "Psychosocial evaluation of organ transplant candidates: A comparative survey of process, criteria, and outcomes in heart, liver and kidney transplantation," *Psychosomatics* 1993;34 (4): 314–23.

11. Annas, "Prostitute," 189.

12. Atterbury CE, "The alcoholic in the lifeboat: Should drinkers be candidates for liver transplantation?" *Journal of Clinical Gastroenterology* 1986;8 (1): 1–4; Moss AH, Siegler M, "Should alcoholics compete equally for liver transplantation?" *JAMA* 1991;265: 1295–98; Ubel PA, Transplantation in alcoholics: Separating prognosis and responsibility from social biases," *Liver Transplantation & Surgery* 1997;3 (3): 343.

13. See, e.g., Segev DL, "Evaluating options for utility-based kidney allocation," *American Journal of Transplantation* 2009;9: 1513–18; Ladin K, Hanto DW, "Rational rationing or discrimination: Balancing equity and efficiency considerations in kidney allocation," *American Journal of Transplantation* 2011;11: 2317–21; Ross LF, Parker W, Veatch RM, Gentry SE, Thistlethwaite JR Jr., "Equal opportunity supplemented by fair innings: Equity and efficiency in allocating deceased donor kidneys," *American Journal of Transplantation* 2012;12: 2115–24. A review of surveys of physicians is given by Tong A, Jan S, Wong G, et al., "Rationing scarce organs for transplantation: Healthcare provider perspectives on wait-listing and organ allocation," *Clinical Transplantation* 2013;27 (1): 60–71.

14. Neuberger J, "Public and professional attitudes to transplanting alcoholic patients," *Liver Transplantation* 2007;13 (11 suppl 2): S65–68.

15. Sears SF Jr, Marhefka SL, Rodrigue JR, Campbell C, "The role of patients' ability to pay, gender, and smoking history on public attitudes toward cardiac transplant allocation: An experimental investigation," *Health Psychology* 2000;19 (2): 192–96.

16. Johri M, Ubel PA, "Setting organ allocation priorities: Should we care what the public cares about?" *Liver Transplantation* 2003;9: 880.

17. Ubel PA, Baron J, Asch DA, "Social responsibility, personal responsibility, and prognosis in public judgments about transplant allocation," *Bioethics* 1999;13: 57.

18. Ibid., 58.

19. Ubel PA, "The challenge of measuring community values in ways appropriate for setting health care priorities," *Kennedy Institute of Ethics Journal* 1999;9: 263–84.

20. Ibid., 263.

21. National Organ Transplant Act (NOTA), Public Law 98-507, Oct. 19, 1984, 98 Stat. 2339.

22. See, e.g., Ubel PA, Loewenstein G, "The efficacy and equity of retransplantation: An experimental survey of public attitudes," *Health Policy* 1995;34 (2): 145–51; and Ubel PA, Arnold RM, Caplan AL, "Rationing failure: The ethical lessons of the retransplantation of scarce vital organs," *JAMA* 1993;270: 2469–74.

23. Lenaghan J, New B, Mitchell E, "Setting priorities: Is there a role for citizens' juries?" *British Medical Journal* 1996;312 (7046): 1593. The authors reference Cooper L, Coote A, Davies A, Jackson C, *Tackling the democratic deficit in health* (London: Institute for Public Policy Research, 1995).

24. See, e.g., O'Doherty KC, Burgess MM, "Engaging the public on biobanks: Outcomes of the BC biobank deliberation," *Public Health Genomics* 2009;12 (4): 203–15; Lemke AA, Halverson C, Ross LF, "Biobank participation and returning research results: Perspectives from a deliberative engagement in South Side Chicago," *American Journal of Medical Genetics* 2012;158A: 1029–37; and Rychetnik L, Carter SM, Abelson J, et al., "Enhancing citizen engagement in cancer screening through deliberative democracy," *Journal of the National Cancer Institute* 2013;105 (6): 380–86.

25. Longstaff H, Burgess MM, "Recruiting for representation in public deliberation on the ethics of biobanks," *Public Understanding of Science* 2010;19 (2): 212–24.

26. Trotter G, "Bioethics and deliberative democracy: Five warnings from Hobbes," *Journal of Medicine & Philosophy* 2006;31: 235–50; and Kim SY, Wall IF, Stanczyk A, De Vries R, "Assessing the public's views in research ethics controversies: Deliberative democracy and bioethics as natural allies," *Journal of Empirical Research on Human Research Ethics* 2009;4 (4): 3–16.

27. Burdick JF, Turcotte JC, Veatch RM, "General principles for allocating human organs and tissues," *Transplantation Proceedings* 1992;24: 2226–35.

Chapter 17

A General Moral Theory of Organ Allocation

Once organs are procured, they must be allocated among the hundreds or thousands of potential recipients. In the United States there is a legal federal mandate that the allocation system must take into account both efficiency and equity.[1] In chapter 2, we set out a general ethical theory and suggested that efficiency and equity are code words for two major principles in ethical theory: maximizing utility, and distributing consequences justly. Maximizing utility, in turn, will take into account the need to follow two principles: to produce benefit, and to avoid harm. The technical names for these principles are, respectively, *beneficence* and *nonmaleficence*—the notions that an action is morally right if it produces benefit and/or avoids harm.

In some cases efficiency and equity are both served at the same time by the same allocation. They come together, and their implications for an allocation decision are clear. But often the concepts are ambiguous and, once their meanings are clarified, efficiency and equity can come into conflict. Moreover, there are additional ethical considerations that are not accounted for by the principles of utility maximizing and justice in distribution. Western society is committed to respect for persons, including respect for their autonomy; to keeping commitments to them, and to dealing honestly with them. Overwhelmingly, we are committed to avoiding the killing of humans, even in cases where people are willing, indeed eager, to end their lives. We refer to these notions as the principles of autonomy, fidelity, veracity, and avoiding killing. Together with utility and justice, they make up the core ethical principles.

An ethically acceptable allocation must conform to the requirements of these principles. Because any resulting policy will need to take many moral and practical concerns into account, we need a formula that integrates these multiple concerns in a concrete way. The systems used to allocate organs in the United States should reflect these moral principles. Each element in an allocation formula can be seen as being incorporated into the formula because it is a marker for one or more moral concerns. For example, we include human leukocyte antigen (HLA) tissue typing in the kidney allocation formula because we believe that an HLA match is an empirical predictor of the likelihood of graft survival. Tissue typing is included because it predicts good outcomes, which are what the ethical principle of beneficence requires. By contrast, points for time on the wait list are included because we believe that treating people equally requires that we do something to respond to the needs of those who have waited the longest. This is a manifestation of the principle of justice. There is no reason to assume that those who have waited the longest will do better or get more benefit from the available organs. In some situations this may be the case, but time on the wait list is a factor in allocation because of our concern for justice. Assuming that most will consider both utility and justice—efficiency and equity—to be relevant, we need to examine the factors that might come into play in an allocation formula.[2]

Social and Medical Utility

It is obvious that we are interested in organ transplants because we are convinced that they can be very beneficial to those in need of organs. There is utility in transplants. The utility is not limited, however, to the medical benefits to the recipients. There is also a broader social utility. Saving people's lives leaves them potentially able to return to society as productive citizens, which can produce social utility.

A pure social utilitarian would take all the envisioned benefits of alternative uses of organs into account in deciding how to allocate organs. If giving the organ to the president of a company (or a nation) would do much more good than giving it to a homeless, unemployed person, this is the kind of information a utilitarian would find morally relevant. A straightforward utilitarian allocation policy would rank potential recipients on the basis of the amount of good that would result from receiving organs.

However, as we saw in the last chapter, this ranking of recipients can become very controversial. It might require generating some interpersonal agreement on the amount of good that can be expected to be produced by each use of an organ. It was the original policy approach to the allocation of hemodialysis machines in the 1960s, when they were still scarce resources. Shana Alexander has provided a detailed account of the chaos that resulted at the University of Washington when the dialysis selection committee tried to pick patients based on their social worth.[3] As we discussed in the previous chapter, this situation generated significant controversy as those involved tried to determine who was the most socially valuable when picking patients from among a business executive, a poet, and the parent of three small children.

For various reasons there is widespread agreement that the social worth of organ recipients should be excluded from the organ allocation process. Utilitarians might argue that the very process of ranking recipients would be so controversial that there would be net disutility in opening the doors to such considerations. One can envision investigators doing background checks on those on the organ wait list. Even on utilitarian grounds, it may not make sense to consider social utility in organ allocation.

Of course, those who focus more on justice would have their own reasons for excluding social worth from the allocation decisions. If they believe in the equal moral worth of all people regardless of their social contribution, they would reject such considerations in principle, even if it were easy to determine something called "social worth."

Even if social utility is ruled out of bounds, the utilitarians are not finished using their approach in making allocation decisions. Considering *medical utility* receives much better press coverage. Clearly, the goal of transplants is to save lives, or at least make them more tolerable. If a transplant can be predicted to be very likely to do a great deal of medical good for one recipient but has almost no chance of helping if given to another patient, that medical fact seems relevant. Just as there is a consensus against using social utility, there is also a consensus that medical benefit is morally relevant. Calculating the expected medical benefit of a transplant, however, can be a very difficult task. Several different factors have seemed relevant.

Patient and Graft Survival

The most obvious medical benefit from a transplant is saving a life. Of course, not all transplants are lifesaving. It is often claimed, for example, that a kidney transplant is more about improving life's quality by sparing the patient from dialysis than about lifesaving. Even under this assumption, in some cases, such as those in which veins become inaccessible for dialysis, it could truly be lifesaving. We have, however, known since the late 1990s that a kidney transplant is, statistically, a lifesaving intervention. The death rate for patients on dialysis on the transplant wait list is 6.3 per 100 patient-years, whereas that of those who have received transplants is 3.8.[4] Hence, even kidney transplants should be thought of as saving lives.

Even if we agree that patient survival is an enormous benefit, it can present serious problems for utilitarians when calculating the benefit of a transplant. Not only is there the complicated scientific question of predicting graft survival, there is also the more theoretical problem of whether each life saved should count as an equal benefit. However, this is not the "social worth" question revisiting us—although that could become an issue. The first problem is whether it is the fact of a life saved that counts or whether we should, instead, count years of life added from transplants. Does saving a fifty-year-old from imminent heart failure, leaving the beneficiary with a twenty-year life expectancy, count the same or half as much as saving a thirty-year-old, leaving that person with a forty-year life expectancy? There is no factually correct answer to the question of whether it is lives saved or years of life added that should be counted. Both seem important, but deciding which is more important and how much to weigh each in a formula is a serious problem for utilitarians.

If life-years added is the criterion, the utilitarian will need to face some awkward situations. It seems common sense that, other things being equal, giving a transplant to a young person will add more life-years than giving a transplant to an older person. In the case of kidneys, giving transplants to twenty- to twenty-nine-year-olds adds sixteen years of life, whereas giving transplants to sixty- to seventy-four-year-olds adds only four years.[5] Also, men do not do as well as women when it comes to years of life added because of a kidney transplant—twelve years for females, but only nine years for males.[6]

This story is made even more complicated by the facts that people do not die just because organs fail, and that not all organ failures lead to death. We measure both graft survival and patient survival. Particularly for a kidney transplant, a graft failure merely puts one back on dialysis and back on the wait list for another organ. Even in the case of more obviously life-prolonging solid organs, a graft failure could lead to a second transplant, although the case would certainly be a more urgent one.

Other things being equal, it is clear that a graft failing is a bad thing even if the patient survives. At best, it will mean another transplant, and the consumption of another scarce organ from the donor pool.

The problem for a theory of allocation is how much weight one should give graft survival as compared with patient survival. Should the calculation of the medical utility of a transplant take both into account? If so, should the attention focus on the straight measure of expected years of graft survival, or should it also take into account the expected impact of retransplanting on those on the wait list, on the insurance system, and on the patient and his or her family? Insofar as we are concerned about medical utility, it seems that the proper criterion, at least to begin the analysis, is the predicted number of years of life added. For each organ available, we should consider each potential recipient's years of life expectancy both without and with a transplant. The difference between these two numbers of years, taking into account the probability of a successful graft, would be the expected number of years added for each candidate. We shall start the consideration of medical utility with the assumption that the goal, insofar as medical utility is concerned, is to give the organ to the person expected to gain the greatest number of years of life from its transplanting.

A new kidney allocation algorithm was proposed in 2011 that, with some modification, will go into effect in late 2014 and that incorporates a two-stage allocation method, which has been referred to as the 20/80 model. The top 20 percent of the kidneys available (determined by using ten criteria known to affect graft survival) will be allocated to the top 20 percent of candidates (determined by six criteria known to affect patient survival), whereas the remainder of the kidneys will be allocated using an algorithm based mainly on time spent on dialysis. The details of this new algorithm are further explored in chapter 20. We raise it here to point out that the first stage of the algorithm was designed to ensure that those kidneys with the expected longest graft survival rate would be allocated to those candidates with the longest graft survival expectancy, in order to avoid "death with a functioning graft," which has been considered one of the main pitfalls of the current allocation method.[7]

The Psychological State of the Patient and the Quality of Life

Saving lives and minimizing graft failure are not the only medical goods resulting from a successful transplant. Patients also normally see a dramatic improvement in their psychological well-being and quality of life. A serious utility calculation would need to take these into account as well. But measuring such benefits is difficult, and to use these benefits in allocation, we would need to determine the differential psychological benefit for different people on the wait list.

The more serious problem, however, is deciding how much weight to give changes in psychological well-being compared with the reality of saving a life. A strategy for comparing the value of the quality of well-being with that of the saving of a life that is used in health planning is calculating what is called a quality-adjusted life-year (QALY).[8] This measure discounts the number of expected years of life by their quality by asking people to compare years of life in a particular compromised state (e.g., being on dialysis) with a shorter number of years in good health. Using responses, tables can be created that, for example, might view ten years on dialysis as the equivalent of eight healthy years. A year on dialysis then equals 0.8 QALYs. This ingenious strategy permits the integration of data measuring years of life with estimates of the quality of that life. Some utilitarians believe that the best health policy is the one that maximizes QALYs. Thus, for each candidate for an organ transplant, we would estimate the number of additional years of life added (taking into account probabilities) and then adjust the estimate for the quality of the added years as well as the changes in the quality of the years that the patient would have lived without the transplant. Thus, QALYs are the criterion for determining the expected medical utility that would result from giving the organ to each candidate. Because both the quality and quantity of added life expected will vary as a function of the status of the donor (given the donor's HLAs, blood type, etc.), these estimates would have to be made anew for each organ that becomes available.

The calculation of QALYs as a health planning tool has been criticized because it discriminates against hard-to-treat patients. These critics consider this approach to violate the principle of justice.[9] A more basic problem for organ allocation, however, is that no one has ever claimed that such strategies can be applied at the micro level—at which, say, the individual patients on a wait list can be compared. At best, these statistics could be used to compare organ transplants for different diagnoses or different candidate groups. The result would be, at best, an approximation of the amount of good done by transplanting an organ into a typical or average patient in a particular diagnostic category. To simplify the allocation decision, defenders of the criterion of maximizing expected medical utility favor basing the allocation on certain empirical factors that are known to correlate with various medical outcomes. These empirical factors become crude surrogates for predicting the number of QALYs each candidate can expect from an available organ. The factors need to be considered individually.

Immunologic Factors

For kidney transplants, the degree of HLA match is a predictor of graft survival. Although the science is not completely understood, it is known that each person has at least three pairs of HLA antigens (called A, B, and DR). Because there are many possible antigens of each type, there are literally thousands of possible combinations. With six antigens for donor and recipient, there is a maximum match or mismatch of six antigens. It is common to report HLA by the degree of mismatch rather than the degree of match, thus making zero mismatch the best status. This is done in part because not all six antigens can be identified in all patients. If not all six antigens are identified, either an antigen is present but unidentifiable or there is a homozygous pair (two copies existing of the same antigen). By reporting the degree of mismatch, it is as if we are assuming that missing antigens are present in duplicate. If, in fact, an unusual antigen is present but not identified, reporting mismatches provides a slight advantage to those with unidentifiable antigens while reporting the number of matches would provide a disadvantage. Hence, racial minority groups, who are more likely to have antigens that cannot be identified, would be disadvantaged if priority were based on degree of match, but are advantaged if priority is based on degree of mismatch. Back in 1997, the overall graft survival rate based on degrees of antigen mismatch varied by as much as 5.3 percent one year, and 15.0 percent by five years, with zero-antigen mismatch having the longest survival (89.9 percent and 72.4 percent respectively) and six-antigen mismatch having the lowest (84.6 percent and 57.4 percent respectively).[10]

Thus, the degree of match (or mismatch) was a predictor of graft survival in the 1990s. If the goal were to get as many life-years as possible per graft, giving priority to recipients with the smallest number of mismatches with the particular donor would make sense. Points were therefore awarded based on the number of mismatches. Logically, the points should be assigned in proportion to the influence of the particular mismatch on graft survival. If there are no mismatches, to this day, as a matter of current policy, there is a mandatory priority, even if this involves sharing the organ with some other organ procurement organization or even some other region of the country. Beyond these mandatory shares, in the 1990s points were awarded as follows: 7 points if there are no D or DR mismatches, 5 points if there is 1 B or DR mismatched, and 2 points if there is a total of 2 mismatches at the B and DR loci (these points are on a scale that is somewhat open-ended, depending on various factors, e.g., HLA, time on the wait list, blood type, and whether one has previously been an organ donor).[11]

In 2014 matching or mismatching still makes a difference. In fact, the difference at one-year survival is slightly greater (5.9 percent), although the difference at five-year survival is smaller (13 percent). According to the website of the United Network for Organ Sharing (UNOS), zero-antigen and six-antigen mismatched kidneys transplanted between 1997 and 2004 respectively had a one-year graft survival rate of 94.6 percent versus 88.7 percent and a five-year graft survival rate of 78.7 percent versus 65.7 percent.[12] Today, priority continues to be given to zero-antigen mismatches, but only for those candidates who are at least modestly sensitized (panel-reactive antibodies, PRA > 20). The reason for this is that the vast majority of zero-antigen mismatches occur in white recipients, and it was felt to further the disparity of access for minorities (a concern that is about fair distribution and not about utility). Points are only given for HLA–DR matching, but not for other matching due to the relative importance of these different HLA sites in graft survival.

There is much more to be learned about the science of tissue matching. At some point in the future, we are likely to know much more. Therefore, the formula and the points assigned are likely to change. From the point of view of the theory of allocation, this raises questions about the legitimacy of using factors that we know are only crude approximations. Moreover, what HLA is predicting is graft survival, something already on our working list of factors that would interest a utilitarian. In the end, what a utilitarian would want is a complex formula that assigns consideration based on the percentage of variance explained by each factor known to predict graft survival (or, more accurately, the number of QALYs expected to be added). We are only part way toward being able to construct such an algorithm.

Age

Age is another factor that predicts graft survival. Younger patients are believed to have more resiliency when facing major surgery. A good utilitarian would want to take this into account, giving more priority to younger patients on the wait list. Chronological age, however, is not a perfect predictor of physiological age, in which utilitarians would really be interested. This, of course, poses problems for deciding how to incorporate age into a utilitarian calculus for predicting the overall benefit from a transplant.

There are further complications. If we are using predicted years of patient survival as our criterion of medical utility, younger patients will not only have better results from their surgery; they will also have more years of future expected life. In a world where antirejection medications were completely effective, many organs might survive until the patient's death. The older one is, the shorter the patient survival, and therefore the fewer the predicted years of benefit from the graft. This is another reason why a consistent utilitarian would give greater weight to younger patients.

Finally, in the case of kidney transplants, age plays another role. Small children cannot only be expected to have their organs survive longer, they may get greater benefit from the transplant.[13] Small children in kidney failure experience growth problems and neuro-logical damage that is not completely controlled by dialysis.[14] Thus, a utilitarian would want to give small children extra consideration over and above the belief that the surgery will go better and the expectation that they will get more years of graft use from their organ. This is one reason why the old kidney allocation formula awarded extra points to children (four additional points for children under age eleven, and three for those older than eleven but less than eighteen). Under the newly adopted kidney allocation formula, all pediatric patients (patients under eighteen years) would be prioritized ahead of adults for the best-quality kidneys. This is, in part, because of these utilitarian considerations (but we shall suggest that there are also nonutilitarian reasons for this).

The Availability of Alternative Treatments

Another factor that a utilitarian would want to consider is the availability of alternative treatments. Other things being equal, we would want organs to go to those who had no alternative. The net good of such a policy would be greater because more lives would be saved. Hence, most patients in end-stage renal failure have dialysis available. The few for whom veins are not accessible for dialysis would get priority, not only because they are in greater need (a fact that would be of concern to those committed to justice in allocation) but also because more net good will be done.

Structuring a Utilitarian Allocation Formula

The project for a utilitarian who wanted to allocate organs according to the strategy of maximizing the net good from the transplant program, regardless of the distribution of the good, would be to construct a formula that adequately took into account all these factors in their proper proportion. We have seen that a consistent utilitarian would need to factor in the social good that could come to society from each life saved (unless one could successfully argue that the disutilities of making these comparisons outweighed any benefits). When considering medical goods, one would first need to establish the overall outcome goal. Would it be the short-term patient survival of the transplant (i.e., the avoidance of acute rejection), the expected years of life added to the patient, the expected years of graft survival, or the improvement in the quality of the patient's life?

Integrating these goals into a single formula is a formidable task. In principle, the medical utility maximizer's goal should be to give an organ to the one who will predictably gain the greatest number of QALYs from the organ. Assuming that this goal can be identified, the next task would be to determine which specific factors—HLA matching, age, diagnosis, the availability of alternative treatments—should be taken into account. The ideal formula would be one that includes every factor known to explain some of the variance in the outcome measure upon which we have decided. Because there are several different outcome goals, we can expect that there will continue to be disputes among utilitarians over exactly what the proper formula should be.

In February 2011 the UNOS Kidney Committee released a paper titled "Concepts for Kidney Allocation."[15] Its stated objectives were to make clear that a major goal was the more efficient production of good from the limited supply of organs—that is, in the language of ethics, utility maximizing. These objectives were to:

▶ Better approximate graft longevity and recipient longevity so that the potential survival of every transplanted organ can be realized within biological reason and acceptable levels of access for those on the waiting list:
  • Foster or promote graft survival of the kidney transplant for candidates with longest post-transplant survival who are likely to require additional transplants due to early age of [*end-stage renal disease*].
  • Minimize loss of potential functioning years of deceased donor kidney grafts through improved matching of recipient and graft survival.
▶ Improve offer system efficiency and organ utilization through the introduction of a new scale for kidney quality, called the kidney donor profile index.
▶ Make comprehensive data better available to patients and transplant programs to guide them in their renal replacement choices.
▶ Reduce differences in transplant access for populations described in the National Organ Transplant Act (e.g., candidates from racial/ethnic minority groups, pediatric candidates, and sensitized candidates).[16]

All these goals except the last one were driven by the ethical goal of utility maximizing. Moreover, when one examines the details of the paper, there are elaborate analyses to show the new algorithm's efficiency, whereas there is essentially no attention to the goal of reducing differences in access among candidate groups. More detail about the new kidney allocation formula is provided in chapter 20.

The Issue of Justice

The major problem for the utilitarian solution to the allocation problem is not the determination of the formula. The real issue is whether such a formula, even if it could be determined, would be fair or just. It is the essence of utilitarianism that it ignores the pattern of the distribution of the good being allocated.[17] Thus we have already seen that utilitarians would be inclined to discriminate against the elderly. Moreover, they would discriminate against any hard-to-treat group (e.g., those with concomitant disease or those who have had previous transplants). The available data suggested, at least in the

1980s, that some racial groups matched the donor pool better than others and therefore predictably did better. The data also suggested that one gender did better than the other, and one socioeconomic group better than another. Before one knows which sociological groups would be advantaged, it would be good to confront the critical question in the abstract.

With the knowledge that predicted success may correlate with race, gender, age, and income level, would it be acceptable to take these sociological facts into account in allocating organs? A good utilitarian would do this, once it is known that these variables predict success. It would be consistent to base allocation on these predictors of success, even though it may be impossible to identify exactly which people in the various groups will do better.

It turns out that, statistically, in the 1980s and 1990s young, white, middle-class males did best, at least with kidney transplants. We have already seen why age is relevant. Socioeconomic status probably has to do with having an intact support network available to help in recovery and the capacity to follow a proper follow-up regimen. It is also relevant to the ability of recipients to comprehend and follow instructions about how to maximize the maintenance of the organ once transplanted. Gender is perhaps related, at least in part, to PRA, which we shall take up below. There is, however, some recent evidence that women now actually do better than men. The moral issue then is whether, assuming that we have reliable sociological data for predicting which groups will do better with a transplant, these data should be used to maximize the aggregate net benefit from the limited supply of organs—even if it could mean providing more limited access to those of certain races, ages, genders, or income groups.

The concern of people committed to the moral principle of justice is that the allocation be fair or equitable. Because efficiency and equity sometimes conflict, the most efficient system for maximizing the good resulting from a transplant system may well not be the fairest. Conversely, the fairest system may need to be inefficient. Depending on how one trades off the principles of utility and justice, one will give more or less weight to concerns about distribution.

In the abstract the focus of any theory of justice is not on the amount of good done but on the pattern of the distribution of the good. Several factors have been proposed as the criteria for the proper pattern of distribution. Most modern theories of justice, however, are egalitarian. They consider a pattern of distribution to be just insofar as it contributes to giving people opportunities for equality of outcome. In health care this often means targeting those who are medically worst off in order to give them the opportunity, insofar as possible, to become as healthy as other people. Because most allocation theories consider both need and utility, the result of defining justice in terms of medical need does not need to lead to an allocation whereby the members of some group who are terribly sick with an incurable disease command all the resources. The point is merely that, insofar as the principle of justice is concerned, we will strive to give the worst-off patients opportunities to improve their situation.[18] Still, identifying exactly what we mean by being medically worst off is a complex task.

At least three factors must be taken into account. We call them present need, urgency, and need over a lifetime.

The Factor of Present Need

Existing organ allocation often takes into account the potential recipient's present medical status. The idea of the principle of justice, interpreted in an egalitarian way, is that all people should have an opportunity to be as well off as others, insofar as possible. This means that those who are the sickest or otherwise worst off deserve first consideration. And this is the idea behind the historical organ allocation policies that gave priority to those in the hospital over those at home who were up and around and gave further priority to those in intensive care over those who were otherwise hospitalized.

Sometimes those who are the sickest will also benefit the most by receiving a transplant. (If a life is saved from inevitable decline toward death, that is a substantial benefit as well as saving someone who is plausibly considered to be among the worst off.) If transplanting organs to the sickest does more good than to those who are healthier, the utilitarian as well as the egalitarian would also give these people priority. However, some people are so ill that, although they are the sickest, they will predictably not get as much benefit from a transplant as those who are healthier. They may be so sick that they have a higher chance of dying, regardless of treatment, or they may simply have a condition that will be only partially ameliorated by the transplant. For example, persons with co-morbidities (e.g., diabetes) in organ failure may not get as much benefit from transplant as some nondiabetic persons who are healthier. This is because the person with diabetes (or other co-morbidities) may die sooner, regardless of the transplant.

It is these cases where the worst-off patient cannot be expected to get as much benefit from a transplant as can better-off patients that pose the most important moral conflict—that between utility and present need, between efficiency and equity. Someone giving justice the priority will still want the sickest patient to get the organ if only one is available. Someone who affirms both utility and justice will strive to combine both considerations into the allocation formula.

The idea is that the sickest person has the greatest need and, when justice is considered, needs to be given priority. This has not been a major factor for kidney transplants because it has been believed that these persons can usually be maintained indefinitely on dialysis. As we realize that patients in kidney failure do not do as well on dialysis as with a transplant, this assumption is changing.[19] For more obviously lifesaving organs such as the heart and liver, how sick one is seems like a plausible indicator of need. This is a measure of current medical need. This notion of how sick a patient is at the present time has been the definitive notion of need reflected in the allocation policies of the national Task Force on Organ Transplantation and UNOS. However, it is not the only way one can think about medical need.

The Factor of Medical Urgency

Harvard University philosopher Frances Kamm deserves credit for increasing the sophistication of the discussion about the ways of thinking about medical need and urgency.[20] She defines urgency as "how soon someone will die without a transplant."[21] The crucial point here is that some patients on the wait list may urgently need a transplant, even though they are not presently among the sickest categories of patients.

In the allocation of livers, a patient with fulminant liver failure with a life expectancy without a liver transplant of less than seven days is considered status 1A, the highest priority.[22] This is followed by similarly urgent cases involving chronic illness and then by the Model of End-Stage Liver Disease (MELD) score, a score that uses objective medical data to determine a patient's risk of dying while waiting for a liver transplant. The MELD score ranges from less than 9 (with a three-month mortality risk of 1.9 percent) to greater than 40 (with a three-month mortality risk of 40.1 percent).[23]

The liver allocation formula generally gives higher priority to patients with the greatest short-term mortality risk. Among those patients who are not presently the most ill, some may still have claims of justice because they are particularly urgent cases, that is, we can predict they will be among the worst off in the future if they are not given transplants soon. We should take into account the fact that some people who are not presently the sickest may eventually become the worst off if they are not treated. A justice-based allocation formula would give priority to someone who is presently healthy but who will not have another chance to avoid becoming the sickest over someone who is presently sicker but who is stable and will not decline to be as poorly off. Two different kinds of cases of urgent need can be identified.

Expected Imminent Decline

Consider, for example, a patient with a newly diagnosed primary cancer of the liver. Some transplant centers treat such cancers, if detected early, with a liver transplant. Such persons may not feel terribly ill. They may be at home or even getting about in the community. However, they may decline very rapidly to the point where a transplant is no longer feasible. They may, in fact, die within months if they do not receive a transplant. Such a transplant has an urgency in spite of the fact that presently he or she is in relatively good condition. Urgency, as we are using the term, classifies transplant candidates on the basis of how long they can be expected to live without the transplant. This could be measured in QALYs, but insofar as we are concerned about identifying who has a claim of justice (rather than a claim based on medical utility), we are not focusing on the expected number of QALYs added by the transplant but rather on who has the smallest number of QALYs expected in the future—that is, who is worst off from a "future QALYs" perspective.

Often, the patients who are presently the sickest will also have the greatest urgency, but this need not be the case. It seems that, if we want to identify those on the wait list with the greatest medical need, we should seek out those who will have the smallest number of expected future QALYs without a transplant, not necessarily those who are presently the sickest.

The Likelihood of Finding a Suitable Organ in the Future (PRA, Blood Type, and Wait Time)

There is a second way in which a patient who is not presently among the sickest might be said to have a particularly urgent need. Some who do not have a rapidly progressing disease such as liver cancer may nevertheless be in urgent need because it can be predicted that there is a lower probability that they will have another chance at getting an organ.

High panel-reactive antibodies. This distinction is important in taking into account PRA among the factors in an allocation formula. Some candidates for organ transplant have antibodies in their system from being previously exposed to foreign tissues—PRA. This may be true for people who have received a graft earlier. It may also be true of anyone who has received a blood transfusion and for women who have ever been pregnant. These antibodies stemming from these conditions may react to tissues in the transplant, causing a rejection.

It is possible to measure antibody levels and then cross-match the potential recipient with the specific donor to see if the antibodies are likely to cause a rejection. Under the old kidney allocation system, anyone with a PRA above 80 percent was considered at particularly acute risk for such rejection and was not permitted to receive an organ from a donor who is a positive cross-match. Those with a high PRA would thus face a difficult time in finding a suitable cross-match negative donor. Because of this, in kidney transplants, they were given 4 bonus points. The reason is not that people with a high PRA can be expected to do particularly well. Rather, the concern has been that, if a cross-match negative organ becomes available, chances are greater that it will be the only suitable organ to become available for a long time. Out of fairness—the likelihood of finding another organ—high-PRA patients are, therefore, given special consideration. Recently, it has been found that only patients with a much higher PRA (on the order of 98 percent) need to be given special priority in order to find a suitable organ. Thus, in the new kidney allocation formula, only those with the highest PRA are given special priority. Nevertheless, they are placed at the top of the list, even though they will not do better. In fact, they may well do worse, but they still have a strong moral claim when a suitable organ becomes available because it is unlikely another one will appear.

Blood group. For some organs, such as kidneys, the candidate must be blood group compatible with the donor. Hence, an O-blood-group candidate can receive an organ only from an O-blood-group donor, while an O-group donor could donate to anyone. By contrast an AB-blood-group donor could donate only to an AB-recipient. A-group and B-group donors could donate to their own group or to an AB-recipient.

When an O-blood-group organ becomes available, it could go to the next person on the wait list regardless of blood type; but if it went to someone other than an O-group recipient, eventually the supply of O-donors will be exhausted and some O-recipients would be left without any organs available. Thus, there is a sense in which there is greater urgency in transplanting the O-recipient. This person will have less of a chance of getting a suitable organ in the future and thus has a shorter life expectancy if not transplanted with the presently available organ. Therefore, to be fair to O-recipients, they need to get priority for O-donor organs.

Since the early 2000s, however, candidates in blood group B have had an even longer wait, on average, than those in blood group O. The new kidney allocation model takes this into account by giving priority to candidates of blood type B for O-organs over candidates of other blood groups when no O-organ candidate is available.

In liver transplantation, ABO-identical recipients have significantly better outcomes than ABO-compatible, meaning that it is not the case that an O-donor liver does as well in an A-blood-type or B-blood-type candidate as it does in an O-blood-type candidate. However, ABO-incompatibility is more tolerated, particularly for candidates in acute liver failure.[24]

Since the implementation of MELD in 2002, status 1A and 1B candidates matching the liver donor's blood group have been awarded 10 points, blood-group-compatible recipients have been awarded 5 points, and ABO-incompatible recipients have been awarded no additional points—although all are eligible for the liver. If no status 1 candidates are available, O-blood livers are made available only to those on the wait list of O-blood type or, because B-blood candidates also have long wait times, to B-blood candidates with MELD or Pediatric End-Stage Liver Disease (PELD) scores greater than or equal to 30 (i.e., candidates who have a high three-month mortality risk.)[25]

Because relatively healthy O-blood-type candidates (e.g., those with a low MELD score) statistically will have some opportunity to get another O-organ, the rule that gives status 1 candidates of other blood types priority over lower-status O-candidates is a workable approximation. Nevertheless, the result will inevitably be a statistically longer wait time for O-blood candidates. According to the UNOS database, candidates of blood type O listed in 1999–2000 had a median wait time of 1,314 days, double that of any other blood type. However, since the implementation of MELD/PELD, the disparities have decreased. Candidates of blood type O listed in 2003–4 have a median wait time of 457 days, which is the longest wait (compared with 350, 231, and 76 days for candidates, respectively, of blood types A, B and AB).[26] However, it is much shorter than it was before the implementation of MELD. Because liver recipients with long waits increase their risk of dying while waiting, this rule of thumb will necessarily discriminate against those with O-blood type. It could be argued that, because being status 1 is, in some sense, a random event and being of O-blood type is more genetically determined, need based on blood type should be given more consideration than it is presently. There have been no proposals, however, to do this; rather, all revisions continue to give highest priority to those of status 1.

The Question of Wait Time

If the goal of the allocation system is to be fair to all on the list, we should be concerned if some people must wait inordinately long times for transplants. In some cases, this may be unavoidable. In the case of a kidney transplant, for example, the O-blood-group person who has a high PRA and unusual size requirements may simply require a long time to find a suitable organ. Conversely, the delay could be caused by the fact that others on the list have a better HLA match or have identical rather than merely compatible blood types. Neither a poor HLA match nor a compatible rather than identical blood group is a disqualifier for a transplant, however. If this person has been waiting a very long time, we might want to take that long wait into account, so that eventually the long wait overrides the HLA or blood-typing considerations. Hence, all organ allocations in one way or another take wait time into account. The new kidney formula, for example, relies on wait time to rank candidates within each category.

It can be argued that, no matter what adjustments have been made for these other factors, if someone still must wait an inordinately long time, he or she has a claim for special consideration. Following the rule that ties go to the person waiting longest seems reasonable. Adding more consideration merely for the fact that one has been waiting the longest seems to be a fair way of taking into account other factors that may not otherwise be considered.

Need Over a Lifetime

There is still a third way that need can be conceptualized. Some persons may not have extraordinary present need or even great urgency in getting transplanted, but may nevertheless be expected to lead lives that we would consider undesirable. If offered these lives, we might say that those leading them are particularly poorly off and that therefore we would not want to "trade places" with them.

The Role of Age

Consider, for example, whether we would view two persons with end-stage liver disease to have lives that are equally desirable if one develops her disease at age eighty and the other develops it at age thirty. Even if the two persons were equal in their present need and had equal urgency (i.e., had the same number of predicted future QALYs without treatment), we are likely to have little difficulty concluding that the person getting her disease at eighty has a much better life, overall, than the one who develops it at age thirty. One might plausibly say that the thirty-year-old is much needier than the eighty-year-old. This can be referred to as "over-a-lifetime need."[27] The needier person is the one who will end up with fewer QALYs if not given a transplant.

We have seen that utilitarians might insist that younger patients deserve priority over older patients, even when the two are equally sick. The younger person may have a better chance of responding to the surgery and may live longer if the graft is successful. This has raised cries of unfairness among the advocates for the elderly. Although this has the makings of a fight between the efficiency people and the equity people, it turns out that there is also a strong case to be made in the name of justice or equity for giving allocational priority to younger people. It is also possible to make the case that priority for younger people is more fair as well as more efficient.

At present, this over-a-lifetime notion of need is almost never taken into account in organ allocation. This seems strange. However, rather than incorporate this over-a-lifetime notion of need into the present chapter, we devote all of chapter 20 to this perspective.

Conversely, there are many other allocational factors that some people would take into account, especially if they want to promote medical utility, which those committed to justice will oppose.

First versus Repeat Transplants

Another variable that raises justice problems is the appearance on the wait list of some people who have had previous grafts that have failed. Some argue that it is unfair to give these people a second shot at an organ while others are still waiting for their first turn.

Moreover, there is evidence that people do not do as well with their second grafts. For kidneys, the one-year graft survival rate is 91.9 percent for first transplants and 89.7 percent for those with previous transplants. For five-year survival, the gap is more than 5 percent (72.0 percent vs. 66.8 percent).[28] For livers the one-year survival rate difference is greater—83.3 percent compared with 68.7 percent. For hearts the numbers are 87.1 percent and 81.8 percent.[29] This difference in each case is getting smaller, but it still remains. For reasons of both efficiency and equity, the case has been made that repeat transplant candidates deserve lower priority. However, there are convincing arguments that repeat candidates do not deserve to be downgraded. These are explored in chapter 19.

Geography

One final factor raises problems of justice. Presently, as a general rule organs are distributed on a basis by which they go first to those on the wait list of the local organ procurement organization (OPO). (There are fifty-eight federally designated OPOs in the United States and its territories.) Then, if no one is available locally, they go next to the region, of which there are eleven. Finally, if no one suitable is found at the local or regional level, the organ is allocated nationally. There are exceptions—cases that command priority regardless of region. In the new kidney formula, for example, highly sensitized patients, those with 0 AB–DR mismatch, and candidates who were prior living donors take precedence over geography; but these are rare cases. This means that in most cases a rather healthy potential recipient locally will get priority over a very critical patient on the regional list, and the healthy patient on the regional list will get priority over the very critical patient on the national list. Moreover, some OPOs have a relatively small potential for donor organs in comparison with their number of potential recipients, but others have a more generous supply of donor organs. Recently, people have asked whether this local priority is fair. A federal regulation mandates that UNOS revise its formula to make it fairer.[30] Some transplant surgeons and UNOS itself have responded by claiming that reducing local priority may be a less efficient way to allocate organs. The feud between the advocates of efficiency and those of equity involving geography is explored in detail in chapter 22.

Respect for Persons

The federal mandate for a national organ procurement network requires that the allocation system consider both efficiency and equity, but we saw earlier in this chapter that many ethical theories also include a number of moral principles that can be grouped under the rubric of *respect for persons*. This includes the principles of autonomy, fidelity, and veracity, perhaps along with the avoidance of killing. It seems clear that these moral principles are also very relevant to a systematic organ allocation theory.

In organ allocation, the principles grouped under the rubric of respect for persons can often be fully satisfied. This differs from utility and justice, which seem often impossible to satisfy fully. A system that fully maximized utility or one that was perfectly just seems utopian. Conversely, one that completely avoids killing people, lying to them, or breaking promises is conceivable. It may be that the fact that these respect-for-persons principles can be fully satisfied has led lawmakers to presume they are a prior constraint on the organ allocation system. The philosopher Robert Nozick has introduced the term *side constraint* to refer to the demands of respect for freedom.[31] The idea is that certain requirements of morality are prior conditions that constrain whatever policies are adopted. Whatever we do to reconcile the conflict between efficiency and equity, these side constraints must be satisfied. Thus, at least until recently, we have generally accepted the dead donor rule.[32] No one is to be killed in order to procure an organ, even if that person volunteers for the execution. Likewise, any competent person who wishes to decline a transplant has a right to do so, even if that person would get the most benefit from the organ and would therefore be the first candidate from the point of view of medical utility. By the same reasoning, we might conclude that no organ procurement or allocation system should be built on lies or deception—even if the lies or deceptions would increase the overall good that would come from a transplant program. (This insight stands behind our opposition to presumed consent programs, as discussed in chapter 10.) Finally, we might conclude that if someone has been promised an organ, he or she has a special claim to it, independent of consideration of either utility or justice. We saw earlier in this chapter that many theoreticians hold that, when ethical principles conflict, especially deontological ethical principles, no one principle will always automatically deserve priority. Hence, we could imagine a situation where the promise of an organ could be trumped by the realization that it would be grossly unfair to keep the promise. In that case, justice would take priority over promise keeping. The point, however, is that if a promise has been made, it is morally relevant and, other things being equal, there is a duty to keep it. It is unusual that promises will be a crucial factor in the morality of organ allocation, but the case could arise.

The principle of respect for autonomy raises especially important problems for a theory of organ allocation. It deserves special consideration in several contexts.

Free Exchanges among Autonomous Individuals

The moral principle of autonomy holds that people have a right of noninterference with choices they make based on their own life plans as long as these choices do not impose harms on other parties. We saw in chapter 11 that this raised an important problem for the marketing of organs. The straightforward implication of the principle of autonomy and its correlate of self-determination would be that people should have the right not only to donate their organs but also to sell them. We suggested that it is difficult to reject the logic behind this view, but that such a policy is open to the charge that a market for organs might be exploitative. It would be if those who would do the buying had it in their power to address the problems in life that would make it rational for people in a desperate situation to sell their organs in order to get basic needs met for themselves or their family members.

A similar question arises with regard to organ allocation. We could adopt a policy of permitting people to buy organs—either from individual vendors or from the organ allocation system. The attractiveness of the free market system to those in modern Western culture cannot be doubted. Those following the logic of Adam Smith believe that there is greater overall utility in a society if the free market is allowed to function. The real issue is whether a free market that would permit the buying of organs is also just or fair. Once again, one issue is whether it could be considered exploitative. In the case of individual vendors, if those doing the buying had it within their power to address the concerns of those desperate enough to sell their organs, they would have a moral duty grounded in justice to do so. Presumably, if they have the resources to buy an organ, they might have that ability.

The problem is more complex if the system is the vendor—if, for example, UNOS acquired all organs and then sold them. Here organs would be procured, but then sold to the highest bidder. Because the seller would not be in a desperate situation, the buyer would not be in a position to be accused of exploitation. But once again the issue of justice arises. If there is a national procurement network that receives organs by gift from individuals and families that altruistically want to help their fellow citizens, then this public organization would surely have a duty to allocate the organs in a way that gives people a chance to receive the organs in proportion to their need rather than on the basis of wealth. Although a private organ allocation system might tolerate a free market for organs, a national, public system cannot. Hence, in the United States we have a law prohibiting markets for organs.[33]

Directed Donation

A related problem is whether, under the principle of autonomy, those members of the moral community who are motivated to make a gift of their organs can choose to whom they will make the gift. Can they direct the gift to anyone they choose—an individual, an organization, or a social group?

Normally, according to the ethics of gift giving, one is permitted to give away anything of one's own to whomever one chooses. The choice of the recipient is up to the donor. But organs raise special problems. In the first place we have seen that individuals have only a "quasi–property right" over their bodies. They can only make a limited range of choices about what they can do with their bodies. Moreover, just as they cannot sell their body parts, they are restricted somewhat in choosing to whom they may make a gift of an organ. We have sympathy for someone who wishes to make a gift of an organ to a fellow family member or close friend. The law permits us to make a gift to a named individual.

It also permits us to make a gift to a named hospital or health organization. This is a bit more controversial. The law was written before the emergence of OPOs. There is the possibility of a conflict between an individual transplant hospital and the OPO if the donation is made to the hospital. The OPO might rightly claim that such a gift circumvents the organ allocation system that has been carefully crafted to make sure organs in the area are allocated efficiently and equitably. Some might claim that after the hospital receives the organ, it is bound by its relationship with the OPO to turn the organ over to the OPO for allocation according to the standard criteria.

Conversely, some donors may have long-term ties and loyalty to certain hospitals. They may feel a duty of loyalty to give to that one hospital, just as they might feel duty-bound to give to a family member. This occurs so infrequently that it seems that little harm will be done by permitting a hospital to receive such a gift and transplant it in any responsible manner that it sees fit to do. A hospital that turns the organ over to its

OPO for allocation according to preestablished criteria of efficiency and equity would be commended, however.

What would be unacceptable would be directing the donation by sociological group to unnamed members of a particular ethnic, racial, religious, or gender group. The arguments for this are discussed in detail in chapter 23.

Voluntary Health-Risky Behaviors

There is one final way in which the ethical principle of autonomy may come into play in a theory of allocation organs. Any society that is committed to the principle of autonomy will permit individuals to engage in certain behaviors even though it is known that these behaviors are risky to one's health. These behaviors—smoking, drinking in excess, leading a sedentary lifestyle, and so on—may increase the likelihood that those engaging in them will need an organ for transplant. In some cases, such as that of an alcoholic, the person who engages in the behavior and thereby comes to need a transplant will be competing directly with others who need an organ because of genetic or other reasons beyond their control. The issue is, if we permit people to engage in voluntary, health-risky behavior, do those who do so have an equal claim on organs as those who need an organ through no fault of their own?

This issue is contentious, is hotly debated in both transplant and public circles, and is the only topic about which the two authors could not come to agreement. The controversy, including four possible policy options, is discussed in chapter 18.

Conclusion

This completes our discussion of a general moral theory of organ allocation. We began with the premise that such a theory will be dependent upon some more general theory of ethics. Holders of specialized moral theories of various religious or secular traditions will logically tease out the implications of their ethics for organ allocation. What has been constructed here is a theory grounded in the common moral premises of the tradition of Western liberal political philosophy. These are views that seem quite compatible with the mainstream Judeo-Christian ethics of our heritage. What has been suggested is an ethic that includes considerations of both utility and justice. Our preference is for an ethic that gives justice a priority over utility, focusing on making those who are worst off among us more equal insofar as possible—that is, on giving the sickest the opportunity to recover their health, even if that means a less efficient system for allocating organs. We acknowledge, however, that not everyone in our society sees this as the proper relationship between utility and justice. In a democratic society, some political compromise may be necessary. The compromise that has emerged is one in which organs are allocated on the basis of a formula that gives weight to both justice and utility. A good case can be made using democratic political theory that, although some would prefer utility and others justice, the appropriate political compromise is to give them equal weight in organ allocation. This was the position taken by the UNOS Ethics Committee in the 1990s.[34] At least it seems clear that no allocation formula will be acceptable that is driven exclusively by utility, whether that includes social utility or merely medical utility.

Several different approaches would permit operationalizing the notion of giving equal weight to utility and justice. One strategy would be that, in order to incorporate both utility and justice into a common metric, we should give chances for an organ to be transplanted in proportion to need. This would give the worst off the best chance at getting an organ, but would refrain from giving them absolute priority. This is an egalitarian variant on Dan Brock's proposal to assign chances in a lottery for organs in proportion to expected benefit, a strategy that would give relatively more, but still not absolute, priority to those with the greatest expected benefit.[35]

There is another strategy for integrating utility and justice that more plausibly would give them equal weight. We could standardize measures of expected medical benefit so that the candidate with the most expected benefit would get a full or maximum number of points for medical benefit. Then all the other candidates would be assigned lesser numbers of points in proportion to their expected medical benefit from the particular organ being allocated. Finally, we could standardize measures of medical need (taking into account present need, urgency, and, as we argue in chapter 20, age), with the most needy person receiving a maximum number of "justice points" and others who are less needy receiving lesser numbers of points in proportion. If we were to give equal weight to (medical) utility and justice, we suggest, this would require an equal maximum number of points of each type, that is, an equal maximum number of utility and justice points. The points of each type would then need to be allocated based on empirical evidence of how various factors are related to their target. For example, when considering medical utility for a kidney transplant, we would assign HLA points in proportion to how the various antigens influence outcome. Likewise, when it comes to allocating justice points, they would be assigned to such factors as degree of illness, likelihood of being in imminent need, PRA, blood type, and time on the wait list, in proportion to how these variables were believed to be related to being poorly off when expected QALYs were considered.

We have argued, however, that utility and justice are not the only principles at stake. Whatever the proper compromise between utility and justice, the allocation system must be embedded into an arrangement whereby the principles related to respect for persons—autonomy, fidelity, veracity, and avoidance of killing—become side constraints that must never be violated just because it would be more efficient to do so. There may be rare cases in which these respect-for-persons principles need to be balanced against justice. We are open to that, in theory. However, it seems unlikely that this will be necessary in many real-life cases. Now we turn to a series of more specific organ allocation problems.

Notes

1. National Organ Transplant Act, Public Law 98-507, Oct. 19, 1984, 98 Stat. 2339.

2. The lists of utilities to consider and factors related to justice that follow are taken from the report of the UNOS Ethics Committee Organ Allocation Subcommittee, of which one of us (RMV) was the chair and primary drafter. See Burdick JF, Turcotte, JG, Veatch RM, "General principles for allocating human organs and tissues," *Transplantation Proceedings* 1992;24 (5): 2227–35.

3. Alexander S, "They decide who lives, who dies," *Life Magazine* 1962;53: 102–25. Also see Jonsen AR, *The birth of bioethics* (New York: Oxford University Press, 1998), 211–13.

4. Wolfe RA, Ashby VB, Milford EL, et al., "Comparison of mortality in all patients on dialysis, patients on dialysis awaiting transplantation, and recipients of a first cadaveric transplant," *New England Journal of Medicine* 1999;341 (23): 1725–30.

5. Ibid.

6. Ibid.

7. Organ Procurement and Transplantation Network, Concepts for Kidney Allocation, February 2011, 4, http://optn.transplant.hrsa.gov/SharedContentDocuments/KidneyConceptDocument.PDF.

8. Zeckhauser R, Shepard D, "Where now for saving lives?" *Law and Contemporary Problems* 1976;40: 5–45; Acton JP, "Measuring the monetary value of lifesaving programs," *Law & Contemporary Problems* 1976;40: 46–72; Williams A, "The value of QALYs," *Health and Social Service Journal*, July 18, 1985, 3–5; Cubbon, J, "The principle of QALY maximisation as the basis for allocating health care resources," *Journal of Medical Ethics* 1991;17: 185–88.

9. For the various arguments pertaining to the problem of justice in the use of QALYs, see Hastings Center, Institute of Society, Ethics and the Life Sciences, "Values, ethics, and CBA in health care," in *The implications of cost-effectiveness analysis of medical technology*, ed. Office of Technology Assessment (Washington, DC: Office of Technology Assessment, US Congress, 1980), 168–85; Veatch RM, "Justice and outcomes research: The ethical limits," *Journal of Clinical Ethics* 1993 (3): 258–61; Broome J, "Good, fairness and QALYs," in *Philosophy and medical welfare*, ed. Bell JM, Mendus S (Cambridge: Cambridge University Press, 1988), 57–73; Wagstaff A, "QALYs and the equity-efficiency trade-off," *Journal of Health Economics* 1991;10: 21–41; Kappel K, Sandoe P, "QALYs, age and fairness," *Bioethics* 1992;6: 297–316; Faden R, Leplege A, "Assessing quality of life: Moral implications for clinical practice," *Medical Care* 1992;30 (5 suppl): MS166–75; Lockwood M, "Quality of life and resource allocation," in *Philosophy*, ed. Bell, Mendus, 33–55.

10. "Graft survival rates for years 1988–96 from UNOS *1997 Annual Report*, table 26. See also Connolly JK, Dyer PA, Martin S, Parrott NR, Pearson RC, Johnson RW, "Importance of minimizing HLA-DR mismatch and cold preservation time in cadaveric renal transplantation," *Transplantation* 1996;61: 709–14; Zhou YC, JM Cecka, "Effect of HLA matching on renal transplant survival," *Clinical Transplantation* 1993, 499–510; Pirsch JD, Ploeg RJ, Gange S, Allessandro AM, et al., "Determinants of grant survival after renal transplantation," *Transplantation* 1996;61: 1581–86; Terasaki PI, Gjertson DW, Cecka JM, Takemoto S, "Fit and match hypothesis for kidney transplantation," *Transplantation* 1996;62: 441–45.

11. UNOS, Policy 3.5.9.2, from the UNOS website.

12. Organ Procurement and Transplantation Network, "Kaplan-Meier graft survival rates for transplants performed: 1997–2004," from OPTN data as of March 28, 2014, http://optn.transplant.hrsa.gov/latestData/step2.asp.

13. Tejani AH, Sullivan EK, Harmon WE, et al., "Pediatric renal transplantation: The NAPRTCS experience," *Clinical Transplantation* 1997, 87–100; Ettenger RB, Blifeld C, Prince H, et al., "The pediatric nephrologist's dilemma: Growth after renal transplantation and its interaction with age as a possible immunologic variable," *Journal of Pediatrics* 1987;111 (6 pt. 2): 1022–25; Davis ID, Bunchman TW, Grimm PC, et al., "Pediatric renal transplantation: Indications and special considerations—a position paper from the pediatric committee of the American Society of Transplant Physicians," *Pediatric Transplantation* 1998;2 (2): 117–29.

14. See, e.g., Johnson RJ, Warady BA, "Long-term neurocognitive outcomes of patients with end-stage renal disease during infancy," *Pediatric Nephrology* 2013;28 (8): 1283–91; Moser JJ, Veale PM, McAllister DL, Archer DP, "A systematic review and quantitative analysis of neurocognitive outcomes in children with four chronic illnesses," *Paediatric Anaesthesia* 2013;23 (11): 1084–96; Jung HW, Kim HY, Lee YA, et al., "Factors affecting growth and final adult height after pediatric renal transplantation," *Transplantation Proceedings* 2013;45 (1): 108–14; Mohammad S, Alonso EM, "Approach to optimizing

growth, rehabilitation, and neurodevelopmental outcomes in children after solid-organ transplantation," *Pediatric Clinics of North America* 2010;57: 539–57; and Copelovitch L, Warady BA, Furth SL, "Insights from the chronic kidney disease in children (CKiD) study," *Clinical Journal of the American Society of Nephrology* 2011;6: 2047–53.

15. Organ Procurement and Transplantation Network, "Concepts for kidney allocation," Feb. 16, 2011, http://optn.transplant.hrsa.gov/SharedContentDocuments/KidneyConceptDocument.pdf.

16. Ibid., 4.

17. Utilitarianism has, of course, at least since the days of John Stuart Mill, taken into account what is known as decreasing marginal utility. Hence, if a utilitarian is allocating money or food or some other good and can choose between someone who already has a lot of the item and someone who has little, the assumption is that often (but not always) giving the resource to the person who has less will produce more utility. Frances Kamm has brought this notion to bear on the question of organ allocation by arguing that the same notion might apply to life. Hence, she suggests that one might direct organs to younger transplant candidates on the grounds that the years of life one could add to the younger person would be of greater value than the same number of years added to an older person who has already had many of life's experiences. See Kamm, FM, *Morality, mortality, volume I: Death and whom to save from it* (New York: Oxford University Press, 1993), 237. This is not the concern of those dealing with justice. "Justice," as used here, focuses on the fact that some people have had less well-being than others. The focus is on producing greater fairness in the distribution of well-being, not on the amount of additional well-being a transplant will bring.

18. There is another possible interpretation of the idea of treating people equally. Generally, liberal political theory is premised on the egalitarian notion that all human beings are equal in their moral worth; that is, even though they may vary widely in how useful they are to others, they all count equally as human beings who are to be treated as ends in themselves, as moral beings with claims to equality. This could be interpreted as implying not that the worse off have claims to be made more equal to those who are better off, but rather that everyone who is in need of a lifesaving intervention has an equal claim to get that intervention. That view was suggested by Dan Brock; see Brock D, "Ethical issues in recipient selection," in *Organ substitution technology: Ethical, legal, and public policy issues*, ed. Mathieu D (Boulder, CO: Westview Press, 1988), 93. It has long been recognized that either a strict lottery or the principle of first-come/first-served would approximate this strict notion of equality. Unfortunately, for organ allocation, this would ignore many factors, e.g., HLA tissue match, age, organ size, blood type, and geography as well as degree of urgency. If we could provide equal opportunity while permitting some degree of matching based on these factors, the allocation system could be more efficient while still being fair. In a world in which both efficiency and fairness are taken into account, we might be even more inclined to depart from strictly equal claims on organs.

The main problem with allocation on the basis of equal claims for all potential recipients is that it would—in the name of fairness—give the relatively well off equal claim to that of the sickest. Another interpretation of fairness or justice is the one followed here: that all should have equal claim to opportunities for equality of well-being. That, in effect, means that the worst off have the strongest claims of justice rather than giving all persons equal claim regardless of how well off they are.

19. Wolfe et al., "Comparison."

20. Kamm, *Morality*, esp. 233–65.

21. Ibid., 234. Kamm actually distinguishes two types of urgency: urgency^T and urgency^Q. "T" stands for time, referring to how soon someone will die without a transplant; and "Q" stands for quality, indicating how badly off someone will be without a transplant. We have followed the approach of combining length of life and quality of life into a single measure, the quality-adjusted life-year, or QALY. Hence, we refer to urgency in terms of how soon one will die without transplant measured in QALYs.

22. Organ Procurement and Transplantation Network, "Policy 3.6: Allocation of Livers"; see 3.6.4.1, "Adult candidate reassessment and recertification schedule," Oct. 31, 2013, http://optn .transplant.hrsa.gov/PoliciesandBylaws2/policies/pdfs/policy_8.pdf.

23. Wiesner R, Edwards E, Freeman R, Harper A, et al., "Model for End-Stage Liver Disease (MELD) and Allocation of Donor Livers," *Gastroenterology* 2003;124: 91–96.

24. Yilmaz S, Aydin C, Isik B, Kayaalp C, et al., "ABO-incompatible liver transplantation in acute and acute-on-chronic liver failure," *Hepato-Gastroenterology* 2013;60 (125): 1189–93; Mendes M, Ferreira AC, Ferreira A, et al., "ABO-incompatible liver transplantation in acute liver failure: A single Portuguese center study," *Transplantation Proceedings* 2013;45 (3): 1110–15; Song GW, Lee SG, Hwang S, et al., "Successful experiences of ABO-incompatible adult living donor liver transplantation in a single institute: No immunological failure in 10 consecutive cases," *Transplantation Proceedings* 2013;45 (1): 272–75.

25. Organ Procurement and Transplantation Network, "Policy 3.6"; see 3.6.2, "Blood type similarity stratification/points."

26. Organ Procurement and Transplantation Network, "Liver Kaplan-Meier median waiting times for registrations listed: 1999–2004."

27. Veatch RM, "Distributive justice and the allocation of technological resources to the elderly," in *Life-sustaining technologies and the elderly: Working papers, volume 3—legal and ethical issues, manpower and training, and classification systems for decisionmaking* (Washington, DC: Office of Technology Assessment, US Congress, 1987), 87–189; Veatch RM, "How age should matter: Justice as the basis for limiting care to the elderly," in *Facing limits: Ethics and health care for the elderly*, ed. Gerald R, Winslow GR, Walters, JW (Boulder, CO: Westview Press, 1993), 211–29. Frances Kamm has more recently given considerable attention to this interpretation of the concept of need, indeed, specifying in her work that this should be the primary notion of need. See Kamm, *Morality*, 234, where she says, "I shall use the term 'need' so that it correlates with how much a person will have had by the time he dies."

28. Organ Procurement and Transplantation Network, "Kidney Kaplan-Meier graft survival rates."

29. UNOS Staff, *1997 Annual Report of the Scientific Registry and the OPTN* (Washington, DC: United Network for Organ Sharing, 1998), tables 26, 30, and 34.

30. US Department of Health and Human Services, Organ Procurement and Transplantation Network: Final Rule, 42 CFR 121, *Federal Register* 1998;63 (April 2, 1998): 16296–16338.

31. Nozick R, *Anarchy, state, and utopia* (New York: Basic Books, 1974), 29.

32. Miller, FG, Truog, RD, *Death, dying, and organ transplantation* (New York: Oxford University Press, 2012).

33. National Organ Transplant Act.

34. Burdick, Turcotte, Veatch, "General principles."

35. Brock, "Ethical issues."

Chapter 18

Voluntary Risks and Allocation

Does the Alcoholic Deserve a New Liver?

A*s we saw in chapter 17,* one of the implications of the moral principle of autonomy is that people who are substantially autonomous agents should be free to live their own lives even if, on occasion, they make choices that are not in their own interest. Some of these choices jeopardize their own organs and can eventually lead to the need for organ transplants. If justice requires that we give people *opportunities* for medical well-being, should we view these people as having had that opportunity but having squandered it? If so, does this mean that people who choose to take such risks deserve a lower priority in the organ allocation system?

The behaviors involved may include the consumption of alcohol, smoking cigarettes, eating fatty foods, and failing to exercise. The jump from these behaviors to the conclusion that people needing livers, lungs, or hearts deserve a lower priority is, however, a huge one. This chapter looks at the role of purportedly voluntary, risky lifestyle choices in organ allocation. We focus on alcoholism and liver failure as the primary example, but also consider a range of other possible behaviors that increase the need for organs. As will be obvious, the authors have agreed to disagree.

The Theory of Voluntary Health-Risky Behavior

Let us assume for the time being that we can identify certain health-risky behaviors that increase the likelihood that organs will be needed for transplant. How would those who hold the various moral views discussed in the previous chapter use that information in planning an organ allocation system? It turns out that those committed to maximizing aggregate net utility may reach different conclusions than those committed to an egalitarian interpretation of the principle of justice.

Utility

In developing the general moral theory of organ allocation in chapter 17, we distinguished between those utilitarians who consider the social impact of giving organs to one recipient or another and those who limit their utilitarian judgments to the expected medical benefit of the transplant. We saw that, for one reason or another, almost everyone agrees that the social impact of transplanting to one recipient rather than another—the social value of the transplant—is excluded from consideration in the organ allocation. That may be for utilitarian reasons (that the disutilities of determining who is a more worthy recipient outweigh the expected gains by picking the most valuable recipient) or for deontological reasons (that it is unethical to include social worth in the calculation). The utilitarian question that is on the table is which candidate will get the most medical benefit from the organ.

If the concern is who will get the most medical benefit, the history of the medical problem may be irrelevant. In the case of alcoholism, for instance, whether one did in one's liver by consuming alcohol or has cirrhosis from some other cause may turn out to be irrelevant. The utilitarian who is trying to determine the likelihood of medical benefit is interested in the prognosis, not the history. In fact, if one examines the prognosis of a liver transplant as a function of diagnosis, alcoholic cirrhosis patients apparently do quite well—better than some with other diagnoses.[1] The utilitarian is concerned about graft survival or patient survival, not whether one has voluntarily engaged in some behavior that may have created the need for the transplant.

Some sophisticated utilitarians might not completely accept this analysis, however. They may probe further to ask whether a policy of taking voluntary health-risky behaviors into account might create incentives to discourage the behavior. It could be that one of the consequences of letting voluntary behavior count against getting an organ would be reducing the demand on the organ supply, thus leaving more organs for those needing organs for nonvoluntary reasons as well as improving the health of the risk takers. However, depending on how wide we make the claim on voluntary behavior (overeating and obesity and its impact on liver failure; noncompliance with diet and exercise and its impact on heart failure; noncompliance with hypertensive medications and its impact on heart failure and/or kidney failure; smoking and its impact on heart failure and/or lung failure), it may turn out that the vast majority of candidates could be downgraded, and this could cause a backlash against the whole organ transplant system.

These are, of course, quite speculative claims. In fact, utilitarians who participate actively in the allocation debate have taken the position that a history of voluntary risks such as alcohol consumption should not count for allocation priority. As we have seen, physicians traditionally think in utilitarian terms. Hippocratic physicians considered benefit to the patient to be the only criterion of moral practice. When physicians took on the more social ethical question of allocation, in great numbers they continued to reason as utilitarians. In the United Network for Organ Sharing's (UNOS's) Ethics Committee's Subcommittee on Allocation, when the issue of voluntary health-risky behavior was debated in the 1990s, one of the authors (RMV) recalls that there was a perfect division, with all the physicians taking the utilitarian stance and opposing such considerations, while all the nonphysicians took a more deontological position, seeing some legitimate relevance to the cause of the organ failure in the allocation.[2]

The Deontological View: Concerns of Justice

Still assuming for the moment that some truly voluntary behaviors can be identified that lead to increasing the risk of organ failure and thus the need for a transplant, deontologists may see matters differently. They believe strongly in the right of individuals to make autonomous choices according to their own lifestyle, and to accept the consequences of these choices. Moreover, they are committed to a principle of justice that is not automatically swayed by the course of action that will maximize future outcomes. They are more concerned about equality of opportunity for well-being. If we are dealing with medicine, this often means medical well-being.

For one of us (RMV), the logical implication of a commitment to equality of opportunity is that if two people are equally needy because of a medical problem and one has previously had the opportunity to avoid the problem, the one who has not had that opportunity has a stronger claim. Conversely, if the need is not dependent on behavior that is truly voluntary, one committed to egalitarian justice would insist that persons have an equal claim to the organ even if it turned out to be inefficient to grant access. This means that it will be crucial to the deontologist to determine whether the health-risky behaviors are truly voluntary.

The other author (LFR) disagrees, from an alternative deontologic framework. She argues that commitment to a fair distribution of resources need not incorporate history, but instead could focus on current needs. In this vein two individuals with the same medical problem are equally needy and equally deserving, regardless of how each one got there.

Voluntarism versus Determinism

The entire question of voluntary health-risky behaviors is moot if it turns out that we cannot establish whether the behaviors in question are really voluntary. If alcoholism, smoking, and any other behaviors related to organ need are not really voluntary—are genetically determined, can be traced back to toilet training or some other psychological phenomenon of childhood, or are due to the social environment in which one was raised at the family and community levels—then holding the needy patient responsible is nothing more than "blaming the victim."

The literature on voluntary health-risky behavior is filled with this controversy. Left-wing critics of the 1970s tended to claim that behaviors affecting health were adversely correlated with socioeconomic status and thus were, in effect, economically determined.[3] For instance, they saw alcoholism as a response to socioeconomic oppression and therefore as not the alcoholic's fault. Rather, it was the fault of the broader, oppressive society. Of course, not all alcoholics are from lower socioeconomic classes, but their claim was that this was a factor, an important factor, and that making such behaviors a factor in allocating organs would simply transfer the oppression of society further onto people who were suffering because of social causes.

Others interpreted these behaviors the way a behavioral scientist would. They viewed them as conditioned responses to stimuli in these people's lives that were trained into them through an environment that was beyond their control. Freudian psychologists might differ with the behaviorists in the details of the causal mechanism, but they share the view that behavior is determined, not chosen. Still others believed that the behavior should not be seen as voluntary because genetics had a significant causal role in the disease.

All these deterministic accounts—whether they involve economic, psychological, or genetic determinism—need to be taken seriously. There is probably some truth in each of them. The issue, however, is whether they provide complete accounts of the behaviors in question. If they do, then the human is totally devoid of freedom of choice. We are creatures of forces outside us, to the point that voluntary behavior choices are impossible.

According to one author (RMV), this is a tragic view of human behavior that, carried to the extreme, makes all ethics impossible. Ethics is the discipline of moral evaluation of human conduct, practices, and character. To the extent that these are determined by economics, psychology, or genetics, such evaluation is meaningless. We simply must continue to operate on the assumption that all human behavior is, to some degree, free and open to choice. Of course, economics, psychology, the environment, and biology are important as well. They set certain limits on our choices. But there must be an element of freedom in behavior if life has any meaning. It is necessary to gamble on the assumption that there is some degree of choice in behavior, at least for adults who are deemed to be substantially autonomous.

The exact proportion of behavioral choices that can be attributed to voluntary choice is probably impossible to determine. It will surely vary from one situation to another and one medical condition to another. It seems, however, that the only assumption that is compatible with human morality is that at least some behaviors have at least some voluntary component and, if we are to treat people with dignity and respect, we will acknowledge that their behavior is significantly voluntary. The corollary of this assumption is that people ought to be held responsible for their voluntary actions. Answering the question of whether this has implications for organ allocation policy will require additional work.

The other author (LFR) disagrees. She believes that attempting to determine degree of causality for different factors and proximate cause is both too intrusive on privacy and fraught with too many known and unknown cofactors. But even if it could be determined easily, this author would reject this determination of degree of causality on the grounds that we would not want to place physicians in the position of trying to do so, as it would be inconsistent with their obligation to their patients. A physician trained in the Hippocratic tradition would educate his or her patient not to divulge this information, lest the physician have the obligation to disclose it to UNOS, thereby promoting dishonesty, and even distrust, in the doctor–patient relationship. A utilitarian-based physician would act similarly because he or she seeks to maximize outcomes and knows that the transplant outcomes are equivalent. Even a physician who holds a deontologic perspective would argue against this responsibility on the grounds that physicians must treat all patients as equals, deserving of equal respect, even though some are ill through no fault of their own, and others are causally responsible.

This approach can be criticized in that it ignores both autonomy and the actual outcomes of voluntary choices. It does, but this is only relevant if we define fairness to include the outcomes of voluntary choices. If we define fairness to require equal regard and treatment of all patients, then we are required to meet people's claims of need, regardless of how the need came about. In this approach the role of autonomy is limited to the patient's decision to be listed only if he or she accepts the restrictions imposed by transplant programs (e.g., smoking cessation, alcohol abstinence). This is consistent with the main theme of this book, which is that allocation policies are mainly focused on a balance between equity (justice) and efficiency (utility). Clearly a patient could volunteer not to be listed or to have a lower priority on the grounds that he or she perceives himself or herself to be "at fault"; but according to the author who is opposed to taking previous voluntary choices into account (LFR), the transplant community should not give him or her lower priority. According to the author who believes that justice requires taking previous voluntary choices into account (RMV), the transplant community should give at least some lower priority.

Linearity: Fairness in Holding People Accountable

If voluntary health-risky behaviors are relevant to organ allocation, they will, at a minimum, need to meet certain tests. One is that there needs to be a predictable relationship between the amount of the behavior and the degree of risk. This has been referred to as the criterion of *linearity*.[4] The degree of risk should be proportional to the amount of the behavior. One of us (RMV) believes that the health risks of certain key behaviors for organ transplants, including alcohol consumption and smoking, probably meet the linearity criterion. The other (LFR) does not. Like Benjamin and Cohen and the Ethics and Social Impact Committee of the Transplant and Health Policy Center, she is unwilling to include past behavior based on doubts about comparative degrees of voluntariness, which makes it impossible to pass judgment fairly and consistently.[5] In part her position is pragmatic because it would require a large degree of intrusiveness on the part of the health care team to determine how "responsible" any particular individual is. This position is held by a number of deontologists interested in health care allocation. Harald Schmidt, writing in a symposium about Norman Daniels's book *Just Health Care*, summarizes Daniels's position: "He rejects attempts at making 'people bear the cost of risky lifestyle choices' (p. 67) for several reasons: assessing someone's causal contribution is practically unfeasible (p. 67n53); corporate sector activities and environmental factors complicate responsibility attribution (p. 148); risks that might seem avoidable from some people's perspective are often part of conceptions of what makes life worth living for the persons concerned (p. 68); assessing responsibility is administratively burdensome, costly, intrusive, demeaning, liberty and privacy infringing, (p. 68); and we may 'victim blame' already disadvantaged groups (pp. 68, 148)."[6]

The other author (RMV) agrees that it is very difficult to identify which behaviors are voluntary and that the social, psychological, economic, and environmental factors are important, but insists that there is some residual element of voluntarism in alcohol, tobacco, and calorie consumption and that this voluntary element should show up as a small factor in allocation algorithms.

Responsibility Rather Than Moral Judgment

The author willing to downgrade the alcoholic (RMV) emphasizes that it is important to realize that the position outlined here is not that behaviors such as alcohol consumption and smoking are morally bad—vices—and that those who engage in them are therefore to be given a low priority for the allocation of organs. It is widely agreed that public health policy will have a very difficult time getting into the business of providing moral evaluations of behaviors. In a pluralistic society, it is unlikely that we could reach such agreement in any case. What is at stake here is whether people are responsible for their behavior and the impact of that behavior on social policy, including organ allocation.[7] If it is correct that there is a significant voluntary element in certain behaviors, then those engaging in them must be held responsible for them. The critical variable is not whether the behavior is moral or immoral, but whether one could have knowledge of the risks involved and voluntarily choose whether to engage in the behavior. To the extent that one knows the risk and chooses to take it, in principle, one should be responsible for the consequences.

The other author (LFR) accepts the argument that some individuals are responsible for some of their health problems, in the sense that their actions were based on degree of "conscious choice." However, she adopts Scanlon's position that "a judgment of substantive responsibility depends on more than this." As Scanlon explains, "To justify the claim that a person who has done A has a certain obligation, or that someone who has done A has to bear the consequences (and that others are not obligated to share this burden) it is not enough to point out that this person chose to do A. One must also consider the costs that this assignment of responsibility imposes on a person who does A, the alternatives to A that are available to a person in this situation, and the implications, for this person and others, of assigning responsibility in some other way."[8] That is, even if the action (e.g., drinking to excess) is at least partly voluntary and therefore it is fair to hold the individual responsible in the sense of acting out of free will, that is necessary but not sufficient to assign responsibility as liability—that is, to claim that one can therefore place the individual lower on the transplant wait list.

It is important to make clear that the author who is willing to hold alcoholics responsible (RMV) asserts that he is not trying to make a moral judgment. It is not how evil or sinful the behavior is, but rather how serious the impact is on the health care system. Theoretically, there could be a behavior that we do not consider ethically suspect in the slightest but that nevertheless poses a significant risk for a person needing an organ. Think of mountain climbing, if it should ever turn out that mountain climbing becomes a significant risk for organ damage resulting in the need for a transplant. We could probably agree that mountain climbing is a significantly voluntary behavior. We do not think of it as substantially determined by our genetic makeup or toilet training. We would not consider someone blameworthy simply for climbing a mountain. Nevertheless, it seems that one should be held responsible for the foreseeable consequences.

The other author (LFR) thinks the choice of example is important. When the mountain climber falls, as a number do in any given year on any given mountain, rescue teams are often sent out, even in conditions that may place the rescuers at risk. But no one would suggest that we not try to help on the grounds that the risk was voluntary. And though these searches do not require scarce organs, they require extensive financial and personnel resources, for which the climber is not held responsible. This is relevant because this author (LFR) believes that if we are going to hold some people responsible for their health choices, fairness requires that we hold all people responsible for those choices that can be labeled voluntary. Otherwise, it does begin to suggest that we disvalue and are willing to penalize some health actions more than others.

One author (RMV) agrees that we should hold all responsible for those choices that can be considered voluntary, but that because voluntariness is so hard to determine, he would make this only one factor in organ allocation—one small factor. He poses the situation in which two people engage in voluntary risky behaviors—one of which is quite benign but poses a significant risk of damaging organs, while the other is generally regarded as morally outrageous but poses essentially no risk. If someone were engaging in the immoral, almost risk-free behavior and, through some unexpected freak accident, irreversibly damaged an organ, it would seem wrong to take the behavior into account in organ allocation. Conversely, the benign but risky behavior would imply holding the person responsible for the consequences of the behavior, including, perhaps, adjusting the organ allocation formula because of the personal responsibility. The objective is not even to discourage the behavior (as it might be if we were in the business of labeling behaviors as vices and punishing their practitioners). Thus, one of us (RMV) is simply suggesting that if one is free to engage in these risky behaviors, one must be prepared to take responsibility for the consequences, even if the consequences happen to be a lower position on the organ wait list.

Exemptions for Socially Noble Behavior

Although what has been said thus far suggests that, insofar as one takes voluntary behavior into account at all, it is responsibility for actions rather than moral assessment of persons that is the relevant factor in voluntary health-risky behavior, there is an exception. Some behaviors for which we are responsible are important to society. Society wants to encourage the behavior, not discourage it. A good example might be professional fire-fighting. Surely this is the quintessential socially noble behavior. It is in society's interest that firefighters take chances. Normally, they take these chances knowing the risks and voluntarily choosing to take them. If a firefighter is injured in such a way that it would require an organ transplant—for instance, if a firefighter aspirated hot smoke to the point that his or her lungs were irreversibly damaged and a lung transplant were to become necessary—we would not want to penalize the firefighter for taking that risk. Even though he or she knew the risk and voluntarily chose to take it, society should see such behavior as noble. If we are debating the question of whether voluntary risk takers should bear the consequences of their behavior, the firefighter should be exempt. If we are debating the question of whether voluntary risk takers should have their behavior influence organ allocation, it certainly should not lower the firefighter's claim on an organ. Perhaps it should even raise it. The other author (LFR) agrees that socially noble behaviors should not lower the firefighter's claim, but argues that this example shows that the activities for which we are willing to ascribe responsibility are those we devalue.

Alcohol and Liver Transplants

Everything said thus far is meant to be general and theoretical. If behavior can be seen as significantly voluntary and humans should be held responsible for the consequences of their actions, then they may be responsible for the need for an organ resulting from these voluntary behaviors. Furthermore, if justice requires opportunities for equality, then those who voluntarily choose to engage in health-risky behaviors should be seen as having had an opportunity and should be placed in a somewhat subordinate position when it comes to allocating organs. This has nothing to do with whether the behavior is moral or immoral, a virtue or a vice. It is rather a matter of being responsible for the consequences of one's behavior.

Now it may turn out that even though all this holds in theory, it is of no significance for organ transplants. This will depend upon whether there are significantly truly voluntary behaviors in which those who choose to participate can reasonably expect to understand the organ-threatening consequences of their behavior. Because alcoholism and liver transplants are the primary examples of this kind of problem, this section of the chapter looks at the question of how plausible it is to treat alcoholism as a voluntary health-risky behavior and whether this reality should be taken into account in liver allocation policy.

The Empirical Data

There is increasing evidence that alcoholism has a genetic component.[9] In addition, behavioral patterns appear to be learned, so offspring and siblings may not only inherit tendencies toward alcoholism but also develop alcohol consumption patterns from role models starting at a very early age. Both these factors are sometimes cited as a basis for claiming that alcoholism is a disease rather than a voluntary behavior and that, therefore, alcoholics should not be held responsible for their behavior. One author (LFR) points out that even if one rejects the idea that alcoholism is a disease, one may still argue that alcoholics should not be held responsible because both genetics and social factors are critical for the development of alcoholism and both are beyond the individual's control.[10] An additional factor against holding alcoholics responsible is the fact that alcoholics often show co-morbid disorders, such as a personality disorder, schizophrenia, and social phobia. Indeed, many alcoholics have two or more mental disorders.[11]

What Would It Take for Alcoholism to Be Considered Nonvoluntary?

Given all these data, it is still not clear what the implications for allocation policy ought to be. We still need to know whether we should view alcoholism as having a significant voluntary component and, if so, whether that should count in deciding organ allocation priorities.

We should begin by asking what it would take to declare alcoholism nonvoluntary. Even if we assume that there is a significant genetic component in alcoholism, we need to understand what this could mean. It could mean that alcohol is metabolized differently because of some genetic variant. This could lead to some neurological event that makes alcoholics unable to exercise the judgment that would enable them to stop their alcohol consumption, so they tend to end up drunk once they start. But even if all this could be shown to be a true account of why alcoholics get drunk and damage their livers, it does not show that starting a bout of drinking is involuntary. Quite to the contrary, if the genetic factor changes the metabolism once the alcohol is consumed, this would suggest that the effect occurs after the drinking has started. This first drink would, to some extent, be independent of the genetic effects on the metabolism of the alcohol. But if the first drink were to occur when one is still a minor, as is the case with most alcoholics, then the behavior may still be judged involuntary from the standpoint of causal responsibility.

Another possibility is that alcoholics become psychologically dependent on alcohol, so that even that first drink is beyond their voluntary control. This sounds closer to an involuntary behavior. But there are two problems with this account. First, we have suggested that even those conditions that have a strong psychological component in their causation should nevertheless be seen as under voluntary control to some degree. Can it truly be said that any behavior is psychologically determined to the point that it is totally beyond the influence of the will? It is hard to imagine what evidence one could mount in support of such a claim. Second, even if after a while one becomes so psychologically dependent on alcohol consumption that it is truly nonvoluntary, was the development of the psychological dependence also involuntary? Could the alcoholic have seen the dependence coming and avoided it? If, for example, one realizes that one's parent is an alcoholic, should that be a warning of a potential risk that should lead one to voluntarily take steps to avoid developing the dependence oneself?

The answer is dependent upon how this psychological dependence develops. If, for example, it emerges in adolescence before one is substantially autonomous, then perhaps we should say it really is significantly involuntary. Conversely, if it emerges in adulthood, the ability to see it coming may increase the likelihood that one could have exercised some voluntary constraint before the dependence develops. But it may also be the case that it developed in an adult along with other psychiatric co-morbidities that were inadequately addressed but may seriously constrain the voluntariness of the alcoholic's behavior.

Logically analyzing these issues will be very difficult. Some will undoubtedly conclude that we are so uncertain about the casual chains leading to alcoholism that we cannot presume that one could voluntarily control it. This would mean that liver allocation should ignore the history of alcoholism, even for one who accepts the general premises of the voluntary health risk position sketched above. Conversely, one of us (RMV) concludes that even though alcoholism has nonvoluntary components related to genetics, psychology, and social status, it also contains significant opportunities for voluntary decision making. If the alcoholic had the opportunity for any significant choice, he or she should be held responsible for the consequences, including the consequences for liver damage.

This author (RMV) insists that his position is not meant to be a vindictive policy of punishment for alcoholism. One can be held responsible for the consequences of one's behavior without believing that one should be punished for it. Moreover, it seems that even if there is a voluntary component, there certainly are also nonvoluntary elements. This should mitigate any claim that there is a dramatic difference in the status of alcoholics compared with others who may need livers. The other author (LFR) disagrees and does perceive it to be an issue of blame, which becomes particularly obvious as we contrast alcoholism with other activities that cause health problems. Willem Martens of the Netherlands explains:

> A large number of studies show that there is a strong relationship between Type A behavior and coronary heart disease. . . . Because their risk-taking behavior is socially acceptable, these patients are rarely blamed for their heart failure, although they are in

fact responsible for it. Compared with the medical treatment of this type of heart patient, who is responsible for his disease, the treatment of the alcoholic patient who is not responsible for his disease is frequently less pleasant and more biased and denouncing, even if they receive the same medical priority. In many hospitals there is an unjustified bias against alcoholic patients because of their supposed responsibility for their alcohol abuse and related health problems, and this is, of course, not tolerable.[12]

The Role of a History of Alcoholism in Allocation Policy: Four Options

Although the analysis of alcoholism raises many controversial, contentious issues about which there is little agreement, the options for public policy may present decisions that are more manageable. In the 1990s the UNOS Ethics Committee considered four options.[13] Although, in the end, it could not reach a consensus on these questions, it came closer to a consensus than many expected. Two rather extreme policies were first considered and ruled out. Then two more moderate policies were debated.

Option One: Banning All Alcoholics from Liver Transplant

The first policy one might consider is to ban all alcoholics from any liver transplants. Stressing the voluntary component—perhaps along with manifesting a serious streak of vindictiveness—some have suggested that no organ resources should be used for alcoholics at all. Perhaps exceptions would be made for alcoholics who had never been mentally competent; but adults who are presumed to have made some voluntary choices along the way would simply be excluded from access.

This proposal probably rests on a moral judgment about the person as much as or more than a judgment about justice and opportunities for health. In this crude form, it is hard to defend. It seems we could agree that, at least in the case in which an organ was available that would otherwise go to waste, the alcoholic should be permitted to receive it. No one on the UNOS Ethics Committee was willing to accept this view.

Option Two: Transplant All Alcoholics, Even Those with Active Alcoholism

A second position was also rejected by the Ethics Committee. It might be defended by someone who considers the history and cause of the liver failure as morally irrelevant. That would be to provide organs to alcoholics, including active alcoholics, without regard to their condition. This proposal, at first, might seem irrational, because it might be argued that the active alcoholic would simply waste another liver, repeating the process in an endless cycle. However, development of full-blown cirrhosis takes considerable time. Certainly, even an active alcoholic would have a chance to get many good years from his or her new liver before causing serious damage.

The active alcoholic might be excluded on the grounds that, as an active alcoholic, he or she would not be able to follow the necessary regimen of immunosuppression and treatment follow-up. That is a legitimate medical reason for excluding the potential recipient, but not all active alcoholics would necessarily fail in their medication routine and follow-up.

Option Three: Transplant Alcoholics Once They Have Demonstrated They Are Reformed

The utilitarians on the UNOS Ethics Committee, including all the physicians, all took a more modest third position supporting transplants for alcoholics. They acknowledged that it was inappropriate to transplant active alcoholics (perhaps because even if the transplant was a success, it was an inefficient procedure because of the risk of follow-up failure and eventual organ damage). However, as was mentioned above, they pointed out that the evidence suggests that alcoholics, once they are off alcohol and reformed for a reasonable period of time, do at least as well as other liver transplant patients. Reasoning from these consequences and committed to seeing the history as irrelevant, these utilitarians defended the view that reformed alcoholics should go into the allocation without regard to their alcoholism. They should in no way be penalized once they were sufficiently reformed. There is some dispute about how long the alcoholic should be dry. Suggestions range from six months to a year.

Option Four: The History of Alcoholism as a Modest Negative Factor in Allocation

By contrast, the nonphysicians on the UNOS Ethics Committee were more willing to ascribe responsibility in their approach to the issue, which constituted the fourth option. They granted that alcoholism was a complex phenomenon with some causal factors well beyond the control of the alcoholic. At the same time they insisted that, to preserve their dignity as human agents, alcoholics must be viewed as significantly responsible for their behavior—that there was a voluntary element in it. Viewing history as morally significant, they wanted this voluntary behavioral choice to be reflected in the allocation of livers.

They were not at all inclined to conclude that this should mean banning alcoholics from the transplant program, even in a world where livers were very scarce. What they concluded was that some small element in the allocation can and should reflect the history of alcoholic cirrhosis. If the liver allocation were based on a point system similar to the kidney allocation, this might suggest a small number of negative points for alcoholic cirrhosis. Thus, now that livers are allocated based on the Model for End-Stage Liver Disease (MELD) score, a history of alcoholism could be reflected by subtracting a point or two. The number would be set in proportion to how important the voluntary component seemed to be. All agreed that it should be small in comparison with other factors such as medical urgency. There are other ways that a history of alcoholism could be taken into account. For example, among candidates of similar status or with a similar MELD score, ties are broken by time on the wait list. This could be modified so that ties are first broken on the basis of whether one has a diagnosis of alcoholism and then by time on the wait list. This would continue to be subordinate to medical urgency; but as a tiebreaker, one of us (RMV) thinks it makes sense.

The Resolution: Agreeing to Disagree

This dispute turned out to be intractable when it was debated by the UNOS Ethics Committee. In the end the utilitarian physicians and the deontological nonphysicians could reach no further compromise between their two moderate positions. The committee had to agree to disagree. The report dealing with the issue simply states the disagreement. What is striking, in reflecting on these debates, is how consistently the physicians insisted that history was irrelevant and that prognosis was all that counted, whereas the nonphysicians considered opportunities forgone as somehow morally relevant. They saw the alcoholic's behavior as complex and not necessarily blameworthy, but nevertheless containing enough of a voluntary component that it deserved to be reflected in some small way in the allocation formula.

Interestingly, this dispute also turned out to be intractable between the two authors of this volume; but in this case, the conflict was not between utility and deontology but instead between two different conceptions of fairness. One of us (RMV) argues that freedom of the will requires us to ascribe responsibility and that this means that health opportunities forgone are morally relevant. The other (LFR) argues that ascribing responsibility in the sense of "voluntary choice" does not mean that we need to ascribe substantive responsibility in the sense of "moral liability." Rather, this author (LFR) objects to the use of moral responsibility as a criterion for listing because (1) "it would undermine the physician–patient relationship and the functioning of medicine in general; and (2) because fairness with respect to organ allocation requires that we meet people's claims of need regardless of how the need came about."[14]

Other Voluntary Behaviors

Although alcoholism is the most visible example of a possibly voluntary health-risky behavior that could damage organs, other behaviors also raise similar questions. The most conspicuous are smoking, which might lead to a lung transplant, and poor diet and exercise patterns, which could lead to the need for a liver, kidney, or heart transplant. Voluntarily failing to maintain a blood pressure reduction regimen might also be seen as a voluntary health-risky behavior leading to the need for a kidney transplant. To the extent that diabetes is the result of a lack of dietary control, it may be another example, this time leading to a pancreas transplant. In what ways do these cases differ from alcoholism and a liver transplant?

Smoking and Lung Allocation

It is now well known that smoking can lead to lung damage—such as lung cancer and emphysema, among other conditions. Should smoking be taken into account in the lung allocation formula, not as a predictor of outcome, but as an indicator of voluntary choice to take a risk?

Lung transplants are much rarer events than either kidney or liver transplants (1,620, compared with 5,372 livers and 9,314 deceased donor kidneys in 2013). Lungs are, thus, less scarce. Moreover, serious cases of lung cancer, at least those with metastases, currently are not treated with transplantation. Nevertheless, some other smoking-related lung diseases may be appropriate for transplants.

The reasoning should be the same as for alcoholism. First, one must determine whether smoking is a significantly voluntary behavior. This is no small task. There are good reasons to believe that tobacco is addicting once one engages in it regularly. In that way, it is little different from alcohol, but tobacco may generate more physical dependency than alcohol. Regardless, the same questions raised about alcohol need to be raised about smoking. Was there ever a time when the smoker was not addicted and could voluntarily choose not to smoke? Moreover, we need an account for the fact that so many former smokers have quit, apparently voluntarily. This implies that, at least for some, the smoking was subject to some degree of voluntary choice. Many people, however, start smoking at such a young age that they cannot be said to be substantially autonomous decision makers when they start. Moreover, we are now learning that they have been subject to exploitative manipulation by very sophisticated advertising and marketing strategies that, at least until recently, no one could have known enough about to consciously resist.

This suggests a final problem for deciding whether smoking should be a modest negative consideration in allocating organs. Not all who have damaged their lungs are in any way like the same position regarding how much they could be expected to have known when they damaged their lungs. Even if it could be argued that today's adult who begins smoking has been given fair warning—by cigarette package warnings, school education programs, and enormous media publicity about tobacco industry practices— that was certainly not the case when today's older generation began to smoke. Many may have done their damage well before the risks were understood by the public. This will make it harder to impose any negative consideration for this behavior at all, because different people are in different positions regarding their knowledge of risk taking when they did their smoking. But it would allow this distinction to be made in another decade or so.

Diet, Sedentary Lifestyle, and Hearts

An even more complicated dynamic exists when we consider whether those who fail to follow proper diet and exercise regimens should have their behavior taken into account in the allocation of hearts and perhaps other organs that they could need. The relationship between these behaviors and organ failure appears to be far more complex than that of alcohol with liver failure and smoking with lung damage. Although almost everyone must have some understanding by now that alcohol and smoking pose risks to livers and lungs, the understanding of the relation of diet and exercise to heart failure is more incomplete. That is in part because the science is less well understood. The public continues to get mixed messages.[15] Cholesterol and triglycerides apparently have complex relations with heart disease. The average citizen cannot understand the relationship as easily as with alcohol or tobacco.

It is not even clear whether diet and exercise meet the criterion of linearity. Some people seem to be able to take in a terrible diet and avoid exercise and not have the effects show up in their coronary health. It is not clear whether this is random or relates to poorly understood genetic and metabolic variations. This suggests that, though the public is beginning to grasp the fact that diet and exercise are related to heart disease and other health factors, the extent to which they can be held responsible for the outcomes is less clear. At least until the dynamics are more fully understood, it will be hard to separate potential recipients of hearts on the basis of whether they have engaged in health-risky behaviors.

Kidneys and Pancreata

The same can be said even more strongly for those who need kidneys because they have failed to maintain blood pressure and those who might need pancreata because they have exacerbated their diabetes with a poor diet. In principle, those who accept the general arguments in the first section of this chapter would be willing to let health-risky behaviors count in some small way against those who have damaged their kidneys and pancreata through voluntary choices. Establishing that these people knew the risks they were taking and voluntarily decided to take them will be much harder here. Given that even the boldest advocates of taking voluntary health-risky behaviors into account in organ allocation favor only a modest, marginal influence on organ allocation, it is likely that, for these latter conditions, the lack of certainty about the risks will lead to a policy of ignoring these factors when it comes to organ allocation.

Of course, one author (LFR) notes that there are also heavy smokers who never develop respiratory disease and heavy drinkers who never develop liver failure. This same concern—lack of certainty—weakens, if not negates, the discussion above about lower rankings for those who smoked and are in need of a lung transplant and for those who drank and are in need of a liver transplant. Until we know why some persons who smoke stay healthy and why some persons who abuse alcohol do not develop liver failure, we cannot truly ascribe moral responsibility. And yet, as this author (LFR) has argued above, even if we could, we should not, because justice requires that we treat all patients according to need, regardless of how the need came about.

Notes

1. De Maria N, Colantoni A, Van Thiel DH, "Liver transplantation for alcoholic liver disease," *Hepatogastroenterology* 1998;45 (23): 1364–68; Neuberger J, Tang H, "Relapse after transplantation: European studies," *Liver Transplantation and Surgery* 1997;3 (3): 275–79; DiMartini A, Jain A, Irish W, Fitzgerald MG, Fung J, "Outcome of liver transplantation in critically ill patients with alcoholic cirrhosis: Survival according to medical variables and sobriety," *Transplantation* 1998;66 (3): 298–302; Stefanini GF, Biselli M, Grazi GL, et al., "Orthotopic liver transplantation for alcoholic liver disease: Rates of survival, complications and relapse," *Hepatogastroenterology* 1997;44 (17): 1356–69.

2. Burdick JF, Turcotte JG, Veatch RM, "General principles for allocating human organs and tissues," *Transplantation Proceedings* 1992;24 (5): 2234.

3. Beauchamp DE, "Public health as social justice," *Inquiry* 1976;13: 3–14.

4. This concept was first developed in Veatch RM, "Voluntary risks to health: The ethical issues," *JAMA* 1980;243: 50–55.

5. Cohen C, Benjamin M, and Ethics and Social Impact Committee of the Transplant and Health Policy Center, Ann Arbor, MI, "Alcoholics and liver transplantation," *JAMA* 1991;265: 1299–1301

6. Schmidt H, "Just health responsibility," *Journal of Medical Ethics* 2009;35: 21–22. Page numbers in the quotation refer to Daniels N, *Just health: Meeting health needs fairly* (New York: Cambridge University Press, 2008).

7. The distinction between responsibility and moral judgment was hinted at by Veatch, "Voluntary risks," and is developed more explicitly and fully in an analysis by Glannon W, "Responsibility, alcoholism, and liver transplantation," *Journal of Medicine and Philosophy* 1998;23: 31–49.

8. Scanlon T, "Justice, responsibility, and the demands of equality," in *The egalitarian conscience: Essays in honour of G. A. Cohen*, ed. Sypnowich C (Oxford: Oxford University Press, 2006), 76–77.

9. Bierut LJ, Dinwiddie SH, Begleiter H, et al., "Familial transmission of substance dependence: Alcohol, marijuana, cocaine, and habitual smoking—a report from the Collaborative Study on the Genetics of Alcoholism," *Archives of General Psychiatry* 1998;55 (11): 982–88; Conneally PM, Sparkes RS, "Molecular genetics of alcoholism and other addiction/compulsive disorders: General discussion," *Alcohol* 1998;16 (1): 85–91; Edenberg HJ, "Genetics of alcoholism," *Science* 1998;282 (5392): 1269; Goate AM, Edenberg HJ, "The genetics of alcoholism," *Current Opinion in Genetics and Development* 1998;8 (3): 282–86; Grau C, "Genetics of alcoholism: An international perspective," *Alcoholism: Clinical and Experimental Research* 1996;20 (8 suppl): 78A–81A; Guze SB, "The genetics of alcoholism: 1997," *Clinical Genetics* 1997;52 (5): 398–403.

10. One of the authors (LFR) would like to thank Walter Glannon for a discussion on these issues.

11. Martens W, "Do alcoholic liver transplantation candidates merit lower medical priority than non-alcoholic candidates?" *Transplantation International* 2001;14: 170–75. See also Sallmén B, Berglund M, Bokander B, "Perceived coercion related to psychiatric comorbidity and locus of control in institutionalized alcoholics," *Medical Law* 1998;17 (3): 381–91.

12. Martens, "Do alcoholic liver transplantation candidates merit lower medical priority," 172.

13. Burdick, Turcotte, Veatch, "General principles."

14. Ho D, "When good organs go to bad people," *Bioethics* 2008;22 (2): 78.

15. Lee I, Paffenberger RS, "Change in body weight and longevity," *JAMA* 1992;268: 2045–49.

Chapter 19

Multi-Organ, Split-Organ, and Repeat Transplants

Daniel Canal's ordeal started when he was eight years old. The Wheaton, Maryland, boy had been born with a defective small intestine. It was twisted and failed to function properly. It gradually caused damage to his pancreas and liver. Eventually, he was placed on the organ wait list for a transplant for all three organs at the University of Pittsburgh Children's Hospital, one of only three hospitals in the country that performed this type of multiple organ transplants. Daniel remained on the wait list for five years, during which time his condition progressively deteriorated:

> In February of 1998 he spoke at a rally in Washington about the issue of basing organ transplants on need rather than geography [an issue we explore in chapter 22]. It was after this speech that his five-year wait gained national attention, and he was then placed on a wait list at Jackson Children's Hospital in Miami. Only three days after being listed, a donor match was found. After the years of waiting, his response was, "Mom, I don't want to go. . . . I'm scared." His mother prevailed, however, and he was flown to Miami by ambulance plane.
>
> He received his transplant on May 15, 1998, by a team of surgeons led by Dr. Andreas Tzakis. The 12-hour operation seemed uneventful, although it was found that Daniel's stomach had deteriorated as well and also needed to be replaced. On May 31, his body had a rare and violent reaction to the small intestine and, because of this rejection, all four organs needed to be replaced. The second transplant occurred on June 2 using donated adult organs, which had to be reduced in size to fit Daniel's body. A hospital spokesperson was quoted as saying, "He's so sick, and we're in such a desperate race against time." They knew the organs were not ideal, but it was an emergency.
>
> This transplant failed because the donated liver failed to function properly. The donor was described as "less than healthy." On June 20th, Daniel received still another set of organs, making twelve in all that he had received. Doctors worked for 19 hours to transplant organs harvested from a young donor in Puerto Rico. This surgery was deemed successful, as Daniel had no adverse reactions. Four months later, he was well enough to have his first solid food in years. It was his request: two pieces of chicken and ten French fries from Burger King. The next spring, he threw out the ceremonial first pitch at a Baltimore Orioles baseball game. His case, however, sparked debate about the fairness of the decision to allocate twelve organs to one person.[1]

One of the most persistent and perplexing problems in organ allocation is what should be done with those who consume more than one of our scarce supply of solid organs. Some have multi-organ failure, needing both kidney and pancreas, heart and lung, or some other combination of organs. Others have had a previous graft that has now failed, so they are in need of another organ. In rare cases, such as Daniel Canal's, patients needing multiple organs find that the first transplant fails, thus requiring repeat multi-organ transplants.

Utilitarian allocators do not look favorably upon those in need of multi-organ or repeat transplants.[2] These potential recipients are sick patients. Those needing repeat transplants find that their new grafts do not do as well as the first one, partly because of the increased risk of antibody reactions. Deontologists who are concerned about fairness and equal opportunity may not look favorably on retransplant cases either, because there is an intuition that fairness requires giving those who have not yet had their first graft a chance before retransplant candidates get seconds.

Conversely, when these cases are successful, they provide some of the most moving testimonies to the marvels of modern medical technology. In May 2012, a Fresno television station reported that Daniel Canal's family was celebrating a milestone as the twenty-seven-year-old graduated with Latin Honors upon receiving his master's degree from Cal State Stanislaus.[3]

Another multi-organ recipient, Robert Casey, received a heart-liver transplant in June 1993 and resumed his position as governor of Pennsylvania in December 1993, leaving office in January 1995 after completing the two-term state limit and surviving for another five years until May 2000. (His case is discussed in detail in chapter 21.)

Although they pose challenges in different time frames, multi-organ transplants and repeat transplants raise some common ethical issues—problems of a single person making such heavy demand on the common and small organ pool, and problems of the fairness issues this demand raises. We look first at multi-organ transplants, then turn to repeat transplants.

Multi-Organ Transplants

Multi-organ transplants are transplants of two or more donor organs into the same patient in the same operation. In Daniel Canal's case, he required four organs: a liver, intestines, a pancreas, and a stomach.

Utilitarian Concerns

It is easy to see why utilitarians are troubled by multi-organ transplants. At their best, they save one life and return one person to a normal life when the same organs could have saved two or more. This makes the utilitarian's mathematics simple. Moreover, for multi-organ transplants, the success rate may be lower than it would be for each of the organs transplanted individually, although the success rates have improved greatly in the past decade. For example, the 2010 Scientific Registry of Transplant Recipients reports that heart-lung recipients have one- and five-year graft survival rates of, respectively,

78.7 percent and 49.0 percent, while heart recipients have one- and five-year graft survival rates of 88.3 and 73.9 percent and lung recipients have one- and five-year graft survival rates of 81.5 percent and 51.2 percent.[4]

Deontologists' Views

The position of the deontologist is more complex. The primary concern is with the fairness of using two or more organs for one person. The analysis of fairness, however, is complicated.

Fairness as Equal Claim on Scarce Resources

For the egalitarian, the deontologist whose understanding of justice is organizing social practices so that people have an opportunity for equality, sometimes fairness means that resources are distributed equally.[5] This approach might work for the distribution of income in a radically egalitarian society or the distribution of food relief during a famine, but it makes no sense to even the most radical egalitarian in the world of health care. Everyone getting the same amount of health care would either mean that those fortunate enough to be healthy would need to needlessly consume and that those with serious ongoing medical needs would need to go without much of what they really need.

One way radical egalitarians have responded to this problem is to emphasize an enriched understanding of resources. They might view resources as including not only money and consumer goods but also one's genetic endowment, inherited social position, and fate in the natural and social lotteries of life. This view suggests that, to the radical egalitarian, when we add up the goods that each person possesses, we include not only material and economic resources but also the health and talents with which one has been endowed. These are sometimes referred to as assets from the "natural lottery." A radical egalitarian might take the position that the goal of social practices such as organ allocation should be equality of opportunity for resources, taking into account what one has received in the natural lottery as well as what one acquires through the "social lottery," that is, through one's family's socioeconomic position, the luck of being born into a favored or disfavored cultural situation, and so forth. This would mean that one endowed with poor health through genetics or culture has a claim on the health care resources needed to get even with those who find themselves through natural and social fortune to be healthier. (As we saw in the last chapter, one of us, RMV, insists that it is only *opportunities* for health to which one is entitled, so that those who squander their opportunities through voluntary lifestyle choices do not have the same standing as those who were shorted in the natural and social lotteries.)

This interpretation of egalitarianism suggests that if someone were endowed with more than one organ that fails (especially if it is not through that person's fault), one has received fewer resources in life's allocation than either those who get a full complement of healthy organs or those who have the misfortune of single-organ failure. If one of the tasks of the social system is to establish practices that continually correct these mal-allocations, then someone who has one organ that has failed is entitled to that one, while those who have more than one in failure are entitled to more and those with a full set of functioning organs, none.

Keep in mind that the holder of the justice perspective is not primarily concerned about the inefficiencies of the system. He or she is concerned with establishing a social practice that will make opportunities more equal. In an ideal world where there are enough organs to go around, everyone would get the number of organs needed to be healthy. But in a less than ideal situation where there is a shortage of organs, all those on the wait list have a claim on the system for an equal chance to get the organs they need. This means that whether someone needs one or several organs, he or she has an equal claim.

Integrating Claims Based on the Number of Organs Needed with Other Claims

There may, of course, be other variables that also influence the justice of claims. One of us (RMV) would argue that voluntary health-risky behavior may be one such factor. Those who have had good organs and have engaged in voluntary behaviors that have ruined them may have somewhat less of a claim. In the chapters that follow, we explore whether age, social status, and race are legitimate variables affecting the legitimacy of claims. Later in this chapter, we consider if retransplants can be such a factor. The point here is that from the justice perspective, the need for multiple organs is not a legitimate factor in deciding one's standing for organs. Thus, two people who each need a kidney have an equal claim, regardless of the fact that one of them may also need a pancreas while the other does not.

The Impact of the Availability of Suitable Organs

There is yet another complication. In chapter 17 we saw that one of the criteria for fair distribution is the likelihood of finding a suitable organ in the future. Because some kidney donors are unable to supply usable pancreata (because of the medical suitability of the organ or the lack of willingness of the donor to consent to pancreas procurement), the recipient needing both organs may actually be given a preference when a donor can provide both organs. It makes sense to transplant the kidney and pancreas from one source at the same time because the chance of another suitable organ becoming available is low, and because organs from separate sources may require additional immunosuppression, which is harmful to the grafts and the patient. It may also require a second surgery and its attendant risks.

Even though there are good utilitarian reasons to place single-organ recipients ahead of those needing multiple organs, in fact, we do not adopt that priority. This suggests that policymakers recognize the wisdom of giving more equal access, regardless of the number of organs needed, and actually give the multi-organ recipient a priority when it is called for by concern for the likelihood of the availability of suitable organs.

The Unequal Demand for Organs

The criticism of Daniel Canal's use of a total of twelve organs raises one final problem. Not all twelve of the organs Daniel received were equally in demand. Two of the organs—the small intestine and the stomach—are not really scarce resources. Very few such transplants are needed. Only 67 intestinal transplants were performed in 1997. Stomach transplants are so rare that statistics are not even kept. In March 1999, 445 were awaiting a pancreas transplant, which made it scarce, but not as scarce as the liver. The only organ in really high demand that Daniel received was the liver. Moreover, the second transplant he received was not medically ideal. It is doubtful whether it would have been used on anything other than an emergency basis. That means that Daniel really only received two organs that were in great demand, the two good-quality livers. Daniel's case is rather similar to one where a patient was a candidate for a second liver after the first had failed. Although some have suggested that repeat transplant candidates deserve lower priority than first-time recipients, such proposals are controversial. No one is advocating a complete prohibition.

Repeat Transplants

Daniel Canal needed not only multiple organs, but also repeat transplants. Retransplants pose a somewhat different set of problems for both utilitarians and deontologists.

Utilitarian Concerns

Utilitarians seek to maximize medical utility. Simplistically, one would think they would object to permitting retransplantation because of lower graft survival; yet failure to permit retransplantation could lead to less willingness to accept marginal organs, and therefore to lower overall utility.

The Direct Relevance of Retransplants

The fact that some potential transplant recipients have already had grafts that failed is not a direct concern of utilitarians who are trying to maximize medical utility. By the time a graft has failed and the recipient needs a new organ, as long as there is an organ shortage, only a fixed number of transplants can take place. Only one life can be saved with the second organ. Whether it is the same person who has already had a previous graft or is a new candidate makes no direct difference to someone who is not concerned about the distribution of a good but only with the aggregate total. A life is a life. Because utilitarians are not concerned about the distribution of goods but only the aggregate amount of good, especially if we exclude considerations of social worth, it should make no difference to the utilitarian which lives are saved.

Retransplants as an Indicator of Greater Graft Failure

Even though utilitarians have no direct concern about the fact that some potential candidates have had transplants previously, they have an indirect concern. Data reveal that retransplant patients do not do as well as patients receiving a first transplant, and failure rates are greater with each successive transplant. A utilitarian who is striving for maximum benefit regardless of how it is distributed will give priority to those who have not had grafts previously. Other things being equal, the utilitarian will prefer the patient with the better chance of success, which will be the candidate who has not previously had a graft failure. (Of course, other things are often not equal. A true utility maximizer will also take into account the cause of the organ failure, the age of the recipient, and, as we have seen, the race, gender, and socioeconomic status, because they all predict likelihood of success. One who is unwilling to take all these factors into account is probably not a utility maximizer and may come to understand that the slightly poorer success rate of the retransplant candidate is not morally relevant either.)

However, the new kidney allocation algorithm set to go into effect later in 2014 does incorporate the lower survival rates of retransplant candidates in its calculations of estimated posttransplant survival (EPTS), which has a negative impact on whether the candidate will be eligible to receive the best-quality kidneys. This is discussed in greater detail in chapter 20.

Long-Term Implications of Downgrading

Utilitarians may take a more long-term perspective, however. They might ask what the impact would be on a transplant program of giving candidates for a retransplant lower priority. Although many in the public do not realize it, not all donor organs are equal. Some organs are what can be called "marginal." They are less desirable because they come from older donors, have medical characteristics that make them more marginal and less desirable, have been damaged during procurement (e.g., vessels that were cut too short), have long warm-ischemic times, or come from patients who may be at somewhat higher risk for a transmissible disease. Yet none of these organs are totally unacceptable, or they would not be made available to begin with. However, if candidates and their surgeons knew that they had only one chance at a transplant before being relegated to second status in the allocation process, they would have a strong incentive to decline the marginal organ and hold out for the "perfect" one. From a systems point of view, this is not a good incentive to create. Assuming that some of the marginal organs are only slightly less promising and that it is rational to include them in the donor pool to begin with, we do not want potential recipients declining them if they are otherwise suitable (if not perfect) organs. An incentive to reject these marginal organs will undoubtedly lead to organ wastage. Some might be passed along to recipients who are so desperate that they will take the chance, but the delays will cause some harm to all organs and complete wastage to some. They will show up as "discards." Assuming that the organ had a reasonably good chance of success if taken by the first candidate on the list and that there is an organ shortage that will lead to some deaths of patients while on the wait list, these are organs that should be transplanted, preferably to the candidate on the wait list with the highest priority. The reasonable conclusion of the utilitarian might be that the disutilities of giving retransplant candidates lower status outweigh the advantage of giving scarce organs to first-time candidates.

The question of whether downgrading retransplant candidates will lead to greater overall benefit from the transplant system is an empirical question that cannot be answered in the abstract. The answer will depend on the current state of medical science and the relative risk of rejection for first-time and repeat transplants, as well as how much the reduction in status of the retransplant patient will influence the behavior of patients and surgeons.

Deontologists and Retransplants

By way of contrast, deontologists are not as worried about the possibility of a higher failure rate for retransplants or even the incentive to decline marginal organs. Rather, they are concerned about treating the potential recipients on the wait list fairly.

Getting More Than a Fair Share

Some may intuitively feel that there is something unfair about giving someone a shot at a second graft when others are still in line for their first. We all have egalitarian instincts about some distributions. No one gets seconds on dessert until everyone has had firsts.

The assumption for desserts, however, is that "need" is not a critical issue. No one can be said to "need" two desserts. Having received a first portion, the recipient has no particular claim to a second. In the case of organs, however, receiving a graft that fails leaves one in a situation as bad as or worse than someone waiting for the first graft. If "fair shares" are proportional to need, then the person with organ failure from the first graft has a need that is, in general, equal to the need of the first-time transplant candidates on the list.

Retransplants Are at Most Indirectly Relevant

The Ethics Committee of the United Network for Organ Sharing, when it considered retransplants, came to the reasonable conclusion that when people are in organ failure, the crucial issue is not whether one has had a previous graft. The other variables that go into organ allocation—factors such as human leukocyte antigen–match, medical urgency, panel-reactive antibodies, or time on the wait list depending on the organ—are what are morally relevant, not whether one has received a previous graft. Assuming that the candidate for a retransplant was not considered personally responsible for the first graft's failure—through refusal to take antirejection medication or otherwise failure to maintain the prescribed follow-up regimen—the fact that the candidate was the recipient of a previous graft is morally irrelevant to the person concerned with equity in allocation. Just like the multi-organ problem, retransplants are not directly relevant to organ allocation. At most, they will indirectly influence the factors considered relevant, such as the likelihood of success and likelihood of finding another suitable organ.

Although utilitarians might be perplexed about whether to take a need for multiple organs or retransplants into account, deontologists who are committed to equality of opportunity for the resources needed to be healthy will not consider either to be morally relevant. In current policy the deontologists had mostly carried the day. However, the most recent kidney allocation algorithm does include a matching of the top 20 percent of kidneys with the top 20 percent of candidates, defined as candidates with the longest EPTS. One of the factors included in the EPTS calculation is whether a candidate is a former transplant recipient. This means that retransplant candidates will not be ranked in the top 20 percent of candidates, and will only be eligible for the other 80 percent of kidneys, like 80 percent of their peers. (The new allocation system is described in detail in chapter 20.) This is, then, the first allocation algorithm that does give retransplant candidates lower priority but only for the best kidneys. Retransplant candidates remain on an equal footing with the other 80 percent of candidates for the other 80 percent of kidneys to be allocated.

In general, there is also no penalty for being a candidate for multiple organs. In fact, in some cases, multi-organ candidates get priority, which should really perplex the utilitarian. Let us explain why this is so. A person who needs two organs—say, for example, a liver and a heart—will be placed on both lists; and when he or she is offered an organ from either list, he or she will be offered both organs from the same donor. The justification for doing this is efficiency—it makes no sense to give one organ if the person needs two lifesaving organs, because unless he or she gets both, he or she will die. If a heart becomes available, then he or she will get both organs, even if it means skipping ahead of the liver wait list. Governor Casey of Pennsylvania (who is discussed in detail in chapter 21) needed this combination—a heart and a liver.

But we also allow patients to get both organs, even if one is not lifesaving. Consider, for example, the patient with diabetes who is listed for a kidney and a pancreas. Now the patient could do well enough with a new kidney and remain on his insulin regimen, but given the policy that both organs are given when the patient gets an offer for either organ because he or she has made it to the top of that wait list, the patient with diabetes who is offered a pancreas (which is the organ with the shorter wait time) will get both a kidney and a pancreas from the same donor. Now the pancreas wait list is shorter, and pancreatic grafts must come from relatively "healthy" deceased donors. Thus, the multi-organ transplant candidate will get a high-quality kidney faster than most because he gets to jump ahead on the kidney wait list.

Public Opinion

Although there is not a large literature on public attitudes about organ allocation in the United States and internationally, what data do exist show mixed attitudes about focusing exclusively on utility or fairness. And though we could not find any empirical survey data about public opinion about the fairness of multi-organ transplants, we did find a number of surveys that examined public opinion about retransplantation.

In a study of attendees at the Pittsburgh Botanical Gardens annual flower show, Peter Ubel and George Loewenstein surveyed 138 individuals about how to distribute scarce deceased donor livers. In one group, the subjects were told that a candidate had either a 70 percent or 30 percent chance of surviving based on a "blood marker"; in the second group, the same odds were given, but they were based on the fact that primary transplants have a better prognosis than retransplants. They found that subjects answering the retransplantation survey trended toward giving preference to the better prognostic group (although it was not statistically significant). They also found that fewer than one-fifth of all respondents were willing to give all the available organs to the better prognostic group, expressing some interest in benefiting those who were "worst off."[6]

Ubel and Lowenstein concluded that their study confirmed other health policy research that found that the public does not act strictly in a utilitarian fashion. However, they also argued that their data supported the "public's preference that retransplant status be taken into consideration as an allocation criterion."[7] How much of a consideration, however, is debatable. First, the survey suggested that the difference in outcome between primary and retransplantation was 40 percent survival, which was an exaggeration even back in the early 1990s. For the decade 1988–96, the liver one-year graft survival rate was 79.1 percent for the first transplant and 55.0 percent for the retransplant.[8] Second, even with a 40 percent survival difference, 19 of 71 (27 percent) respondents given the retransplant survey thought the livers should be allocated equally between the two groups, and only 18 percent thought that all the kidneys should be allocated to primary transplant recipients.

Like Ubel and Loewenstein, Julie Ratcliffe in the United Kingdom (2000) looked at public preference in the allocation of liver transplantation by inviting a convenience sample of academic and nonacademic employees of a British university to participate in a survey in which they were asked to allocate 100 donor liver grafts between two groups of 100 individuals.[9] The survey manipulated various efficiency and efficacy factors: length of time spent waiting, life-years gained following transplantation, age, personal responsibility for their illness, and whether they were primary or retransplant candidates. Of 303 completed questionnaires, only 2 respondents (0.7 percent) consistently gave all organs to highest expected survival; and 7 (2 percent) were allocated in a strict egalitarian fashion. Everyone else balanced efficiency and equity. Of the five factors, the issue of primary transplant versus retransplant was ranked either fourth or fifth in importance by 70.6 percent of respondents. "Survival and benefit" was ranked first, followed by younger age, longer wait time, and naturally occurring liver disease.[10]

In 2006 Chan and colleagues surveyed participants from Hong Kong households regarding the allocation of deceased donor livers. They used the same five criteria as Ratcliffe in the United Kingdom and found that survival and benefit and younger age were the most important factors and that first transplant over a retransplant was the least important. Interestingly, though 91 percent of their respondents agreed or strongly agreed that priority should be given to those most likely to survive and benefit from a transplant, when the participants were asked to allocate a finite number of donor livers, they preferred giving priority to patients who had waited the longest, again showing their preference to balance equity with efficiency.[11]

Thus, two conclusions follow from the diverse public opinion surveys regarding organ allocation: (1) whether a wait list candidate needs a primary versus a retransplant is not that important; and (2) the principle of efficiency alone is not adequate for an organ allocation policy.

Splitting Organs and Combining Organs

One final issue needs to be taken up in this chapter. It is an issue closely related to multiple and repeat transplants. We now know that, just as we can procure a liver or lung lobe from a living donor, we can also divide these organs when procured from deceased donors. We, in effect, can decide to give a deceased donor liver to one large recipient or two smaller ones. The traditional split liver gave the larger graft to a small adult and the smaller graft to a child. This has been instrumental in reducing pediatric mortality on the deceased donor wait list.[12] However, there is controversy in the literature whether the outcome for the adult is as good as it would have been if the adult had received the whole liver graft.[13] Outcomes when livers are split to create two grafts for smaller adults are not as good,[14] and such transplants are often characterized as experimental, but they do help two adult individuals and so the overall benefit is greater.[15] For example, the data by Aseni and colleagues found 63.3 percent survival for each of the two adult split liver recipients, compared with 83.1 percent for the whole liver recipient. In the United States, the rate of split liver transplants remains at less than 5 percent of all liver transplants, and these are mainly transplants involving a child and an adult.[16]

At the other extreme, we know that at the extremes of ages, kidneys may be allocated as a pair (it is called en bloc in infants because they are procured together, and dual kidneys in the elderly). The data show that the youngest kidneys and older kidneys have a lower graft survival rate when allocated and procured as single kidneys. The data show that pediatric en bloc kidneys from donors older than one year of age have excellent outcomes, comparable to living donor kidney transplants.[17] For donors older than one year, some argue that all the kidneys should be allocated as single kidney transplants because this increases overall community graft survival in that it gives a kidney to two candidates rather than giving both kidneys to one candidate, even though each of the two candidates gets a kidney with a lower graft survival than the one candidate who would otherwise receive the en bloc kidneys.[18] Others argue not to divide kidneys procured en bloc because the excellent outcomes will encourage transplant surgeons to use these kidneys rather than discard them due to fears of primary graft failure in small kidneys.

Similar arguments are given about allocating dual kidneys from older donors, particularly those older kidneys that are from donors who are very old or sicker at the time of procurement. Dual kidney transplants from these more "marginal donors" appear to have outcomes similar to other expanded criteria donor kidneys (in contrast to en bloc young kidneys, which are comparable to the best deceased donor kidneys if not to living donor kidneys). Again, the argument in favor of giving two kidneys to one candidate is to encourage the use of these marginal kidneys rather than see them discarded. Currently, however, there is no strict policy about how the very young and very old kidneys are procured and/or allocated. A policy that delineated specific criteria about when to procure kidneys en bloc and when to allocate them to one or two candidates would have the advantage of providing equal circumstances for all candidates and would not leave the decision to the whim of a particular organ procurement organization or transplant team.

The moral analyses for split livers and dual kidney transplants are quite similar to those provided for multiple and repeat transplants. From the point of view of the utilitarian, the payoff from dividing deceased donor organs, when it is technically feasible to do so, is about 150 to 175 percent, compared with transplanting these organs to a single recipient. From the utilitarians' perspective, there is good reason to increase the expected benefit when a scarce organ is allocated.

From the point of view of the deontologist, however, such a policy raises serious questions of fairness. If two candidates are on the wait list, each of whom needs a life-saving organ such as a liver, the principle of justice requires that, other things being equal, they deserve an equal opportunity to receive the organ. Hence, among those in the same category for degree of urgency, the same blood type, and the like, allocation would either have to be made on the basis of time on the wait list or by some random method such as flipping a coin. From the point of view of the individuals who both want to live, giving advantage to one recipient because he or she is smaller seems unfair.

Justice, at least as we have interpreted it, however, requires opportunities for equality of access to organs. We saw in the previous chapter that a principle of equality of opportunity may still leave open the possibility that some people have had their opportunities and not taken advantage of them. So, for example, if two adults were competing for a liver and one candidate had a much larger body mass (large enough so that he would require an entire liver) and the other candidate was sufficiently tiny that a single lobe of the liver would suffice, someone who believed that voluntary lifestyle choices that can contribute to body mass would need to assess whether the candidates' relative size was voluntary and what role these choices played in determining whether they could make do with a lobe rather than a whole organ. If the larger candidate's size were seen as fully within the recipient's control, then in theory they could be said to have had an opportunity to be of a sizc at which only a lobe was required.

It is rather easy to see how problematic such reasoning is in the case of body size. Those doing the allocating must determine the extent to which body size was voluntary, as opposed to genetically or psychologically determined. The problems seem insurmountable. Even if we were to decide as a society that certain behaviors (e.g., alcoholism) are sufficiently voluntary that they should count against a candidate in an organ allocation, it seems even more troublesome to apply this approach to matters of body size. Certainly some large people are large because of voluntary behaviors (e.g., overeating, inadequate exercise, drinking), whereas others are large due to factors beyond their control (e.g., genetics). Deciding which people should be given lower priority on the basis of body size would pose overwhelmingly difficult problems.

If that is the case, then deontologists will be firm in their conclusion that all people with an equal need for an organ should have an equal opportunity to obtain one, regardless of the fact that some will need an entire organ while others can make do with only part of one. This is simply one more case where we choose to make our organ allocation formulas somewhat less efficient in order to make them more fair. The appropriate policy seems to be one in which, when an organ becomes available, it is allocated on the basis of a standardized formula that takes both equity and efficiency into account. If the organ goes to an adult who needs the whole organ, that ends the story. If it goes to an adult who needs only part of an organ, it could be split, with the second portion going to the next available person on the wait list who could use a split organ.

A related problem exists in deciding whether to allocate an organ to an adult or a child. There may be good moral reasons why children deserve priority, independent of the fact that they could use only a part of an organ, thus making the transplant system produce more aggregate benefit. Before determining whether children deserve priority for a liver lobe over an adult who would need the entire organ, we need to examine the role of age in allocation, to which we now turn.

Notes

1. Based on Frazier L, "Wheaton family's dream comes true: After a five-year wait, 13-year-old gets a multiple-organ transplant," *Washington Post*, May 17, 1998; Frazier L, "Wheaton boy's transplants

fail," *Washington Post*, June 3, 1998; Goldstein A, "13-year-old undergoes history-making surgery: Boy gets 3rd multiple-organ transplant," *Washington Post*, June 23, 1998; and Pressley SA, "Recovery leads to fast-food heaven: After multiple transplants, Md. teen is finally able to eat again," *Washington Post*, Oct. 11, 1998.

2. Menzel PT, "Rescuing lives: Can't we count?" *Hastings Center Report* 1994;24 (1): 22–23.

3. "One North Valley man is beating the odds after facing a medical condition that almost cost him his life," Fresno, CA: KFSN-TV/DT, May 24, 2012, http://abclocal.go.com/kfsn/story?section = news/local&id = 8675721.

4. *HRSA SRTR Scientific Registry of Transplant Recipients*, source OPTN/SRTR data as of Oct. 1, 2010: table 13.10, "Unadjusted graft survival, heart-lung transplants survival at 3 months, 1 year, 5 years and 10 years"; table 11.10, "Unadjusted graft survival heart transplants survival at 3 months, 1 year, 5 years and 10 years"; table 12.10, "Unadjusted graft survival, deceased donor lung transplants survival at 3 months, 1 year, 5 years and 10 years." Conversely, one- and five-year graft survival of kidney-pancreas is 93 percent and 79.9 percent, which is better than one- and five-year survival of all deceased donor kidney transplants with one- and five-year survival of 91.7 percent and 70.8 percent. Table 5.10C, "Unadjusted graft survival, deceased donor kidney transplants survival at 3 months, 1 year, 5 years, and 10 years," but equivalent at one year to non-ECD kidney transplants (a fairer comparison as pancreata can only be procured from non-ECD donors). Non-ECD kidneys have a one- and five-year survival of 92.8 percent and 73.2 percent; table 5.10a, "Unadjusted graft survival, deceased donor non-ECD kidney transplants survival at 3 months, 1 year, 5 years, and 10 years." These data are much better than pancreas-transplant-alone transplants; table 6.10, "Unadjusted graft survival, pancreas transplant alone (PTA), transplants survival at 3 months, 1 year, 5 years and 10 years."

5. Dworkin R, "What is equality? Part 1: Equality of welfare," *Philosophy and Public Affairs* 1981;10 (3): 185–246; Dworkin R, "What is equality? Part 2: Equality of resources," *Philosophy and Public Affairs* 1981;10 (4): 283–345; Veatch RM, *The foundations of justice: Why the retarded and the rest of us have claims to equality* (New York: Oxford University Press, 1986).

6. Ubel PA, Loewenstein G, "The efficacy and equity of retransplantation: An experimental survey of public attitudes," *Health Policy* 1995;34: 145–51.

7. Ibid.

8. US Scientific Registry for Transplant Recipients and Organ Procurement and Transplantation Network, *1997 annual report of the US Scientific Registry for Transplant Recipients and the Organ Procurement and Transplantation Network: Transplant data, 1988–1996* (Richmond and Rockville, MD: United Network for Organ Sharing and Division of Transplantation, Office of Special Programs, Health Resources and Services Administration, US Department of Health and Human Services, 1996), table 30.

9. Ratcliffe J, "Public preferences for the allocation of donor liver grafts for transplantation," *Health Economics* 2000;9 (2): 137–48.

10. Ibid.

11. Chan HM, Cheung GMY, Yip AKW, "Selection criteria for recipients of scarce donor livers: A public opinion survey in Hong Kong," *Hong Kong Medical Journal* 2006;12: 40–46.

12. Hong JC, Yersiz H, Busuttil RW, "Where are we today in split liver transplantation?" *Current Opinion in Organ Transplantation* 2011;16: 269–73.

13. The data are summarized by Hong et al., "Where are we today," who refers to split livers for an adult and child recipient as "conventional split-liver transplantation" to distinguish from adult-to-adult split liver transplantation. On p. 269, Hong cites references that show that the results seem to depend on whether the study uses pooled registry data or only examined results from specialized centers. See also ibid., data on p. 272, table 2, where conventional split-liver transplantation data are presented.

14. Aseni P, De Feo TM; De Carlis L, et al., on behalf of Split-Liver Study Group, "A prospective policy development to increase split-liver transplantation for 2 adult recipients: Results of a 12-year multicenter collaborative study," *Annals of Surgery* 2014;259: 157–65.

15. See Aseni et al., "Prospective policy development"; Hong et al., "Where are we today."

16. Berg CL, Steffick DE, Edwards EB, et al., "Liver and intestine transplantation in the United States 1998–2007," *American Journal of Transplantation* 2009;9 (part 2): 907–31.

17. Bhayana S, Kuo YF, Madan P, et al., "Pediatric en bloc kidney transplantation to adult recipients: More than suboptimal?" *Transplantation* 2010;90 (3): 248–54; Sharma A, Fisher RA, Cotterell AH, King AL, Maluf DG, Posner MP, "En-bloc kidney transplantation from pediatric donors: Comparable outcomes with living donor kidney transplantation," *Transplantation* 2011;92 (5): 564–69.

18. Sureshkumar KK, Patel AA, Arora S, Marcus RJ, "When is it reasonable to split pediatric en bloc kidneys for transplantation into two adults?" *Transplantation Proceedings* 2010;42 (9): 521–23.

Chapter 20

The Role of Age in Allocation

In this chapter we consider what legitimate role age should play in allocation. It is widely believed that there are utilities in allocating organs to younger people, but some believe that fairness also is a relevant issue and would proscribe a categorical exclusion of older candidates. Many have held that fairness requires giving older persons equal consideration for an organ, even if efficiency does not. And yet equal consideration does not necessarily mean that older persons must be offered the same organs as their younger counterparts, and it leaves open the possibility of some degree of age matching of donors and recipients. Here we present a new argument suggesting that justice or fairness actually requires differential treatment of the elderly in allocating organs. We also address the question of whether it is equitable to give children special priority for organs.

The Moral Norms for Allocation

In chapter 17, we suggested that there are basically three general criteria for allocating any good including organs: efficiency, incorporating the principle of utility; equity, incorporating the principle of justice; and the right of refusal, incorporating the principle of autonomy. The National Organ Transplant Act of 1984 specifically required that organ allocation achieve both efficiency and equity, and this mandate was reaffirmed in the Final Rule that was promulgated by the Department of Health and Human Services on March 16, 2000, to "establish a regulatory framework for the structure and operations of the Organ Procurement and Transplantation Network."[1] With respect to the allocation of organs, section 121.8 requires that the Board of Directors establish "policies for the equitable allocation of cadaveric organs among potential recipients."[2] The allocation policies were to be designed to avoid wasting organs, to avoid futile transplants, to promote patient access to transplantation, and to promote the efficient management of organ placement—that is, they were to consider both equity and efficiency. Autonomy played a minor role, mainly in the context of declining an organ.

Efficiency (Utility)

As we have seen, most physicians are implicitly committed to a kind of utilitarian perspective. They believe the morally relevant feature of a choice is its consequences. They are often Hippocratic in their concern about consequences. They include only consequences for the patient; but when they are forced into a role in social policy questions, they continue to take the utilitarian perspective, simply shifting to the goal of maximizing aggregate consequences, taking into account all affected parties.

This utilitarian perspective leads to the conclusion that organs should be allocated in the way they will do the most good. Although some try to take into account the social benefits of alternative uses of organs, we have seen that for transplants, most people agree to limit their attention to medical benefits. Age can be important in assessing medical benefits.

The Consequentialist Argument for Taking Age into Account

The most obvious relevance of age in predicting benefit is that an organ, if transplanted into an elderly person, will produce time-limited medical benefit. Even if the graft does not fail, other medical problems will predictably lead to death. However, death with a functioning graft is not only a problem for the elderly kidney transplant recipient but also for all patients over the age of forty years.[3] In fact, in kidney allocation, the only group for which the leading cause of graft loss was not death was that consisting of patients younger than forty years, for whom the main cause of kidney graft loss was chronic allograft nephropathy. Coronary vascular disease was the primary cause of death in all age groups, followed by infection. In liver transplantation, using livers procured by donation after circulatory death (DCD), recipient age of greater than fifty-five years was associated with graft failure and patient mortality.[4] In heart transplantation, three recipient factors were found to be associated with one-year graft failure in a multivariate model: older age, increasing serum creatinine, and mechanical ventilation before heart transplant. "Moreover, each decade increase in recipient age was associated with a 20 percent increase in odds of one-year graft failure (odds ratio, 1.02; 95 percent confidence interval, 1.01 to 1.04; $p = 0.005$)."[5]

These data clearly do not support the conclusion that transplants into old people are doomed to fail, but only that these recipients do worse statistically. If one believes that our scarce organ resources should be allocated so they will do the most medical good, a case can be made that old age should count against a patient. At least if medical good is defined as we did in chapter 17—as maximizing the expected number of quality-adjusted life-years per organ transplanted—then targeting younger recipients will produce more medical good.

The Consequentialist Argument against Taking Age into Account

At this stage of the argument, a sophisticated consequentialist may point out that there are also predictable disutilities of preferentially allocating organs to younger patients. Some elderly patients may actually do quite well. Moreover, if we know that the organ allocation formula is designed to discriminate against the elderly, those who have elderly relatives will be distressed at the thought that their loved ones will be forced to die for a lack of organs. In fact, we ourselves may worry about our future old age, knowing that we will not be able to get the organ we need. These factors should count against excluding the elderly from the organ allocation system.

The problem with this counterargument is that although some elderly patients may do well, we have seen that statistically they will not do as well and for as long as younger persons would with the same organs. And though we might be distressed at the thought of excluding the elderly, we should also be distressed at least as much at the thought of young persons dying because the available organ went to an older person.

A second counterargument against discriminating against the elderly for deceased donor transplants is that this may lead to more older candidates seeking living donors. It is more likely that the living donor will be a younger relative, given that older candidates are often excluded from living donation due to co-morbidities. From a justice perspective, a living donor graft does not deprive other candidates on the wait list, so this is not a problem. And yet, from a utility perspective, the elderly do not need living donor grafts, which have the longest graft survival rates, and so this exposes living donors to risks, even though their recipients cannot get the full benefit of the organ.

The problem with this counterargument is that living donors are not a public good but a private good over which society has no control. And yet, data show that when policies change with regard to deceased donor allocation, the policies have an impact on living donor practices. The clearest example in this regard was Share 35, a policy that gave children younger than eighteen years of age priority for deceased donors younger than thirty-five years. The implementation of this policy led to fewer living donations to children younger than eighteen years.[6] So a policy that increases deceased donation to young adults may lead to fewer living donors to this age group, an age group that currently receives more than 50 percent of its organs from living donors.

On balance, medical utility does support some degree of discrimination against the elderly, although this is mitigated by the potential unintended consequences that such a practice may have. At most, age is a morally relevant factor, but it should be a relative and not an absolute contraindication against the allocation of organs to the elderly.

Equity (Justice)

Equity in organ allocation refers to fairness in allocation. It may or may not be in tension with efficiency (maximizing graft and/or patient survival).

The Case That Equity Requires Avoiding Discrimination against the Elderly

The case for nondiscriminatory organ allocation to older persons is often made in terms of equity or justice. It is derived from a more general concern about the injustice of discriminating against the elderly.[7] The argument is that even if it would be more efficient to give the organs to younger persons, doing so would be unfair. The elderly deserve "equal treatment." To do otherwise would be "ageism"—immoral, unfair treatment of the elderly. Those who suggest that equity requires nondiscrimination against the elderly claim that justice requires treating similarly situated people equally and that those who are the sickest deserve priority, even if it is not always the most efficient use of resources. They claim that all persons who are equally sick deserve equal treatment, regardless of age.

The Case That Equity Requires Discrimination against the Elderly

Although the justice-based argument in favor of equal treatment of the elderly comes easily, recent scholarship on the ethics of age has suggested that the picture is more complex. Whether these more complex, justice-based arguments in support of allocating organs preferentially to younger people succeed is a matter of considerable current controversy.

It should be apparent that the claim that justice requires giving the elderly who are equally needy equal access to organs depends on what in chapter 17 we called "present need" or perhaps "urgency." The results turn out to be quite different if we introduce the concept of "over-a-lifetime need." The arguments here are worth examining, and at least three different arguments have surfaced—suggesting that to be *fair*, one should take age into account in allocating organs.

THE NOTION OF A NATURAL LIFE SPAN

Daniel Callahan, the former director of the Hastings Center, has gained considerable notoriety for his advocacy of the view that humans have a natural life span and that it is hubris to strive to prolong life indefinitely beyond its natural endpoint with expensive, exotic medical technologies.[8] He would include organ transplants in this group of technologies that merely postpone the inevitable, depriving others of what they need to merely get up to their normal years.

He stresses that those who have completed their life span should still be treated humanely—they should receive pain-relieving medications; compassionate, high-quality care; and simple treatments for acute illness—but he would draw the line at expensive, resource-consuming treatments for chronic illnesses, such as those requiring an organ transplant. It is not that transplanting organs is inefficient for the elderly, although it may be. It is rather that continuing to pursue more days of life misunderstands our natural limits and is unfair to others who have not yet reached their natural end.

Even for those like Callahan who accept the notion of a natural limit to the life span, this approach raises some problems. For one, as a practical matter, if we were to incorporate this notion into our organ allocation policy we would need to set a specific, recognizable point when one is no longer eligible for organs. Callahan has variously put this point at age seventy-five and in the late seventies or early eighties.[9] But that is not specific enough to establish a cutoff point for entitlement to organs. We would need a specific, sharp line, but one that results in a much too dramatic change, so that the day before one's critical birthday one would have full entitlement, but the next day one would have none. That cutoff point would be arbitrary, would be hard to enforce, and would have the appearance of being unfair.[10] Moreover, this notion of a natural life span does not seem to provide any theoretical basis for continuing to provide treatment for acute illness, pain relief, and good nursing while expensive treatment for chronic illness is excluded.

THE PRUDENTIAL LIFE SPAN ACCOUNT

Norman Daniels, a philosopher at the Harvard University School of Public Health, developed a second justice-based argument for allocating health resources based on age that can be adapted to justify organ allocation with priority for younger persons.[11] He points out that allocating resources among different age groups can be reconceptualized as allocation to a single person among different stages of his or her life span. Assuming we live a full life span, we each pass through each of life's stages. It is unrealistic to assume that we are entitled to the same kinds of health care resources at the various stages of our lives. What is needed for adolescence may be less important for middle-aged adults; treatments crucial for these ages may not be as fitting for old age, while other services may be more essential. For instance, young adult females who are infertile and wish to become pregnant seem obviously to have a different claim on health insurance for infertility treatment than do postmenopausal women with a similar desire.

Daniels claims that it is a matter of prudence how we allocate our resources among the various stages of our lives. As long as all with similar needs at a particular stage are treated equally, it is not unfair that our entitlements change from one stage to another.

Daniels's account goes a long way toward overcoming the problems not only with utilitarian-based rationing by age but also those growing out of a notion of a natural life span. Still, it raises problems. Most critically, Daniels does not directly tell us which age groups have claims and what kinds of claims they have. In fact, he suggests that this is a matter of mere prudent judgment, rather than there being some intrinsic moral reason to choose one age group over another. On the contrary, there may be sound moral reasons why one *ought* to give priority to younger persons.[12] Moreover, he assumes that all persons pass through all the life stages. In fact, people who are candidates for a major organ transplant may not all have an opportunity to live through all life stages if they do not receive the transplant. We need an account that explains which age groups have which claims—in particular, which have claims to transplantable organs.

THE JUSTICE-OVER-A-LIFETIME ARGUMENT

In the first edition of this book, it was suggested that another approach to allocation by age be used, one from the perspective of justice that focuses on benefiting the worst off and how we determine who is worst off. It emphasizes that there are two different ways of thinking about who is worst off. The first, which can be called the "slice-of-time perspective," asks who is worst off at a given moment of time. This is the view taken by those who advocate equal access to organs for those who are equally sick, regardless of age. This can also be called the "present need" view.

But there is a second way to think about who is worst off. We call this the "over-a-lifetime perspective."[13] Others have referred to it as the "fair innings" argument.[14] It so dominates Frances Kamm's approach that she uses it as the only meaning of need.[15] It asks who is worst off considering peoples' whole lives. From the slice-of-time perspective, a forty-year-old and a seventy-year-old both dying of heart failure are equally poorly off; but considering their entire lives, who could deny that the one who has been healthy enough to make it to seventy is much better off? To be fair, we need to allocate our resources so that the forty-year-old has a chance to make it to seventy. From this over-a-life-time perspective, justice requires that we target organs to these younger persons who are so poorly off that they will not make it to old age without being given special priority. Therefore, the younger the age of the person needing an organ, the higher his or her claim to it. Moreover, in contrast to the utilitarian principle, which would give attention to physiological age, this justice-based perspective would focus on chronological age, something that is much easier to determine.[16]

Autonomy

On the question of the role of age in allocation, autonomy plays a small but growing role. When autonomy is interpreted to refer to "liberty rights"—that is, the right to be left alone or to refuse to participate in a transplant—then patient autonomy supports the right of patients to decline organs if they consider themselves too old to endure the surgery. It also supports the right of patients to refuse organs from donors whom they consider to be too old.

Autonomy has also been used to refer to individual choice, which has taken on growing importance given the greater willingness in the past decade to procure older organs, which have a higher rate of graft failure. The allocation method for kidneys that was in place at the time that this book was being written divided kidneys into two categories: standard criteria donors (SCDs) and expanded criteria donors (ECDs). An ECD was defined in 2001 as any kidney whose relative risk of graft failure exceeded 1.7 when compared with a reference group of ideal donor kidneys. ECD kidneys include all kidneys from donors older than sixty years and kidneys from donors fifty to fifty-nine years with two of the following co-morbidities: hypertension, terminal serum creatinine greater than 1.5 milligrams per deciliter, or death from cerebrovascular accident. All wait list candidates are registered for SCD kidneys. The United Network for Organ Sharing (UNOS) implemented the ECD category in 2002. Whereas some US transplant centers initially listed all patients on the ECD wait list, UNOS policy requires that patients consent to such listing. At some institutions, very few older candidates are listed for ECD, whereas in other centers, virtually all older candidates are listed. The difference depends in part on the attitudes of the transplant team and in part on the average wait time. Ideally, such a decision is reached through a shared decision between a candidate and the transplant team and would reflect a number of factors, including human leukocyte antigen (HLA), *panel reactive antibodies*, blood type, life expectancy on dialysis, and life expectancy with a transplant, as well as personal factors such as quality of life on dialysis and how urgently one wants the transplant. In 2006 Schold and Hall showed that older patients, who have a higher risk of dying on dialysis, do better accepting an ECD kidney rather than waiting for an SCD organ.[17] Other individuals who are doing poorly on dialysis may also benefit from listing for an ECD kidney.[18]

Allocation to Minors

Within several years of the development of the UNOS registry in 1987, children were being given priority points for kidney allocation. Initially children under six years of age received 2 points and children under eleven years received 1 point. Over the intervening two decades, additional priority has been given to children, and the age of minority has expanded to include all individuals younger than eighteen years. In 2005 UNOS implemented the policy known as Share 35, which gives all minors younger than eighteen years priority for kidneys from deceased donors younger than thirty-five years that are not shared mandatorily for zero HLA-mismatching, for combined renal/nonrenal organ allocation, or locally for prior living organ donors. The impact of Share 35 has been shorter wait times for children, who now receive some of the most ideal SCD organs, although it has also had the unintended consequence of decreasing HLA-matching and decreasing living donations to children so that overall efficiency has improved less than it could have.

There are two reasons why giving priority to children can be justified. First, medical utility justifies giving priority to children because they would get the benefit for a longer time than many adults. Giving priority to children can also be justified on both interpretations of benefiting the worst off. Children are worst off with the over-a-lifetime argument because they developed end-stage organ failure at a younger age. And from the slice-of-time perspective, children are worst off because organ failure interferes with neurological development, which they can never make up.[19]

Allocation algorithms for other organs also give significant advantage to minors. The Model for End-Stage Liver Disease (MELD), adopted in 2002, has a parallel model for children called Pediatric End-State Liver Disease (PELD). Both MELD and PELD estimate the risk of ninety-day wait list mortality in order to allocate organs in a way that minimizes death on the wait list. Today, minors get priority for liver allocation in three ways. First, PELD gives greater priority to children because the same MELD and PELD scores receive the same priority for a liver, even though the score in an adult indicates a greater mortality risk. Second, pediatric candidates younger than twelve years get priority to receive livers from pediatric donors younger than eighteen years over adults with the same score. And third, individuals can be granted exception points in cases of chronic liver disease because these cases are poorly captured by PELD scores alone. For example, children with metabolic liver disease may have a low PELD score, and yet liver failure interferes with their growth and development. MELD/PELD and the exception points have successfully benefited children, who are now less likely to die on the wait list.

Splitting deceased donor organs is another way to increase the number of pediatric liver candidates who get a liver graft in a timely fashion. Current UNOS policy (as of June 2013) permits transplant centers to decide whether to participate in segmental transplantation and allows candidates to elect whether to receive a segmental transplant. Of course, in allocation, not only willingness but also the size of the candidate are requirements to avoid small-for-size syndrome (portal hyperperfusion). These priorities for children make sense from both utility and justice perspectives.

Allocation to Older Persons

As we have said, the system of kidney allocation in place until the implementation of the new formula late in 2014 distinguishes between two classes of kidneys, SCD and ECD. Because the wait list for ECD is an opt-in decision, any candidate can be listed, although it is often encouraged for older candidates and discouraged for younger individuals unless they have other health conditions that make it important to get an organ quickly (e.g., poor venous access), or if they are highly sensitized and may find it very difficult to be matched to any kidney. Nevertheless, the vast majority of those who opt in for the ECD wait list are older candidates, which has the unintended consequence that older candidates are more likely to get a deceased donor kidney because they are listed twice—once for an SCD and once for an ECD.[20]

The ECD system in the United States is based on autonomy because one chooses whether to be listed for an ECD kidney. In contrast, in Europe the only kidneys offered to older candidates are older kidneys. The Eurotransplant Senior Program allocation policy, established in January 1999, allocates organs from donors sixty-five years and older to candidates who are sixty-five years and older, and does not permit candidates sixty-five years and older to receive younger kidneys.[21] The policy was based on justice, using an over-the-lifetime perspective. The old-to-old practice has the advantage of allocating older kidneys with shorter long-term graft survival rates to older adults, thereby minimizing the need for retransplant that might occur if older donor kidneys were transplanted into younger recipients. Though restricting older candidates to the Eurotransplant Senior Program also restricts their autonomy, age matching does promote other principles of allocation—utility and justice—that may justify such a restriction.

New Formulas for Taking Age into Account

Although allocation programs such as the separate ECD wait list and the Eurotransplant Senior Program take extreme ages into account, they create artificial, false dichotomies about age. An allocation that takes an over-a-lifetime approach to allocating organs would incorporate the notion that age is one of the morally relevant factors in allocating all organs. The ideal formula would take age into account without making it dominate the allocation.

At the time of this writing, there is considerable interest in new kidney allocation formulas that take age into account without letting it completely dominate. At the UNOS Board of Directors meetings on June 24 and 25, 2013, the proposal from the UNOS Kidney Committee was adopted and is scheduled to take effect in late 2014. We consider this newly adopted proposal and two others in order to provide a context for examining the ethics of age-based allocation. Although one of these proposals has been adopted, our main concern is gaining an understanding of the ways that age can affect the efficiency and equity of allocation formulas. Hence, we consider all three: an earlier UNOS Kidney Committee formula, from February 2011; one we have published previously, which we refer to as "equal opportunity supplemented by fair innings"; and the 2012 Kidney Committee proposal, adopted in June 2013.

The UNOS Kidney Committee's February 2011 Formula

In February 2011 the Kidney Transplant Committee of UNOS proposed a new kidney allocation model colloquially named the 20/80 plan, a proposal that was subsequently abandoned. Here it is useful to examine this plan in some detail.

The Role of Age in the 20/80 Plan

This proposal would have retained Share 35 for the allocation of deceased donor kidneys to children and would still have given special priority to zero-antigen mismatches and prior living donors. Otherwise, candidates and kidneys would have been classified in the top 20 percent or the remaining 80 percent. Candidates would have been classified as in the top 20 percent based on estimated posttransplant survival (EPTS) and, in fact, will be so classified under the newly adopted program discussed below. EPTS is calculated using four criteria: candidate age, length of time on dialysis, any prior organ transplant, and diabetes status. Deceased donor kidneys would have been classified based on a kidney donor profile index (KDPI) that includes ten characteristics: age, race/ethnicity, hypertension, diabetes' creatinine, cerebrovascular cause of death, height, weight, donor after cardiac death, and hepatitis C. The proposed allocation was two tiered; the top 20 percent of kidneys would have been allocated to the top 20 percent of adult candidates, and the remaining 80 percent of kidneys would have been allocated to the remaining 80 percent of recipients using an age-matching formula whereby recipients would have been eligible for kidneys from donors in an age range from fifteen years younger than the recipient to fifteen years older (i.e., ± fifteen years).[22]

The impetus for this proposal was the inefficiency of the kidney allocation system in place at the time. This system mainly focused on the equity principle of queuing based on wait time and what amounts to a lottery among all SCD organs. It included some efficiency considerations (e.g., ABO and HLA matching), but wait time dominated the allocation. As the gap between demand and supply grew, many people felt there was a greater need to make every organ count maximally. The Kidney Committee showed that this model would have improved the life span benefit per transplant from 4.9 to 5.4 years.

Although the justification for the proposal was to increase efficiency, the Kidney Committee noted that a pure age-matching proposal would have actually provided a slightly better life span benefit per transplant, 5.5 years. However, they argued in favor of the 20/80 concept for "greater flexibility."[23]

A Critique of the Proposal

The main problem with the 2011 20/80 proposal—and also with the newly adopted plan scheduled to take effect in late 2014, which also relies on a similar identification of the top 20 percent of donors and recipients—is that it is justified solely on the basis of its efficiency. The issue of equity was not mentioned in the 2011 report, thus violating both the National Organ Transplant Act and the Final Rule, which require that one consider both equity and efficiency concerns. To evaluate equity in the 20/80 proposal, one must consider the top 20 percent and the remaining 80 percent separately, because each component has a different impact on allocation. Even more fundamentally, such an analysis should begin with an explanation from the Kidney Committee of why it chose to have two different rules and how it chose 20/80 versus 25/75 or any other division ratio.

THE TOP 20 PERCENT

When one analyzes the individual components, the rules that establish the 20 percent are inequitable for a variety of reasons. First, the criteria used to determine EPTS single out diabetes as the only health condition that reduces an individual's chance of being ranked in the top 20 percent of candidates. Even though cardiovascular disease is known to have a greater impact on EPTS, UNOS does not have all the data it would need to include cardiovascular disease, and therefore the Kidney Committee chose to ignore it. This is unfair, given that some who are classified in the top 20 percent are known to be less healthy than some who are excluded. It is also problematic, because it discriminates against young individuals who frequently have type 1 diabetes, a genetic condition that they develop through no fault of their own. One could argue that individuals in need of a kidney who also have type 1 diabetes are the "worst off" because they are doubly disadvantaged and furthermore have suffered a health problem since a young age. Egalitarian forms of justice require that any changes in allocation benefit those who are worst off, whereas the way EPTS is defined, the 2011 proposal directly harmed them.

A second problem with the criteria that establish the top 20 percent is that the KDPI is calculated independent of recipient characteristics, although it is known that "the impact of donor risk varies dramatically with respect to recipient race, primary diagnoses, and age."[24] In particular, higher donor risk kidneys are better tolerated by older diabetic and African American recipients, and lower donor risk kidneys have a significantly different graft survival rate, based on different recipient characteristics.

A third problem with the 20 percent portion of the 20/80 proposal is that it is arbitrary in its categorization of the top 20 percent of kidneys and candidates. The methodologies cannot distinguish between a 19 percent and 21 percent kidney or candidate. Even supporters of the system admit that the EPTS calculation will get it right only about 70 percent of the time. (The calculation has a c-statistic estimated to be 0.693, which means that the model is only accurate about 70 percent of the time.) So 30 percent of the time, individuals will be miscategorized. The impact of being placed in the 21st percentile rather than 19th percentile of EPTS is the difference between being eligible for the top 20 percent of kidneys or not. Thus, those in the top 20 percent are more likely to be offered a kidney because they are eligible for 100 percent of kidneys, whereas those who do not make the top 20 percent are only eligible for the remaining 80 percent.

A fourth problem with the 20 percent portion of the 20/80 proposal is that it is based on local candidates being offered the best local kidneys, whereas the data show that both the allocation system that currently exists and the 2011 and 2012 UNOS proposals would be more efficient and more equitable if kidneys were allocated nationally, not locally.[25]

THE REMAINING 80 PERCENT

The policies affecting the group making up the remaining 80 percent also pose problems. In the 2011 proposal the allocation within the 80 percent would have been based on an age-matching rule, which means that younger kidneys would have been matched with younger candidates and older kidneys with older candidates. The rule promotes efficiency by giving younger (a proxy for healthier) kidneys to younger (a proxy for healthier) candidates. By matching young with young and old with old, the rule would have avoided giving a young kidney to an elderly candidate who would die with a functioning graft. The rule also would have promoted equity, whether understood as fair innings, prudential life span equity, or justice over a lifetime. It is fair to give the younger (aka healthier) kidneys to younger candidates, provided that all younger candidates are treated similarly at different stages of life. That is, age matching can be ethically justified on the over-a-lifetime perspective in that younger individuals need a kidney that will last longer given that they have longer expected longevity.

However, a problem with age matching as an exclusive allocation principle is that there is currently a severe mismatch between the age of donors and age of candidates (see figure 20.1). This means that under the age-matching proposal, older candidates would have been offered significantly fewer kidneys than younger candidates, leading to a significant mismatch in opportunity. This would have been efficient but inequitable, to the extent that one believes that all individuals who are ill deserve an equal chance of getting treated.

The Department of Health and Human Services' Criticism of Age Matching

Although many criticized the 20 percent component of the 20/80 rule proposed in 2011, the Department of Health and Human Services' Office of General Counsel and its Office

Figure 20.1   Deceased Donor Kidney Transplants (DDKT) by Donor Age and Wait List Candidates (WLC) by Candidate Age

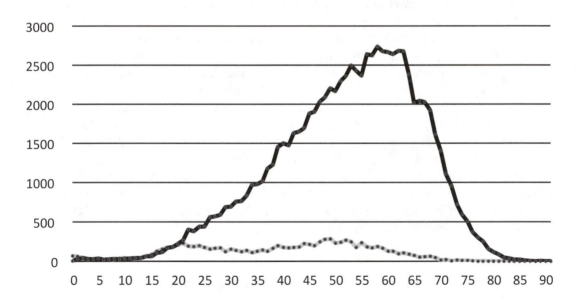

DDKT in 2010 versus WLC on 12/31/2010 by age

<!-- legend -->
▬▬▬ # of DDKT per donor age in 2010   ▬▬▬ WLC per candidate age on 12/31/2010

Note: Discrepancy between age of deceased donors versus age of candidates. Annual number of deceased donor kidney grafts is fairly constant between the ages of 18–55 years, with slight peak at approximately 21 years due to trauma and at approximately age 50 due to cerebrovascular disease. However, there are far fewer young adult candidates (18–35 years) than older candidates (>35 years) up to age 70 years. Thus allocating younger deceased donor kidneys to younger candidates—such as proposed by the algorithms in the UNOS Kidney Concept Paper—without correcting for the mismatch in age distribution of donors and candidates is age discriminatory because it disproportionately allocates deceased donor kidneys to young candidates.

Source: This figure and legend are reprinted with minor modifications with permission from Wiley Publishers, from Ross LF, Parker W, Veatch RM, Gentry S, and Thistlethwaite JR, Jr., "Equal opportunity supplemented by fair innings: Equity and efficiency in allocating deceased donor kidneys, plus appendix," *American Journal of Transplantation* 2012;12: 2115–24, at 2116.

of Civil Rights expressed concern that the use of a ± fifteen-year age matching algorithm, as described in the Kidney Committee proposal (either as the sole algorithm or in combination with the 20/80 proposal), did not meet the requirements of the Age Discrimination Act of 1975.[26] At this point the UNOS Kidney Committee abandoned this proposal. However, James Bowman of the federal government's Division of Transplantation did explain that "according to the stipulations in the act, age may be used if it is a proxy for medical variables."[27]

The UNOS Kidney Committee's September 2012 Formula

In September 2012 the Kidney Committee issued a proposal for another allocation system that was distributed for public comment.[28] This proposal was then adopted by the UNOS Board of Directors in June 2013 and is scheduled to go into effect in late 2014. In this version the Kidney Committee stated that although the existing system's use of wait time may be perceived as fair (i.e., equity as queuing), "it does not strive to minimize death on the wait list nor maximize survival following transplant" (two different ways of evaluating the efficiency of the allocation system).[29] In effect, the committee was restating the complaint that, even if the current allocation was equitable, it failed to be efficient.

The Main Features of the Proposal

The 2012 proposal classifies deceased donor kidneys into four categories based on the quality of the donor kidneys, as measured by the KDPI score. The kidneys are classified as the top 20 percent, the next 15 percent, the next 50 percent, and the poorest 15 percent. These four groups are called sequences A through D, with sequence D being the worst. (The allocation for each sequence is shown in table 20.1.)

The proposal also takes into account several other factors. One is the degree of sensitization to foreign tissues. This is an important equity issue, because highly sensitized candidates find it very difficult to find a suitable kidney match. The allocation in each sequence follows a similar pattern, with distribution first to those candidates who are most highly sensitized.

Another factor taken into account is the extent to which donor and recipient antigens match (a predictor of likelihood of organ rejection). In each sequence, after the highly sensitized candidates, priority goes next to those who have a zero-antigen mismatch with the donor. Giving priority to those candidates who have the best antigen match with the available organ makes the system more efficient by increasing the likelihood of graft survival.

The next factor in priority is whether the candidate is a prior living donor himself or herself. It seems fair to give priority to those who have previously given a kidney, but the priority could also be defended on efficiency grounds if it is likely to increase the likelihood of living donation.

After these considerations, in sequences A and B, minors younger than eighteen years are the next group to be offered a kidney. After minors, in sequence A, the next group to receive a kidney is adults in the top 20 percent EPTS. In sequences B–D, all adult candidates are classified by a point system similar to the current policy, with the qualification that dialysis time is substituted for wait list time (a change discussed below).

Table 20.1 Kidney Allocation According to UNOS, 2012

Sequence A KDPI <= 20%	Sequence B KDPI > 20% but < 35%	Sequence C KDPI >= 35% but <= 85%	Sequence D KDPI > 85%
Local CPRA 100	Local CPRA 100	Local CPRA 100	Local CPRA 100
Regional CPRA 100	Regional CPRA 100	Regional CPRA 100	Regional CPRA 100
National CPRA 100	National CPRA 100	National CPRA 100	National CPRA 100
Local CPRA 99	Local CPRA 99	Local CPRA 99	Local CPRA 99
Regional CPRA 99	Regional CPRA 99	Regional CPRA 99	Regional CPRA 99
National CPRA 99	Local CPRA 98	Local CPRA 98	Local CPRA 98
Local CPRA 98	Zero mismatch	Zero mismatch	Zero mismatch
Zero mismatch (top 20% EPTS)	Prior living organ donor	Prior living organ donor	Local + regional National
Prior living organ donor	Local pediatrics	Local	
Local pediatrics	Local adults	Regional	(All categories in
Local top 20% EPTS	Regional pediatrics	National	sequence D are
Zero mismatch (all)	Regional adults		limited to adult
Local (all)	National pediatrics		candidates)
Regional pediatrics	National adults		
Regional (top 20%)			
Regional all			
National pediatrics			
National (top 20%)			
National (all)			

Note: KDPI = kidney donor profile index; CPRA = calculated panel-reactive antigen (degree of sensitization); EPTS = estimated posttransplant survival.

Source: "Proposal to substantially revise the national kidney allocation system," Sept. 21, 2012, http://optn.transplant.hrsa.gov/PublicComment/pubcommentPropSub_311.pdf.

A Critique of the Proposal

Like the 2011 Kidney Committee proposal, the 2012 proposal does not offer an analysis of what equity principles will guide allocation, nor which efficiency considerations will be given greater priority. Again, this is a violation of both the National Organ Transplant Act and the Final Rule. Reading between the lines, it is clear that the Kidney Committee is focusing on efficiency, as defined by maximizing survival, given the fact that sequence A perpetuates the policy of giving the top 20 percent of kidneys (as defined by KDPI) to the 20 percent of candidates who are predicted to have the longest posttransplant survival time.

The report that supports the 2012 proposal does not provide any systematic analysis of equity—how fair the allocation is. It fails to consider what this new policy will do to those candidates on the wait list, who will predictably be less efficient to treat. For example, older candidates and candidates with diabetes have a higher mortality rate on dialysis. Because they will be excluded from the top 20 percent of EPTS, they are now competing for 80 percent of the kidneys, when they were previously competing for 100 percent of deceased donor kidneys; thus the new policy may increase the death rate because those candidates now remain on the wait list.[30]

From an equity perspective, the main problem with the 2012 proposal (the one that will go into effect in late 2014) is the retention of the 20 percent rule, which was discussed above in the September 2011 proposal. In the newly adopted proposal, all the efficiency gains are achieved by this component, without consideration of equity.

Although the report supporting the recently adopted proposal also fails to discuss what equity factors, if any, were considered in the development of the new allocation program, the new one does incorporate two allocation rules that promote two distinct forms of equity. First, in each sequence, consideration is offered to highly sensitized individuals, allowing them to be considered first for all organs. Although the report does not explore the justification for this policy, highly sensitized individuals are very unlikely to find a match; so to give them any fair chance of finding a match, it is critical that they be considered for a wide range of organs. This allocation rule promotes the equity principle of equal opportunity. Second, although candidates with the top 20 percent EPTS are given priority for kidneys with KDPI in the top 20 percent and children are given priority for kidneys with KDPI in the top 35 percent, most other candidates are selected by using dialysis time, a new criterion that replaces wait list time.

Both wait list time and dialysis time can be considered to be criteria grounded in equity. They are both versions of queuing—first come, first served. We now know, however, that wait list time can introduce unfairness in allocation. Currently, wait list time for a deceased donor kidney is defined as the length of time that a candidate is on the wait list. The candidate begins to accrue time from the moment he or she is listed on the deceased donor wait list. Dialysis time, the alternative being proposed, would begin the clock the moment the patient needs renal replacement therapy and/or has a glomerular filtration rate of less than or equal to 20 milliliters per minute, even if the individual does not get listed for weeks or months. These points will now be retroactively awarded at the time of listing. The change from wait list time to dialysis time improves the equity of the queuing rule, given the barriers that many young and minority patients face when attempting to get listed for a deceased donor kidney.[31] This change to dialysis time is incorporated into the adopted 2012 proposal.

The 2011 20/80 proposal and the more recent adopted 2012 allocation plan are both designed to increase efficiency by getting the best organs to the candidates who will predictably do best with those organs. In the 2012 plan, equity is accounted for by giving priority to highly sensitized patients and by relying on dialysis time; but as in the 2011 proposal, the Kidney Committee has provided no formal equity analysis in the 2012 plan. The Kidney Committee did not justify why it chose to use an efficiency component for 20 percent of the candidates and an equity component for the remaining 80 percent; nor did it provide a moral justification for doing so. Serious public criticism has been voiced about this proposal. Nevertheless, it has been adopted and, at the time of this writing, is scheduled to go into effect in late 2014.

The EOFI Proposal

The Kidney Committee's decision to dismiss age matching due to potential age discrimination concerns failed to consider how age could be ethically incorporated (e.g., if it is a proxy for other medical factors). This has led us, together with colleagues, to propose an alternative that we call "equal opportunity supplemented by fair innings," or EOFI. We agree with the Office of Civil Rights that pure age matching would be discriminatory if used as a solitary allocation principle given the current distribution of deceased donors and candidates. The age-matching algorithm in the original 2011 Kidney Committee proposal would have discriminated against candidates over age sixty. However, the statement by the Office of Civil Rights did leave open the possibility of using age, if it is employed as a proxy for other medical variables.[32] Moreover, good arguments, such as the fair innings (over-a-lifetime fairness) one, suggest that an allocation program that ignores age would actually be unfair. The benefit of using an age-matching type of algorithm is that it can be justified ethically on the grounds of over-a-lifetime equity, and it simultaneously increases efficiency.

The Basics of EOFI

In August 2012 we were part of a research team that published EOFI, an algorithm developed to equitably allocate deceased donor kidneys to adults. (We would leave Share 35 as the allocation policy for pediatric candidates.) The proposal would allocate kidneys following a two-step procedure—with the first step designed to assure equal opportunity to get an organ for all candidates in end-stage renal disease (ESRD); and the second step designed to ensure that those with the greatest medical need for high-quality organs get them based on "fair innings" considerations.

Step One: Equal Opportunity

The first step in the EOFI procedure, equal opportunity, maintains that individuals of all ages should have an equal chance of getting a kidney. The algorithm is designed to give adult wait list candidates of different ages the same chance of getting an organ in any given year. In order to deal with local allocation realities where few candidates of any one particular age may exist, all candidates on the wait list are grouped into candidate age groups. Deceased donor organs are also divided into age-based groups in such a way that any candidate for an organ has the same chance of getting one, regardless of which age group he or she is in. We suggested that the size of the age groups could vary depending on other goals.

Step Two: Fair Innings

The second step in the EOFI procedure, fair innings, maintains that those developing ESRD at younger ages are worse off than those developing ESRD when older because they have had fewer healthy life-years. This second step would direct the better deceased donor kidneys to younger recipients. We proposed using donor age as a proxy for a better kidney.[33] Thus, in step two, kidneys from younger donors are assigned to the younger candidates. We would ensure that recipients in different age groups have the same probability of receiving a kidney by restricting the number of kidneys that are offered to candidates in each candidate age group. Although there is wide variability of donor ages for candidates in each candidate age group in the current system, under EOFI, younger kidneys would be consistently distributed to younger candidates (see figure 20.2).

EOFI is similar to age matching but is more accurately described as age mapping. One difference between age matching in the earlier 2011 Kidney Committee proposal and the age-mapping proposal in EOFI is that the kidney offered to a thirty-five-year-old individual in the age-matching proposal is a kidney from a donor age twenty to fifty years, whereas under age mapping, all thirty-five-year-olds will be offered kidneys from donors younger than thirty-five years (because there are more of these younger donors available and fewer younger candidates). Thus, depending on the size of the donor age group in age matching, young candidates may receive some less optimal kidneys. In contrast, under age mapping, all young candidates will be offered young deceased donor kidneys (where age is a proxy for healthy). Thus, age mapping (younger to younger) is more efficient because the youngest candidates (where age is used as a proxy for the healthiest) are only allocated the best kidneys (kidneys from donors aged eleven to thirty-four). In fact, 90 percent of the kidneys allocated to candidates under fifty years also derive from donors aged eleven to thirty-four.

Now it is the case that some thirty-five-year-old deceased donor kidneys are better than others. Under the 2012 Kidney Committee proposal—the one now adopted by the UNOS Board of Directors—kidneys would be allocated by KDPI rather than age alone. KDPI was designed to reduce the variability in kidney quality, such that the top 20 percent of candidates would get the kidneys that were expected to have the longest expected survival rates. The problem, as we saw, is that KDPI does not include all the important factors that correlate with kidney graft health and ignores all recipient characteristics. Thus, the randomness of kidney quality in KDPI is a limitation of the KDPI calculation, which is a critical component of the model. In contrast, in our EOFI age-mapping proposal, a kidney from a donor of any given age is intentionally assigned randomly—by lottery.

EOFI is a multiprincipled allocation algorithm that gives lexical priority to equity but also improves efficiency. EOFI improves efficiency by allocating younger organs to younger recipients and older organs to older recipients. But unlike the 2011 Kidney Committee proposal, it does so in an equitable way, treating all individuals as having equal worth and deserving of an equal chance for a kidney, even if not the same quality of kidney. Second, the allocation of kidneys using age mapping—a modified, less random approach—can be justified by two conceptions of equity: (1) the principle of fair innings, whereby younger candidates are worse off and should receive younger (using age as a proxy for better) kidneys, to give them the greatest chance of achieving some full life span (per the over-a-lifetime perspective); and (2) the principle of prudential life-span equity, whereby candidates should expect age-matched kidneys because those are similar to the kidneys that they would have had if they had not developed ESRD.

The Limitations of EOFI

EOFI is not yet ready for implementation. There are other issues affecting both equity and efficiency that need to be addressed and would require serious mathematical computation to help make policy decisions. These issues include (1) how to deal with the

Figure 20.2 Percent DDKT by Donor Age under Two Allocation Methods

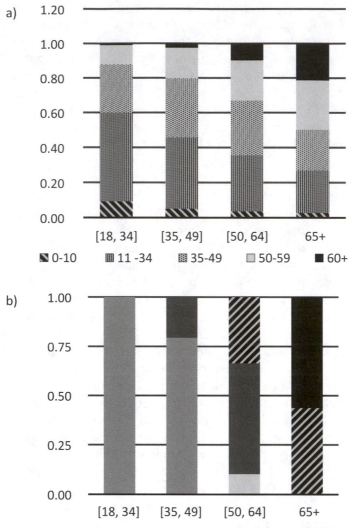

Note: This figure demonstrates the age distribution of deceased donor kidneys to each of the candidate age groups for the year 2010 under two distinct allocation methods. Figure 20.2A shows how organs were actually allocated in 2010 using UNOS data. Note that kidneys of all ages are allocated to WLC of all ages. In contrast, Figure 20.2B demonstrates that Equal Opportunity Fair Innings (EOFI) methodology assigns DD kidneys based on their Donor Age Range (DAR). In the EOFI 2010 projection, all candidates between the ages of 18 and 34 years would have received a DD kidney from a donor younger than 35 years (equivalent to deceased donor kidneys that are allocated under Share 35), and candidates over the age of 65 would have received all of their DD kidneys from donors over the age of 50 years. Note that even for candidates >65 years, 45 percent would come from donors 50–59 such that the average donor age for all kidneys allocated to candidates >65 years would be 59.7 years.

Source: This figure and legend are reprinted with minor modifications with permission from Wiley Publishers, from "Equal opportunity supplemented by fair innings: Equity and efficiency in allocating deceased donor kidneys. Plus Appendix," by Ross LF, Parker W, Veatch RM, Gentry S, and Thistlethwaite JR Jr., *American Journal of Transplantation* 12 (2012): 2115–24, at 2117.

youngest kidneys (e.g., kidneys from donors younger than five years, which have lower graft survival rates and are comparable to some ECD kidneys);[34] (2) how to deal with sensitized patients, former living donors, and zero-antigen mismatches; and (3) what sizes to make the age groups of the transplant candidates and the age ranges of the donors. A strength of this proposal is that these can be varied depending on the size of the groups. If one were to allocate nationally, the age ranges could be very small, but they would need to be enlarged as the area of distribution was reduced. Given improvements in graft function, even with longer cold-ischemia times, allocation based on a larger geographical area would greatly improve equity (an issue discussed further in chapter 22) with minimal impact on efficiency.[35]

Over-a-Lifetime Need versus Present Need

If we are right, using an age-based allocation method is an equitable way to allocate scarce resources. Organs other than kidneys, however, must also take into account the issue of urgency or present need, and we have not yet addressed, in an overall allocation formula, how much weight should be given to present need and how much to age and other over-a-lifetime considerations. This lack of consideration of present need is due, in part, to our focus on kidney allocation, where it receives little attention because dialysis offers a very successful bridge that removes the urgency for transplant except for children, due to the neurological harms of dialysis, and for the rare adult who lack appropriate venous access.

In liver transplantation, however, urgency cannot be ignored. What, for instance, should be done if there are two candidates for a liver: one a twenty-two-year-old who has a MELD score of 25 and the other a sixty-six-year-old who is status 1 (the most urgent status)? On the grounds of present need, the older patient has a higher claim. Furthermore, that person would get the clear preference based on today's allocation formula. However, it is not clear that this is the correct policy. Surely, the fact that the sixty-six-year-old has already had three times the opportunities for living as the twenty-two-year-old is not irrelevant. Yet it is beyond the capacity of this analysis to determine exactly what the relative weights should be for age and medical urgency. If we used the criterion of justice requiring opportunities for equality of quality-adjusted life-years, then the younger patient would have a strong claim, even if his or her healthier status would mean that he or she could be expected to live several more years without a transplant. It is unlikely that he or she would be a liver transplant candidate if he or she had a life expectancy of forty-four years without it.

A subjective judgment will need to be made by policymakers to determine the relative importance of present need, over-a-lifetime need, and medical utility. We would want to give over-a-lifetime need (i.e., age) at least half of the needs-based consideration, but we are unwilling to fully ignore urgency and present need based on the equity principle of equal worth.[36]

Notes

1. Public Law 98-507, Oct. 19, 1984, National Organ Transplant Act, 98 Stat. 2339;"Title 42: Public Health: Chapter 1, Public Health Service, Department of Health and Human Services, Subchapter K,

Health Resources Development, Part 121: Organ Procurement and Transpantation Network," www
.ecfr.gov/cgi-bin/text-idx?c = ecfr&tpl = /ecfrbrowse/Title42/42cfr121_main_02.tpl.

2. Ibid.

3. Morales JM, Marcén R, del Castillo D, et al., "Risk factors for graft loss and mortality after renal transplantation according to recipient age: A prospective multicentre study," *Nephrology Dialysis Transplantation* 2012;27 (suppl 4): iv39–iv46.

4. Mathur AK, Heimbach J, Steffick DE, et al., "Donation after cardiac death liver transplantation: Predictors of outcome," *American Journal of Transplantation* 2010;10: 2512–19.

5. Kilic A, Weiss ES, Arnaoutakis GJ, et al., "Identifying recipients at high risk for graft failure after heart retransplantation," *Annals of Thoracic Surgery* 2012;93 (3): 712–16.

6. Thistlethwaite, JR Jr, Ross LF, "Potential inefficiency of a proposed efficiency model for kidney allocation," *American Journal of Kidney Diseases* 2008;51 (4): 545–48.

7. Churchill LR, "Should we ration health care by age?" *Journal of the American Geriatrics Society* 1988;36: 644–47; Kilner JF, "Age criteria in medicine: Are the medical justifications ethical?" *Archives of Internal Medicine* 1989;149: 2343–46.

8. Callahan D, *Setting limits: Medical goals in an aging society* (New York: Simon & Schuster, 1987).

9. Ibid., 174.

10. Kamm, FM, *Morality, mortality, volume I: Death and whom to save from it* (New York: Oxford University Press, 1993), 247. One of us (RMV) developed this critique of the life-span account in the 1980s, well before Frances Kamm took up the subject. We note, however, that she reaches essentially the same conclusion. In considering a plan similar to Callahan's (but without citing Callahan) that gives equal status to all ages up to some cutoff at the end of the normal life span, she says, "I find this an odd result."

11. Daniels N, "Am I my parents' keeper?" in *Securing access to health care*, vol. 2, ed. President's Commission for the Study of Ethical Problems in Medicine and Biomedical and Behavioral Research (Washington, DC: US Government Printing Office, 1983), 265–91; Daniels N, *Am I my parents' keeper? An essay on justice between the young and the old* (New York: Oxford University Press, 1988); Daniels N, "Am I my parents' keeper?" *Midwest Studies in Philosophy* 1982;7: 517–40.

12. See Kamm, *Morality*, 247. Again, our view that the preference for the young is morally required rather than a matter of mere prudence converges with Kamm's position, which she appears to have developed independently.

13. Veatch RM, "How age should matter: justice as the basis for limiting care to the elderly," in *Facing limits: Ethics and health care for the elderly*, ed. Winslow GR, Walters JW (Boulder, CO: Westview Press, 1993), 211–29; Veatch RM, "Justice and valuing lives," *Life span: Values and life-extending technologies* (San Francisco: HarperSanFrancisco, 1979), 197–224; Veatch RM, *The foundations of justice: Why the retarded and the rest of us have claims to equality* (New York: Oxford University Press, 1986).

14. Harris J, "Does justice require that we be ageist?" *Bioethics* 1994;8: 74–83; Harris J, *The value of life: An introduction to medical ethics* (London: Routledge & Kegan Paul, 1985), chap. 5; Kappel K, Sandoe P, "QALYs, age and fairness," *Bioethics* 1992;6: 297–316; Kappel K, Sandoe P, "Saving the young before the old: A reply to John Harris," *Bioethics* 1994;8: 84–92; Williams A, "Intergenerational equity: an exploration of the 'fair innings' argument," *Health Economics* 1997;6 (2): 117–32. Cf. Rivlin MM, "Why the fair innings argument is not persuasive," *BMC Medical Ethics* 2000;1 (1), www.biomed central.com/1472-6939/1/1.

15. Kamm, *Morality*, 234.

16. There is an interesting theoretical problem with giving priority based on chronological age. Consider two candidates for a liver who are in all respects equal (equal in disease and equal in life expectancy without an organ but also standing to gain the same number of years if they get the organ). If their age difference is smaller than the predicted additional years gained from the transplant, then

giving the organ to the younger person simply reverses the age-based justice claims. If the candidates are thirty-five and thirty-eight years of age respectively, and whoever gets the organ is expected to gain six extra years, then giving it to the thirty-five-year-old will give him a life expectancy of forty-one years, thus making the thirty-eight-year-old disadvantaged by three years. In a purely egalitarian world, this would be as unacceptable as the original inequality.

Kamm, *Morality*, 276, discusses an ingenious, if purely theoretical, response. She refers to it as "lending organs." If it were technically feasible, we could "lend" the younger patient the organ until he achieves the age of the older competitor and then take it back when the candidates have equal claim, assigning it by some random process, e.g., drawing straws. In fact, precisely this would be feasible for allocating a scarce device such as a hemodialysis machine. We could give the machine to the younger until age parity is established and then allocate randomly. Doing so, of course, comes up against the moral notion that those already receiving a treatment have "dibs" on it until they do not need it any more. That is precisely the moral view that many people take regarding intensive care unit beds. If a patient once occupies the bed, he or she has it until it is no longer needed—even if another patient comes along at a later time who could benefit more or who could stake a claim because of a worse off condition.

Because, technically, organs cannot be lent (and the disutilities of repeated surgery would preclude the arrangement), this is of no more than theoretical interest. In the meantime, it seems clear that the egalitarian would strive to benefit the person who is worst off (who has the smallest number of expected life-years without the organ). The alternative would be to produce an even greater inequality, for example, producing in our example life expectancies of thirty-five and forty-four years, respectively. Assuming we will not give the organ to the thirty-five-year-old and then remove it and discard it after three years, this is the best a strictly egalitarian allocator can do.

17. Schold JD, Hall YN, "Enhancing the expanded criteria donor policy as an intervention to improve kidney allocation: Is it actually a "net-zero" model?" *American Journal of Transplantation* 2010;10: 2582–85.

18. Merion RM, Ashby VB, Wolfe RA, et al., "Deceased-donor characteristics and the survival benefit of kidney transplantation," *JAMA* 2005;294: 2726–33.

19. Falger J, Latal B, Landolt MA, Lehmann P, Neuhaus TJ, Laube GF, "Outcome after renal transplantation, part I: intellectual and motor performance," *Pediatric Nephrology* 2008;23 (8); 1339–45. See also Icard P, Hooper SR, Gipson DS, Ferris ME, "Cognitive improvement in children with CKD after transplant," *Pediatric Transplantation* 2010;14 (7): 887–90.

20. Ross LF, Parker W, Veatch RM, Gentry SE, Thistlethwaite JR Jr., "Equal opportunity supplemented by fair innings: Equity and efficiency in allocating deceased donor kidneys," *American Journal of Transplantation* 2012;12: 2115–24.

21. Frei U, Noeldeke J, Machold-Fabrizii V, et al., "Prospective age-matching in elderly kidney transplant recipients: A 5-year analysis of the Eurotransplant Senior Program," *American Journal of Transplantation* 2008;8: 50–57.

22. United Network for Organ Sharing (UNOS) and Organ Procurement and Transplantation Network (OPTN), Concepts for Kidney Allocation, Richmond, Feb. 16, 2011, http://optn.transplant .hrsa.gov/SharedContentDocuments/KidneyConceptDocument.PDF.

23. Ibid., 29.

24. Heaphy ELG, Goldfarb DA, Poggio ED, Buccini LD, Flechner SM, Schold JD, "The impact of deceased donor kidney risk significantly varies by recipient characteristics," *American Journal of Transplantation* 2013;13: 1001–11.

25. Kasiske BL, Snyder JJ, Skeans MA, Tuomari AV, Maclean JR, Israni AK, "The geography of kidney transplantation in the United States," *American Journal of Transplantation* 2008;8: 647–57.

26. OPTN/UNOS Kidney Transplantation Committee (chair, John Friedewald; vice chair, Richard Formica), "Report to the Board of Directors," Nov. 14–15, 2011, Atlanta, http://optn.transplant.hrsa.gov/CommitteeReports/board_main_KidneyTransplantationCommittee_11_17_2011_17_29.pdf.

27. Ibid.

28. "Proposal to substantially revise the national kidney allocation system," Sept. 21, 2012, http://optn.transplant.hrsa.gov/PublicComment/pubcommentPropSub_311.pdf.

29. Ibid., 5.

30. The top 20 percent of candidates for kidneys get a chance to receive the top 20 percent of kidneys, but also all other kidneys. By contrast, the remaining 80 percent of the candidates as a practical matter only get a chance at the inferior, remaining 80 percent.

31. Danovitch GM, Cohen B, Smits JMA, "Waiting time or waster time? The case for using time on dialysis to determine waiting time in the allocation of cadaveric kidneys," *American Journal of Transplantation* 2002;2: 891–93.

32. US Department of Health and Human Services, OPTN, Kidney Transplantation Committee, "Meeting summary," Aug. 2011, http://optn.transplant.hrsa.gov/CommitteeReports/interim_main _KidneyTransplantationCommittee_9_15_2011_10_35.pdf.

33. We also suggest reclassifying donors who were minors younger than ten years as equivalent to fifty-year-old kidney donors due to their graft survival.

34. In fact, how to classify all kidneys from donors younger than ten years needs to be clarified. Data from Opelz and Dohler suggested that these kidneys function more like fifty-year-old kidneys; see Opelz H, Dohler B, "Pediatric kidney transplantation: Analysis of donor age, HLA match, and post-transplant non-Hodgkin lymphoma—a collaborative transplant study report" *Transplantation* 2010;90: 292–97. However, some data suggest that their function may depend on whether they are allocated en bloc (two kidneys transplanted into one candidate) or as single kidney transplants; see Bhayana S, Kuo YF, Madan P, et al., "Pediatric en bloc kidney transplantation to adult recipients: More than suboptimal?" *Transplantation* 2010;90: 248–54.

35. Kayler LK, Srinivas TR, Schold JD, "Influence of CIT-induced DGF on kidney transplant outcomes," *American Journal of Transplantation* 2011;11: 2657–64; Kayler LK, Magliocca J, Zendejas I, Srinivas TR, Schold JD, "Impact of cold ischemia time on graft survival among ECD transplant recipients: A paired kidney analysis," *American Journal of Transplantation* 2011;11: 2647–56.

36. If we understand her correctly, Kamm, *Morality*, 252, would give almost absolute precedence to how much life an individual will have lived when he or she dies over how urgent the medical need is, that is, how soon one will die if not given a transplant. That, in effect, gives almost absolute priority to young age over the seriousness of the patient's current medical condition. In the terms we have presented, this means she is willing to give strong weight to opportunities for future life and very little weight to the fact that someone is in an immediate crisis. She—like any rational, systematic analyst—is willing to take a very long-term view. We are sympathetic to her perspective, but less willing to discount as totally as she the unique moral appeal of the urgency of a moment of crisis. We are not convinced that it is irrational to spend more to save an identifiable life in crisis (the child in the well) than to save a statistical life in a cool hour. We know of no sound theoretical basis for arguing for any particular formula that would establish exactly what the proper ratio should be for considering present need and over-a-lifetime need. We are convinced, however, that for transplants, the over-a-lifetime perspective is legitimate.

Chapter 21

The Role of Status

The Cases of Mickey Mantle, Robert Casey, Steve Jobs, and Dick Cheney

Certain transplants to high-status figures capture a great deal of public press, often with the suggestion that they have received some form of special treatment so that they jumped to the head of the wait list and received organs faster than ordinary citizens. The liver transplant of Mickey Mantle and Steve Jobs and the heart transplant of Dick Cheney come to mind, as does the heart-liver transplant of former Pennsylvania governor Robert Casey. Getting special priority because of one's status is ethically controversial. In this chapter we look at these cases and ask whether this actually occurs and can ever be morally justified.

Mickey Mantle and Liver Priority

The liver transplant of former baseball star Mickey Mantle, on June 8, 1995, captured a great deal of publicity. We could have encountered his case briefly in chapter 18, because his liver damage was a result of a long history of alcohol consumption. Many at the time raised the question of whether it was fair for him to receive a liver under those circumstances. It turns out that he also had metastatic cancer, from which he died two months later. It thereby raised the question of whether he was already too sick from the cancer to be eligible for a deceased donor liver. Finally, the case generated controversy because, even though there were 4,657 people in the United States waiting for a liver and the average wait was 130 days in the Dallas area, where Mantle was hospitalized, an organ was found for him the next night after he was listed. Many hinted that they suspected that, because he was a folk hero, he received special treatment, that he was moved to the top of the list, jumping over four thousand more ordinary, nameless souls who were just as eager to get a transplant. This case provides a context for examining the role of status in organ allocation.

Mickey Mantle: The Real Facts

As a member of the United Network for Organ Sharing (UNOS) Ethics Committee at the time, one of us (RMV) was contacted by many of the press reporters who were eager for an ethicist to condemn the organ procurement organization (OPO) or the national organ network for letting a celebrity get special treatment. As longtime advocates for the rights of the ordinary patients, either of us would have been pleased to be able to make such a criticism—if we thought it were true.

The liver allocation formula in use at the time was readily available. It should have been used to allocate any liver that became available. Statistics about how many people were on the wait list were also available. After a review of the data, it seems reasonable to conclude that, once one understood the rules for allocation in place at the time (they have changed since then), it turns out to be very plausible that Mantle got a liver so soon after he was listed. It raises questions about whether the allocation formula was morally proper, but it is hard to raise the issue of Mantle's status if the OPO merely gave him an organ by following the same rules that would have applied to everyone else, the rules in place at the time.

The single most important factor is that the rule in place at the time required that a liver procured first go to anyone on the local OPO wait list, no matter how sick the person was or how long the person had been waiting. In Mantle's case, he was competing for an organ with others on the waiting list of the Southwest Organ Bank, the OPO serving the Dallas area. Only if no one locally could use the liver would those beyond the local group have been given access. In that case, it would have gone first to those in the region (i.e., one of 11 geographical areas in the US organ transplant system). Finally, if no one in the region could have used the organ, it would have been made available nationally. This three-tier geographical arrangement is very controversial. UNOS was ordered to adjust its allocation formula to alleviate potential unfairness from this geographical priority. It has since made some adjustment so that the sickest (status 1) candidates regionally have priority over less sick local candidates. This controversy is the subject of chapter 22. The locals-first priority plan in place at the time, however, was what clearly applied to all candidates on the liver wait list, including Mantle.

The geographical requirement that local candidates get priority meant that Mantle was competing with 140 other people on the wait list of the Dallas OPO. This reduces the number from 4,657 to 141, considerably reducing the odds. Next, the OPO must consider blood type and height and weight characteristics. As we discussed in chapter 17, priority goes to persons of identical blood type over those with compatible blood. Mantle was of O-blood group, as was the organ donor. Generally, 50.9 percent of those on the recipient list are of the O-blood group. If that percentage existed in the Dallas wait list, Mantle was now one of about 70 people competing for the liver based on blood-type criteria. Additional candidates would probably have been eliminated based on size criteria.

Finally, at the time organs were allocated on the basis of degree of medical urgency. The categories have changed since the time of the allocation of Mantle's organ, but at the time patients were divided into four groups: Status 1 included patients in the hospital intensive care units (ICUs). Status 2 was for those in the hospital, but not in an ICU. Status 3 was for patients who are not hospitalized but homebound. And status 4 for others still up and about. The liver allocation rule was governed by what appears to be the principle of justice, that the sickest get first priority. Mantle was in the hospital, but not in the ICU—in what was called status 2. Thus if there were any patients in the ICU, they should have had priority over Mantle, but Mantle should have had priority over those who were still healthy enough to be living at home. Moreover, among those in the same category, the tiebreaker is time on the wait list, so anyone in the hospital in status 2 longer than Mantle should have also received priority. In order for Mantle to be first, there should have been no one in the ICU and no one in the hospital longer than Mantle who had O-blood type and was otherwise eligible for the organ.

In the Dallas area 0.45 percent of those on the liver wait list were in status 1. This means that there should have been about 0.45 percent of the 70 O-blood type patients in the ICU. And this suggests that, statistically, there should have been between zero and one in the ICU with the right blood type and size. The claim that there was none is not surprising.

There were normally about 1.9 percent of those waiting for a liver in status 2, that is, perhaps one, maybe two, people. The claim that Mantle was the only one in the hospital is quite plausible. The claim that Mantle was first in line for an O-blood type liver in the Dallas area is, thus, consistent with what one might expect, knowing the details of the allocation formula.

Updated Liver Allocation and the Possibility of Advantage from High Status

Under the liver allocation formula in place now (in 2014), it is likely that Mantle would not have done as well. There is no reason to believe he would have been classified as status 1 under the current classification (which would require that he have fulminant liver failure with a life expectancy of less than seven days). This means that any candidate in the region in status 1 would be given priority. Mantle today would be allocated a liver based on his Model for End-Stage Liver Disease (MELD) score (which we cannot calculate without having his medical data). Depending on his score, some regional candidates with higher MELD scores might have taken precedence. This suggests that Mantle could well have had to wait longer for his transplant if his case arose today. Nevertheless, he would still have taken precedence over even the sickest status 1 candidates beyond the region. This continues to raise fairness issues, which we discuss in chapter 22.

Does all this imply that Mantle's status played absolutely no role? It is impossible to know for sure. It is clear to anyone who knows how OPOs function that they feel very strongly about making the allocation system work fairly. There are very strong incentives for them to do so. An OPO that intentionally diverted an organ to someone because of the candidate's status or because the candidate was a favorite patient could be in very serious trouble. Moreover, there are many players on the scene who would have a strong incentive to scream if there were any gaming of the system. Surgeons, with their historical Hippocratic conditioning, are militantly committed to their patients. Moreover, they like to do transplants, and their income may be dependent on them. Any surgeons who had O-blood-group patients in a hospital in the Dallas area for longer than a day waiting for a transplant would have known that their patients were bypassed. They would have been morally bound to protest and would have had the self-interest to do so. Moreover, surgeons have the personality to do so. That no one protested after the enormous publicity given this case reinforces the conclusion that Mantle could reasonably have been the only O-blood-group patient in the hospital in the Dallas area awaiting a liver.

There is still the possibility that Mantle's status gave him some advantage. To one who understood the liver allocation system at that time, there were some actions a surgeon could have done to advantage his or her patient. First, a surgeon could have placed his or her patient on the wait list earlier than is medically indicated, realizing that it is likely to be some time before the patient's number comes up in the allocation. By that time, the patient might be more nearly ready for the transplant. Second, if the surgeon hospitalized the patient when that patient actually could be at home, using the categories in place at the time, the patient would have moved from status 3 to status 2, helping the patient step over almost everyone on the wait list. The current allocation system of 2014 is probably harder to manipulate in this way. It is based on the seven-day death prognosis for status 1 and on laboratory data for calculating MELD scores.

Could Mantle have been advantaged by listing or hospitalizing him earlier than necessary? In theory, yes—but it would be difficult. There are criteria for listing a patient. There is considerable camaraderie among fellow physicians in a community, as well as considerable competition. Although most might be Hippocratic enough to consider fudging the data for their patient, most would have the integrity and fear of being caught that would incline them to resist. There is no way to prove that Mantle's physician did not list this famous and likable patient sooner than was necessary. It is apparent, however, from Mantle's rapid demise that he was a very sick patient. There is no reason to believe he was listed prematurely.

Once the patient is listed, if he were placed in the hospital prematurely, many people—fellow physicians, residents, nurses, and others—would see it. Although we cannot rule out the possibility that Mantle was listed too early or that he was hospitalized before he needed to be, there is no evidence that either of these things happened. The fact that he died so soon after the transplant helps support the conclusion that he was a very sick man.

Was Mantle transplanted when he had a cancer that should have disqualified him? This is another way in which his status could have influenced his care. If the surgeon knew his cancer had metastasized before the surgery, he should not have received the transplant. The surgeon claimed that he did not know about the metastasis in advance. There is no evidence that he did or should have. It is hardly doing a patient a favor to inflict the rigors of transplant surgery on him in the final weeks of his life. If the physician knew his patient had metastatic cancer, it seems unlikely that he would have hidden that fact in order to get him a transplant that would have done nothing to address the underlying cancer.

The conclusion seems reasonable that, even though Mantle was a national hero, there is no evidence that his status helped him get an organ. The real issue raised by his case is whether UNOS is right in giving priority to any local and regional patients, no matter how ill, over others in the nation who may be in greater need. Surely there was someone nationally who was in status 1 who could have used that organ, but such a person would, even today, still have a lower priority than regional candidates with high MELD scores. Of course, this is in no way a criticism of the Dallas OPO, which seems to have followed the rules in place at the time. In chapter 22 we explore the controversy over the change to a national list.

Governor Casey's Case

Governor Robert P. Casey of Pennsylvania, at sixty-one years of age in 1993, suffered from amyloidosis, an inherited condition characterized by abnormal protein deposits (amyloid) in organs and tissues. He had had a heart attack in 1991 and had undergone quadruple bypass surgery. By 1993 his condition had deteriorated. In the previous four years some fifteen patients had undergone liver transplant for amyloidosis, fourteen of whom had survived. Many had seen a major improvement. Six patients had undergone a more experimental heart-liver transplant, most of whom had died within a few months.[1]

Casey was placed on the wait list for a heart-liver transplant at the University of Pittsburgh Medical Center the night of June 12, 1993, and received his transplants in less than a day. It is reported that the median wait time for a liver was 67 days; and for a heart, 198 days. According to Howard Nathan, executive director of the Delaware Valley Transplant Program—the OPO for Eastern Pennsylvania, southern New Jersey, and Delaware (the neighboring OPO to the Pittsburgh area)—in the five years before Casey's transplant, his OPO had overseen 479 heart transplants, of which 12 were within 24 hours of listing. It had been involved in 356 liver transplants, 22 of which were less than 24 hours after listing. Six patients were ahead of Casey on the wait list for a heart, and two for a liver.[2] As with the Mantle case, the rapid transplant for this first citizen of the state where his surgery was performed led to suspicions that his prominence as the governor of the state had gotten him special treatment. The fact that this Democratic governor, famous for the legal case against abortion bearing his name, received the heart and lung of a black, long-jobless, victim of a drug gang merely added to the controversy.[3]

The allocation rules were not as clear in this case as in Mantle's, where we saw that even if there were people who had been on the wait list longer, they could have been excluded because they were the wrong blood type, were not as sick, or were not local. Casey was reportedly in the sickest category for a heart transplant and the second category for a liver. From the numbers we used for Mantle, we can see why so few patients were ahead of the governor. Still, critics were troubled by his rapid access to organs and his apparent priority over those who appeared to be ahead of him.

In this case, the real issue is whether those needing two organs should be taken ahead of those needing only one. We suggested in chapter 19 that there is a good case for such a priority, because it could be a long time before two suitable organs would again become available simultaneously. If patients needing two organs are given priority, it is easy to see why Casey was chosen.

UNOS did not have a clear policy dealing with multi-organ allocations for cases involving a heart and liver. Transplants of this combination of organs are extremely rare. However, apparently, the University of Pittsburgh Medical Center had such a policy, which gave priority to multiple-organ transplants. John Armitage, then the director of adult cardiac transplantation at the University of Pittsburgh Medical Center, was also quoted as saying, "the governor's life was in imminent danger."[4]

Following this episode, the US Department of Health and Human Services asked UNOS to clarify its policy on priority for multi-organ transplants. The UNOS Board adopted a policy that, if a patient is on the wait lists for both a heart and a liver, he or she must be ranked first on the wait list for at least one of the organs. If first on the list for one of the organs, the patient will be offered the other organ or organs at the same time.[5] This does not give actual priority to multiple-organ transplant candidates until they rise to the top of one of the lists. It does ensure, however, that the candidate will get both organs at the same time. Even if the Pittsburgh program did not precisely follow this policy (which was written after Casey's transplant), its procedure of giving priority to multiple-organ transplant candidates for whom both organs were acceptable is not outside the bounds of reason.

It seems that a plausible explanation is available for the governor's rapid transplant, but the situation was ambiguous. The rules were not made clear in advance. It is situations such as these where the status of the patient can exert an influence. Of course, no organ network can have a rule in place for every possible situation. About all that can be said here is that there was no obvious favoritism shown. The current rule requiring the candidate to rise to the top of the list for at least one of the organs seems plausible, even though the need for one of the organs may not be urgent because simultaneous transplants spare the patient multiple major operations and avoid exposure to two versions of foreign tissues.

Since the writing of the first edition of this book, two additional high-status patients have gained considerable publicity while receiving organs, raising questions about whether their status gave them special priority. We turn to these now.

Steve Jobs's Liver

Steven Paul "Steve" Jobs (1955–2011) was the cofounder, chairman, and chief executive of Apple, Inc. In January 2009 he took a leave of absence from his responsibilities at Apple for what we now can presume was liver failure. He had been diagnosed with a pancreas endocrine tumor in 2003, which was treated surgically following a nine-month delay, during which time he tried alternative therapies. He underwent a liver transplant at Methodist University Hospital Transplant Institute in Memphis in April 2009.[6]

Because he lived in Palo Alto, California, the fact that the transplant took place in Memphis might, at first, seem odd. Receiving a transplant outside the vicinity of one's home is rare. There is reason to believe that he was multiple-listed at two, perhaps more, hospitals in different donor service areas. This would not be illegal, and would significantly increase his chances of getting an organ. The fact that Tennessee had an unusually short wait time for livers probably explains why Jobs was listed there. Tennessee had a median wait time of 2.0 months, whereas the national wait time was 11.8 months.[7]

There is no evidence that Jobs's enormous financial resources (reportedly, he was worth more than $8 billion in 2010) led to any illegal actions to gain advantage. It seems clear, however, that Jobs used those resources to gain a favorable position. Whether he was also listed at other transplant centers is unclear, but doing so would involve even more expense. The medical workup to be listed for a transplant is not inexpensive. And further follow-up to keep listings up to date would add to the costs. It would be reasonable for typical health insurance to pay for this at only one institution. In addition, someone who is multiple-listed would need to be available on short notice wherever listed, a cost insurance would not cover. Only those with substantial private resources could afford to be listed at more than one institution.

If there is an unfairness with the extremely wealthy being able to gain advantage by using their economic and other resources, it would appear to come primarily from the failure to have a national wait list. The present allocation plan for livers, which gives local and regional priority for even relatively healthy liver transplant candidates, makes possible a system whereby Jobs and others with similar resources can get organs more quickly. If organs were allocated with higher priority to a larger area, at least the unequal wait times could be largely neutralized. Those with wealth might still gain some advantage with multiple listings—gaining more chances to find an organ or suitable blood type, size, and human leukocyte antigen characteristics, for example—but at least the unequal wait times would not be present for the wealthy to take advantage of. It probably would not be necessary to have a completely national list. A good analyst should be able to devise an allocation system that makes wait times more equal while still minimizing cold ischemia time. This issue is taken up in chapter 22.

Dick Cheney's Heart

One final case involving a high-status transplant recipient is worth exploring. Former vice president Dick Cheney has a long, well-known history of heart problems.[8] By December 2009 a series of serious cardiac events was occurring: an arrhythmia, requiring his implanted defibrillator to shock his heart back to more normal rhythm; six weeks later, bleeding that required surgery to stop; by the end of February, chest pain, requiring emergency helicopter transportation; in May shortness of breath, requiring ICU admission; and by the end of June, fluid retention. By the first week in July, Cheney required emergency surgery to implant a left ventricular assist device (LVAD), typically used as a bridge to a transplant while awaiting the availability of a heart. It was implanted by Nelson Burton, who had extensive experience implanting LVADs and is a surgeon at INOVA Fairfax hospital's Heart and Vascular Institute in suburban Washington. In Cheney's case, he survived with the LVAD until March 24, 2012, when a suitable heart was located for him.

At the time there were more than 3,100 people on the national wait list for heart transplants. Just over 2,300 heart transplants had been performed the previous year. And 330 people had died the previous year while awaiting a transplant.[9]

These numbers suggest that there was nothing unusual about Cheney's access. The only thing that is notable is that not many hearts go to those over age sixty-five, and Cheney was seventy-one when he received his. That being said, 332 people over sixty-five had received hearts the previous year.

It would not be surprising if a famous political figure received some special attention. For example, it is notable that the best cardiac surgeon in the area interrupted his stay on the Outer Banks of North Carolina to return to Washington to implant the LVAD. There is no evidence, however, that Cheney received any favorable treatment in getting access to a heart for transplant. The fact that he waited twenty months suggests that he did not. And the fact that he was on an LVAD would make him status 1B, the second-highest status for heart allocation.[10]

Social Worth versus Social Status

For all the celebrity transplants described above, the real issue is: Would it have been wrong if preference had been given in any of these cases? And if not, why? There are differences in these cases that are worth examining.

Governor Casey and Social Worth

The governor of a state is in a position of enormous responsibility. Thus getting Casey healthy again as quickly as possible not only served his interests; it served those of the other citizens of Pennsylvania as well. Can we argue that the common good is so important in his case that a special priority was justified, even if he would not have qualified according to the normal allocation rules?

The Utilitarian Position

In chapter 17 we saw that most utilitarians take medical utility into account and ignore social utility in organ allocation. Here we examine whether utilitarians might be persuaded to take social worth into consideration for exceptional cases.

Utilitarian Acceptance of Social Worth

Classical social utilitarians would make allocational decisions by asking about the net benefits for all parties affected for each of the alternatives that are available. That means that they would try to envision the effect on all parties of giving the organs to Casey or to others who are waiting on the basis of what we have called their "social worth." They would take into account all the population affected by restoring the governor to health compared with how they are affected if some other person received the organs.

This, of course, is the assessment of the social worth of the candidates that we indicated in chapter 17 was excluded by almost everyone in the transplant world. Now, however, we encounter the question of whether there may be special exceptional cases. Strictly hypothetically, transplant policymakers have asked what should be done if the president of the United States needed an organ. There is a great temptation to say that there should be rare, exceptional cases.

A Possible Utilitarian Case for Excluding All Social Worth Judgments

Conversely, the counterarguments are powerful. First, especially with political leaders, there will be enormous controversy over the amount of good the politician would do if restored to functioning by a transplant. There will always be those who believe the leader is making the wrong decisions and thus doing more harm than good. Trying to reach an agreement on how to estimate the benefits and harms will be as difficult in these cases as in choices between less-well-known wait list candidates. The quantification of the amount of good done would lead to endless controversy.

Second, even if, in principle, the quantification problems could be solved for the exceptional case, how would we know when and how often to make such exceptions?

Would it be only for the president, or would governors qualify as well? What about other politicians? And why only politicians? As we suggested above, there may be more disutilities in the utility-calculating enterprise than benefits.

There is a third concern with making these calculations in exceptional cases. Some utilitarians believe that it is wrong, in principle, to make these calculations on a case-by-case basis. They are what are called *rule-utilitarians*.[11] They hold that ethics is a matter of calculating benefits and harm, but these calculations should not be done in the individual case. Rather, they should be done only when choosing the rule by which conduct is to be governed. They will compare the utilities of the rule that "social worth" should be excluded from consideration with two other possible rules: the rule that would routinely take it into account, and the rule that would permit it to come into play only in exceptional cases. Taking social worth into account in every case would have the enormous disutility of forcing those involved to identify the social worth of every candidate on the list, something that would paralyze the transplant program. Taking it into account only in exceptional cases would have the added disutility of causing controversies about just who is so socially worthy that the exception should be made.

It is not clear whether a rule-utilitarian would permit exceptions or would, as we suggested in chapter 17, simply rule out all such social value judgments. Perhaps the exceptional case would be ruled out, just as more routine social worth determinations were. At most one could imagine a general policy of excluding social worth considerations, but leaving open the possibility of an exception for the extreme case—perhaps one of major international importance. It is at least as plausible to adopt a flat policy of no exceptions.

The Deontologists and the Problem of Justice

Whether utilitarians would make use of the arguments about the disutility of social worth judgments or adopt a rule-utilitarian stance, most deontologists have their own reasons for resisting social worth as an allocational criterion. Insofar as they include egalitarian justice among their principles, their goal is equality of opportunity. It is hard to imagine how egalitarians would favor making an exception for the governor or anyone else based on social worth.[12] They might use other criteria unrelated to maximizing good consequences (e.g., promises made or the voluntary health-risky behavior discussed in chapter 18), but not the mere fact that one of the transplant candidates was socially useful.

The net result seems to be ambivalence if the utilitarian perspective is taken—some arguments in favor of taking social worth into account, and some against. However, justice theorists would seem to come down squarely against a social worth exception. One who is committed to considering both utility and justice (efficiency and equity) would thus combine a factor that is quite ambivalent with another that is strongly opposed when it comes to considering social worth. The end result would seem to be clear opposition.

Jobs, Cheney, and Social Worth

The relation of social worth to the case of Steve Jobs is more complex. One might argue that he has great social worth because he is a key figure in a major corporation and that his health is important to the welfare of the employees and other benefactors of Apple. It is clear, however, that this would be controversial. If Jobs can claim priority, what about the executives of other major corporations? What about lower-level managers? A defense of Jobs's special access to organs because of his financial ability to be multiple-listed would probably need to rest on libertarian arguments that he made use of his talents to generate his enormous fortune and that, in a free market economy, he should be able to use his resources to buy special access. Of course, these libertarian arguments have generally been rejected when it comes to access to organs.

Although one can imagine an argument that a sitting governor, such as Casey, should be an exception because of the social benefits that might accrue, it is harder to make that argument for a retired political leader such as Cheney. Whatever one thinks of his social worth during the time he was an active politician, it is hard to make the case that giving him a heart transplant priority would generate great social benefit now that he is no longer in office. Arguing for priority would need to be based on some other consideration, such as gratitude for his past service.

Mantle and the Duties of Gratitude

If it is difficult to make the case for an exception to the exclusion of social worth consider-ations for the governor of a state—indeed, for the vice president of a nation—it seems likely that it would be even harder to make the case for a long-retired national sports hero. Whatever social value there might have been in Mantle's career as a baseball player, those days were long since past. If there is a reason to give Mantle an advantage, it is not because of the good he will bring to others in the future.

Still, there seems no doubt that some might be tempted to treat him as someone special. The issue is whether any possible case could be made for that treatment. Although utilitarians and other consequentialists are concerned only about the future, nonconse-quentialists, as we have seen so often, consider other dimensions morally important. They consider patterns of distribution; they also consider what happened in the past. This suggests a possible argument for Mantle as well as Cheney.

One of the principles included in some deontological ethics is related to what W. D. Ross calls "duties of gratitude."[13] Ross, and many others, believe that if someone has done something for us in the past, we are in debt to that person. We owe that person something in return. It is the ethic of gift reciprocity; it is captured in the simple gesture of saying thanks, but often requires more, perhaps something of monetary or nonmonetary sig-nificance.[14] If someone has done a favor, other things being equal, a response is called for that can be thought of as a moral duty. The idea of a duty of gratitude is used to explain why, when we have an opportunity to do good for others, but can do the good for only one, if two potential recipients otherwise have equal claims, we may be thought to have a moral duty to pick the one who has previously done something for us.

The idea of a duty of gratitude is not accepted by everyone, but it does explain many of our most basic moral intuitions about repaying favors and showing gratitude. The question, however, is whether it could possibly justify allocating an organ to a national sports hero or a retired politician. Even if we grant that many people received great joy from Mantle's baseball skills, can we express our gratitude by depriving another transplant candidate who otherwise is equally entitled to an organ? We should at least have to ask whether there are similar or even more substantial duties of gratitude to others on the wait list.

There are several reasons to suspect that applying the concept of a duty of gratitude to organ allocation will be difficult. First, duties of gratitude normally are understood to apply to close friends or family members who have done something very personal that leaves us with a moral sense of owing something in return. It normally does not apply to famous talents who have given us satisfaction in such an impersonal way. Arguably, it could apply to a famous politician who has served a long period of time; but even then, the case would be difficult and controversial.

Second, even if the duty of gratitude applies to famous talents, it is not clear that Mantle's "gift" to the public is really one that generates such a duty. The controversial nature of Cheney's public service raises similar questions. We might imagine a public duty of gratitude for national war heroes who have made a great sacrifice or for socially noble heroes whose works of supererogation are inspiring. Mother Teresa may generate a duty of gratitude, but hardly an athlete who combines luck and natural physical ability to repeatedly accomplish physical feats that are modestly entertaining. National celebrities, at most, might deserve a round of applause—not a lifesaving organ at the expense of others.

If Mantle, Cheney, or Jobs did receive any special consideration, it is more likely that it resulted from some psychological phenomenon other than gratitude. Some people may, out of intimidation or some psychological inadequacy, feel compelled to show deference to status. It is this same feeling that might lead to permitting prestigious, high-status individuals to avoid long waits in lines. It may result from feeling some degree of pride from being associated with the famous. This does not imply that such deference is justified. Surely, there is no possible legitimate reason for giving a folk hero such as Mantle any priority over others on the wait list for an organ just because he is famous or because he accomplished much in his chosen sport. The cases of Jobs and Cheney are only slightly more credible. If Mantle got his organ over others on the wait list because of such factors as blood type and medical urgency, he was deserving (at least according to the rules in place at the time); if he got it because he could run and hit a baseball, that is not possibly justifiable. Neither social worth to others nor social status can play any legitimate role in organ allocation, unless it is a matter of international urgency and the rule providing for the exception is articulated publicly in advance.

Notes

1. This account is based on information in "Controversy about allocation of organs for transplantation: The case of Governor Casey," *BioLaw Update*, Oct. 1993, U303–5; Russakoff D, "The heart that didn't die," *Washington Post*, Aug. 9, 1993; Menzel PT, "Rescuing lives: Can't we count," *Hastings Center Report* 1994;24 (1): 22–23; Belkin L, "Fairness debated in quick transplant," *New York Times*, June 16, 1993; and Colburn D, "Gov. Casey's quick double transplant: How did he jump to the top of the waiting list?" *Washington Post Health* 1993;9 (June 22): 8–9.

2. "Gov. Casey's quick double transplant," 8.

3. *Planned Parenthood of Southeastern Pennsylvania v. Casey*, US Supreme Court, *Supreme Court Reporter* 1992;112 (Jun 29—date of decision): 2791–2885.

4. "Controversy about allocation."

5. UNOS, "UNOS clarifies multi-organ allocation policy," News Release, July 2, 1993, cited in "Controversy about allocation." At the July 31, 1998, UNOS Board of Directors meeting, a change in policy 3.9.3 was proposed so that these same procedures will also be followed for multiple-organ transplants involving the lung as well as the heart and liver, although there are minor technical differences regarding payback if the policy leads to organs being moved beyond the local OPO. These changes are now in place. UNOS Policy 3.9.3, http://optn.transplant.hrsa.gov/PoliciesandBylaws2/policies/pdfs/policy_11.pdf.

6. Isaacson S, *Steve Jobs* (New York: Simon & Schuster, 2011), 484. For a summary of Jobs's life, including his health issues, see "Steve Jobs," *Wikipedia*, http://en.wikipedia.org/wiki/Steve_Jobs#Health_issues.

7. Charlier T, "Disputes erupt over Memphis-area transplant change," *Commercial Appeal*, May 11, 2012, www.commercialappeal.com/news/2012/may/11/disputes-erupt-over-transplant-changes/.

8. Cheney D, Reiner J, with Cheney L, *Heart: An American medical odyssey* (New York: Scribner, 2013); Cheney D, *In my time: A personal and political memoir* (New York: Threshold Editions, 2011).

9. "Cheney receives heart transplant," Fox News, March 24, 2012, www.foxnews.com/politics/2012/03/24/cheney-recovering-from-heart-transplant-surgery/.

10. UNOS, Policy 3.7, http://optn.transplant.hrsa.gov/PoliciesandBylaws2/policies/pdfs/policy_9.pdf.

11. For a good, if somewhat dated, discussion of the concept see Lyons D, *Forms and limits of utilitarianism* (Oxford: Oxford University Press, 1965).

12. There is one possibility. Some justice theorists accept the idea of taking into account effects on other parties while nevertheless rejecting the technique of aggregating the beneficial effects on these parties. For example, assuming John Rawls's "difference principle" could be applied at this level of specificity (see chapter 23 for a discussion of this assumption), he would permit practices that consider the benefits to another person of giving a differential advantage to someone who is already well off. He would permit this provided the other party who was indirectly benefited was among the worst off. For example, if it could be successfully claimed that giving Governor Casey priority for an organ would improve the lot of the worst-off citizens of Pennsylvania, then someone who would apply the difference principle at this level of specificity would support the special consideration. Frances Kamm seems to have something like this in mind when she suggests that there may be special exceptions to the policy of excluding consideration of social contribution. She says, "There may be exceptions, for example, for those who can complete projects that have truly exceptional social importance." She goes on, however, to qualify this apparent exception. She would not permit social importance from "aggregation of small gains to each individual in society." This is the mark of a deontologist's concern for giving special advantage based on the claim that doing so will produce greater social good in aggregate. This is seen by Rawlsians and other defenders of the difference principle as morally different from giving a special advantage in order to help some individual who is even worse off than the one given the advantage. According to them, justice might permit this kind of exception while mere aggregate net benefit would not. In chapter 23 we question the legitimacy of even this very limited endorsement of special favoritism. See Kamm FM, *Morality, mortality, volume I: Death and whom to save from it* (New York: Oxford University Press, 1993), 260.

13. Ross WD, *The right and the good* (Oxford: Oxford University Press, 1930), 21–23.

14. Titmuss RM, *The gift relationship: From human blood to social policy* (New York: Random House, 1971); Mauss M, *The gift: Forms and functions of exchange in archaic societies*, trans. Cunnison I, and introduction by Evans-Pritchard EE (Glencoe, IL: Free Press, 1954).

Chapter 22

Geography and Other Causes of Allocation Disparities

Before the advent of cyclosporine in the early 1980s, organ transplant survival rates were low and only a few programs existed. The passage of the National Organ Transplant Act (NOTA) in 1984 greatly expanded organ transplantation because it required funding for regional organ procurement agencies, mandated Medicare/Medicaid funding for transplants, established the national Organ Procurement and Transplantation Network (OPTN) to facilitate the procurement and distribution of organs, and called for a task force to further study organ allocation.[1]

The first contract from the US Department of Health and Human Services (HHS) to operate the OPTN was awarded to the United Network for Organ Sharing (UNOS), a nonprofit entity that has held the contract since 1986. Due to a lack of consensus on the UNOS organ distribution committee, UNOS adopted preexisting point systems—one for kidneys and another one for extrarenal organs—that had been developed and used by the University of Pittsburgh, which conducted one of the largest transplant programs at the time.[2] The Pittsburgh allocation protocols provided that organs should be allocated first locally, then regionally, and finally nationally so that a relatively healthy local candidate would get priority over a more distant patient in desperate need. (That is part of the reason why Mickey Mantle received his liver so quickly, which is discussed in detail in chapter 21.)

Taking the liver as an example, as the number of transplant programs expanded rapidly (from 4 programs in 1983,[3] to 25 in 1985,[4] to 58 in 1987, and to 112 in 1993[5]), programs like Pittsburgh saw their share of deceased donor liver grafts drop dramatically, and Pittsburgh urged a change in allocation that would abandon this strict local priority and focus on medical urgency in order to promote greater equity (with the intended effect that, because Pittsburgh had large numbers of sicker patients, it would probably get more organs).

Through political maneuvers, the liver allocation issue was referred to then secretary of HHS Donna Shalala. When HHS issued the OPTN Final Rule on April 2, 1998, it had three components: (1) minimal listing criteria for wait list candidates, (2) priority given to medical urgency, and (3) standardized and objective medical criteria for assessing medical urgency.[6] Many (but not all) transplant programs and key stakeholders voiced concern that this would require a single national list. There was also concern that (1) a "sickest first policy" could result in decreased survival rates unless it considered potential benefit as well, (2) that small transplant centers would be forced to close, (3) net outflow of donor livers from high-procurement areas would be a disincentive for them to procure organs, and (4) HHS was assuming a policymaking role that many believed should be the purview of the medical community.[7] The 1999 Omnibus Spending Bill included an amendment that delayed implementation of the Final Rule by one year and mandated that the Institute of Medicine (IOM) conduct an independent investigation into the "potential impact of a pending new federal regulation (the 'Final Rule') on the system of organ procurement and transplantation."[8] The IOM's report supported the recommendations of the Final Rule, which was then adopted one year later with publication of the revised Final Rule.[9] This regulation gave the OPTN the authority to enforce its policies.

This chapter reviews the controversy surrounding the Final Rule in terms of the equity/efficiency conflict with a focus on the geographic disparities that local-first algorithms create and that the Final Rule was designed to amend. We then look at other disparities in organ allocation—race/ethnicity, socioeconomic, and gender—and how different allocation algorithms exacerbate or ameliorate them.

The Role of Geography in Allocation

The role of geography in organ allocation has been a point of controversy since the earliest days. We start with the pattern at the time NOTA was passed and in the years before 2000.

Before 2000

NOTA did not specify policies or procedures regarding the distribution of donor organs, but stipulated the creation of a task force that would help develop these policies and procedures. The Task Force on Organ Procurement and Transplantation was a forty-member multidisciplinary panel led by Olga Jonasson. It recommended the use of medical criteria that were transparent, that were developed by a broadly representative group that considered both need and probability of success, and that were fairly applied.[10] In the case of a tie, the task force recommended selection based on wait time.[11] The task force also rejected the use of candidate social worth in the allocation plan. It emphasized that organs are a "national resource" that should be used for the public good and that the public "must participate in the decisions of how this resource can be used to best serve the public interest."[12]

The earliest algorithms adopted by the OPTN, however, were not developed by a multidisciplinary committee because of a looming deadline, but instead were taken verbatim from the Pittsburgh protocols, with its emphasis on local allocation in order to (1) incentivize procurement and (2) to minimize cold ischemia time.[13] When there was no suitable local candidate, the organs would be allocated regionally and then nationally. With the expansion in the number of transplant programs after the passage of NOTA, the University of Pittsburgh was instrumental in having the federal authorities review the allocation process and propose the recommendations that are now known as the Final Rule. The Final Rule criticized the current allocation system, which was "heavily weighted to the local use of organs instead of making organs available on a broader regional or national basis for patients with the greatest medical need consistent with sound medical judgment."[14] The Final Rule noted that technological advances have made it possible for organs to tolerate longer cold ischemia times that would permit them to be allocated to a broader geographic region, but the system did not at the time yet take full advantage of this capacity. It also noted that the criteria used for listing were not uniform, which made it difficult to compare the medical needs of patients in different transplant centers. As a result of both the local preference in allocation and the lack of standard medical criteria, wait times for organs were much longer in some geographic areas than in others. The statute envisioned a national allocation system, based on medial criteria that would result in a more equitable treatment of transplant patients.[15]

The IOM report focused on the disparities in the allocation of livers, because liver transplantation "was the center of the debate leading to this study."[16] The IOM committee noted that "one of the most visible and contentious issues regarding the fairness of the current system of organ procurement and allocation is the argument that it results in great disparities in the total amount of time a patient waits for an organ, . . . depending on where he or she lives."[17] It proposed larger regions for organ sharing for liver allocation to increase the number of organs allocated to the most urgent candidates, which at the time were referred to as status 1 candidates (candidates with fulminant liver failure with a life expectancy of less than seven days) and status 2 candidates (defined at the time as hospitalized patients). Status 2 candidates were further categorized as 2A or 2B, depending upon whether the candidate was in the intensive care unit (2A) or not (2B). The recommendation would reduce the number of organs allocated to status 3 candidates (candidates in need of continuous medical care but not meeting status 2).

In response to the Final Rule and the IOM report, UNOS made one adjustment to the liver allocation algorithm: It gave priority to regional status 1 patients above local status 2 patients. Otherwise the algorithm was not changed. Not surprisingly, then, despite the Final Rule, geographic disparities in organ allocation persisted. Although the newest liver allocation algorithm, from June 2014, continues to expand liver allocation regionally (for those with a Model for End-Stage Liver Disease, or MELD, score > 35, it remains the case that status 1 candidates outside the region get lower priority than many not-so-ill liver transplant candidates (candidates with a MELD score as low as 15).[18] In addition, other disparities also exist and persist, including those due to race/ethnicity, socioeconomic status, and gender. We begin by evaluating the current policies and examine the impact of these policies on utility (understood in terms of urgency) and equity (understood in terms of equal opportunity for an organ transplant regardless of one's geographical location). After an evaluation of the reasons for geographic disparities, we then evaluate the impact that the various allocation policies have on racial/ethnic, socioeconomic, and gender disparities.

Current Policies

UNOS revises its organ allocation policies in light of best evidence as well as political considerations (see the case of Sarah Murnaghan, discussed in detail in this subsection).

Allocation for each organ weighs factors relevant to medical need, medical urgency, and fairness differently, as we explore here.

The Kidney

In the summer of 2013 UNOS passed a new kidney allocation system policy that is expected to go into effect in late 2014. Although more nuanced details were described in chapter 20 and are taken up again later in this chapter, the crux of the algorithm is based on two features: (1) a kidney donor profile index (KDPI) score, an indicator of expected donor kidney quality; and (2) an estimated post transplant survival (EPTS) score of candidates, a measure of expected longevity.[19] The goal is to increase efficiency by matching better kidneys with patients who have a greater expected longevity. Thus, after giving priority to highly sensitized candidates, zero-antigen mismatched candidates, prior living donors, and minors, the algorithm allocates the top 20 percent of kidneys as defined by KDPI to the top 20 percent of candidates locally. If no such candidate is found, then the kidney is allocated to local candidates with an EPTS greater than 20 percent, and only if no candidate is found locally is it allocated to a regional candidate in the top 20 percent EPTS, and if no such candidate is found, to a national candidate in the top 20 percent EPTS. The preferential allocation of kidneys procured in one area to candidates of lower EPTS in that area rather than to regional candidates in the top 20 percent EPTS is surprising, given that the Kidney Committee states its focus is on increasing efficiency. It ignores the Kidney Committee's own data, which show that both the current and proposed allocation systems would be more efficient and more equitable if kidneys were allocated using a broader primary geographic sharing plan.[20]

The remaining 80 percent of kidneys will be allocated in a way that is similar to the previous point system, except that wait time will be replaced by dialysis time, an important change given the barriers to getting on the wait list, which have led to racial/ethnic and socioeconomic disparities in kidney transplantation. However, kidneys allocated under this new algorithm still give preference to local candidates over regional and national candidates, even though these other candidates may have more points. Thus despite the mandate of the Final Rule to assure that allocation of scarce organs will be based on common medical criteria, and "not on the basis of accidents of geography," the new kidney allocation algorithm has a very strong local allocation preference.[21]

Pancreata

Pancreata, which are sometimes transplanted along with a kidney, are allocated using the same geographical priority as kidneys. Again, highly sensitized candidates with a zero-antigen mismatch get highest priority, with a first pass for local, then regional, and then national allocation.[22] If there are no such candidates, then the local organ procurement organization (OPO) has discretion in allocating pancreata to its patients needing an isolated pancreas, a kidney–pancreas combination, or a combined solid organ–islet transplant. Although some might debate whether low mismatches for isolated pancreata should come before combined pancreas–kidney transplants, for instance, the real issue of controversy is why, except for the zero-antigen mismatch case in highly sensitized candidates, all local candidates, even those who predictably would get another chance at a graft, should take precedence over any regional or national candidate, even if that more distant candidate has a good antigen match, has been waiting a long time, is of the identical blood group, and/or has a modest degree of sensitization.

Liver

Until the change following the passage and adoption of the Final Rule, livers were allocated locally to status 1 candidates in descending point order, then to local status 2A candidates, local status 2B candidates, and local status 3 candidates, all in descending point order. The first change made after the adoption of the Final Rule was to prioritize regional status 1 candidates before allocating to local status 2 candidates.

Whereas earlier liver transplant algorithms gave many points for wait time, in 2002 UNOS adopted the MELD / Pediatric End-Stage Liver Disease (PELD) score approach, which attempts to prioritize the "sickest first" into its liver algorithm.[23] MELD is calculated using three laboratory parameters—serum creatinine, bilirubin, and international normalized ratio (INR) for prothrombin time—and uses these laboratory data to stratify patients according to their disease severity, defined as the risk of dying in the short term (three months) on an objective and continuous ranking scale. The new liver allocation algorithm maintained status 1 for those with fulminant liver failure and life expectancy of less than one week, and in response to the Final Rule, gave priority to status 1 regional candidates before other less ill local candidates. After status 1 local and regional candidates, priority is given to local candidates based on descending MELD score, and the organs are not offered to a regional candidate unless there is no local candidate. The MELD-based liver graft allocation policy has led to a reduction in listing of low-MELD candidates, a reduction in mortality, shorter wait times, and an increase in transplants, without altering overall graft and patient survival rates after transplantation.[24]

In 2005 the MELD-based organ distribution policy was revised to incorporate a rule known as Share 15, which expanded regional sharing even further based on what is now known as "survival benefit."[25] Merion and colleagues analyzed data from the Scientific Registry of Transplant Recipients and showed not only that liver transplants for candidates with low MELD scores were associated with less transplant survival benefit than those with higher scores, but that candidates with a MELD score below 15 had a higher risk of death with the transplant than did similar candidates who remained on the wait list.[26] In response to this finding, in 2005 the liver allocation rules were changed so that regional candidates with MELD scores greater than 15 outside the local area were given access to offers before local candidates with MELD scores less than or equal to 15.[27]

One additional change was implemented in 2013, and this is to give priority to sicker local and regional candidates. After status 1 candidates, livers are allocated to candidates with a MELD score greater than 35. The offers are made by descending MELD scores first made locally then regionally (i.e., local, 40; regional, 40; local, 39; regional, 39) to ensure allocation priority to those most in need.[28]

The current liver allocation algorithm also gives exception points for seven diagnoses, including a diagnosis of hepatocellular carcinoma without metastases for whom resection is not an option and cystic fibrosis. Candidates who do not meet these standard MELD exception criteria or have other complications of liver disease that may warrant additional exceptional priority can submit a petition to a regional review board.[29]

From a justice perspective, the new liver allocation algorithm does incorporate a broader geographic distribution system than it did before the Final Rule was implemented (local and regional priority for status 1, followed by local and regional allocation for each MELD score 35 and higher). However, the algorithm still allocates livers to candidates with lower MELD (between 15 and 35) locally before regional candidates and before the sickest national candidates (status 1 and MELD 35 or greater). Even greater equity and efficiency could be achieved with broader geographic sharing.[30]

Other Organs

The current allocation algorithms for thoracic organs (hearts and lungs) continue to give priority to local candidates. One argument in support of this practice is the shorter cold ischemia time that thoracic organs tolerate. In this framework, allocation is delineated by five zones of concentric circles, with the donor hospital at the center: starting at zone A, with a radius of 500 nautical miles; and moving to zone B, 1,000 nautical miles; and then to zones C and D, 1,500 and 2,500 nautical miles respectively before moving to zone E, which involves all transplant hospitals more than 2,500 nautical miles from the donor hospital.[31]

Local heart candidates of status 1A and 1B get first priority for a deceased donor heart, followed by those in status 1A and 1B, who are in zone A, followed by local status 2 candidates, before the heart is offered to zone B status 1A and 1B candidates.[32]

Adult lung candidates get a lung allocation score, which is based on all the following: (1) the waiting list urgency measure, which is the expected number of days a candidate will live without a transplant during an additional year on the wait list; (2) the posttransplant survival measure, which is the expected number of days a candidate will live during the first year posttransplant; and (3) the transplant benefit measure, which is the difference between the posttransplant survival measure and the waiting list urgency measure.[33] Until June 2013, adult lung organs were allocated locally to candidates more than twelve years of age according to the lung allocation score in descending order, first to ABO identical and then to ABO-compatible candidates. Only after these categories have been exhausted do they offer to candidates in zone A in the same order, followed by zone B, and so on.

In May 2013, the parents of Sarah Murnaghan, a ten-year-old child with cystic fibrosis, challenged the current policy of not allowing children under twelve access to adult deceased donor lungs. They first sought an exception from the Organ Procurement and Transplantation Network, but when that failed, Sarah's parents went to court, and they won a temporary injunction on June 5, 2013.[34] The case was not heard as Sarah received her first of two sets of adult lungs on June 12, 2013. Meanwhile, the Organ Procurement and Transplantation Network passed a temporary, one-year appeals process for children under the age of twelve whose doctors believe that they may benefit from adult lungs. This policy was made permanent on July 1, 2014.[35]

The Reasons for Local Priority

The support for this local priority practice has been very strong within UNOS and the organ procurement organizations. The question is why. The reasons involve both moral concerns and program self-interest.

Moral Reasons

There are both moral reasons and reasons of self-interest why local priority has been defended. First, considering moral reasons, some believe there is a duty to serve one's own community. There are also efficiency-based reasons.

Serving One's Own Community First

The most obvious reason is probably because it is natural for each community to feel it should serve its own members first. If a program is organized to develop an organ donation system that covers a metropolitan area, the members of that community who are being called upon to donate organs like to think that they are helping their neighbors. For example, Nancy Kay, who is the executive director of the South Carolina Organ Procurement Agency, was quoted as saying, "Our work is based on the giving of South Carolinians. . . . We like to take care of our neighbors here."[36] Oklahoma's governor, Frank Keating, is quoted complaining that the federal government is trying to "suck organs" from states such as his.[37]

The concern about keeping local organs for local folks had become so great that by the mid-1990s four states (Louisiana, South Carolina, Wisconsin, and Oklahoma) had passed laws requiring locally procured organs to be used within the state if a patient in the state could use them. Although passage of the Final Rule preempted these state laws, UNOS can grant variances to allow various donor service areas (DSAs) to incorporate rules not otherwise permitted.[38] UNOS has granted two statewide sharing variances: one to Florida, in June 1991, entailing four DSAs; and one to Tennessee, in November 1992, entailing two DSAs that continue to be enforced. Statewide sharing first offers a procured kidney to the procuring DSA but then allocates the kidney to the other DSAs within the state before regional and national allocation.[39]

Statewide sharing has its limitations. Many OPOs, for example, serve metropolitan areas that cross state lines. This means that, under such laws, even locally procured organs could cross a state line. For example, there is only one active liver transplant program within the Washington Regional Transplant Community. It is at a hospital in the District of Columbia, which is identical to the City of Washington. A patient in suburban Maryland needing a liver who wanted to go to the nearest liver transplant program would go to the District of Columbia. Passing a law in Maryland requiring that Maryland organs go first to Maryland programs would require the organs to go to Baltimore, guaranteeing that they would go outside the area of Maryland residents in the Washington suburbs and away from the hospital that would most naturally serve these Maryland residents. Furthermore, the District of Columbia could retaliate by insisting that its organs be used for its own residents, thus prohibiting suburban Marylanders from getting access.

Even if one becomes convinced that a local priority makes sense, the allocation should not be based on state lines. Requiring that OPOs retain local priority would serve the goal of keeping local organs for local people much better. This would keep organs within a metropolitan area rather than using state boundaries, which often do not reflect metropolitan areas. As we shall see below, however, there is a strong moral case to be made for removing the priority for local allocation and going to some version of a national list—or at least a larger geographical area based on medical urgency.

Increasing Efficiency

Those within the transplant community may give more technical reasons for local priority as well as the notion of loyalty to the local community. They may claim that a system with local priority is more efficient. This could be for several reasons. First, it is believed that after a certain point that varies for each organ, delays in implanting organs increase the risk of graft failure. Although a kidney can last 24 hours or more, a heart must be transplanted much more quickly. A local allocation not only eliminates travel time or keeps it to a minimum; it also eliminates the delay from having to negotiate communication between OPOs and between the OPOs and UNOS. Local allocation results in a faster, simpler system.

It is difficult to interpret the data supporting the claim that longer waits between procurement and transplant (cold ischemia times) lead to worse outcomes. They vary for each organ and change as better preservation techniques are developed. Data for kidneys, for example, show delayed graft function, but long-term function does not seem to be affected.[40] In contrast, the pancreas may be the most susceptible abdominal organ to ischemia reperfusion injury, but there are inadequate data for the best retrieval strategy and optimum perfusion solution.[41]

It is not clear, however, how many kidney transplants would need to be delayed beyond some organ-specific standards and/or whether or how much advantage is gained by transplanting very quickly. Because transportation within the United States is not likely to take more than a few extra hours, the impact on kidney graft survival of a national list would be modest at most. Nevertheless, for other organs, additional delays may be more important.

Second, it is postulated that local organ priority increases organ procurement. Starzl and colleagues asserted that people might be more willing to donate in a time of crisis if they know that the organs are likely to be used locally.[42] However, there are no data to support this claim.[43] In fact, as Ubel and Caplan explain, "Studies of donors' motivation show no evidence that donors or their families ask whether organs will be distributed locally or nationally."[44]

Another claim is that hospital personnel may be more inspired to initiate procurement activities (raising the issue with families or, preferably, contacting the OPO, so that those skilled in procurement can take over) with local priority. Also, local transplant surgeons may be more willing to take the lead in developing educational and counseling programs to stimulate organ procurement if they believe there is a good chance that the organs may come to them to do a transplant. In actuality, these responsibilities have now been taken over by organ procurement organizations because of the inconsistent and ineffective approaches to donation requests by many hospital personnel.[45]

The Self-Interest of Transplant Programs

The interest in local priority is not entirely altruistic. Transplant programs, hospitals, and health professionals involved in transplants all have important self-interests at stake in maintaining local priority for organ allocation. Transplants are big business for hospitals and surgeons. Keeping the organs locally may mean significant income for both the hospital and the surgeon.

Of course, with local priority, other OPOs outside the local area will also have these incentives to keep their organs for themselves. In the long run, on average, surgeons will do about the same number of transplants and hospitals will receive about the same income if everyone agrees to share. The only costs of sharing nationally will be modest coordination and transportation costs, plus any decrease in donations resulting from donor family awareness that the sharing takes place on a national basis rather than within the local metropolitan area.

There may be another self-interest for local transplant programs, however. Surgeons must meet minimal criteria in order to establish and maintain their credentials. Also, transplant centers that function as training programs must ensure that their trainees perform a certain specific number of transplants. A program that just barely meets the minimum number risks losing its certification or its training program if it exports organs that could have been used locally, at least if it will not import a comparable number. Other than for training, there are no minimal number requirements imposed nationally, but local and state requirements (e.g., for certificates of need) may impose such minimums.

The shift to any allocation that increases exports could jeopardize the interest not only of the hospitals and surgeons involved but also of the patients. If an area has only one heart transplant program and it is in jeopardy of losing it, then the patients in that community would need to travel elsewhere to get their heart transplants. This is difficult for patients, family members, and friends. Follow-up would be increasingly difficult. Of course, if patients can expect that their program doing a marginal number of transplants is inferior to the large program elsewhere, these patients may have a reason to want to have the local program closed down in favor of the larger, more experienced program.

Determining the relation between program size and quality, however, is difficult and may vary by organ. The 1997 "Center-Specific Graft and Patient Survival Rates" report examined these issues. It calculated expected survival rates for each transplant program in the United States for each organ transplanted, adjusting for the risk level of the patients. It then compared actual survival rates, flagging those at which actual survival rates were significantly lower than expected rates. It pointed out, however, that larger differences between actual and expected rates were nearly always seen in programs that reported relatively few transplants.[46] The report's authors point out that this is, in part, a statistical artifact, because large variations in survival rates in small programs can be produced easily. The authors are sensitive to the indignation shown by some small programs when it is assumed that small volume necessarily means poor results. Nevertheless, the 1997 report repeated the conclusion of an earlier study of cardiac transplantation that "the risk of mortality at earlier and intermediate time points is higher in low-volume cardiac transplant centers," a finding that the report points out has been demonstrated for other surgical procedures as well.[47] Although some small programs may produce very good results, there are reasons related to both outcomes and economies of scale to question the appropriateness of continuing to fund very-low-volume programs. More recent data continue to show strong evidence that greater volume correlates with better results in thoracic transplant programs.[48] The more recent data are mixed with respect to liver transplantation, with some studies showing a correlation between volume and outcomes, and other studies not showing any correlation.[49]

On balance, many people have an interest in keeping local programs running. That could be part of the explanation for why many people want local organs to be used locally. Still, utilitarians have a hard case to make to defend the claim that more aggregate benefit accrues from sustaining many local programs. It is not clear that the number of organs procured would go down if local programs exported organs based on a national allocation. It is also not clear what the impact would be on the survival rates and other measures of patient benefit. If the imports to an OPO equal the exports (as they would on average), the result will be about the same. The utilitarian must rest his or her case on claims about changes in procurement rates, patient benefit from receiving a transplant nearer to home, and the quality of small programs.

The controversy over the liver allocation illustrates why small, local programs fear they may suffer a net loss of organs if the United States goes to a national list. Throughout the 1980s and 1990s, the University of Pittsburgh Medical Center's liver transplant program was the dominant program in the United States. In 1988, before many cities had developed their programs, the University of Pittsburgh did 406 of the 1,713 liver transplants in the United States, and Children's Hospital of Pittsburgh, which is affiliated with the Medical Center, did another 99 of them.[50] When it was one of the very few programs, it built its reputation not only as *the* place to get a liver transplant but also as the place where surgeons went to train to become liver transplant surgeons. As long as there were few other programs, organs would be sent by other OPOs that could not use them. But as those surgical trainees completed their course of training, they gradually moved on to other communities seeking to begin liver transplant programs, and all wanted livers to be allocated for their own local patients. Because there was local priority for the allocation of livers, the small programs across the country had a claim on organs that they used to transplant into their relatively healthy patients while Pittsburgh's wait list grew. Hence the reason that Pittsburgh was so eager to have the allocation system changed.

The Demand for a National List

The inequities created by local liver allocation led to a cry for a national list for allocating organs, or at least for one that covers much larger geographical areas. The concern is, in part, a moral one; as we show below, wait times vary greatly from one center to another, and patients are much sicker at some centers than others. The obvious solution seems to be to go to some version of a national list based on such factors as degree of medical urgency and time on the wait list. If the current UNOS allocation formulas were maintained as they are, but the priorities for local and then regional allocation were eliminated, the problem would be solved—or so the argument goes.

The HHS Mandate

This is more or less what Donna Shalala, the US secretary of HHS, concluded when she faced the issue in the mid-1990s. Urged by intense lobbying from the University of Pittsburgh, she issued an order directing the OPTN—that is, UNOS—to revise its organ allocation policies. It mandated that the allocation fairly and equitably give every citizen access to organ transplantation, requiring the OPTN to create a policy that places medical need as the foremost criterion. It also called for reducing disparities across the nation by, at least to some extent, taking geography out of the equation. In addition to criteria for allocation based on medical urgency rather than geographic proximity, the rule calls for the development of uniform criteria to decide when to place a patient on the wait list and what status he or she holds there.[51] The mandate was introduced to equalize wait times across the entire country; to give every individual equal opportunity for a transplant, no matter where he or she lives or is registered; and to ensure that all criteria are uniform and fair.[52] But as we have seen, most organ policies still place great emphasis on local candidates.

The Case for a Modified National List

Although a single national list may require many adjustments to address logistical issues, a reasonable proposal consistent with the principle of justice described in this book would be to allocate organs to the sickest class of patients (status 1, in the case of the liver) first locally, then regionally, and finally nationally. Then organs would go to patients in the next sickest class (MELD greater than 35) locally, then regionally, and then nationally. But this has not happened, as the algorithm moves to allocation by MELD scores 35 or greater locally and regionally, then to local candidates with MELD scores all the way down to 15, before offering the organs to the sickest (status 1) national candidates.

Cold ischemia time is least important in the case of kidneys, and yet the kidney algorithm is focused on local allocation. And yet, in designing the newest allocation method, the UNOS Kidney Transplant Committee presented data that compared a plan called life-years following transplant, with and without geographic boundaries. The plan without boundaries added 32 percent more life-years from transplants than the same plan based on current boundaries (an additional 34,026 life-years versus an additional 25,794 life-years compared to the baseline).[53] In contrast, the newly adopted plan scheduled to go into effect in late 2014, with its local allocation, is only expected to provide an additional 8,380 life-years.[54]

It is hard to imagine how to devise a fair and equitable allocation system that eliminates geographical differences without going to some version of a national list. There are, of course, technical questions requiring scientific knowledge that are relevant to deciding how to allocate organs—questions of organ deterioration during cold ischemia, relative graft and patient survival for patients at various stages of their illness, and so forth. But in the end, the real issues in the debate over a local or more national allocation are moral. Assuming that there may be some losses in efficiency in reducing disparities (and going to something like a national list), deciding whether to trade off efficiency to make the allocation more fair is fundamentally not a technical medical question. It is a question of the relative moral priority of efficiency and equity (of maximizing aggregate utility and distributing the utility equitably). Although our personal moral theory would give priority to equity over efficiency, we recognize that there is no consensus in favor of this view. We continue to support the compromise developed in the UNOS Ethics Committee during the time when one of us (RMV) served as chair of its Organ Allocation Subcommittee. That compromise, as described in chapter 17, endorsed giving efficiency and equity equal weight. That suggests a modified national list that may not be perfectly equitable (at least if something close to equal wait times for equally sick people can be developed that is significantly more efficient), but it will at least be considerably more equitable than the present system.

Moral Reasons for a National List

Although many of the defenders of the local priority claim that it increases organ procurement, improves quality due to shorter ischemia times, and is necessary to support local transplant centers so that patients will be able be transplanted close to home, defenders of the national list also can point to benefits that they believe would accrue by going to the national list.

One moral reason for a national list is that it increases efficiency (utility). Defenders argue that some small programs are marginal in quality as well as quantity. They suggest that some of them going out of business might mean greater efficiencies of large-scale operations at the societal level and improved outcomes for patients who would get transplants in programs with more experience. As we have seen, there is some controversy about the accuracy of this claim.

The defenders also point to the benefits that would come from getting organs to sick patients who might die soon if they do not get transplanted. They suggest that, in the case of livers, for example, small programs that have few patients on a wait list may get organs from the local priority policy that end up going to patients with quite low MELD scores who are still up and around and relatively healthy. This suggests that these patients could wait for their organs with little loss. In fact, some data show that some liver transplant recipients may be receiving transplants too early, so that their life expectancies are actually shorter than if they had not been transplanted.[55] That is, if those organs go to sicker patients in other areas, the good they receive could exceed the harm to the patients with low MELD scores in the area where the organ is procured.

A second moral reason for a national list is that it increases equity. The real claim of defenders of the national list often has nothing to do with increasing expected benefits. They are concerned instead with increasing the equity of the organ transplant system. They say it is patently unfair to have a national organ transplant system maintained by federal funds in which patients in one OPO have average wait times for lifesaving organs that are much greater than those in another OPO. Secretary Shalala illustrated the claim of unfairness in wait times in her testimony to Congress in June 1998: "For example, the median waiting times for the two major liver transplant centers in Kentucky were vastly different—38 days at one center, 226 at the other. Similarly, in Louisiana, the median waiting time at one center was reported to be 18 days, whereas at another it was 262 days. In Michigan, the numbers were 161 days and 401 days. Although these numbers do not tell the whole story, they certainly reflect that unacceptable disparities in waiting times exist, even within States. I believe that basic fairness to patients demands that these disparities be substantially reduced and that the transplant community should ultimately develop the means to this end."[56]

To be sure, people can transfer their registration to another center that has a shorter expected wait time for an organ. They can even register at more than one transplant center, thus having two or even three chances at getting an organ and shortening the expected wait time. Shifting to another center is not easy, however. It would need to be in another metropolitan area (because other transplant programs in the same area would involve the same wait list with the same poor odds). Getting registered in another community would mean moving to that area or at least traveling there often enough to establish a medical relationship. When receiving the transplant, not only would the patient need to travel to the new community for the operative and postoperative period; family members who are to become the support system would also need to do so. All this takes money, time, and mobility—commodities available more readily to the more wealthy. Registering in more than one center likewise takes extensive resources. Many insurance programs would not fund the repeat testing and medical workups. Shifting to a program with a shorter wait list and double-listing are options more likely to be available to the wealthy.

The bottom line is that local priority makes the transplant program inequitable. People who are equally sick, who have equal entitlement to a transplant, and who are equally good candidates will have significantly different probabilities of getting an organ. Because many people die while on the wait list, a delay in getting an organ equals an increased risk of death. The moral principle of justice requires that people who are equal are entitled to be treated equally. This is referred to by theorists as the "formal" criterion of justice, the most general and most widely accepted element of the concept of justice.

Defenders of the egalitarian version of the principle of justice go further. They not only claim that equals deserve equal treatment but also go on to state which group deserves priority: the worst off. They are offended by a system that is designed to let a relatively healthy person—a person with a MELD score in the high teens in the case of a liver transplant candidate—get an organ with priority over a much more critical status 1 patient just because the healthier patient happens to live in an area that has a large supply of donated organs compared with the demand for those organs. Such an arrangement leaves the acutely ill patient in fulminant liver failure (status 1—the highest status) to die simply because he or she happens to live in a location where the supply of organs is disproportionate to the number needing them.

Both supply and demand can be determined by utterly arbitrary variables. The supply will be contingent on such factors as the socioeconomic status of the residents of the community, the quality of the highway construction, and the religious persuasion of the community members. The demand may be great simply because a high-quality transplant center attracts many out-of-towners to register, increasing the competition for the organs. Defenders of the egalitarian version of the principle of justice claim that the inequity in wait times for people with equal severity of illness is the essence of an unfair system. If we had a national organ system, wait times would be evened out, and the sickest patients would have first claim (even if it turned out to decrease the efficiency of the system).

Political/Economic Reasons for a National List: Pittsburgh Politics

It also cannot be denied that the movement for a national list has economic and political dimensions. Donna Shalala did not simply dream up the idea of mandating that UNOS change its organ allocation system to make wait times more equal. Groups with an interest in this outcome worked very hard to see that the issue was brought to her attention and that she saw the arguments for making the change.

The University of Pittsburgh was instrumental in organizing testimony in favor of allocations that would create pressure to challenge the locals-first priority. Of the 106 individuals scheduled to testify at the December 1996 hearings, which provided the background for the issuing of the departmental rule, at least 20 were associated with the University of Pittsburgh, including surgeon John Fung; Mark A. Joensen, from CONSAD Research Corporation in Pittsburgh (which is associated with the university); at least ten University of Pittsburgh transplant recipients; four transplant candidates; two relatives of deceased University of Pittsburgh transplant recipients; one relative of a current candidate; and an attorney with ties to university-affiliated organizations and Pittsburgh's organ procurement organization. In addition, Pittsburgh was instrumental in encouraging others to testify. (We know, because one of us, RMV, was phoned by personnel associated with the University of Pittsburgh urging that he testify.)

Other Advocates for a More Nationally Oriented List

At the same time, others beyond Pittsburgh have concluded that some version of a national list is morally equitable and the right thing to do. Clive Callender, the head of the transplant program at Howard University and an outspoken defender of greater equity in organ allocation, is one of the few leaders of UNOS other than those from Pittsburgh who supported the HHS call for a fairer national allocation system.[57] He has long been aware that sometimes the most efficient allocation system is not the fairest. He has, for example, criticized excessive emphasis on human leukocyte antigen (HLA) tissue typing in kidney transplants, pointing out that tissue typing works to the disadvantage of blacks and other minorities whose HLA antigens do not match the donor pool as well as the Caucasian majority.

The Ethics of the Conflict over Geography

As demand for transplants continues to grow faster than supply, the question of geography remains the elephant in the room. In a book on the ethics of transplantation, it is appropriate to look at the ethics of this conflict.

The Inconclusiveness of the Utility Argument

Utilitarians may come out of this conflict about geography perplexed. The defenders of local priority have couched their arguments in utilitarian terms: shorter ischemia times, better-quality organs, more willingness to donate, and the preservation of local programs with more convenient care for local patients. However, we have seen that defenders of the national list can mount utilitarian arguments as well: more lives saved with modest burdens on patients in OPOs with short wait lists who lose organs to sicker patients elsewhere. The defenders of local priority counter by suggesting that a national list will simply force local patients in areas with short wait lists to wait until they are as sick and as hard to treat as those who are going to get the new priority claims on organs.

It is not immediately obvious which side wins the utilitarian debate. We may not have all the data we need. Moreover, utilitarian disputes have a way of depending on nonempirical questions such as how we quantify outcomes. This debate may hinge on such nebulous, hard-to-quantify issues as how bad it is to make a very sick person travel to another town to get multiple-listed and transplanted. It is not only the mortality rate that is at stake; it is also the quality of life of patients as they are on the wait list.

Perhaps the defenders of the existing local priority win the utilitarian argument, but it seems to be a complicated, close call. The utilitarian analysis is about a draw.

The Clear Implications of the Justice Argument

Conversely, the justice analysis, especially if it is carried out from the egalitarian perspective that we defended in chapter 17, seems overwhelmingly to favor a national list. There are gross inequities in making people who in all morally relevant respects are equal wait radically different lengths of time for desperately needed organs. There are even greater inequities in directing organs to healthier patients by priority over those who are desperately ill (local and regional candidates with MELD scores in the high teens before status 1 national candidates in the case of liver transplant) simply because of the morally irrelevant variable of where one happens to live.

If justice takes priority over utility, as we have consistently claimed in this book, some version of a national list seems to be a moral necessity—perhaps with modifications that nevertheless result in approximately equal wait times for similar candidates. But even if one makes the rather common move in moral theory (as was seen in the UNOS Ethics Committee) to claim that conflicts between utility and justice must be resolved by considering the weightiness of each principle and balancing the competing claims, a modified national list seems to carry the day. The utilitarian calculation leads to a standoff, whereas the principle of justice is weighted strongly on the side of some version of a national list (or at least one in which enough organs cross local area boundaries to offset existing inequities).

Only a pure, uncompromising utilitarian seems to be left perplexed. He or she is pulled between the claims of the smaller programs that have been pointing to the purported benefits of the local priority and the claims of the advocates of a national list who point to new benefits to be expected from the change to a national perspective. It is not clear where the pure utilitarian will come out. It is clear, however, that adopting the pure utilitarian position requires the belief that justice is irrelevant as a moral principle.[58] We argued in chapter 17 that accepting the utilitarian principle of utility maximizing has horrendous implications that are so offensive to the moral senses that they must be rejected.

Even if one is unwilling to accept this as a moral conclusion, one is still confronted with the legal reality that in the United States, federal law requires taking into account both equity and efficiency—that is, both justice and utility. When one principle (utility), with implications so evenly balanced that it is hard to tell which allocation it supports, is balanced against another that overwhelmingly supports one of the allocation options, then that option, on balance, must carry the day. Anyone committed to giving justice and utility equal consideration needs to support a single national list. And anyone who gives justice priority over utility must be even more convinced of this conclusion.

The Nation as a Moral Community

Another dimension of the controversy must be confronted that leads to the same conclusion. Defenders of local lists, especially shortsighted politicians in those states that have attempted to pass laws prohibiting the export of organs when they can be used within the state, adopt the moral position that the residents of the local area constitute a moral community that has a prior claim on citizens' loyalty before "outsiders" deserve any benefit. Only in cases where none of the members of the in-group can benefit will exports outside the group be accepted.

This is a troublesome view about the nature of the moral community. First, there is an obvious problem of whether people are supposed to be loyal to the citizens of their state or the citizens of their metropolitan area (their OPO) when they donate their life-saving organs. More seriously, we must ask why it is that we ought to feel morally bound to be loyal to human beings of our particular state or metropolitan area over those of other parts of the country. Is there some reason why we need to be so parochial in our identification with the needs of our fellow humans that a stranger a few score miles from us counts more morally than one a few hundred or thousand miles away?

In the United States the organ procurement and transplant program is a national one. In the case of kidneys, it is funded almost entirely by Medicare. For other organs, some of the funding is national—the organs funded by Medicare, Tricare (the military health care program), and other public insurance systems. Even most private health insurance systems have a national perspective. The transplant program is established by Congress. It is administered nationally. It is hard to see how nearby transplant candidates have a moral claim over those in more distant communities.

There is something to be said for the provision in the Uniform Anatomical Gift Act that permits donation of an organ to a member of one's own family who is in need. That law also permits donation to friends, to a hospital with which one has had an ongoing relationship, or to a transplant surgeon whom one knows. It is widely accepted that there are special duties of loyalty to one's family and friends. A mother with very limited resources confronted with her own child in need and a stranger child in equal need will undoubtedly pick her own child for favored treatment. We would be shocked if she did not. Family bonds of loyalty are strong and command priority over strangers.

It is hard to see why the same should be said for one's state or metropolitan area, why the people in that geographical area have any claim of loyalty over others, equally needy, in some other state or metropolitan area. Cultural maturity requires recognizing the irrationality of preference based solely on geographical proximity.

In the case of states like Louisiana or Oklahoma that once attempted to pass laws restricting the exporting of organs, the parochial restriction may not even be in the citizen's self-interest. Without examining the data, it is hard to know whether Louisiana is a net importer or exporter of organs. Ethics requires the principle of reciprocity. If it is morally correct for Louisianans to restrict exports, it must also be acceptable for other states to restrict shipments of organs into Louisiana. If Louisiana happens to be a net importer at the present time, its citizens will lose in their efforts to be ethnocentric.[59] Even if restriction turns out to be a winning policy—that is, if they happen to be exporters once a national list is adopted based on principles of fairness and equal treatment— morality cannot support such an irrational preference for one's own kind over outsiders.

The difference between being a Louisianan in heart failure and being a Mississippian similarly in heart failure is really not all that great. Taking a moral point of view, there can be no basis for each state giving its own citizens priority over the citizens of the other, especially in a national program where all are asked to participate as equals.

A full-blown ethic of organ transplantation would press on to ask similar questions about the morality of giving priority to the citizens of one's own country over those of another. This question raises complexities, no doubt. It would be particularly problematic to hold that morality requires sharing organs with nations that themselves have resisted developing organ procurement programs. (Conversely, it seems strange to hold those citizens who need organs responsible for their nation's objections to organ procurement, at least if the one needing the organ was not opposed to a procurement program.) For purposes of the present discussion, the least we can conclude is that the residents of the United States form a moral community with a single organ transplant practice. There can be no reason why organs should be restricted solely on the basis of geographical proximity between the donor and the recipient, except in those cases where medical necessity prohibits transport of the organ in a way that would maintain viability. Even then, the moral claim of all potential recipients similarly situated with regard to medical urgency, blood type, and time on the wait list is the same. This means that we have to have a single national list for allocating organs modified only in ways that increase efficiency without significantly sacrificing equity.

Did the Final Rule Achieve Equity?

The Final Rule, and the IOM report that affirmed its aims, focused on geographic disparities. It is a serious disparity that persists because the allocation revisions have been incremental and continue to promote more local priority than is necessary.

There are also other disparities—racial/ethnic, socioeconomic, and gender disparities—which have been documented since the early days of organ transplantation, and which persist today.[60] It is to these disparities that we now turn. We begin by evaluating other aspects of the organ allocation systems and their revisions that either intentionally or unintentionally have an impact on these other disparities.

Kidneys

As mentioned above, kidney allocation has morphed a great deal in the past three decades. The first standardized allocation system, as developed by Starzl, awarded points to candidates based on HLA matching, wait time, degree of presensitization, medical urgency, and logistical factors (including distance from the transplant center).[61] The Terasaki modification adopted in 1989 deleted the proximity to transplant center and urgency factors and placed even greater emphasis on HLA matching.[62] In addition, in November 1987, UNOS mandated that deceased donor kidneys having a recipient six-antigen match (or a zero-antigen mismatch) be shared on a national basis. This policy was instituted based upon the reported 10 percent graft survival advantage of zero-antigen mismatched kidneys when compared with less-well-matched kidneys, and the results were significant, despite the longer cold ischemia times.[63] Although this policy can be lauded for sharing nationally, the policy also mandated a "payback system." To prevent a net loss or gain of kidneys by any OPO, the OPO that accepts such a kidney must then "pay back" a kidney to a common national pool. That is, kidneys were still considered local resources. This policy was criticized by the Office of the Inspector General in 1991, quoting a transplant surgeon who ran an OPO: "Establishing a payback system also creates the illusion that a kidney is the property of a given OPO. Clearly, we need to foster the notion that organs for transplantation are a national resource which should be used in the most efficient and successful manner possible. They are not anyone's individual property."[64]

From a utility perspective, allocating kidneys to zero-antigen mismatch candidates was historically justified on efficiency grounds because better-matched kidneys had greater graft and patient survival, but more recent data show that the differences are less significant.[65] It was also noted early on that it puts African American transplant candidates at a significant competitive disadvantage.[66] By the early 1990s transplant researchers were noting that the amount of additional benefit from a zero-antigen mismatch was not so significant when compared with 1 and 2 antigen mismatches, and the differences continue to decrease given improvements in immunosuppression.[67] Thus the special status given to a zero-antigen mismatch can no longer be justified, particularly because a policy of nationally distributing zero-antigen, mismatched organs exacerbates racial and ethnic disparities, given that white candidates were more likely to have a zero-antigen mismatch than any other racial or ethnic group.[68] Also, the policies at the time required OPOs to "pay back" kidneys that were accepted for national sharing, further exacerbating the wait times of minority candidates in areas where white candidates were able to skip the queue with a zero-antigen mismatch.

The impact of the zero-antigen mismatch has been muted since a June 2012 policy revision that restricted national sharing of zero-antigen, mismatched kidneys to sensitized candidates (those with an elevated calculated panel reactive antibody who are more difficult to match). This will lead to many fewer organs shared at a national level, but it will reduce the inequities caused by zero-antigen mismatching. Although whites are more likely to have zero-antigen mismatches with potential donors, many of the whites are preemptively listed and are often nonsensitized, so they will not be allocated these organs. As such, the restriction of national sharing of zero-antigen mismatches to highly sensitized individuals will reduce the number of such kidneys shared and the disparities that they exacerbate. And the lost efficiency is quite small, given that zero-antigen mismatches really do not do much better than 1- or 2-antigen mismatched kidneys.

Another important component of the new kidney allocation algorithm is the switch from wait time (time spent on the wait list) to dialysis time. Dialysis time refers to the time on dialysis, whether or not one has succeeded in getting listed. Many studies show that there are many barriers for women, minorities, and those of low socioeconomic status to getting onto the wait list.[69] By using dialysis time, these candidates will accrue points even before they finish the process. However, the new system is actually not just dialysis time but dialysis time or a poor glomerular filtration rate (GFR < 20 mL/min/ 1.73 m^2). This means that individuals can accrue points when they have chronic kidney disease but still have enough function so they do not need dialysis. These individuals can get a transplant preemptively (before they begin renal replacement therapy). The data show that whites with private insurance are more likely to be listed preemptively and to get a preemptive transplant (based on zero-antigen mismatch), such that the new algorithm's tolerance of preemptive listing limits the equity that it might have otherwise obtained.[70]

But the new allocation system creates new inequities that should not be overlooked. The characterization of individuals in the top 20 percent EPTS (those who are matched to the best kidneys) uses four criteria: age, previous dialysis, previous transplant, and diabetes. First, setting the cutoff at 20 percent was arbitrarily chosen without any moral justification as to why it was 20 percent rather than 18 percent or 22 percent. Second, the 20 percent rule only evaluates candidates on one health condition—diabetes—that adversely affects life span. Now it is the case that diabetes is associated with shorter life expectancy, but so is cardiac disease, and that is not considered, mainly because we do not have good measurements in the UNOS database. Thus, the new algorithm discriminates against one disease, and one disease only. Egalitarians will find this offensive, given that individuals with diabetes are often considered some of the "worst off" individuals in kidney failure because of how poorly they do on dialysis and the other co-morbidities associated with diabetes.[71]

Liver

As mentioned above, the liver allocation algorithm has also evolved significantly since the passage of the Final Rule. The first step was small: The initial UNOS response to Shalala and the Final Rule was to retain the status quo with one exception—it gave status 1 regional candidates higher priority than less severely ill local candidates. The Share 35 policy was introduced in June 2013, and it further promotes regionalization. In addition to local and regional priority for status 1, the Share 35 policy requires local and regional priority for all candidates with a MELD score greater than or equal to 35. However, the algorithm still gives priority to local candidates with MELD scores greater than or equal to 15 before national sharing for candidates in status 1.

Another major change in the liver allocation process was the adoption of MELD and PELD in 2002. Although MELD/PELD has led to a reduction in mortality on the liver transplant wait list, the new algorithm is not without its critics. First, there are conditions that are not properly accounted for by the MELD score, either because (1) they are not accounted for properly by the variables included in the score or (2) the disease may progress more rapidly than others with the same MELD score, such that the focus on the risk of dying fails to account for the risk of disease progression that leaves individuals transplant-ineligible—for example, hepatocellular carcinoma (HCC).[72] To address the latter issue, candidates with HCC (and six other conditions) are given extra points. Although justice would support these algorithm variations to ensure that all candidates have a fair chance at getting an organ, some express concern that these extra points may be too great for some conditions. For example, data show that candidates with HCC have better outcomes than other candidates on the wait list, which has led some to advocate downgrading of their priority.[73]

Criticisms about the MELD score take one of two forms: (1) that there are additional objective criteria that could be incorporated and would improve its accuracy and (2) that the algorithm exacerbates disparities. Among the prognostic factors that could be incorporated into the MELD formula in an attempt to improve its reliability, hyponatremia (low sodium levels) has received the broadest attention. The biggest problem is that it is easily manipulated by simple therapeutic maneuvers, such as diuretic administration, plasma volume expansion, or hypotonic fluid infusion.[74] Another factor is serum albumin, which improves prognostic accuracy and is less easily manipulated.[75]

Myers and colleagues found that the MELD-based allocation system disadvantages women because of the use of serum creatinine in MELD. As Cholongitas and colleagues suggest, "A simple increase of points should be instituted for women awaiting liver transplant when MELD is used or in other formulae that use creatinine as it leads to unequal access.[76] Also, it is not only gender disparities that persist, despite so-called objective criteria.[77] Studies show that there are significant racial/ethnic and socioeconomic disparities in access to liver transplantation.[78]

Disparities: Root Causes

The disparities seen in kidney and liver transplantation are not solely caused by the algorithms used. Rather, the data show that disparities occur along the entire spectrum—from the timing of referral to subspecialists and the education obtained about the benefits of transplantation to undergoing the workup and getting listed.[79] There are also social barriers that often correlate more with socioeconomic status but may delay or hinder listing; these include inadequate or unstable health insurance, a lack of a care partner, an inability to obtain transportation and lack of a reliable way to contact the patient (low educational and health literacy level and/or a language barrier).[80]

Whether we are discussing racial, ethnic, or gender disparities in kidney or liver transplantation, two issues remain the same. First, the number of organs is finite, so not all candidates will receive one. Second, any allocation system will need to balance efficiency (maximizing aggregate utility) and equity (fair distribution). Although our personal moral theory would give priority to equity over efficiency, we recognize that there is no consensus in favor of that view.

This crucial choice involves how a society should affirm that it is a moral community of equals and how much it should sacrifice maximum efficiency in adding years of life in order to add them more equitably. This is fundamentally not a question for transplant professionals; nor is it a question for any other single interested stakeholder. Rather, it is a choice that all of us must make. Public trust demands as much.

Notes

1. National Organ Transplant Act, October 19, 1984, PL 98-507.

2. Starzl TE, Hakala TR, Tzakis A, et al., "A multifactorial system for equitable selection of cadaver kidney recipients," *JAMA* 1987;257: 3073–75; Starzl TE, Gordon RD, Tzakis A, et al., "Equitable allocation of extrarenal organs: With special reference to the liver," *Transplantation Proceedings* 1988;20 (1): 131–38.

3. Four programs were reported by Gunby P, "Media-abetted liver transplants raise questions of 'equity and decency,'" *JAMA* 1983;249: 1973.

4. There were twenty-five liver transplant programs in 1985 according to the *Health Care Financing Administration*; see Office of Organ Transplantation, American Council on Transplantation and Pancreas Transplantation Registry, as cited in table I-1, p. 17. US Department of Health and Human Services, Office of Organ Transplantation, Task Force on Organ Transplantation, *Organ transplantation: Issues and recommendations* (Washington, DC: US Government Printing Service, 1986).

5. The data from 1987 and 1993 are given by Norman DJ, "Letter to the editor: The distribution of organs for liver transplantation," *JAMA* 1994;272: 848.

6. US Department of Health and Human Services, "Organ Procurement and Transplantation Network: Final Rule," 42 CFR Part 121, *Federal Register* 63 (April 2, 1998): 16296–338.

7. Barshes NR, Hacker CS, Freeman RB Jr, Vierling JM, Goss JA, "Justice, administrative law, and the transplant clinician: The ethical and legislative basis of a national policy on donor liver allocation," *Journal of Contemporary Health Law & Policy* 2007;23 (2): 118.

8. Committee on Organ Procurement and Transplantation Policy, Division of Health Sciences Policy, Institute of Medicine, *Organ procurement and transplantation: Assessing current policies and the potential impact of the DHHS Final Rule* (Washington, DC: National Academy Press, 1999), 1.

9. US Department of Health and Human Services, Health Resources and Services Administration, 42 CFR Part 121 Organ Procurement and Transplantation Network, *Federal Register* 64 (202) (October 20, 1999): 56650–61.

10. US Department of Health and Human Services, Task Force on Organ Transplantation, *Organ transplantation*, 9–10.

11. Ibid.

12. Ibid., 9.

13. Starzl, Gordon, Tzakis, et al., "Equitable allocation," 132–33.

14. US Department of Health and Human Services, "Organ Procurement and Transplantation Network: Final Rule," 16296.

15. Ibid.

16. Committee on Organ Procurement and Transplantation Policy. Division of Health Sciences Policy, Institute of Medicine, *Organ procurement and transplantation*, 5.

17. Ibid., 1.

18. UNOS, "Policy 9: Allocation of livers and liver-intestines," effective date July 3, 2014, http://optn.transplant.hrsa.gov/ContentDocuments/OPTN_Policies.pdf#nameddest = Policy_09.

19. UNOS, "Policy 8: Allocation of kidneys," effective date July 3, 2014, http://optn.transplant.hrsa.gov/ContentDocuments/OPTN_Policies.pdf#nameddest = Policy_08.

20. A more complete discussion of these issues is given by Hippen BE, Thistlethwaite JR Jr., Ross LF, "Risk, prognosis, and unintended consequences in kidney allocation," *New England Journal of Medicine* 2011;364: 1285–87; and Ross LF, "Is the new kidney allocation proposal fair?" *US News & World Report*, Nov. 12, 2012, 14, 15, www.usnews.com/opinion/articles/2012/11/12/new-kidney-allocation-proposal-is-ethically-unacceptable.

21. US Department of Health and Human Services, "Organ Procurement and Transplantation Network: Final Rule," 16298.

22. UNOS, "Policy 11: Allocation of pancreas, kidney-pancreas, and islets," effective date July 3, 2014, http://optn.transplant.hrsa.gov/ContentDocuments/OPTN_Policies.pdf#nameddest = Policy_11.

23. Bernardi M, Gitto S, Biselli M, "The MELD score in patients awaiting liver transplant: Strengths and weaknesses," *Journal of Hepatology* 2011;54 (6): 1297–1306.

24. Smith JM, Biggins SW, Haselby DG, et al., "Kidney, pancreas and liver allocation and distribution in the United States," *American Journal of Transplantation* 2012;12: 3191–3212.

25. Merion RM, Schaubel DE, Dykstra DM, Freeman RB, Port FK, Wolfe RA, "The survival benefit of liver transplantation," *American Journal of Transplantation* 2005;5: 307–13.

26. Ibid.

27. Merion RM, "Current status and future of liver transplantation," *Seminars in Liver Disease* 2010;30 (4): 411–21.

28. United Network for Organ Sharing, "Talking about transplantation: Questions and answers for transplant candidates about liver allocation policy," July 15, 2013, www.unos.org/docs/Liver_patient .pdf.

29. UNOS, "Policy 9: Liver and liver-intestine."

30. Gentry SE, Massie AB, Cheek SW, et al., "Addressing geographic disparities in liver transplantation through redistricting," *American Journal of Transplantation* 2013;13: 2052–58.

31. UNOS, "Policy 1: Administrative rules and definitions," effective date July 3, 2014, http://optn .transplant.hrsa.gov/ContentDocuments/OPTN_Policies.pdf#nameddest = Policy_06.

32. UNOS, "Policy 6: Allocation of hearts and heart-lungs," effective date July 3, 2014, http:// optn.transplant.hrsa.gov/ContentDocuments/OPTN_Policies.pdf#nameddest = Policy_06.

33. UNOS, "Policy 10: Allocation of lungs," effective date July 3, 2014, http://optn.transplant .hrsa.gov/ContentDocuments/OPTN_Policies.pdf#nameddest = Policy_10.

34. *Janet and Francis Murnaghan v. United States Department of Health and Human Services, Kathleen Sebelius*, US District Court for the Eastern District of Pennsylvania, www.paed.uscourts.gov/ documents/opinions/13D0477P.pdf.

35. OPTN/UNOS Board of Directors, Proposal for Adolescent Classification Exception for Pediatric Lung Candidates, approved, effective date July 1, 2014, 11–14, http://optn.transplant.hrsa.gov/Content Documents/OPTN_Policy_Notice_07-01-2014.pdf.

36. "States wanting to prevent residents' donated organs from crossing state lines," *Topeka Capital-Journal*, July 15, 1998, http://cjonline.com/stories/071598/new_stateorgans.shtml.

37. Ibid., citing Frank Keating.

38. See, e.g., Jacobbi LM, McBride V, "Evolution of a statewide organ donation, recovery and allocation program: 'A Louisiana perspective,'" *Oschner Journal* 1999;1 (1): 19–26.

39. Davis AE, Mehrotra S, Kilambi V, et al., "The effect of the statewide sharing variance on geographic disparity in kidney transplantation in the United States," *Clinical Journal of the American Society of Nephrology (CJASN)*, Jun 26, 2014, ii, CJN.05350513, citing US Department of Health and Human Services, Organ Procurement and Transplant Network, *Catalogue of all current OPTN member variances*, April 2010.

40. Kayler LK, Srinivas TR, Schold JD, "Influence of CIT-induced DGF on kidney transplant outcomes," *American Journal of Transplantation* 2011; 11: 2657–64; van der Vliet JA, Warle MC, "The need to reduce cold ischemia time in kidney transplantation," *Current Opinion in Organ Transplantation* 2013;18 (2):174–78.

41. Maglione M, Ploeg RJ, Friend PJ, "Donor risk factors, retrieval technique, preservation and ischemia/reperfusion injury in pancreas transplantation," *Current Opinion in Organ Transplantation* 2013;18: 83–88.

42. Starzl, Gordon, Tzakis, et al., "Equitable allocation," 132–33.

43. Ubel PA, Caplan AL, "Geographic favoritism in liver transplantation: Unfortunate or unfair?" *New England Journal of Medicine* 1998;339: 1323.

44. Ibid.

45. Mandell MS, Zamudio S, Seem D, et al., "National evaluation of healthcare provider attitudes toward organ donation after cardiac death," *Critical Care Medicine* 2006;34: 2952–58; Siminoff LA, Agyemang AA, Traino HM, "Consent to organ donation: A review," *Progress in Transplantation* 2013;23 (1): 99–104; Siminoff LA, Arnold RM, Caplan AL, Virnig BA, Seltzer DL, "Public policy governing organ and tissue procurement in the United States: Results from the National Organ and Tissue Procurement Study," *Annals of Internal Medicine* 1995;123: 10–17.

46. Lin H-M, Kauffman HM, McBride MA, et al., "Center-specific graft and patient survival rates: 1997 United Network for Organ Sharing (UNOS) Report," *JAMA* 1998;280: 1158.

47. Ibid., 1160, quoting Hosenpud JD, Breen TJ, Edwards EB, Daily OP, Hunsicker LG, "The effect of transplant center volume on cardiac transplant outcome: A report of the United Network for Organ Sharing Scientific Registry," *JAMA* 1994;271: 1844–49.

48. Shuhaiber JH, Moore J, Dyke DB, "The effect of transplant center volume on survival after heart transplantation: A multicenter study," *Journal of Thoracic Cardiovascular Surgery* 2010;139 (4): 1064–69; Russo MJ, Iribarne A, Easterwood R, et al., "Post–heart transplant survival is inferior at low-volume centers across all risk strata," *Circulation* 2010;122 (suppl 1): S85–91; Pettit SJ, Jhund PS, Hawkins NM, et al., "How small is too small? A systematic review of center volume and outcome after cardiac transplantation," *Circulation: Cardiovascular Quality and Outcomes* 2012;5 (6): 783–90; Scarborough JE, Bennett KM, Davis RD, et al., "Temporal trends in lung transplant center volume and outcomes in the United States," *Transplantation* 2010;89: 639–43.

49. Macomber CW, Shaw JJ, Santry H, et al., "Centre volume and resource consumption in liver transplantation," *HPB: The Official Journal of the International Hepato Pancreato Biliary Association* 2012;14 (8): 554–59. Other studies, in contrast, did not show a correlation between volume and outcome. See, for example, Tracy ET, Bennett KM, Aviki EM, et al., "Temporal trends in liver transplant centre volume in the USA," *HPB: The Official Journal of the International Hepato Pancreato Biliary Association* 2009;11 (5): 414–21; and Reese PP, Yeh H, Thomasson AM, Shults J, Markmann JF, "Transplant center volume and outcomes after liver retransplantation," *American Journal of Transplantation* 2009;9: 309–17.

50. "Transplant Recipient Characteristics 1988-1996," Liver Recipients from the UNOS Annual Report for 1997, table 21.

51. Some other provisions of the regulation include a basic definition of the make-up of the OPTN, the procedure for the HHS to review OPTN policies, better availability to center-specific data about transplant centers, and authority to approve the OPTN wait list registration fee.

52. US Department of Health and Human Services, "Organ Procurement and Transplantation Network: Final Rule."

53. UNOS Kidney Transplant Committee, slide set titled "Proposal to substantially revise the National Kidney Allocation System," Sept. 2012, slide 9. The slide can be found at www.annanurse.org/download/reference/health/activities/unosWebinar_11_7_12.pdf, 5.

54. Ibid. The additional life years of 8,380 was reaffirmed by another report. See UNOS Kidney Committee, "Proposal to substantially revise the National Kidney Allocation System," Sept. 21, 2012, http://optn.transplant.hrsa.gov/PublicComment/pubcommentPropSub_311.pdf.

55. Merion et al., "Survival benefit"; and Merion, "Current status."

56. Testimony on organ donation allocation by the honorable Donna E. Shalala, secretary, US Department of Health and Human Services, before the Senate Labor and Human Resources Committee and also before the House Committee on Commerce, June 18, 1998, http://www.hhs.gov/asl/testify/t980618a.html.

57. Statement of Clive Callender, MD, Howard University Medical School, Hearings of the Department of Health and Human Services, Bethesda, MD, December 1, 1996.

58. Utilitarians may not accept this claim without a fight. They may refer to the British utilitarian, John Stuart Mill, who pointed out in chapter 5 of his *Utilitarianism* that even a utilitarian will recognize that more equality in the distribution of benefits is likely to lead to more aggregate benefit because usually giving a resource to a person who is poorly off will produce more good than giving it to one who is well off. This is normally the case with food or money, for instance. Giving food to someone who is starving does much more good than giving the same amount of food to someone who is already satiated. Giving $100 to a pauper may produce more good than giving it to a millionaire. This is the economist's notion of "decreasing marginal utility." Transplantation (and many other medical allocation problems), however, are interesting precisely because it is not obvious that giving the medical resource to the sicker person will do more good than giving it to the healthier one. In some cases, allocation will reflect decreasing marginal utility, just as it does in many economic problems. In some cases, however, giving the resource to the worse-off persons will actually do less good. They may already be so ill that they will predictably get less benefit from the resource than someone who is healthier. In that case, the utilitarian who is honest will accept the implications and defend the proposition that utility requires directing resources away from the worse off. Those in the worst-off category, unfortunately, will simply lose out. They will die from lack of an organ. Utilitarians will insist they did not set out intentionally to exclude the person so sick he is inefficient to treat. They will, in all honesty, say that it simply turns out when the numbers are crunched that more overall good is achieved if the organs go to those who are healthier.

59. Determining whether a state is a net importer or exporter is more difficult than it may appear. We cannot simply count the organs imported to the state's OPOs and the number exported. As we have seen, many OPOs cross state lines so it is not easy to track whether an organ procured in one state is moved to a part of the OPO in another state. Moreover, patients do not always get transplanted in the state in which they live. For example, Louisiana residents who have become listed for a transplant in another state would have their interests jeopardized by a rule requiring Louisiana organs to stay in Louisiana. To determine whether Louisiana is a net importer or exporter, we would have to learn how many Louisianans import organs within their bodies that they have received in out-of-state transplant centers.

60. Council on Ethical and Judicial Affairs, American Medical Association, "Black-white disparities in health care," *JAMA* 1990;263: 2344–46. Gaston RS, Ayres I, Dooley LG, Diethelm AG, "Racial equity in renal transplantation: The disparate impact of HLA-based allocation," *JAMA* 1993;270: 1352–56; Held PJ, Pauly MV, Bovbjerg RR, Newmann J, Salvatierra O Jr., "Access to kidney transplantation: Has the United States eliminated income and racial differences?" *Archives of Internal Medicine* 1988;148: 2594–600; Kjellstrand CM, "Age, sex, and race inequality in renal transplantation," *Archives of Internal Medicine* 1988;148: 1305–9.

61. Starzl, Gordon, Tzakis, et al., "Equitable allocation," 132–33.

62. Gaston et al., "Racial equity."

63. Takemoto S, Carnahan E, Terasaki PI, "A report of 504 six antigen-matched transplants," *Transplantation Proceedings* 1991;23 (1 Pt 2): 1318–20; Burlingham WJ, Munoz del Rio A, Lorentzen D, et al., "HLA-A, -B, and -DR zero-mismatched kidneys shipped to the University of Wisconsin, Madison, 1993–2006: Superior graft survival despite longer preservation time," *Transplantation* 2010;90: 312–18.

64. US Department of Health and Human Services, Office of Inspector General, *The distribution of organs for transplantation: Expectations and practices 8*, Report OEI-01-89-00550 (Washington, DC: US Government Printing Office, 1991), quoting a letter from Dr. Raben Kirkman, medical director of the New England Organ Bank.

65. Hata Y, Ozawa M, Takemoto SK, Cecka JM, "HLA matching," *Clinical Transplantation* 1996: 381–96; Su X, Zenios SA, Chakkera H, Milford EL, Chertow GM, "Diminishing significance of HLA matching in kidney transplantation," *American Journal of Transplantation* 2004;4: 1501–8.

66. Greenstein SM, Schechner R, Senitzer D, Louis P, Veith FJ, Tellis VA, "Does kidney distribution based upon HLA matching discriminate against blacks?" *Transplantation Proceedings* 1989;21 (6): 3874–75; US Department of Health and Human Services, Office of Inspector General, *Distribution of organs*.

67. Su et al., "Diminishing significance."

68. Gaston et al., "Racial equity"; Held PJ, Kahan BD, Hunsicker LG, et al., "The impact of HLA mismatches on the survival of first cadaveric kidney transplants," *New England Journal of Medicine* 1994;331: 765–70.

69. Joshi S, Gaynor JJ, Bayers S, et al., "Disparities among blacks, hispanics, and whites in time from starting dialysis to kidney transplant waitlisting," *Transplantation* 2013;95 (2): 309–18.

70. Kutner NG, Zhang R, Huang Y, Johansen KL, "Impact of race on predialysis discussions and kidney transplant preemptive wait-listing," *American Journal of Nephrology* 2012;35: 305–11; Grams ME, Chen BP, Coresh J, Segev DL, "Preemptive deceased donor kidney transplantation: Considerations of equity and utility," *Clinical Journal of the American Society of Nephrology* 2013;8: 575–82.

71. Guerra G, Ilahe A, Ciancio G, "Diabetes and kidney transplantation: Past, present, and future," *Current Diabetes Reports* 2012;12 (5): 597–603; Reutens AT, "Epidemiology of diabetic kidney disease," *Medical Clinics of North America* 2013;97 (1): 1–18; Helve J, Haapio M, Groop PH, Gronhagen-Riska C, Finne P, "Comorbidities and survival of patients with type 1 diabetes on renal replacement therapy," *Diabetologia* 2011;54 (7): 1663–69; Haapio M, Helve J, Groop PH, Gronhagen-Riska C, Finne P, "Survival of patients with type 1 diabetes receiving renal replacement therapy in 1980–2007," *Diabetes Care* 2010;33 (8): 1718–23.

72. Bernardi, Gitto, Biselli, "MELD score."

73. Ibid.; Huo TI, Wu JC, Lin HC, et al., "Determination of the optimal model for end-stage liver disease score in patients with small hepatocellular carcinoma undergoing loco-regional therapy," *Liver Transplantation* 2004;10: 1507–13; Pomfret EA, Washburn K, Wald C, et al., "Report of a national conference on liver allocation in patients with hepatocellular carcinoma in the United States," *Liver Transplantation* 2010;16: 262–78; Washburn K, Edwards E, Harper A, Freeman R, "Hepatocellular carcinoma patients are advantaged in the current liver transplant allocation system," *American Journal of Transplantation* 2010;10:1643–48.

74. Bernardi, Gitto, Biselli, "MELD score."

75. Myers RP, Shaheen AA, Faris P, Aspinall AI, Burak KW, "Revision of MELD to include serum albumin improves prediction of mortality on the liver transplant waiting list," *PLoS ONE* 2013;8 (1): e51926.

76. Cholongitas E, Marelli L, Kerry A, et al., "Female liver transplant recipients with the same GFR as male recipients have lower MELD scores—a systematic bias," *American Journal of Transplantation* 2007;7: 685–92; Lai JC, Terrault NA, Vittinghoff E, Biggins SW, "Height contributes to the gender difference in wait-list mortality under the MELD-based liver allocation system," *American Journal of Transplantation* 2010;10: 2658–64; Mindikoglu AL, Regev A, Seliger SL, Magder LS, "Gender disparity in liver transplant waiting-list mortality: The importance of kidney function," *Liver Transplantation* 2010;16 (10): 1147–57.

77. Mindikoglu et al., "Gender disparity."

78. Mathur AK, Schaubel DE, Gong Q, Guidinger MK, Merion RM, "Racial and ethnic disparities in access to liver transplantation," *Liver Transplantation* 2010;16 (9): 1033–40; Yu JC, Neugut AI, Wang S, et al., "Racial and insurance disparities in the receipt of transplant among patients with hepatocellular carcinoma," *Cancer* 2010;116 (7): 1801–9.

79. Institute of Medicine, *Unequal treatment: Confronting racial and ethnic disparities in health care* (Washington, DC: National Academies Press, 2003); Joshi et al., "Disparities." See also Ladin K, Rodrigue JR, Hanto DW, "Framing disparities along the continuum of care from chronic kidney disease

to transplantation: Barriers and interventions," *American Journal of Transplantation* 2009;9: 669–74; and Schold JD, Gregg JA, Harman JS, Hall AG, Patton PR, Meier-Kriesche HU, "Barriers to evaluation and wait listing for kidney transplantation," *Clinical Journal of the American Society of Nephrology* 2011;6 (7): 1760–67. Kutner NG, Zhang R, Huang Y, Johansen KL, "Impact of race on predialysis discussions and kidney transplant preemptive wait-listing," *American Journal of Nephrology* 2012;35 (4): 305–11; Purnell TS, Hall YN, Boulware LE, "Understanding and overcoming barriers to living kidney donation among racial and ethnic minorities in the United States," *Advances in Chronic Kidney Disease* 2012;19 (4): 244–51.

80. Flattau A, Olaywi M, Gaglio PJ, Marcus P, Meissner P, Dorfman EBL, Reinus JF, "Social barriers to listing for adult liver transplantation: Their prevalence and association with program characteristics," *Liver Transplantation* 2011;17 (10): 1167–75. See also Wong LL, Hernandez BY, Albright CL, "Socioeconomic factors affect disparities in access to liver transplant for hepatocellular cancer," *Journal of Transplantation* 2012: 870659, www.hindawi.com/journals/jtrans/2012/870659; and Hook JL, Lederer DJ, "Socioeconomic barriers to lung transplantation: Balancing access and equity," *American Journal of Respiratory & Critical Care Medicine* 2012;186 (10): 937–39.

Chapter 23

Socially Directed Donation

Restricting Donation by Social Group

Although the possibility of donating an organ to a specific individual who needs it—a family member or friend—has been recognized since the beginning of organ transplants, recently some people have attempted to direct organs to a specific social group—for example, to a group defined by race, religion, ethnicity, gender, or sexual orientation. This chapter examines how organ transplant programs should respond to such attempts. The goal here, however, is not merely to spell out our current national policy regarding this socially directed donation but also to tease out its surprisingly radical implications for some major questions in ethical theory—in particular, the theory of justice and what it means to have a just or fair social practice. The implication is that by careful consideration of our considered moral intuitions about a specific policy, we will not only discover a better understanding of the morally correct practice but may also be able to advance more fundamental work in ethical theory, a development that could have implications well beyond transplantation. The suggestion is that practical ethics may turn out to be a two-way street. Not only do we move from ethical theory to practical problem solving, but we may also move the other way—from clear, considered moral judgments to a more sophisticated and precise ethical theory.

Two Examples of Socially Directed Donation

As we have seen in earlier chapters, if organs are donated, normally they go to the individual selected by an allocation formula that, depending on the organ, takes into account such factors as human leukocyte antigen (HLA) tissue histocompatibility, time spent on the wait list for organs, blood type, degree of medical urgency, and geography. In the United States the selection is made by a computer that is independent of the wishes or knowledge of the family of the deceased. It can be claimed that this computer allocation system is procedurally fair. Once the patient is listed in the system, it is virtually impossible for either the patient or a physician to manipulate the system for a special advantage.[1] The computer does not take into account race, gender, socioeconomic status, or other social classification.[2] In this sense the computer allocation system could be considered fair and impartial. Two examples may help frame the issues.

Thomas Simons: Organs to Whites Only

When Thomas Simons, a resident of Florida, died as a result of being shot in a $5 robbery, he became a potential source of organs for transplant. Members of his family were approached by the organ procurement officials. But then the family made an unusual request. Simons had been a sympathizer of the Ku Klux Klan. Three Klan cards were found in his wallet. His family offered his organs, but stipulated on the donation form "donation to white recipients only."[3] Similar requests for "socially directed donation" have been reported that direct organ donation to members of a specified race, religion, gender, sexual orientation, or disease group. Some have considered directed donation in favor of a specific hospital or surgeon, for or against people with liver disease as a result of alcoholism, and so forth.

Those within the transplant community have been almost unanimously unsympathetic to socially directed donation. They support the allocation based on a formula because it is likely to provide organs that have a good chance of survival and/or allocate organs fairly. When families persist, however, the question arises whether this kind of directed donation should be accepted with the limits set by the donors rather than intentionally losing a set of organs that have the potential of saving several humans lives and improving the quality of lives of others.

The organ procurement agency in the Simons case agreed to the family's conditions on the donation. That decision generated considerable controversy. The Ethics Committee of the United Network for Organ Sharing (UNOS)—the US national body responsible for allocating organs—has, without opposition, adopted the position that donation directed to a particular social group (race, religion, or gender) is morally unacceptable. And since the Simons case, the State of Florida has passed legislation making socially directed donation illegal in that state.[4] The Washington Regional Transplant Community, the group responsible for producing and allocating organs in the Washington metropolitan area, has banned donations directed by social group. But some people, including a number of transplant surgeons and advocates for groups that presently do not get organs in proportion to their numbers in the recipient pool, have argued that it is wasteful to refuse lifesaving organs even if they come with discriminatory conditions. They have proposed that society tolerate a directed donation in cases where the family members, after attempts to persuade them to the contrary, persist in making a donation with discriminatory limits attached.

Directing Donation to the Military

The example of restricting donation to Caucasians sounds blatantly offensive. In order to give a fair hearing to the arguments for socially directed donation, however, it is useful to also consider proposals for socially directed donation that are more intuitively attractive. One such proposal has surfaced recently. Under this proposal, families asked to donate the organs of a loved one might be given the opportunity to donate one of the kidneys (and perhaps more of the organs) to a current or former member of the military. The logic seems to be that such individuals have served their country and deserve special consideration, especially if their need for an organ is the result of an injury suffered in battle or otherwise as a consequence of their military service. Should families be invited to make such a restricted gift? If not, should procurement organizations accept gifts of organs from deceased donors if the deceased or the family of the deceased attaches such a restriction?

The Concept of Socially Directed Donation

These two examples—donations directed based on race or on military service—are instances of what we will call "socially directed donation" or "conditional donation." The donation is restricted, but not to a named individual or institution. Rather, the restriction is to a sociological category—race, religion, gender, sexual orientation, age, or occupation. Someone might want to donate preferentially to children or to a member of their religious group. There have been cases where living individuals may want to donate their organs nondirectedly, but to specify that the organ not be given to someone who smokes or drinks (i.e., who brought on liver failure through voluntary actions) or a Buddhist who requested that her organs not be given to someone in a "killing vocation" (e.g., a hunter, fisherman, or military person).[5]

We distinguish, then, between donations directed to a sociologically defined group—such as a member of a certain race, religion, employment group, or age group—and those that are directed to a named individual or institution, even though the donor did not know the individual in any way before establishing a relation for the purposes of donation. Current law permits directing a donation not only to a named person (typically, a relative needing an organ) but also to a hospital. This appears to be left over from the days before there existed a systematic organ allocation system in the United States. If a donation is directed only by specifying a sociological category, it would normally need to rely on the organ procurement organization to match the donor's organ or organs with the specified class of recipients. If directing to a named individual or institution, the process will normally rely on provisions in the law that permit people to donate organs to named individuals or institutions, thus avoiding the involvement of procurement organizations. In this chapter, then, we limit our attention to socially directed donations to sociologically defined groups.

Moral Arguments about Socially Directed Donation

The justification to support socially directed donations is usually based in utility, although some sophisticated utilitarians might decide that the benefits are not worth the risk of an angry public. Similarly, some forms of egalitarianism may support socially directed donation to the extent that it offers some benefit to those who are worse off. In this section we discuss these moral arguments.

Utilitarian Considerations

Even though the UNOS Ethics Committee adopted its position to proscribe socially directed donations without opposition, there continues to be a moral division of opinion in UNOS, in the transplant community, and among donor families over what is the morally preferable policy. At first it appears that the surgeons and others who favor tolerating socially directed donation do so on utilitarian grounds. Some have recommended a policy of having the procurement personnel explain the reasons why it would be preferable to donate to the person at the top of the list, without regard to social group. The allocation algorithms are finely tuned, complex formulas that take into account many variables—the probability of success, likelihood of getting an organ in the future, time on the wait list, blood type, HLA, age, geography, and many other factors. The algorithm represents a collective judgment about what constitutes a fair balance between equity and efficiency in the use of a precious, scarce resource. By contrast, directing the organ to a specific social group circumvents this algorithm and directs the organ to someone with a weaker claim to it.

Let us assume that the national policy should be that the procurement organization should attempt to persuade a family wanting to direct a donation to a specific social group that it would be preferable to make an unrestricted gift. The question is what should happen if the family refuses to agree and continues to insist that the donation be directed to a specific social group. Many surgeons have suggested that we should reluctantly accept the restricted gift.

If some plausible assumptions are made, it appears that more lives will be saved and more years of organ graft survival can be expected with a policy that tolerates socially directed donation than one that simply wastes the organs that are donated conditionally. Surgeons are often known to be moral consequentialists. They might hold that they should choose the policy on donation that will maximize the aggregate net benefit from the organs that are available. If they did, they would be utilitarians.

If that were the basis for evaluating a socially directed donation, it seems that some social categories could prove more problematic than others. Donations restricted to children or the military, for example, may not be as likely to produce a backlash. This suggests that as a matter of social policy, we should evaluate which groups are likely to produce the problem of turning people against the transplant endeavor.

Could we then create a list of permissible conditional donations? Children do much worse on dialysis than adults because it affects their growth and cognitive development. Some would argue that this justifies giving them extra priority in the deceased donor kidney wait list, and might justify allowing conditional donations to children. Others, however, rely on the "fair innings" argument we developed in chapter 20 to claim that children would still be worse off even if they did not suffer more serious growth and development problems. Wayne Arnason has argued in favor of permitting conditional donations by black deceased donors to black recipients, given the longer wait that black candidates have. He compared it with the practice of retaining blood type O organs for blood type O candidates, even though any candidate could benefit from the donation.[6]

Interestingly, the public supports some conditional donations. Aaron Spital has shown that the majority of individuals support allowing a donor who wants to donate to a child, but most do not support the donor who wants to donate based on race or religion.[7] However, he also found that of those who would consider donating to a stranger, more than 90 percent would still donate, even if they could not choose the type of recipient.[8] Peter Ubel has shown that the public does not want to donate deceased livers to those who drink and smoke, suggesting that some conditional donations may be more acceptable to the public than others.[9]

Trying to categorize acceptable and unacceptable social groups, however, could itself be controversial. There are probably disutilities in undertaking to establish which donations are acceptable and which are not. This has led some—on utilitarian grounds—to favor a policy of excluding all socially directed donations. One organ procurement organization was once asked to restrict a donation to a "good Catholic." Clearly, the organization wanted nothing to do with deciding who qualified as a good Catholic. There is likely to be some degree of opposition to any imaginable social category. Trying to decide who is acceptable and unacceptable is perhaps not worth the effort.

Nonutilitarian Considerations

Opponents of socially directed donation, when asked, offer an array of reasons for their opposition. Occasionally, a sophisticated utilitarian may oppose socially directed donation, claiming that the overall transplant endeavor could be jeopardized if a dramatic socially directed donation case, such as that of the Ku Klux Klan member or of a donation limited to a gay recipient, turned the public against the organ transplant system.

However, based on the existing literature opposing socially directed donation and the Florida law that has made donation directed to a sociological group illegal, many opponents, when asked why they oppose socially directed donation, will respond with the statement that it is unfair, inequitable, or unjust.[10] The policy is one that would take a carefully crafted policy judgment producing an algorithm that yields a computer-generated priority list of recipients and replaces it with a policy permitting individual donors to circumvent the algorithm. Doing so would pluck a recipient out of the middle of the wait list—based solely on factors such as race, gender, or religion—to give that person a lifesaving advantage. In general, the dispute has the appearance of a feud between utilitarians, who tolerate socially directed donation, and egalitarians, who are committed to the principle of justice, and who thus oppose it even at the expense of losing some valuable organs. This would be yet another example of a commitment to justice meaning sacrificing efficiency for equity.

The analysis, however, must be more complex. Utilitarian aggregate net benefit maximization is not the only plausible defense of a policy that accepts or tolerates socially directed donation. One of the most respected versions of the principle of justice also seems to provide a case for socially directed donation—the theory of American twentieth-century philosopher, John Rawls. In his seminal work, *A Theory of Justice*, Rawls claimed that justice should take precedence over utility in the establishment of basic social practices.[11] His interpretation of justice, however, includes a rationale for permitting certain inequalities. In particular, inequalities are tolerated when favoring the advantaged group ends up benefiting the worst off. For example, rewarding talented elites would be acceptable, provided that this was necessary to encourage those with such talents to use them to help those who are among the worst off. The goal of the Rawlsian understanding of justice is to maximize the well-being of those with the minimum (even if it requires further advantaging those on the top). For this reason, it is often referred to as a "maximin" view—the goal is to maximize the minimum. This understanding of justice is also referred to as the "difference principle," because it attempts to justify different levels of benefit for people when accepting such differences helps the worst off.

The Rawlsian maximin difference principle, to the extent it can be applied at this level of specificity, also provides a basis for supporting socially directed donation.[12] After showing that the maximin has the potential of supporting socially directed donation, we consider alternative theories of justice that are less supportive.

Organ allocation in the United States is made on the basis of formally developed algorithms designed to integrate the goals of fairness and efficiency.[13] With socially directed donation, one person is given what is easily seen as an unfair and undeserved lifesaving advantage.[14] He or she is taken from the middle of the ranked priority list and given an extremely scarce and valuable good—a human organ. This constitutes unequal treatment based on a morally irrelevant consideration—race, gender, or religion. But this is a very special kind of advantage. It is realistic to say that, at least if the organ would otherwise be discarded, no one is disadvantaged by the privileged position of the designated recipient. In fact, those above him or her on the wait list are left exactly where they were before the socially directed donation, assuming that the alternative to discriminatory allocation is letting the organs go to waste.

The intriguing thing about socially directed donation is that everyone below the privileged recipient is actually made better off because of the discrimination. They all move up one position on the wait list.[15] This is a pure example of a case where tolerating the unequal treatment of one person by permitting discrimination based on factors such as race or religion is to the advantage of everyone who is worse off (lower on the list) and to the disadvantage of no one.

The maximin principle holds that inequalities are justified when (and only when) they are to the benefit of the least well off. Because the worst off are made somewhat better off if they are discriminated against, the maximin principle seems to support socially directed donation. The moral basis of that support converges with the utilitarian's basis, although the claim is a different one. The maximin supports socially directed donation because it benefits the worst off, not because it maximizes the aggregate good of the transplant endeavor.

However, the Rawlsian maximin theory of justice is not the only interpretation of what justice requires. Some justice theorists, who can generally be referred to as "true" or "radical" egalitarians, criticize Rawls insofar as he is providing a defense of inequality (when inequality helps those who are worst off). True or radical egalitarians find that an odd implication of a theory of justice. They understand justice to require not only the equal treatment of people who are equal in their relevant characteristics but also policies that give people opportunities to be more equal with others.[16] The controversy is over how one should evaluate the moral situation when an action can benefit the worst off, but in the process make people less equal. This is what happens when we follow the Rawlsian strategy of giving a significant advantage to an already-well-off person in order to help those worst off (even if they are helped less than the already-advantaged one). The result is helping the one on the bottom but, in the process, making the difference greater. This is precisely the case when, through socially directed donation, someone who is already fairly well off (e.g., someone fairly far up on the wait list) is advantaged unfairly (moved to the top of the list) and the justification is that doing so helps those on the bottom. Although Rawlsians would consider this to be fair, true or radical egalitarians would not. Thus, socially directed donation seems to be a real-life case in which a max-imin version of the principle of justice leads to a significantly different conclusion from a true egalitarian version.

The Inadequate Case for the Maximin

Rawls is very much aware of the difference between the maximin and what we call true egalitarianism. He suggests the rather strange notion that egalitarianism "admits to degrees," so that in some forms of egalitarianism, disparities are permitted.[17] Thus, according to this view, some equalities are more equal than others. In a critical section of *A Theory of Justice*, he addresses the reasons for supporting the maximin difference prin-ciple version over the idea that justice requires allocating resources so as to produce opportunities for equality of well-being as far as possible.[18] In the context of socially directed organ donation, this should be seen as a defense of favoring one already-advantaged candidate when doing so means those in other social groups will not be given equal treatment.

Rawls's Grounding of Strict Egalitarianism in Envy

Rawls apparently views the principle of true egalitarianism—of striving for opportunities for equality of outcomes—as grounded in envy. He begins the analysis with the plausible presumption that envy is to be "avoided and feared" and that the principles of justice should not be influenced by this trait.[19] He is quite committed to showing that his princi-ples of justice need not be based in envy, but in the process posits that strict egalitarianism can only be founded on it. Note in the following passage his movement, without argu-ment, from the claim that strict egalitarianism "conceivably" derives from envy, to the view that this strict egalitarianism would be adopted only on the basis of this psychological propensity. He begins by attempting to defend the maximin version of equality from the foundation in envy, differentiating his version from strict egalitarianism in the process: "To be sure, there may be forms of equality that do spring from envy. Strict egalitari-anism, the doctrine which insists upon an equal distribution of all primary goods, *conceiv-ably* derives from this propensity. What this means is that this conception of equality would be adopted in the original position only if the parties are assumed to be sufficiently envious" (emphasis added).[20]

Of course, Rawls is correct that envy could be the basis for a striving for greater equality, whether he has in mind the strict or the maximin version. This amounts to saying that those who are not the beneficiaries of a socially directed donation *may* oppose it because they are envious. But is there any basis for his statement that strict egalitari-anism would be adopted only if the parties are sufficiently envious?

Rawls posits that rational people are not envious. He can think of no reason why rational people behind a veil of ignorance (i.e., if they did not know their own position in society[21]) would see moral significance in pursuing equality per se. It is only getting the worst off as well off as possible that has moral significance. Often this can be achieved by transferring assets from the well off to those who are worse off, which would shrink the gap between the two groups. But it is not the shrinking of the gap itself that is morally significant; it is the raising of the floor (even if the only way to do so is to increase the gap between the haves and the have-nots). In the context of organ donation, it is not equality of access to donated organs per se that is morally important; it is getting an organ to those at the bottom of the list as soon as possible.

Problems with Grounding Strict Egalitarianism in Envy

There are some serious problems with this position that grounds strict or true egalitarianism in envy, however. For one, it seems to assume that it is only those who are the have-nots (or think from the perspective of the have-nots) who would favor strict egalitarianism. In fact, it is often the elites, the well off, who have a moral sense of justice that supports greater equality, other things being equal. Thus, for example, many of the most vocal defenders of a strict egalitarian prohibition on socially directed donation of organs come from the groups (e.g., the white liberal intelligentsia) whose members are precisely the ones who would be most favored by certain socially directed donations.

Without envy, Rawls claims, no one would favor equality as an interpretation of the principle of justice.[22] They would favor inequalities when necessary to benefit the worst-off groups. What this interpretation cannot explain is why those in the most favored groups (e.g., white liberals) also favor strict egalitarianism.

This grounding of support for equality in envy must be challenged. What is at stake is our understanding of what Rawls calls the "sense of justice." According to him, those imagining their interests if they happened to be among the well off would never favor equality; they would only support boosting the floor out of empathy for the worst off. In the case of organ donation, they would favor whatever policy got an organ to those on the bottom of the wait list, even if it meant giving others an unfair advantage. Yet many who have cultivated a sense of justice who are well off in fact feel discomfort when they contemplate inequality. It is surely not envy that would lead them to favor equality.

Of course, it is not acceptable to assume that this discomfort is automatically evidence for the existence of some moral force grounded in equality. The discomfort could result from other psychological phenomena, such as the long-held cultural belief that inequalities were ethically suspect or were disapproved of for other reasons. For example, if it were only the worst off who experienced this discomfort, Rawls's explanation based on envy might provide an adequate account.

That a "Sense of Justice" May Perceive Opportunities for Equality to Be Inherently Right Making

However, the widely experienced discomfort throughout all sectors of the population when one experiences an undeserved advantage (when one gets moved to the head of the wait list for organs based on social group) casts doubt on the envy hypothesis. One possibility is that a properly cultivated "sense of justice" would see moral rightness in equality of opportunity as well as in improving the lot of the worst off.

What is missing from the Rawlsian sense of justice is any notion of community solidarity. Some have such an empathy for their fellow humans that they have a moral sense of revulsion at a lack of opportunities for equality, regardless of whether they are among the best or worst off. For example, parents, contemplating the life outcomes for their children, may not be content with the utilitarian arrangement that would maximize the sum total of net well-being for all their children by making one do particularly poorly. They might not even favor a maximin arrangement, whereby inequalities among their children would be accepted provided they served the interests of the worst off. They might hope for some similar amount of well-being for each. They might, in fact, purposely arrange their resources so as not to maximize either the aggregate total well-being or the well-being of the worst off, but rather to give each child a fair opportunity for equality of well-being. This orientation seems particularly plausible when the improvement in the lot of the worst off would be small and the inequalities large. Rawls's account does not seem to be able to account for this aspect of the sense of justice.

Likewise, persons who have a well-developed sense of justice, complete with sympathy for their fellow humans, might see moral rightness in arrangements that provide opportunities for equality of well-being. They might consider it morally right to arrange resources to accomplish this end (other things being equal). That could include opposition to a policy that would extract someone from the middle of a wait list to give that person an organ just because that person is a member of a particular social group.

Egalitarian Justice as a Prima Facie Principle

Thus, there is an alternative that is a much simpler and more straightforward conception of the principle of justice: To view justice as a right-making characteristic of actions that strives for equality of opportunity for well-being. Doing so seems much more straightforwardly an understanding of the notion of equality that drives egalitarian notions of justice than the maximin.

There are, of course, problems with this more strictly egalitarian approach to justice. The most obvious is that strictly egalitarian justice would require giving a resource such as an organ to the worst off, even if the advantage to that person was tiny compared with the advantage that could be obtained from it by others. It would seem to require, for example, giving a liver to the worst-off person, even if that person could gain only a few days, whereas some other, better-off patient could gain years.

One response of the egalitarian is to point out that when the advantage to the worst-off person is so minimal, that person might simply waive his or her right of access. In the case of an organ transplant, it would not plausibly be in the candidate's interest to undergo major, painful, risky surgery to gain only a day or two of life. That candidate would rationally decline the organ, even if he or she were entitled to it by the consideration of justice.

Some people might go further. They might say that this worst-off person who could gain only a minimal benefit is not even morally entitled to the resource (and so should not be given the opportunity to refuse it).[23] There are also other lines of argument open to those who would sometimes conclude that following the rule of always giving the organ to the worst-off person is implausible.

Justice as One among Many Prima Facie Principles

Justice is not plausibly going to turn out to be the only moral principle, not even in cases of distribution of benefits and burdens. Other principles may pull simultaneously in other directions by identifying other characteristics of actions that independently make them right. We have seen that current American law requires attention both to efficiency and to equity, utility and justice. The UNOS Ethics Committee adopted a policy that gives these two principles equal weight. This makes true egalitarianism (merely) a prima facie principle, that is, a principle that expresses one characteristic of actions that will tend to make them morally right but that may need to be balanced against other considerations, such as the amount of good done. A morally right distribution of resources would need to take into account other moral principles, including beneficence and autonomy. Rawls, in fact, at some points, makes a similar point; but for some reason, he conceptualizes justice in such a way that considerations of maximizing benefit (for the worst off) are packed into the principle of justice.[24]

Justice as Opportunity for Equality

The alternative is to conceptualize justice more purely as dealing with matters of equality, leaving to the task of resolution of conflict among principles the problem of reconciling conflicts between justice and beneficence or justice and autonomy.[25] True egalitarians face a serious problem at this point, however. It is clear that one easy way to make everyone equal in well-being would be to reduce everyone to the level of the worst off. Everyone with zero well-being (everyone dead) would be pure egalitarianism. But surely that cannot be the goal of any moral system. There is, after all, something to be said for tolerating at least moderate differences in salary if they are necessary to make those receiving the lowest salaries get salaries that are as high as possible. No one favors a medical policy that would reduce everyone to the level of health that is the best that can be achieved for the incurably ill or disabled. Is not the more plausible interpretation the maximin in which the goal is the get the worst off as well off as possible while not reducing the well-being of the better off unless it serves the interest of the worst off?

At the least it is surely better for everyone to be equal at a high level rather than equal at a low level of well-being. That intuition can be explained by the maximin principle, but not by true egalitarianism taken by itself.

Explanations of Tolerance for Inequality: Sacrificing Justice for Other Principles

In this section we consider how to resolve conflicts between justice and other moral principles like beneficence, autonomy, and promise keeping. The practice of tolerating or proscribing socially directed donations offers a good case by which to analyze these conflicting principles.

The Maximin as a Rule to Resolve Conflicts between Justice and Beneficence

There are alternative explanations, however. First, the maximin might be seen as a moral rule that integrates two prima facie principles: justice (in the true egalitarian sense) and beneficence. A full normative moral theory includes several moral principles in addition to justice. Rawls held as much.[26] One of these principles is surely beneficence. How one integrates the claims of (true egalitarian) justice and beneficence is a matter that must be addressed in a moral theory of resolution of conflict among principles.

One hypothesis worth pursuing is that the Rawlsian maximin is, in fact, not a moral principle at all but a proposal for a moral rule that integrates the conflicting claims of the principles of justice and beneficence in situations dealing with the allocation of scarce primary goods. It would hold that, when the goals of maximizing benefit and minimizing inequality come into conflict, the conflict can be resolved by striving for equality unless inequalities redound to the benefit of the least well off. This would incorporate beneficence as a reason to override (egalitarian) justice when (and only when) it increases beneficence to the worst off.

This view of resource allocation involving conflict between egalitarian justice and beneficence easily explains why we would prefer equality at a high level over equality at a low level. Beneficence presses us toward higher levels of well-being. When that can be achieved without sacrificing equality, then beneficence pulls us, without opposition, in favor of the higher level. There is no conflict between the principles.

This suggests that justice should be interpreted in its egalitarian version as a prima facie principle that upon occasion conflicts with a prima facie principle of beneficence. The maximin is a rule for deviating from justice rather than being a principle of justice itself. It is a *specification* of the principles.[27]

Whether the maximin is the best possible rule for resolving conflict between beneficence and justice is controversial. In some cases it seems to lead to quite plausible conclusions; but in other cases it does not. There are other priority rules that may better explain our considered moral judgments.

The socially directed donation example poses a real challenge to the maximin rule interpreted this way. If the maximin rule applies, it seems likely that socially directed donation would have to be accepted. Yet many people find socially directed donation intolerable. The UNOS Ethics Committee, after considerable contemplation, concluded without opposition that socially directed donation was ethically unacceptable. Likewise, government attorneys have held that such a practice would violate current civil rights laws. These commentators have concluded that their considered moral judgment is firm against the practice of directed donation. If the maximin rule is the correct reconciliation of the conflict between justice and beneficence, then why should socially directed donation generate such resistance?

Lexically Ranking Justice over Beneficence While Balancing It against Other Principles

One possible conclusion is that the maximin rule is not the correct rule, at least in all cases. In some cases it appears that holding out for a right to an opportunity for equality is preferable to tolerating inequalities merely to improve somewhat the lot of the worst off. Socially directed donation may be one such case. If so, socially directed donation would not be made acceptable merely because it raises the worst off one notch on the wait list.

A more plausible rule for reconciliation of conflict may be that egalitarian justice is lexically ranked over beneficence and therefore equality is always a more weighty claim when only those two principles come into conflict. (This is the reconciliation between these two principles that we outlined in chapter 2.) If other prima facie principles can constrain egalitarian justice (even though beneficence cannot), then it may be possible to explain a certain social acceptance of inegalitarian outcomes without permitting beneficence to compete with justice. Other principles, such as respect for autonomy and promise keeping, may provide a more limited and more plausible basis for overriding egalitarian justice upon occasion without opening the floodgates to permit beneficence to offset it.

If inequalities are to be tolerated in the name of the maximin, it seems to make a difference whether it is the worst off who are making the case for the toleration of the inequality or it is those who will be given unique, unjustified advantage. Rawls himself acknowledges as much, but the defenders of the Rawlsian version of the maximin cannot explain this sense that it makes a difference who proposes tolerating the inequality.[28] Those who favor a lexical ranking of egalitarian justice can easily explain it. If the worst off have a claim to equality ranked above the principle of beneficence, then they could have the right grounded in autonomy to waive this claim. If they waive it, then there would be no moral imperative to pursue equality. If the advantages gained are great in comparison with the amount of inequality created, then they could plausibly exercise their autonomy to waive their right to equal treatment. Beneficence would then run free to permit maximizing the well-being of the worst off by increasing inequality. If the worst off do not exercise their waiver, then the unequal advantage created by socially directed donation would not be acceptable.

Likewise, promises made could provide a counterclaim to justice in a way that does not permit beneficence to run amuck. Consider, for example, a case where an equitable health care system promised certain benefits, such as transplantable organs, to certain groups of people. For example, the present allocation promises children a special advantage in obtaining kidneys over their older colleagues on the wait list. If persons are promised an advantage, they may have some moral claim to it, even if fulfilling the promise will tend to produce inequality.[29]

The True Egalitarian Alternative

Our purpose here is to explain why socially directed donation has generated such resistance in spite of the fact that it helps those who are worst off, in the sense that they predictably have the longest wait times to get an organ. We have suggested that the concepts that would support socially directed donation are either utilitarian or maximin and that both are morally problematic. We have suggested that the maximin is not a formulation of a basic principle, but rather is a rule for resolving conflict between the principles of justice and beneficence (interpreted as requiring maximization of aggregate net well-being). If so, then a different priority rule could give a different resolution of this conflict if one lexically ranked the other principles over beneficence. If justice (taken as requiring true egalitarianism) is lexically ranked over beneficence, then only if the requirements of justice are waived by the least well off or if other prima facie principles (beyond beneficence) override justice could socially directed donation be morally acceptable. Because in many cases the least well off are not in a position to exercise such a waiver and in other cases it would be procedurally very difficult for them to do so, a general practice of banning socially directed donation in favor of a policy of refusing the organs that can only be obtained by agreeing to discriminate becomes a plausible way to respond as a matter of public policy. A good case can be made that the UNOS Ethics Committee and the local organ procurement organizations that have opposed donation directed by social group are expressing a decision grounded in the priority of true egalitarian interpretations of the principle of justice. They see this as the appropriate resolution of a potential conflict between true egalitarian justice and the maximin.

Conclusion

The case of socially directed donation of organs poses a special problem not only to utilitarians but also to maximin justice theorists who claim to be "relatively egalitarian." The socially directed donation of organs that otherwise would go to waste not only plausibly maximizes the aggregate net utility of an organ allocation system; it also tends to be to the advantage of the worst-off persons while being to the disadvantage of no one. If so, socially directed donation satisfies not only utilitarian but also maximin criteria. Anyone who retains a considered moral judgment opposing socially directed donation must either have some clever way of showing that socially directed donation will not satisfy utilitarian or maximin criteria or must conclude that the utilitarian and maximin allocation principles are unacceptable.

One plausible conclusion is that socially directed donation simply treats people unequally and that, per se, is prima facie unethical, even if it maximizes the position of the least well off. Those who find the true egalitarian position plausible will be skeptical about socially directed donation, along with some sophisticated utilitarians who fear that acceptance of the practice could jeopardize the entire organ procurement system. If socially directed donation is to be seen as acceptable—even in its relatively more attractive forms, such as conditional donations to children or the military—it must pass the test of being approved by a substantial portion of those worst off below the unjustifiably advantaged persons who get an organ before it is their turn.

Notes

1. If manipulation occurs, it is much more likely to come at the stage when the patient is listed, a possibility discussed in chapter 21. A manipulative surgeon, for example, could list a patient before an organ is actually needed, anticipating that by the time the patient's turn comes up, the patient will really need the organ. Physicians treating patients in liver failure might, for example, place their patients in the hospital when not really necessary. As we saw in the discussion of Mickey Mantle's case in chapter 21, at the time of Mantle's transplant, patients in the hospital had a higher priority than those at home. Though we found no evidence of any manipulation of the allocation in the case of Mantle, if it happened, it almost certainly would have had to have come prior to the listing. Even these manipulations in the listing of patients are being eliminated, in part because of the unfairness. Livers are now allocated based on the empirical factors in the Model of End-Stage Liver Disease score, not based on the easier to manipulate basis of whether one is in the hospital. Kidneys are being allocated not on the basis of the manipulatable time on the wait list, but rather on time on dialysis.

2. Of course, income, socioeconomic status, and other social variables can play a role in deciding who gets on the wait list for organs. We know of no one who would claim access to the list is totally impartial or fair. That does not take away from the claim that the stage in the allocation in which organs

are allocated among those on the list is fair. There is also concern that some of the factors that are used in the allocation formula—e.g., HLA; and panel-reactive antibodies (PRA), a measure of exposure to foreign tissues—are indirectly related to race or gender.

3. Testerman, J, "Should donors say who gets organs?" *St. Petersburg Times*, Jan. 9, 1994.

4. Florida Statutes Annotated, 1994, Title XLII: Estates and Trusts, chap. 732, Probate Code: Intestate Succession and Wills, part X, Anatomical Gifts, sec. 732.914.

5. Gohh RY, Morrissey PE, Madras PN, Monaco AP, "Controversies in organ donation: The altruistic living donor," *Nephrology Dialysis Transplantation* 2001;16: 619–21.

6. Arnason WB, "Directed donation: The relevance of race," *Hastings Center Report* 1991;21 (6): 13–19.

7. Spital A, "Should people who donate a kidney to a stranger be permitted to choose their recipients? Views of the United States public," *Transplantation* 2003;76: 1252–56.

8. Ibid.

9. Ubel PA, Jepson C, Baron J, Mohr T, McMorrow S, Asch DA, "Allocation of transplantable organs: Do people want to punish patients for causing their illness?" *Liver Transplantation* 2001;7 (7): 600–607.

10. Arnason, "Directed donation"; Fox MD, "Directed organ donation: Donor autonomy and community values," in *Organ and tissue donation: Ethical, legal, and policy issues*, ed. Spielman B (Carbondale: Southern Illinois University Press, 1996), 43-50, 163; Florida Statutes Annotated, 1994.

11. Rawls J, *A theory of justice* (Cambridge, MA: Harvard University Press, 1971).

12. There is considerable dispute among philosophers over the question of when Rawls's theory should be applied. In this chapter in the first edition of *Transplantation Ethics*, considerable effort was extended to argue that a public policy on organ transplantation is a basic social practice of the sort that Rawls would have in mind when speaking of his theory of justice.

13. This combination of fairness and efficiency is mandated by the US National Organ Transplant Act of 1984. The specification of the exact formula is a task assigned to the Board of Directors of the United Network for Organ Sharing, the designated Organ Procurement Transplantation Network contract holder. This body must reconcile the potentially conflicting moral principles of justice (equity) and utility maximization (efficiency). For kidneys, for example, a formula is endorsed that takes into account both equity criteria (e.g., time on the wait list) and efficiency measures (e.g., extent of histocompatibility). The rank-ordering of potential candidates thus depends on a moral judgment of the board as it decides what is the most acceptable balancing of equity and efficiency.

14. It might be argued that donation of organs is an example of gift giving, which is normally immune from the moral requirement of fairness. Gifts are, by their very nature, undeserved and unfair. This, however, simply calls into question the use of gift giving and donation metaphors to refer to a national organ allocation system. In fact, current national policy specifically authorizes specific donation of organs to named individuals, such as family members or loved ones in need of organs. Such donation to named individuals appears to be conceptually outside the national organ allocation system. When donation is not made to a named individual, however, the organ is being placed into a national allocation system that is quite analogous to allocating other national resources held in common. The "gift" is made to the society, which is then allocated according to statutory and administrative policies legally mandated to be equitable and efficient. The organ is removed from the mode of gift giving and placed into a system in which recipients have rights, specifically a right to fair treatment by the allocation system.

15. Technical matters make this analysis still more complex. The wait list for kidney transplants is generated anew for each donor. The ranking is based not only on time on the wait list, but such factors as HLA tissue compatibility and PRA. For the potential recipient, these factors vary for each donor so someone who ranked below the candidate favored by the socially directed donation on one allocation

could rank above him or her on the next. Still, for any pool of candidates waiting for an organ, certain persons could be described as statistically among the worst off. One who has unusual HLA antigens, O-blood type, and a high percentage of PRA is statistically going to have to wait a long time for an organ. A group of worst-off persons on the wait list can be identified either on a specific wait list or on a statistical basis independent of any given organ. The point made here—that socially directed donation improves the position of the worst off persons—holds whether we identify the worst off on a particular list or identify the worst off on the wait list statistically.

16. Dworkin R, "What is equality? part 1: Equality of welfare," *Philosophy and Public Affairs* 1981;10 (3): 185–246; Dworkin R, "What is equality? part 2: Equality of resources," *Philosophy and Public Affairs* 1981;10 (4): 283–345; Bedau HA, "Radical egalitarianism," in *Justice and Equality*, ed. Bedau, HA (Englewood Cliffs, NJ: Prentice Hall, 1971), 168–80; Nielsen K, "Radical egalitarian justice: Justice as equality," *Social Theory and Practice* 1979;5 (2): 209–26; Nielsen K, *Equality and liberty: A defense of radical egalitarianism* (Totowa, NJ: Rowman & Allanheld, 1985); Arneson RJ, "Luck, egalitarianism, and prioritarianism," *Ethics* 2000;110: 339–49; Veatch RM, *The foundations of justice: Why the retarded and the rest of us have claims to equality* (New York: Oxford University Press, 1986).

17. Rawls, *Theory*, 538.

18. Ibid., 534–41.

19. Ibid., 530.

20. Ibid., 538–39.

21. The concept of the "veil of ignorance" is a device developed and used by Rawls as a way of recognizing that most people believe that ethics requires impartiality. Rawls says that if one wants to know the general principles that would govern social practices, one should imagine what rational people would agree to as the general principles if they did not know their individual position in the social system, that is, if they were behind a "veil of ignorance." This fictional device has the effect of forcing people to try to imagine what people would accept if they could exclude their personal self-interest based on their knowledge of their own gender, income level, age, ethnicity, and the like. Rawls is not claiming that principles were actually created at any real, historical time before people knew their personal positions. His contract is "hypothetical," but it provides a mental exercise for people to try to imagine what would be reasonable from an impartial point of view, that is, a point of view that ignores personal perspectives.

22. As described in note 21, Rawls derives his principles of justice using an imaginary device of thinking how rational people would choose from behind a "veil of ignorance," that is, if they did not know their unique position within the society. From behind a Rawlsian veil of ignorance, rational, self-interested contractors might imagine themselves among the worst off and favor equality of outcomes as a result. That might reflect envy (but not necessarily so). Rawls posits that his contractors should be conceptualized as free of envy.

23. Kamm, FM, *Morality, mortality, volume I: Death and whom to save from it* (New York: Oxford University Press, 1993), 270, 293: Although Kamm is considering a maximin rather than a strictly egalitarian view, she proposes excluding consideration of minimal gains to the worst off. She says "we could minimally change a strict maximin theory in the follow way: Only when what would be gained by the worst off is a gain that makes a real value significant difference to him should we forgo giving the better-off person a much greater gain." She calls this the "Modified Maximin Rule."

24. Rawls, *Theory*, 9, 16, 17, 110, 276.

25. Veatch R, "Resolving conflict among principles: Ranking, balancing, and specifying," *Kennedy Institute of Ethics Journal.* 1995;5: 199–218.

26. Rawls, *Theory*, 9, 16, 17, 110, 276.

27. Richardson HS, "Specifying norms as a way to resolve concrete ethical problems," *Philosophy and Public Affairs* 1990;19: 279–310.

28. Rawls, *Theory*, 231.

29. There are other possible reasons for explaining the priority for children. Both utilitarian and egalitarian reasons have been proposed. Giving children priority for kidneys is utilitarian on two grounds: (1) If children get the kidney, other things being equal, predictably they will get more years from the organ; and (2) because children with end-stage renal disease who are on dialysis have poor growth and cognitive development, making the benefit of transplant to children greater even if the graft survives the same number of years. An egalitarian argument has been made for giving priority to children that is based on a version of the "fair innings" argument. According to it, someone who is in kidney failure early in life is worse off from an "over-a-lifetime" perspective than someone whose kidney failure develops later. In this sense, children can be said to be worse off, and therefore a priority for them could be supported on egalitarian grounds and maximin grounds. Giving them organs makes them more equal to other people, and it improves the lot of the worst off. The point here, however, is that even if one did not accept these utilitarian, maximin, and egalitarian arguments for the priority for children, the mere fact that they have been promised priority is a prima facie moral reason why they have a special claim. The issues of the role of age in rationing are discussed in chapter 20.

Chapter 24

Elective Organ Transplantation

There is a certain degree of hyperbole in the claim that "organ transplantation is a lifesaving therapy for which there are no alternatives." The most common reason for organ transplantation—kidney transplant for end-stage renal disease (ESRD)—has a viable alternative, namely, dialysis. Although a few groups of individuals with ESRD cannot tolerate dialysis (e.g., those who lack venous access), for the most part, kidney transplantation is optional or "elective." Kidney transplants, however, are usually viewed as the preferred option because they reduce morbidity and mortality for all groups of candidates.

Unlike ESRD, many patients with liver failure need a liver transplant, for which there is no therapeutic alternative. But this is not the case for all patients on the liver transplant wait list. Consider, for example, an individual with classic maple syrup urine disease (MSUD), an inherited metabolic disorder that makes the individual unable to metabolize branched-chain amino acids. If untreated, these children experience poor feeding, vomiting, and lethargy, which can progress into neurological deterioration, a coma, and death.

MSUD can be treated with a restrictive diet that must be strictly adhered to for one's entire life. An alternative therapy is liver transplantation. Liver transplantation does not cure the underlying metabolic disorder, because the branched-chain alpha-keto acid dehydrogenase (BCKAD) enzymes are produced not only in the liver but also in the muscles, kidney, and brain. Still, most individuals with MSUD who undergo a liver transplant can liberalize their diet and are freed from the risk of metabolic decompensation and irreversible brain damage that can occur with any stress, illness, or dietary transgression.

Now it turns out that even a heart transplant is elective for some candidates. Consider the diagnosis of hypoplastic left heart syndrome (HLHS), a congenital heart condition in which the left side of the heart is severely underdeveloped. Today there are two therapeutic options: a Norwood multistaged surgical repair or a heart transplant. There are benefits and risks to each therapy; the Norwood procedure involves three separate surgeries, each with its attendant risks. Heart transplantation only requires one surgery but does require lifelong immunosuppression. The data suggest that mortality and morbidity are quite similar.[1] The problem is that slightly more than 100 heart transplants are performed annually in children younger than one year of age, but approximately 20 infants die on the wait list.[2] Thus, one must ask whether children with HLHS should be offered a heart transplant because, if they undergo the Norwood procedures, the heart allografts would be available for infants who have no transplant alternative.

The main ethical issue in transplantation for children with MSUD or HLHS, then, is how to prioritize patients for whom an alternative therapy is available for these patients on the deceased donor wait list compared with individuals who have no alternative. Using MSUD as our case study, we examine the ethical issues of elective transplants.

If Liver Grafts Were Not Scarce

If liver grafts were not scarce, the discussion of whether or not to offer a liver transplant to a child with MSUD would focus on what is in the child's best interest. Here, the benefit of a liver transplant is the ability to liberalize diet and to avoid metabolic decompensation and irreversible brain damage. However, one must concede that a liver transplant does not fully cure MSUD, given that the liver only produces about 9 to 12 percent of the BCKAD activity. Thus these children may still have a small risk of decompensation. In addition, though liver transplantation reduces the risk of decompensation, it does not reverse the changes that have occurred before the transplant. In a case series of fourteen patients with classic MSUD in Pittsburgh who underwent liver transplants between the ages of two and twenty-two years (mean, 11.5 years), twelve of the fourteen required early intervention; nine of the thirteen in school were in special education; and nine of the fourteen had Attention Deficit Hyperdisorder or developmental delays. However, based on neuropsychiatric testing, the researchers found that "liver transplantation minimizes the likelihood of additional central nervous system damage, providing an opportunity for possible stabilization or improvement in neurocognitive functioning."[3] In a larger cohort from the same institution over the same time period (May 2004–December 2009), the authors note 100 percent patient and graft survival in the thirty-seven patients followed at the University of Pittsburgh and 98 percent and 96 percent patient and graft survival in all 54 patients with MSUD who got a liver transplant in the United States during that same period.[4] The authors also show data that provide evidence that "liver transplant may arrest the progression of brain damage, but will not reverse it." Their data show that "the chronic cognitive and motor impairments associated with MSUD reflect structural changes in the brain rather than reversible neurotransmitter deficiencies." Whether neurological protection is sustained over the long term and at acceptable costs may depend on the cause of the neurological deficits.[5]

Furthermore, a liver transplant creates its own risks. Immunosuppression places the child at risk for infection and cancer. Graft failure places the child at risk of imminent mortality, unless another transplant can be arranged. Still, many would argue that the benefits outweigh the risks. Thus, depending on how parents weigh the risks and benefits, the parents could decide that liver transplantation is in the best interest of the child. And for most medical decisions, that is adequate. The principle of beneficence, promoting the patient's best interest, combined with the principle of autonomy, in this case the parents' autonomy to make health care decisions for their child, would support a liver transplant for patients with MSUD, for which a liver transplant is the only therapeutic option.

Elective Liver Transplantation

But livers are scarce, and the main principles guiding organ allocation—justice and beneficence (fairness and efficiency), balanced with one another—require that we make the best use of this scarce resource. Autonomy gets less weight. So the question we must now examine is what impact does listing a child with MSUD for a liver transplant have in terms of fairness and efficiency?

Utilitarianism

As we have seen in other chapters, one way to examine the ethics of allocating organs is to invoke the theory of utilitarianism. The aim of utilitarianism is to maximize aggregate benefit—the efficiency part of the guiding principles. To the extent that some children in need of a liver transplant have no therapeutic alternative and will die without a liver transplant, it would seem that utilitarians would want to give the scarce livers to these children rather than to children who could be treated by dietary means. As such, a strict utilitarian might argue against listing children with MSUD, or at least giving them a lower priority for an organ than children with, for example, biliary atresia, a congenital disease of the liver in which the bile ducts are blocked or absent and that eventually leads to liver failure.

However, the parents of children with MSUD point out that the risk of metabolic decompensation and long-term neurologic sequelae means that children with MSUD will improve their quality of life, if not the number of years that they live with a liver transplant, such that liver transplant gives them more quality-adjusted life-years (QALYs) than dietary restriction. Although the parents are correct, the utilitarian looks at aggregate benefit, and a child who would otherwise die but can live a normal life with a liver transplant gets more years and more QALYs than does a child with MSUD who can live for many years with a good quality of life with strict dietary control. The fact that the individual with MSUD may be unexpectedly adversely affected due to illness or stress, through no fault of the individual, still does not mean that this individual gets as many additional QALYs from a transplant than another child with liver failure who has no alternative treatment. From the perspective of the aggregate or total amount of good done with an available liver, those who would otherwise die statistically can be expected to gain more years and more QALYs. The utilitarian will still give lower priority to the child with MSUD.

The parents make one last claim. They concede that children with MSUD can get dietary treatment, whereas children with biliary atresia do not have a nontransplant alternative, and this means that a liver not allocated to a child with MSUD can be given to an additional child with biliary atresia, one who may have otherwise died on the wait list. However, they argue that it is not only the child with MSUD who has a therapeutic alternative, but the child with biliary atresia as well, given that a living liver donation is feasible for both these classes of children. In fact, a living liver transplant for biliary atresia may have better outcomes than one for MSUD, because the parents of a child with MSUD are obligate carriers of the enzyme deficiency and therefore their livers may be less effective at replacing the enzyme (due to the fact that the liver only provides a small percentage of the body's BCKAD activity). In contrast, because biliary atresia is not inherited, the parent's living donor graft would completely correct the liver failure. As such, the parent of the child with MSUD asks, Why do we judge one alternative (diet) as mandatory for children with MSUD, when many children with biliary atresia could have a living donor and not require a deceased donor's liver?

A strict utilitarian might conclude that a living liver lobe donation by parents of children needing livers for other than MSUD would be the utility-maximizing strategy, assuming not enough livers are available from deceased donors. Technically, however, there may be an even better utility-maximizing organ procurement policy: Adults generally might be seen as having a moral duty to become living donors not only of livers but also of kidneys and perhaps other organs such as lung lobes—particularly when the adult is the parent of the potential organ recipient. Whether a policy of expecting all people to offer their extra body parts when someone else would benefit is utility maximizing, most people would stop short of imposing a moral obligation of this sort.

Requiring parents and others to donate part of their liver or other organs seems to go too far. It is what we would call supererogatory—beyond the call of duty. The risks that it entails and imposes on the donor—the parents and other family members, in the case of children needing livers—are simply beyond what we have a right to expect. The level of harm in requiring third parties to provide organs seems to be so great that most people, even most of those who are generally utilitarians, would not expect it. In fact, one general argument against utilitarianism is that it seems to require too much. It would, for example, require a stranger to become a donor of a kidney or even a liver lobe whenever the benefits to the recipient exceeded the harm to the donor. A living donor graft must be viewed as a supererogatory option, not a universally available alternative. The clearest utilitarian conclusion is that those needing a liver who have no alternative therapy should have priority over those who do have another option. More good would be done in the aggregate.

Deontology

One deontological approach is to focus on justice as fairness. To the extent that all children with liver failure do better with a liver transplant, even if an alternative treatment is feasible, then all children should be eligible for a liver transplant. Unlike in chapter 18, where the authors disagree about whether voluntary behaviors should give an individual less priority for an organ, being born with biliary atresia or MSUD occurs through no fault of one's own.[6]

Now, what if a transplant were not to offer any additional clinical benefit but was merely an alternative therapy. In the case of HLHS, the Norwood procedure and heart transplant are relatively equivalent in terms of morbidity and mortality. Would the deontologist then say that those with congenital heart disease not amenable to surgery are worse off than those with congenital heart disease amenable to surgery (HLHS) and therefore give a higher priority to the former (or a lower priority to the latter)?

Those committed to the principle of justice—interpreted as most modern commentators would do, as requiring opportunities for equality or benefit for the worst off—would not aggregate benefits across patients. They would rather ask which groups of patients are worst off. Thus, when comparing infants with HLHS who have the alternative of the Norwood procedure available with those infants for whom a heart transplant is the only option, they would consider the infants with HLHS to be in a better position. They could live without the heart transplant, but the other infants could not. Egalitarian justice would require giving the hearts to those who will die without them before giving them to the HLHS patients who are in a relatively favorable position without the transplant. It is not that the HLHS patients gain relatively little at best with a transplant rather than other treatment; it is that the HLHS patients are relatively well off compared with the other patients. Those other patients would, according to this justice analysis, have a claim on the available hearts, even if they would, statistically, gain less from them.

A similar analysis applies to livers for MSUD patients. Without a liver transplant, a MSUD patient is surely burdened and medically not as well off as those without this condition. But compared with patients for whom a liver transplant is the only option for survival, the MSUD patients are comparatively well off. The MSUD patients have less of a justice claim for an available liver compared with the child with biliary atresia. But from a fair innings perspective, the child with MSUD may be viewed as worse off than the adult with liver failure, because even though he can get along quite well on a restricted diet, the likelihood of decompensation at a young age looms large. Therefore, the child with MSUD might have a justice claim against adults on the grounds of fair innings and therefore galvanize a split liver transplant, even if this is worse for an average adult candidate who would otherwise get a whole liver transplant.

Do Numbers of Organs Count?

In 2005 the secretary of the US Department of Health and Human Services' Advisory Committee on Heritable Disorders in Newborns and Children adopted the recommendation by the American College of Medical Genetics (now the American College of Medical Genetics and Genomics) for a uniform panel of conditions to be included in mandatory state newborn screening panels. MSUD was included in the recommended panel, and all states have adopted this panel, which means that more children will be diagnosed early and may be diagnosed before any neurological damage occurs. Their parents may decide that a liver transplant is preferable to a restricted diet to avoid the risk of metabolic decompensation. This may lead to greater demand for liver transplants in children with MSUD.

If parents decide that a liver transplant is in their child's best interest, the young child may be eligible not only for a pediatric deceased donor's liver but also for a portion of a deceased adult donor's liver. The practice of "split livers" involves splitting the liver into two portions. This allows for two individuals (usually a small child and a small adult) to get a transplant from one deceased donor liver. In this way, the child does not decrease the number of available deceased donor livers for those who have no nonliver transplant alternative.

Is it ethically permissible to split livers in order to provide children with MSUD with a deceased donor graft? In principle, it seems that benefiting two individuals from one deceased donor's graft would be a win–win solution.[7] However, when one examines outcomes, one finds that the adults who receive the larger portion of the split liver do not have outcomes as good as adults who receive a whole graft.[8] Although two individuals can get livers, and so splitting livers may maximize the number of life-years saved, one must recall that the child could get by with a dietary intervention, and so the number of life-years saved may be greater if an adult is given a whole liver graft.

One interpretation of egalitarian justice would suggest that split liver transplants are morally permissible based on the concept of fair innings—because the child may not make it to adulthood unless transplanted

An alternative way to analyze this is to think about how one would act if one were behind the Rawlsian veil of ignorance. As we argued in chapter 20, children with liver disease can be seen as worse off than adults, so this may allow children to make a claim for a split liver graft, even though the outcomes for an adult receiving a split liver are somewhat worse.

One objection is that the candidate who gets the split liver may not be the same person as the candidate who would have been eligible for the whole liver graft due to size. As such, split livers disadvantage larger adults. Given our organ allocation system, this means that those individuals with a higher priority (who are otherwise at the top of the wait list) may be bypassed when a liver is split, which raises cries of inequity. It is one thing to be bypassed because the graft is too small; it is another thing to be bypassed because the procuring team modified the graft to make it too small. The equity claims of large adults for a whole liver are further complicated by judgments about whether the adult was in any way responsible for being large—the issue we raise in chapter 19. Because at least some component of adult size is surely beyond the control of the individual, and factoring size into an allocation formula is bound to be complex and contentious, many nonutilitarians would take the position that adults who are equally ill and in other respects are morally equal deserve equal access to organs, regardless of size. This mitigates the utilitarian suggestion that splitting a liver for two patients—a child and a small adult—is better than using the whole liver for one adult. If, in fact, some children—those with MSUD—have alternative therapies in any case, a strong case can be made for using adult whole livers for adults. However, from a fair innings perspective, split liver transplantation to the child with MSUD and a small adult may be the fairer option.

Domino Liver

As we have already explained, it turns out that one's liver only makes about 10 percent of the enzyme one needs to digest branched-chain amino acids. In this vein, then, an individual who does not have MSUD but is in liver failure could accept a liver graft from a person with MSUD because they would still get BCKAD activity from other bodily sources (kidney, muscle, and brain) and the MSUD liver would perform the other liver functions normally. We could thus place a deceased donor liver in the patient with MSUD and transplant the MSUD patient's liver to someone on the wait list because of other liver problems. This is called a domino transplant—the patient with MSUD gets a liver graft and in turn provides his or her liver to another person in liver failure.[9] Thus, the parents of a child who has MSUD and gets a liver transplant (whether a pediatric deceased donor, split liver, or even a living donor liver transplant) can also elect to give permission for the use of the child's liver as an organ source. It is not an even trade. The liver the child gets is better because it has 100 percent liver functions, whereas the liver from the child source lacks BCKAD. However, in individuals who make BCKAD in other parts of their body, these livers have been successfully transplanted and the recipients have not required dietary restrictions.[10]

The Pittsburgh group reported that six children with MSUD who received liver transplants between 2004 and 2009 provided a domino liver graft, and all these grafts were doing well at the time of publication.[11] Whether it should be mandatory that the native liver of the patient with MSUD must be available as an organ source for a domino transplant is a separate issue, but the possibility of domino transplant does change the equation as to whether the child is unfairly taking resources that are scarce because the number of other individuals who are transplanted when a child with MSUD gets an organ (and gives one in return) is unchanged The numbers, then, may support liver transplants for children with MSUD, especially if most of the parents are willing to allow the children's resected liver to be used for domino transplantation.

Conclusion

So far we have analyzed the impact of listing children with MSUD for liver transplants with the knowledge that very few procedures have been done to date. The number of children with MSUD is small, and will remain small even with the increased number of diagnosed children given expanded newborn screening. However, as other therapies are developed, liver transplants may become elective for other liver diseases as well. For example, hepatocellular carcinoma is a common cause of liver transplant listing (and in fact, candidates get priority points because if the liver cancer spreads, they become ineligible for a liver transplant). And yet today, both ablation and resection are feasible. Although liver transplantation may have lower morbidity and mortality, the results of these alternative procedures are improving, and one must recall that there are other candidates with liver disease for whom no alternative exists.[12] Given that approximately 1,500 to 1,600 individuals die on the deceased donor liver wait list each year, is it fair to transplant those with small cancers and no fibrosis when others have diseases for which no alternative treatment exists? Again, as with the case of HLHS, patients may have a preference for transplantation rather than ablation or surgical resection, even if the morbidities and mortality rates were statistically equivalent. But as we have argued, justice is the first principle of allocation, and autonomy and patient preferences are given less weight. Thus from a justice perspective, it may be permissible to design an allocation system that gives lower priority to those who have an alternative treatment, even if the alternative treatment has slightly worse outcomes. And yet, when the candidate is a child, arguments from fair innings may suggest that whereas these candidates should get a lower priority than other pediatric candidates with no alternatives, they should get higher priority than adults—based on a fair innings argument—which would lead to split liver transplantation, even if this may be less than ideal from the adult's perspective.

Notes

1. Gordon BM, Rodriguez S, Lee M, Chang RK, "Decreasing number of deaths of infants with hypoplastic left heart syndrome," *Journal of Pediatrics* 2008;153: 354–58; Tibballs J, Kawahira Y, Carter BG, Donath S, Brizard C, Wilkinson J, "Outcomes of surgical treatment of infants with hypoplastic left

heart syndrome: an institutional experience 1983–2004," *Journal of Paediatrics and Child Health* 2007;43: 746–51; Wernovsky G, Chrisant MR, "Long-term follow-up after staged reconstruction or transplantation for patients with functionally univentricular heart," *Cardiology of the Young* 2004;14 (suppl 1): 115–26.

2. US Department of Health and Human Services Organ Procurement and Transplantation Network (OPTN), "Data reports," http://optn.transplant.hrsa.gov/latestData/step2.asp.

3. Shellmer DA, DeVito Dabbs A, Dew MA, et al., "Cognitive and adaptive functioning after liver transplantation for maple syrup urine disease: A case series," *Pediatric Transplantation* 2011;15 (1): 58–64.

4. Mazariegos GV, Morton DH, Sindhi R, et al., "Liver transplantation for classical maple syrup urine disease: Long-term follow-up in 37 patients and comparative United Network for Organ Sharing experience," *Journal of Pediatrics* 2012;160: 116–21.

5. Ibid.

6. One could argue that parents of a child with MSUD could have known prior to conception that they were at risk of having an affected child, particularly if they have a prior child with MSUD. Even in those cases, however, it is not the child's voluntary action that leaves the child in liver failure and therefore no discussion of voluntary behavior should place the child at lesser risk.

7. Cardillo M, De Fazio N, Pedotti P, et al., "Split and whole liver transplantation outcomes: A comparative cohort study," *Liver Transplantation* 2006;12 (3): 402–10; Merion RM, Rush SH, Dykstra DM, Goodrich N, Freeman RB Jr, Wolfe RA, "Predicted lifetimes for adult and pediatric split liver versus adult whole liver transplant recipients," *American Journal of Transplantation* 2004;4: 1792–97.

8. See Merion et al., "Predicted lifetimes"; and Vulchev A, Roberts JP, Stock PG, "Ethical issues in split versus whole liver transplantation," *American Journal of Transplantation* 2004;4: 1737–40.

9. See, e.g., Kitchens WH, "Domino liver transplantation: Indications, techniques, and outcomes," *Transplantation Reviews* 2011;25 (4): 167–77; and Badell IR, Hanish SI, Hughes CB, et al., "Domino liver transplantation in maple syrup urine disease: A case report and review of the literature," *Transplantation Proceedings* 2013;45 (2): 806–9.

10. This is not true for all metabolic liver diseases. For example, primary hyperoxaluria is not a good indication for domino liver transplant because recipients of these livers develop hyperoxaluria and early acute renal failure. See, e.g., Popescu I, Dima SO, "Domino liver transplantation: How far can we push the paradigm?" *Liver Transplantation* 2012;18: 22–28.

11. Mazariegos et al., "Liver transplantation."

12. Zheng Z, Liang W, Milgrom DP, et al., "Liver transplantation versus liver resection in the treatment of hepatocellular carcinoma: A meta-analysis of observational studies," *Transplantation* 2014;97: 227–34.

Chapter 25

Vascularized Composite Allografts

Hand, Face, and Uterine Transplants

Traditionally, organ transplantation has been viewed as a lifesaving therapy. This remains true for individuals with end-stage heart failure or end-stage liver disease who cannot survive without, respectively, a heart or liver transplant. In contrast, composite tissue allografts (now known as vascularized composite allografts)—such as hands, faces, and uteri—are "nonessential" in that they are life enhancing rather than lifesaving. The reason that this is important is that all such allografts still require lifelong immunosuppression, which exposes the individual to risks of infection and cancer along with acute and chronic graft rejection, diabetes, hypertension, hyperlipidemia, and impaired kidney function—all of which make the benefit/risk calculation less obvious.

In spite of the fact that vascularized composite allografts (VCAs) are generally not thought to be lifesaving, but only life enhancing, the stories of some recipients show that the distinction is nuanced. On March 19, 2012, Richard Lee Norris, of Hillsville, Virginia, began a 36-hour operation to replace his face from his hairline to his neck, one of the most extensive face transplants ever.[1] In 1997 he suffered what was reported to be a gun accident when he found that a shotgun that was in a gun cabinet was leaning against the cabinet's glass door. Apparently, when he was opening the cabinet to secure the gun, it fell and discharged, shooting him in the face.

He had lived for fifteen years since the accident so grotesquely deformed that he was living as a recluse. When he went out, he would wear a mask. He faced cruelty from strangers and contemplated suicide. In surgery performed at the University of Maryland Medical Center in Baltimore, he received teeth and an upper and lower jaw. In addition, a portion of his tongue as well as the tissue from the scalp to the base of the neck were transplanted—essentially, all but small areas around the eyes.

Since the surgery, his sense of smell has been restored, and he has partial muscle control of the facial muscles (reportedly 80 percent on his right side and 40 percent on his left). He now says he can go out in public, and those who previously did not know are generally unaware he has had a face transplant. He must take immunosupressants for life, but is doing well, at last report, some fifteen months later.

The concept of VCAs is part of cultural lore. According to Christian traditions, Saints Cosmas and Damian were twin brothers and physicians who grafted the leg of a recently deceased Ethiopian to replace a patient's cancerous leg, a theme that has been portrayed by artists over the centuries. The term "composite tissue allograft" (the precursor to the term "vascularized composite allograft) was first coined by Erle Ewart Peacock Jr.[2] In the mid–twentieth century, Peacock successfully transplanted flexor tendon mechanisms from cadavers to permit finger mobility for those in whom tendon autografts were unsuccessful.[3] He coined the term "composite tissue allograft" to distinguish "these structurally complex grafts of multiple tissue lines from solid organ grafts."[4] More than forty such procedures were done by a handful of clinician investigators, with a reported success rate of 70 percent.[5] Thus the first composite tissue allograft was being performed at the same time that Murray, Merril, and Harrison were performing the earliest kidney isograft (1954) and allograft (1959).

The first modern attempt to replace a human limb occurred in 1964, when a hand transplant was performed in Ecuador. It was amputated two weeks later due to rejection, which was not surprising, given the primitive state of immunosuppression.[6] The next allograft limb attempt in humans would not occur for more than thirty years (1998), during which time immunosuppression therapy improved significantly. In the ensuing sixteen years, other composite tissue transplants have been performed, including bilateral hand transplants, face, larynx, and uterus. In this chapter we review the history of hand, face, and uterine transplants and then examine the ethical issues that they raise.

History

Hand and upper-limb transplants have received significant attention. We begin our account there and then describe other types of VCAs.

Hand and Upper-Limb Transplants

The National Limb Loss Information Center reported that in 2005 approximately 1.6 million people were living with limb loss in the United States, and this number is projected to reach 3.6 million by 2050.[7] Most are lower limbs, but in 2005, 41,000 persons in the United States were living with major upper-limb loss, 62 percent of whom had trauma-related injuries.[8] After the premature attempt in Ecuador, the first human hand transplant was performed in September 1998 by an international team led by Jean-Michel Dubernard in Lyon.[9] The Lyon team beat out a team in Louisville in the United States, which had been preparing for a hand transplant for two years, had developed an institutional review board–approved protocol, had sought external scientific and ethical consultation, and had done much research and practice, including large animal hand transplants.[10] Louisville performed the second unilateral hand transplant in January 1999, and the French team performed the first bilateral hand transplants in January 2000. Unfortunately, the first hand transplant recipient in this contemporary period, Clint Hallam, was not an ideal choice. Although the Lyon team knew that he had lost his hand in an accident, they were not aware that he had lost his hand in an accident while in prison for fraud. Nor were they aware that he had fled his native country in 1996, "facing an arrest warrant in both New Zealand and Australia on fraud charges and earned the label 'King of the Cons.' "[11] Although he initially did well, he did not adjust well psychologically to the graft. He left France after several months against medical advice, and was not compliant with medications and follow-up. He requested to have the hand removed, and the amputation was performed in the United Kingdom in February 2001. His erratic behavior and the adverse result led to increased emphasis on the psychological workup of potential candidates to assess their motivation, willingness to adhere to medical regimens, and ability to adjust to the psychological impact of having another's body part visible to one's self and the world, further compounded by the media scrutiny that these transplants receive.[12] As Dubernard and colleagues write: "Although the results achieved in this first case showed the feasibility of hand allotransplantation, we also learned the great importance of patient compliance to immunosuppressive treatment and physiotherapy as well as his motivation."[13]

In 2002 Dubernard founded the International Registry on Hand and Composite Tissue Transplantation (IRHCTT).[14] It is a voluntary registry, and not all centers report their results. As of 2011 the hand allotransplantation section includes thirty-nine patients corresponding to fifty-seven upper-extremity transplantations (eighteen bilateral and twenty-one single hands) performed at fifteen centers. To date, five grafts have been lost (the first one, as described above, and one involving a bilateral hand and face transplant in which the hands were removed on posttransplant day five due to sepsis, and the patient died on day sixty-five).[15] Two additional deaths have also been reported in the literature. In these two cases there was a triple and quadruple limb transplantation (both arms and legs).[16] The IRHCTT also does not include data from China, where fifteen hand/forearm/palm/digit allotransplantations (five unilateral and one bilateral hand transplantations, three unilateral and two bilateral forearm transplantations, one palm transplantation, and one thumb transplantation) have been performed on twelve patients (eleven males and one female). Seven have lost their grafts due to rejection, primarily as a result of noncompliance or the unavailability of immunosuppression,[17] There have also been two cases of perioperative failure, resulting in reamputations in the United States.[18]

Data from the IRHCTT provide important information about function and morbidity. All the patients have recovered protective sensibility (i.e., they are able to identify sensations that pose a serious risk, like extreme heat) and hand movements that have empowered them to perform most daily activities, including eating, grasping objects, and shaving. The vast majority have recovered tactile sensations (90 percent) and discrimination sensations (82 percent). However, 87 percent of subjects have developed opportunistic infections and more than half have had metabolic complications, such as high sugars, high lipids, and impaired kidney function.[19] Several have elevated creatinine, and one has developed end-stage renal disease. Other complications include osteonecrosis of the hip, posttransplant lymphoproliferative disorder, other endocrine disorders, and one basal cell carcinoma of the nose.[20] The earliest two American unilateral hand transplants are doing well.[21]

Face Transplants

Patients have received facial transplants for trauma, burns, and benign facial tumors (neurofibromatosis—also known as "elephant man" syndrome). As Edwards and Mathes explain, "each type of patient has unique considerations" and the "degree of facial disfigurement does not predict the severity of psychological stress."[22] Other factors influence coping and adaptation, including whether the disfigurement is acute or chronic, and social support.

The first partial face transplant was performed in Lyon in 2005 by a team of surgeons led by Devauchelle and Dubernard.[23] Dubernard describes the recipient: "Isabelle, the first face transplant (2005), was so disfigured that she had to wear a mask in the street. Her body image was totally destroyed. She could not look at herself in the mirror without feeling frightened. Moreover, her functional condition was extremely poor. Not only could she not kiss her children and be kissed by them, she could not speak, drink, or eat. She had to be fed by a gastric tube. Indeed, the graft is not only lifesaving, but life-giving."[24]

Centers across the globe now perform partial face allotransplants. Siemionow of Cleveland performed the first partial face transplant in the United States in 2008, which, as she explained, was based on twenty years of preclinical research.[25] In 2010 two full face transplants were performed in Spain and France. [26] As of June 2013, at least twenty-eight face transplants have been performed, at least two combined with bilateral hand transplants.[27] Most face transplant recipients are satisfied or very satisfied with the graft.[28] As expected, motor recovery has been slower than sensory recovery. For aesthetic purposes, many have required additional reconstruction or revision surgery.[29]

Two of the first seventeen face transplant recipients died: one died sixty-five days after a bilateral hand and face transplant, and the other, in China, after two years. The overall survival rate, then, is, 88 percent.[30] Reportedly, two more have since died.[31] In a review of all cases performed between 2005 and 2010, Siemionew notes that no early graft loss due to technical failure has been reported, although all have reported at least one acute reversible rejection episode.[32] Opportunistic infections and metabolic complications were observed as adverse effects.

Uterus Transplants

Uterine infertility affects millions of women in the United States and more throughout the world. In the United States alone, about 5,000 hysterectomies are performed in women under the age of twenty-four years. In total, nearly 9 million US women of reproductive age have had a hysterectomy. Based on fecundity rates, thousands of these women may be candidates for uterus transplantation.[33]

To date, uterine transplantation has been performed in animals, and a few live animal births have occurred.[34] The first two human uterine transplants were performed in 2000 (Saudi Arabia) using a live unrelated donor who was undergoing a therapeutic hysterectomy, and in 2011 (Turkey) using a deceased donor.[35] The first uterine allograft lasted for three months, but inadequate structural support led to uterine prolapse and necrosis at three months. Eighteen months after the second uterine transplant, the Turkish woman's endometrium was prepared for the transfer of her thawed embryos. She had a positive clinical pregnancy; however, the gestational sac failed to develop on follow-up seven days after the initial examination, and the patient began to have vaginal bleeding. The pregnancy was considered nonviable and was terminated by aspiration and curettage.[36] In 2012 researchers in Sweden performed the first elective living related uterine donor transplants (from mothers and other female relatives, each of whom agreed to undergo an elective hysterectomy of a healthy uterus to donate it to an infertile relative), and newspaper stories report that nine have been performed.[37] In March 2014 the Swedish research team announced that "four Swedish women who received transplanted wombs have had embryos transferred into them in an attempt to get pregnant," and the first birth was announced in *The Lancet* on October 6.[38]

Ethical Issues

Each of the three VCAs described above raises important ethical issues. Here, we evaluate five ethical issues, citing data from one or more of the case studies outlined above. The five issues are: (1) When is innovative surgery ready for first-in-human trials? (2) What is the justification of exposing candidates to immunosuppression for a non-lifesaving transplantation? (3) What specific risks, benefits, and alternatives must be included in the informed consent process? (4) What are ethically relevant inclusion and exclusion criteria for candidates and donors, respectively? (5) What is owed to donors of VCAs? Here we need to consider respect for both deceased donors and, in the unique case of uterine transplants, to what degree of risks is it ethical to expose living donors for a non-lifesaving transplant?

When Is Innovative Surgery Ready for First-in-Human Trials?

One question that recurs with each attempt to expand transplantation to new organs or new composite tissue is: When is an innovative transplant ready to be tested in humans? According to Mark Siegler, a nationally recognized ethicist at the University of Chicago who was asked to evaluate the Louisville protocol before the first hand transplant was performed, the ethical requirements regarding surgical innovation that justify a surgical team to proceed technically in a first-in-human study were enumerated by Francis Moore, a former transplant surgeon at Harvard University: (1) appropriate scientific background, (2) the "field strength" of the team doing the procedure, (3) the ethical climate of the institution itself, (4) open display, (5) public evaluation, and (6) public and professional discussion.[39] Siegler explained that he thought that the Louisville team and the institution had met these criteria. The members of the Louisville team have also published a manuscript in which they show how they have fulfilled these criteria: They described the research on mammals and primates (and explained why the research on large mammals was more relevant particularly with respect to immunosuppression protocols for *composite tissue allotransplantation*; that they had the requisite team and institutional support; that they had sought ethics review external to their institution, created a patient advocate for the potential recipient to protect him from an overzealous team, and made public and professional disclosure of their intention to proceed, seeking public and professional input.

There exists an interesting, more libertarian perspective holding that adequately informed, mentally competent patients should be permitted to take risks when they are convinced that doing so serves their interest and competent clinicians are willing to proceed. For example, an elderly, blind person with a doctorate in biology once reportedly desired to volunteer for avant garde research involving brain implants that someday might restore vision and offered to do so before the normally required nonhuman animal studies had been completed. This person plausibly claimed to be uniquely well prepared for this study and would not live long enough to volunteer after animal studies had been completed. Similarly, one can imagine VCA candidates demanding the right to be human pioneers when they are adequately informed and desperately want to address a problem like infertility for which there is no other solution. In spite of these claims, we assume that normally a plausible case exists for relying on the standards identified by Moore.

Today, only a dozen programs around the world perform VCAs, as would be expected if all judged their ability by Moore's criteria for innovative surgery. Any institution considering VCAs requires significant expertise in many domains, both surgical and medical (i.e., infectious diseases, immunosuppression), as well as in psychiatry, social work, ethics, and rehabilitation.

What Is the Justification for Exposing Candidates to Immunosuppression for a Non-Lifesaving Transplant?

The objection to performing VCAs on non-lifesaving organs such as the hands, face, and uteri is that though the transplant may improve the recipient's quality of life, it may also shorten the quantity of life. The arguments supporting VCAs are based in both utility and patient autonomy. It is widely recognized that benefits in health care are measured considering both the length of life and the quality of life. Concepts such as quality-adjusted life-years incorporate both notions. A transplant that is not going to extend life (barring considerations of suicide prevention) may well improve quality of life so that more quality-adjusted life-years are added with a non-lifesaving transplant. Of equal importance is the appeal to patient autonomy—that competent patients get to decide what risks they are willing to bear, provided they can find a team of physicians willing to perform the surgery.

It is important to appreciate that these VCAs may be "non-lifesaving" in some traditional sense, in that one can live with a disfigured face and also missing hands, but these procedures are not being done merely for aesthetic purposes and are not being offered as an alternative form of cosmetic surgery for those who do not like their nose or the shape of their mouth. Individuals with severe disfigurement—from congenital anomalies, injury, or accident—have two options: facial reconstruction or a face transplant. Reconstructive facial surgery using skin flaps and skin graft is imperfect and can result in a serious loss of function, a lack of facial expression, and a visible difference in the appearance of the face.[40] For some candidates (like Richard Norris), the facial transplant (rather than skin grafting) may be necessary in order to achieve such functions as blinking, chewing, swallowing, speaking, and making facial expressions, all of which are important for quality of life. In addition, the face is critical to social interactions. As such, severe facial disfigurement can perturb both relationships and one's ability to integrate into social settings, leading to significant personal, psychological, financial, and social adversity. But not all individuals with severe facial disfigurement have such negative interactions, and thus, not surprisingly, not everyone with facial disfigurement would be willing to take on the risks of immunosuppression.

Several studies have been done to assess attitudes toward facial transplantation in various populations. Clarke and colleagues report on a public engagement exercise at the Royal Society Summer Science Exhibition in 2004 before the first face transplant was done. More than 90 percent of the attendees were willing to donate a kidney, liver, heart, or lungs, but their willingness lessened to 70.4 and 55.8 percent, respectively, for hand and face graft donation. More than 90 percent of the same respondents were willing to accept a liver, heart, or lungs, and 87.6 percent were willing to accept a kidney. However, only 72.5 and 63.1 percent, respectively, were willing to accept hands or a face.[41] A second study queried a diverse convenience sample of 1,000 Turkish adults, including "patients, doctors, nurses, other medical staff, university students, teachers, secretaries, housewives, and other occupational groups." In this study, only one-third of respondents were familiar with face transplantation, and knowledge correlated with greater acceptance. As part of the study, respondents were shown photographs of severely disfigured faces. Although 203 participants initially refused to support having a face transplant, more than half (57.6 percent) changed their minds after they had seen the photographs, which suggests that education about why candidates may request a VCA may lead to greater support.[42] A Canadian study by Sinno and colleagues surveyed medical students and an internet population regarding face transplantation. They found that if confronted with facial disfigurement, the sample would undergo a face transplant procedure with a 34 percent chance of death and be willing to trade twelve years of their life for a successful graft.[43]

Finally, some studies have focused only on the attitudes of health care professionals. Mathes and colleagues found that only slightly more than one-fourth of plastic and burn surgeons in North America supported VCAs given current immunosuppression, although another fourth would support them with better immunosuppression and another 15 percent would support them if current transplants are viable at ten years. Six percent, however, thought VCAs could never be justifiable and another fourth thought they would only be justifiable if immunologic tolerance could be achieved. More than three-fourths of these same respondents agreed, however, that current techniques do not provide adequate reconstruction for severe facial injuries.[44]

The eligibility criteria for face transplants are rigid, and candidates must have a severe disfigurement. This is not to say that a good quality of life cannot be achieved by people even with severely disfiguring conditions, only that for some individuals, like Isabelle or Richard Norris, it was not possible. Many with severe facial disfigurement talk about the isolation and stigma that they feel. The face is central to social interaction. In that vein, the Louisville team concludes: "By restoring the ability to make facial expressions, enjoy an aesthetically acceptable appearance, and interact comfortably with others, face transplantation could arguably be considered a 'lifesaving' treatment."[45] Similarly, perhaps Richard Norris's face transplant prevented a suicide.

And yet, face transplants are not a viable option for all individuals with severe facial disfigurement. Although different programs may have different criteria, all exclude those who have a poor record of medical compliance and an inability to participate in a strict rehabilitation schedule. There is extensive psychological counseling to ensure that the candidate understands the limitations and risks as well as the benefits, that the person has both individual coping ability and social support for the extensive rehabilitation that the surgery entails, and that the person has the psychological capacity to adapt to a face that is different from the face he or she had preceding the accident or illness. Some individuals will self-exclude; others will be excluded by the program.

A hand transplant is another VCA that is visible and raises important identity issues. Because a hand is in constant view, there is a strong psychological component. As Chang and Mathes explain: "This issue was believed to be the cause of failure for the first Lyon recipient after his hand transplantation. The recipient became increasingly dissociated from his allograft and consequently became noncompliant with his immunosuppression."[46] Because of this experience, hand transplant centers around the world now perform an extensive psychiatric evaluation to screen potential recipients.

Again, those with upper-extremity limb amputation will vary in their willingness to accept life-threatening immunosuppression. It may depend on whether the limb loss is unilateral or bilateral and is the dominant or nondominant hand, and on how well the individuals have adapted to their new body image as well as how much function they can gain from a prosthesis. This is not to suggest that upper-limb loss is anything but "catastrophic." It affects nearly every activity of daily living, leaving patients with substantial disability.[47] Anecdotal data also suggest how important it is for hand transplant recipients not only to get replacement hands in order to resume activities of daily living but also to be able to hug and feel the person in their grasp.

There is some professional uneasiness about hand transplantation because of the immunosuppression, particularly in those who have only had one hand amputated.[48] There is also some objection due to the cost differential between transplants and prostheses. The lifetime cost of a single hand or double hand transplant is about $500,000, in contrast to unilateral and bilateral hand prostheses, which respectively cost about $20,000 and $40,000.[49] This may be an underestimate, given the number of candidates who are evaluated before selection and because the cost and time of surgery were probably underestimated.[50]

One way to reduce the risk of immunosuppression is to perform stem cell transplant along with the VCA in order to minimize the amount of immunosuppression needed. In 2013 Schneeberger and colleagues in Pittsburgh described the "Pittsburgh protocol," in which they performed upper-extremity transplantation followed two weeks later by donor bone marrow cell-based treatment in five patients. The stem cells were collected from nine vertebral bodies. This protocol did not result in complete tolerance, but has resulted in graft survival using only a single immunosuppression agent in all five hand/forearm transplant recipients.

In sum, the justification for immunosuppression in VCAs is that for some candidates who have severe facial disfigurement or are missing a hand, the VCAs allow the candidates to get their lives back, even if they may be life shortening. Still many of the objections to VCAs would be minimized if tolerance of these grafts could be achieved.

The Informed Consent Process for VCAs

In order to be able to give an informed consent to a VCA, candidates must learn about the known and potential risks, the benefits, and the alternatives. The main benefit of both face and hand transplants is the opportunity for the candidate to "be whole" again. Given the experience and data in the IRHCTT to date, transplant recipients can expect both good motor and sensory recovery that continues to improve over time. The risks are also important. First is the risk of death. Because the IRHCTT is voluntary and not all centers outside the United States and Western Europe provide data, the number of deaths is underreported. There have been several deaths reported at conferences or in the literature that have not been reported to the IRHCTT. Then there are the risks associated with immunosuppression and with graft failure. To date, there have been multiple episodes of acute graft failure in both hand and face allografts, but no chronic failures. The saving grace for these VCAs is that rejection of skin is easily recognized and so antirejection treatment (steroids) can begin without delay. However, graft rejection is possible. Although a hand graft failure could leave the candidate back in his or her limb-loss state of being an amputee, facial graft failure could leave the candidate worse off, particularly if he or she does not have bodily tissue that can be used for reconstruction.

The benefit of uterine transplants has not yet been realized, but the goal is to allow a woman to be both a gestational and genetic mother to the children she will rear. For many women, experiencing pregnancy is a central aspect of their identity as women.[51] The risks to the woman are the risks of immunosuppression and the risks of a nonvisible VCA such that early diagnosis of acute rejection is more difficult. There are also risks to the woman of being pregnant with a transplanted uterus and whether it will grow and expand as a native uterus or whether it will expose the woman and/or the fetus to unknown risks and harms. The animal data to date are reassuring about the safety and normal growth and development in a nonnative uterus.

In a uterine transplant, one must also consider the risks and benefits to the child to be. The benefit is a life that might not otherwise have been procreated and gestated. The main risks of immunosuppression to the developing fetus after solid organ transplantation are prematurity and low birth weight.[52] Data from the National Transplantation Pregnancy Registry show that women who have been solid organ transplant recipients and are on immunosuppression do not have increased risk of birth defects (with the possible exception from some of the newer immunosuppressants like mycophenolate mofetil), and the benefits of the various immunosuppressants need to be addressed with all women of childbearing years, whether or not they are actively thinking about childbearing.[53] The additional risks associated with gestating in a nonnative uterus are unknown.

The last factor that candidates need to know about is the alternatives. The alternative options vary significantly among the three types of VCAs under discussion. For face transplants, the alternative is reconstructive surgery, which, as discussed above, cannot always restore all the face's functions and does not always leave a socially acceptable reconstruction.

The alternative to hand transplantation is prosthetics, which continue to improve, and there is even ongoing research to develop prostheses with sensory input. Both hand transplant recipients and prostheses recipients must undergo rehabilitation, which correlates with improved function. Nevertheless, many individuals who experience upper-limb loss reject prostheses. In a study of veterans, McFarland and colleagues evaluated upper-extremity prostheses. They found that rejection varied depending on the type of device. The main reasons for rejection were pain, discomfort, and lack of functionality.[54]

The two alternatives to a uterus transplant are adoption and surrogacy (at least where it is legal), both of which allow for the social demands and rewards of parenthood even if they do not allow for gestational (both) or genetic (adoption) motherhood. Nevertheless, these two options ignore the significance of gestation in many cultures, which explains why women are willing to expose themselves and their fetuses to the risks of immunosuppression and the unknown risks of gestation in a nonnative uterus.

The Selection of Recipients and Donors

It is estimated that 7 million Americans every year would benefit from composite tissue reconstruction owing to oncologic surgery, traumatic injuries, and congenital anomalies.[55] However, the data also suggest that many are not appropriate candidates for VCAs because of the need for lifelong immunosuppression and the rigid rehabilitation protocol. With VCAs of the hand and face, a specific recipient candidate is identified and then a "suitable donor" is found. This is quite different from a solid organ transplant, where donors are routinely sought and only after a donor is identified does UNOS identify the appropriate recipient. One reason for the difference is the attempt to match VCA donors and their recipients in terms of age, gender, ethnicity, and race, because these transplants are visible, and differences may make the allograft more noticeably foreign and complicate the ability of the recipient to accept the graft as his or her own. Matching also makes the graft less visible to the public, thereby reducing social alienation.

Although we have spent decades educating professionals and the public that, for internal organ transplant, there is no valid medical reason to be concerned about transplanting across racial lines, with hand and face transplants almost everyone concedes the legitimacy of striving for a good match of skin tone. This means that transplant personnel, who have the capacity to ignore race, will now operate with an exception if skin tone matching is deemed appropriate for these transplants. It remains to be seen whether this will create tensions. Some civil rights lawyers, for example, have pointed out that taking race or skin color into account in allocating VCAs appears to violate the requirement that all allocations be based solely on medical criteria. And yet given the psychological issues related to these transplants, it may be irresponsible not to include these factors in allocation.

Psychological issues are a major reason to exclude potential recipients. Louisville conducted a mandatory formal psychiatric evaluation to ensure that only ideal candidates from a psychological perspective would undergo hand transplantation. The team interviewed 213 potential hand recipients and found only 9 who were eligible. All 9 clearly articulated that they would have a sense of physical and psychological ownership after a hand transplant. Similarly an Italian program chose only 4 recipients from 534 candidates.[56]

Who should determine what amount of risk is acceptable? Majzoub and colleagues at the University of Louisville studied what risks individuals from four study populations with differing life experiences would accept for a hand transplant. The four groups were healthy individuals, organ transplant recipients, upper-extremity amputee patients, and lower-extremity amputee patients. The authors found that "all populations questioned perceived risk similarly despite their differing life experiences and would accept differing degrees of risk for the different transplantation procedures. Organ transplant recipients were the most risk-tolerant group whereas upper-extremity amputee patients were the most risk adverse, even when considering a single hand transplant. All groups that were questioned would accept a higher degree of risk to receive a double versus a single hand transplant."[57] Approximately one-third of the sample reported a higher level of risk acceptance for a hand transplant than for a kidney, even though the medical community views the former as life enhancing and the latter as lifesaving.[58]

Individuals were willing to accept even greater risk for face transplants. Barker and colleagues at Louisville developed a scale called the Louisville Instrument for Transplantation, known as LIFT. They then recruited three study populations (150 healthy individuals, 42 organ transplant recipients, and 34 individuals with facial disfigurement) to consider the extent to which they would trade off specific numbers of life-years, or sustain other costs, in exchange for receiving seven different transplant procedures. All the groups questioned would accept the highest degree of risk to receive a face or hemi-face transplant, compared with the other procedures, which included kidney, hand, bilateral hand, foot, and larynx transplants. There were differences between groups with respect to face transplants, with the kidney recipients most willing and the disfigured individuals least willing to undergo the procedure. The authors hypothesize that the transplant recipients were most willing to receive a face transplant due to the fact that they are already on immunosuppression. They also hypothesized that the disfigured individuals were least willing due to the fact that some had adjusted to their disfigurement.[59]

Many face transplant candidates are declared ineligible for psychological reasons. In addition, a key part of a face transplant is the active involvement of the patient in treatment and rehabilitation. Exclusion criteria include significant cognitive impairment (related to age, injury, or learning disorder). There is some debate whether blind individuals should be candidates, with the con argument stating that they do not "see" the stigma that they may face and the pro argument stating that they "feel" the stigma that they face, that they can be active participants in rehabilitation, and that it allows them to gain greater reintegration into society.[60]

An early concern was how much the recipient would look like the donor versus the recipient predisfigurement. The results from computer and cadaveric studies show that the final appearance will be a hybrid mainly determined by the recipient's facial skeleton.[61] The face transplants performed to date confirm this. However, most face transplants to date have not involved a facial skeleton that has a significant impact on appearance, as does the resting motor tone of the mimetic muscles. To date no evidence exists that residual donor appearance is a significant problem.[62]

Up until today, VCAs have only been performed on adults. Given their experimental nature, this is consistent with research ethics, whereby risky research is first performed on adults before being performed on children. As VCAs move into mainstream clinical practice, the question arises of what additional safeguards will be necessary before VCAs can be offered to pediatric candidates. The need for lifelong immunosuppression and the risk of rejection over decades make these VCAs even riskier for children, particularly young children. In 2002 a team of surgeons and ethicists in South Africa considered the pros and cons of offering extremity VCAs for two young children, one of whom lost both hands and the other lost all four distal extremities from meningococcal septicemia.[63] The argument in support of proceeding was that children may be the best candidates for rehabilitation. The argument against proceeding was the need for lifelong immunosuppression. The authors also noted that children are often the most able to adapt to changes in body shape and function, and so may not find the transplant as critical for "normal function" as their adult counterparts. After serious reflection, the South African surgeons elected not to perform the procedures. However, if immune tolerance can be achieved, there are a large number of children with congenital birth defects who might benefit from facial transplantation.[64]

Respect for the Donors of VCAs

This is primarily a chapter on the ethics of providing VCAs to recipients, but there are some ethical issues related to donors. In the case of a face and hands, of course, the donors would be deceased. We consider their perspective first. In the case of the uterus, however, a living donor is a possibility. We take up that perspective before concluding the chapter.

Respect for Deceased Donors

Like all organ donation, the procurement of face, hand, and uteri VCAs should follow standard protocols, in which initial screening is done by the local organ procurement organization (OPO). If a prospective solid organ donor appears to be a potential source for a VCA, additional consideration is required to help the family understand the request and to retain trust in the organ procurement process. Agich and Siemionow state: "Addressing how to accommodate the sensitivities of the donor family, the content of donor consent forms, and the consent process are thus a critical ethical concern. The donor family should understand exactly what tissue would be removed, its effect on the presentation of the corpse, and the impossibility of ruling out an identifiable linkage between the donor and the recipient. Defining this protocol is another key requirement for an ethically complete approach to facial transplantation."[65]

We should note that the normal organ and tissue donation forms used by OPOs typically request "all organs and tissues." Donors in advance (and families, if the donor has not specified) are normally given the opportunity to donate or withhold the donation of any particular organ or tissue. In many cases, however, donors will indicate a willingness to donate all usable organs and tissues. Some have claimed that this, in effect, already conveys a consent for OPOs to procure faces, hands, uteri, and literally all body parts. The claim is that all these are nothing more than tissues, and that consent for the donation of tissues has been given.

Although some may claim this is adequate consent for VCAs, we know of no OPO that would accept this reasoning, and it is important morally that they do not. When donors give permission to procure organs and tissues, they reasonably have certain body parts in mind: internal transplantable organs and probably tissues such as heart valves, skin, and bone. Most would be shocked to discover that someone had interpreted their donation to include hands, a face, a uterus, and other body parts. (One of us, RMV, knows of one case where a head was procured preceding cremation, and certainly this was a gross abuse of the consent process.) Traditional consent doctrine requires that people be informed of what they reasonably would want to know before they agree to a proposed course of action. It seems clear that, regardless of what is on the signed consent form, if an OPO wants to procure hands, a face, a uterus, or any other body parts beyond those normally procured in the transplant context, there must be an additional, explicit commitment from the donor. This would also apply for procuring limbs, the spinal cord, or other atypical body parts for research purposes. Hence, we think it is clear that every VCA procurement requires explicit consent from the donor or surrogate regardless of what the consent form says.

One of the main problems in face and hand transplantation is the willingness of families of brain-dead individuals to authorize procurement. The families are often concerned that these donations are visible body parts, which could interfere with funeral plans. Transplant procurement teams need to inform the families that facial masks or prosthetic hands would be created that can give the body the appearance of "wholeness" and allow open casket services.

In addition to routine OPO support, families who donate composite tissue of their loved ones may need to have access to a mental health provider after donation and after the transplant as the family moves through the grieving process. Families should be counseled and reassured that the final result of the surgery is not going to produce someone who looks exactly like their loved one. But as Edwards and Mathes note, "Given the media exposure of facial transplantation so far, families should be counseled that they might inadvertently be made aware of the recipient of their loved one's facial donor tissues."[66]

Risks to Living Donors

Although living donation is permissible, there are limits. We do not allow adults to donate a heart while alive because it would kill them, even if they would be willing to do so. We have also prohibited a father from donating a second kidney to his daughter, even though he could still live on dialysis.[67] Should living uterine donation be permitted? In support, one must acknowledge the minor long-term consequences on donor health from a hysterectomy barring procurement complications. Also, the participation of living donors in VCAs simplifies the timing of the transplant.

One argument against living uterine donation is that in order to make the uterus a good graft, the large blood vessels must be taken with the uterus, which increases the donor's risks. In fact, the first live donor in Saudi Arabia had a ureteric injury.[68] This was particularly problematic because the uterine transplant is not lifesaving. A second argument is that it perpetuates the stereotype that a women is not whole unless she bears and rears her own child, even if it poses serious risk to her and the fetus. In this context, it is critical to confirm that the woman herself expresses a strong interest in undergoing a uterine transplant and that the interest is not coming from her spouse or family members, who may be expressing cultural norms and expectations about what it means to be a woman and wife.

A psychological workup is necessary for both donors and recipients. For the donors, one must explore the meaning of removing the uterus, as data show that some women facing the removal of their uterus through a hysterectomy undergo feelings of loss and damage to their gender identity.[69] For the recipients, counseling will be important, both in selecting appropriate candidates and also during the time that the uterus remains in her body. (The ideal would be to remove the uterus and the need for immunosuppression at the latest after two successful pregnancies.) The candidates need to understand that theirs is not a "typical" pregnancy. First, the uterus will not be innervated, so the woman will not feel the fetus move or feel contractions. (Hormonally mediated effects like morning sickness and fatigue will be preserved.) The lack of innervation may exacerbate feelings of estrangement to the transplanted organ.[70] The fact that the uterus also gestated another's pregnancies may interfere with the recipient's ability to accept it as her own. This may be further complicated when the living donor is a close relative. Second, the transplant recipients must agree to delivery by prophylactic cesarean section because it is unknown how labor would proceed and what its impact would be on maternal or fetal health.

The decision to attempt a living donor uterine transplant in Sweden stems in part from the fact that surrogacy is illegal, so a uterine transplant may be the only option for those women who want to have a biologically related child. Still, it behooves us to consider whether we should focus our energy on a deceased donor uterine transplant because it poses no risks to the donor and removes some of the psychological issues that could arise from the fact that the woman may give birth to a child from the same womb in which she was gestated. The Swedish study of a living donor uterine transplant should not be repeated until the outcomes are known for these women and their infants.

An Update on UNOS Policy and Procedures regarding VCAs

In late 2013 one of us (RMV) was invited to serve on a new UNOS committee that would provide oversight of VCAs. The committee had its first phone meeting in January and its first in-person meeting in February 2014, and it continues to meet regularly. At its February meeting the committee reviewed the results of a survey conducted by the Association of Organ Procurement Organizations regarding current VCA activity in the United States. This survey found that there have been twenty-eight VCA recipients transplanted at eleven different transplant centers and nine patients currently waiting at six different centers. The report also noted that "there are an additional nine transplant hospitals in the planning stages for a new VCA program, with a few close to approving patients, including one children's hospital."[71]

The committee has prepared a "Proposal to Implement the OPTN's Oversight of Vascularized Composite Allografts (VCAs)," which was presented to the OPTN/UNOS Board of Directors in June 2014.[72] The committee unanimously voted that OPOs should "obtain authorization to recover VCAs separately from the authorization to recover other organs for transplant."[73] It is reviewing data elements collected by the OPTN to determine what additional information should be collected for VCAs. Due to timing, the proposal is provisional and will automatically expire in 2015. The committee hopes to seek public comments in the fall of 2014, with more permanent recommendations to be considered by the Board of Directors at its June 2015 meeting.

Conclusion

The ethical issues surrounding VCAs focus on the fact that recipients are exposing themselves to the risks of immunosuppression for a non-lifesaving organ. However, although one can survive without these VCAs, the candidates themselves see the transplant as giving them a new lease on life—whether to fulfill their dream of hugging their loved ones, carrying their child in an arm that has real feeling, or being able to walk into a store and be "anonymous"—unnoticed by other patrons.

We end this chapter by raising one ethical issue not yet addressed: the question of resource allocation between lifesaving and life-enhancing VCAs. The pretransplant VCA hand and face workups are labor intensive, with serious consideration given to psychological adaptation, personal identity, and self-image. The hand and face VCA operations are arduous and exacting, often requiring multiple surgeons for both donor procurement and recipient transplantation. Richard Norris's transplant reportedly involved a team of 150 professionals. The postoperative rehabilitation programs for hand and face VCAs are also long and arduous. Thus, each VCA procedure is expensive in terms of financial costs and health care provider time, and also recipient time and energy. The question of whether and how much we should allocate institutional and professional resources to non-lifesaving VCA programs will only become more pressing if and when immune tolerance is achieved and the millions of individuals with severe facial disfigurement, upper-limb amputation, and uterine infertility seek VCAs as their preferred mode of treatment.

Notes

1. The Norris story was constructed relying on the following public sources: "Face transplant," http://en.wikipedia.org/wiki/Face_transplant; "Richard Norris, face transplant recipient, adjusting to new life June 28, 2013," www.cbsnews.com/news/richard-norris-face-transplant-recipient-adjusting-to -new-life/; James Meikle, "Face transplant man Richard Norris has 'life restored,'" *The Guardian*, March 28, 2012, www.theguardian.com/science/2012/mar/28/face-transplant-man-richard-norris; and Debbie Hall, "Man whose face was reconstructed was from Henry County," *Martinsville Bulletin*, March 28, 2012, www.martinsvillebulletin.com/article.cfm?ID=32599.

2. Tobin GR, Breidenback WC III, Lidstad ST, Marvin MM, Buell JF, Ravindra KV, "The history of composite tissue allotransplantation," *Transplantation Proceedings* 2009;41: 466–71.

3. Peacock EE Jr, "Restoration of finger flexion with homologous composite tissue tendon grafts," *American Surgeon* 1960;26: 564–71.

4. Tobin et al., "History," 467.

5. Ibid.

6. Errico M, Metcalfe NH, Platt A, "History and ethics of hand transplants," *Journal of the Royal Society of Medicine Short Reports*, 2012;3, http://shr.sagepub.com/content/3/10/74.

7. Ziegler-Graham K, MacKenzie EJ, Ephraim PL, Travison TG, Brookmeyer R, "Estimating the prevalence of limb loss in the United States: 2005 to 2050," *Archives of Physical Medicine and Rehabilitation* 2008;89 (3): 422–29.

8. Ibid.

9. Dubernard JM, Owen E, Herzberg G, et al., "Human hand allograft: Report on first 6 months," *Lancet* 1999;353 (9161): 1315–20.

10. Breidenbach WC 3rd, Tobin GR 2nd, Gorantla VS, Gonzalez RN, Granger DK, "A position statement in support of hand transplantation," *Journal of Hand Surgery* 2002;27 (5): 760–70.

11. "Hand-transplant man ran away with his nurse," *Dominion Post*, www.stuff.co.nz/dominion-post/365779.

12. Hartman RG, "Chapter 30: Ethical and policy concerns of hand/face transplantation," in *Transplantation of Composite Tissue Allografts*, ed. Hewitt CW, Lee WPA (New York: Springer, 2008), 429–42.

13. Petruzzo P, Morelon E, Kanitakis J, et al., "Chapter 15: Hand transplantation—Lyon Experience," in *Transplantation of Composite Tissue Allografts*, ed. Hewitt CW, Lee WPA, with Gordon CR (New York: Springer, 2008), 209–14.

14. Petruzzo P, Dubernard JM, "Chapter 22: The international registry on hand and composite tissue allotransplantation," *Clinical Transplants* 2011: 247–53.

15. Ibid.

16. Tintle SM, Potter BK, Elliott RM, Levin LS, "Hand transplantation," *Journal of Bone and Joint Surgery Reviews* 2014;2 (1): e1-9, http://reviews.jbjs.org/content/jbjsrev/2/1/e1.full.pdf.

17. Petruzzo P, Lanzetta M, Dubernard J-M, et al., "The International Registry on Hand and Composite Tissue Transplantation," *Transplantation* 2010;90: 1590–94.

18. Tintle et al., "Hand transplantation."

19. Petruzzo et al., "International Registry."

20. Tintle et al., "Hand transplantation."

21. Breidenbach WC, Gonzales NR, Kaufman CL, Klapheke M, Tobin GR, Gorantla VS, "Outcomes of the first 2 American hand transplants at 8 and 6 years posttransplant," *Journal of Hand Surgery* 2008;33 (7): 1039–47.

22. Edwards JA, Mathes DW, "Facial transplantation: A review of ethics, progress, and future targets," *Transplant Research and Risk Management* 2011;3: 115.

23. Dubernard JM, Lengelé B, Morelon E, et al., "Outcomes 18 months after the first human partial face transplantation," *New England Journal of Medicine* 2007;357: 2451–60.

24. Dubernard J-M, "Hand and face allografts: Myth, dream, and reality," *Proceedings of the American Philosophical Society* 2011;155 (1): 17.

25. Siemionow M, Ozturk C, "Face transplantation: Outcomes, concerns, controversies, and future directions," *Journal of Craniofacial Surgery* 2012;23 (1): 254–59.

26. Siemionow M, Ozturk C, "An update on facial transplantation cases performed between 2005 and 2010," *Plastic and Reconstructive Surgery* 2011;128 (6): 707e–20e.

27. Blake M, "'When I look in the mirror I see myself': Incredible transformation of shotgun victim who had most extensive face transplant surgeons have ever performed," *Mail Online*, June 28, 2013, www.dailymail.co.uk/news/article-2350575/Richard-Lee-Norris-Incredible-transformation-shotgun-victim-worlds-extensive-face-transplant.html.

28. Petruzzo, Dubernard, "Chapter 22."

29. Edwards, Mathes, "Facial transplantation."

30. Siemionow, Ozturk, "Face transplantation."

31. Blake, "'When I look in the mirror.'"

32. Siemionow, Ozturk, "Update."

33. Nair A, Stega J, Smith JR, Del Priore G, "Uterus transplant evidence and ethics," *Annals of the New York Academy of Science* 2008;1127: 83–91.

34. Catsanos R, Rogers W, Lotz M, "The ethics of uterus transplantation," *Bioethics* 2013;27: 65–73; Saso S, Ghaem-Maghami S, Louis LS, Ungar L, Del Priore G, Smith JR, "Uterine transplantation: What else needs to be done before it can become a reality?" *Journal of Obstetrics and Gynaecology* 2013;33 (3): 232–38.

35. Brännström M, Diaz-Garcia C, Hanafy A, Olausson M, Tzakis A, "Uterus transplantation: Animal research and human possibilities," *Fertility and Sterility* 2012;97: 1269–76.

36. Erman Akar M, Ozkan O, Aydinuraz B, et al., "Clinical pregnancy after uterus transplantation," *Fertility and Sterility* 2013;100: 1358–63.

37. "Nine Swedish women receive womb transplants," BBC News, Jan. 13, 2014, www.bbc.co.uk/news/health-25716446.

38. Cheng M, "4 women with new wombs are trying to get pregnant," Yahoo News, March 3, 2014, http://news.yahoo.com/4-women-wombs-trying-pregnant-113219910.html?soc_src=copy. Brännström M, Johannesson L, Bokström H, Kvarnström N, Mölne J, Kähler PD, et al. "Livebirth after uterus transplantation," *The Lancet*, Early Online Publication, 6 October 2014. *doi:10.1016/S0140-6736(14)61728-1. http://www.thelancet.com/journals/lancet/article/PIIS0140-6736(14)61728-1/fulltext#article_upsell*

39. Siegler M, "Ethical issues in innovative surgery: Should we attempt a cadaveric hand transplantation in a human subject?" *Transplantation Proceedings* 1998;30: 2779–82. Siegler cites two of Moores papers: Moore FD, "Three ethical revolutions: Ancient assumptions remodeled under pressure of transplantation," *Transplantation Proceedings* 1988;20 (1 suppl 1): 1061–67; and Moore FD, "The desperate case: CARE (costs, applicability, research, ethics)," *JAMA* 1989;261: 1483–84.

As the Cleveland team prepared for its first Institutional Review Board–approved face transplant, it also used Moore's criteria to justify its readiness for a first-in-man face transplant, although Agich and Siemionow claimed that only Moore's first three criteria were ethically relevant. See Agich GJ, Siemionow M, "Facing the ethical questions in facial transplantation," *American Journal of Bioethics* 2004;4: 3, 25–27. In rejecting Siegler's interpretation, Agich and Siemionow refer to Moore's earlier ethics piece published in 1969: Moore FD, "Therapeutic innovation: Ethical boundaries in the initial clinical trials of new drugs and surgical procedures," *Daedalus* 1969;98 (2): 502–22.

40. Barker JH, Vossen M, Banis J, "The technical, immunological and ethical feasibility of face transplantation," *International Journal of Surgery* 2004;2: 8–12.

41. Clarke A, Simmons J, White P, Withey S, Bulter PEM, "Attitudes to face transplantation: Results of a public engagement exercise at the Royal Society," *Journal of Burn Care and Research* 2006;27 (3): 394–98.

42. Ozmen S, Findikcioglu F, Sezgin B, Findikcioglu K, Kucuker I, Atabay K, "Would you be a face transplant donor? A survey of the Turkish population about face allotransplantation," *Annals of Plastic Surgery* 2013;71 (2): 233–37.

43. Sinno HH, Thibaudeau S, Duggal A, Lessard L, "Utility scores for facial disfigurement requiring facial transplantation," *Plastic and Reconstruction Surgery* 2010;126 (2): 443–49.

44. Mathes DW, Kumar N, Ploplys E, "A survey of North American burn and plastic surgeons on their current attitudes toward facial transplantation," *Journal of the American College of Surgeons* 2009;208 (6): 1051–58.

45. Soni CV, Barker JH, Pushpakumar SB, et al., "Psychosocial considerations in facial transplantation," *Burns* 2010;36 (7): 963.

46. Chang J, Mathes DW, "Ethical, financial, and policy considerations in hand transplantation," *Hand Clinics* 2011;27: 557.

47. Tintle et al., "Hand transplantation," 1.

48. See, e.g., Foucher G, "Commentary: Prospects for hand transplantation," *Lancet* 1999;353 (9161): 1286–87; Herndon JH, "Composite-tissue transplantation: A new frontier," *New England Journal of Medicine* 2000;343: 503–5; and Hovius SE, "Hand transplantation: An opinion," *Journal of Hand Surgery* 2001;26 (6): 519–20.

49. Edwards, Mathes, "Facial transplantation," 557.

50. Chang, Mathes, "Ethical, financial, and policy considerations."

51. Landau R, "Artificial womb versus natural birth: An exploratory study of women's views," *Journal of Reproductive and Infant Psychology* 2007;25: 4–17, cited by Catsanos, Rogers, Lotz, "Ethics."

52. McKay DB, Josephson MA, "Reproduction and transplantation: Report on the AST consensus conference on reproductive issues and transplantation," *American Journal of Transplantation* 2005;5: 1592–99; Mastrobattista JM, Gomez-Lobo V, for Society of Maternal-Fetal Medicine, "Pregnancy after solid organ transplantation," *Obstetrics and Gynecology* 2008;112: 919–32.

53. See, e.g., Deshpande NA, James NT, Kucirka LM, et al., "Pregnancy outcomes in kidney transplant recipients: A systematic review and meta-analysis," *American Journal of Transplantation* 2011;11: 2388–404; Ross LF, "Ethical considerations related to pregnancy in transplant recipients," *New England Journal of Medicine* 2006;354: 1313–16; Armenti VT, Daller JA, Constantinescu S, et al., "Report from the National Transplantation Pregnancy Registry: Outcomes of pregnancy after transplantation," *Clinical Transplantation* 2006: 57–70; and McKay, Josephson, "Reproduction."

54. McFarland LV, Hubbard Winkler SL, Heinemann AW, Jones M, Esquenazi A, "Unilateral upper-limb loss: Satisfaction and prosthetic-device use in veterans and service members from Vietnam and OIF/OEF [Operation Iraqi Freedom / Operation Enduring Freedom] conflicts," *Journal of Rehabilitative Research and Development* 2010;47 (4): 299–316.

55. Gander B, Brown CS, Vasilic D, et al., "Composite tissue allotransplantation of the hand and face: A new frontier in trans plant and reconstructive surgery," *Transplant International* 2006;19 (11): 868–80.

56. For references for the data about the Louisville and Italian programs, see Chang, Mathes, "Ethical, financial, and policy considerations."

57. Majzoub RK, Cunningham M, Grossi F, Maldonado C, Banis JC, Barker JH, "Investigation of risk acceptance in hand transplantation," *Journal of Hand Surgery* 2006;31A: 295.

58. Ibid., 299.

59. Barker JH, Furr A, Cunningham M, et al., "Investigation of risk acceptance in facial transplantation," *Plastic and Reconstructive Surgery* 2006;118 (3): 663–70.

60. Carty MJ, Bueno EM, Lehmann LS, Pomahac B, "A position paper in support of face transplantation in the blind," *Plastic and Reconstructive Surgery* 2012;130: 319–24.

61. Okie S, "Facial transplantation: Brave new face," *New England Journal of Medicine* 2006;354 (9): 889–94; Siemionow M, Agaoglu G, "The issue of 'facial appearance and identity transfer' after mock transplantation," *Journal of Reconstructive Microsurgery* 2006;22 (5): 329–34.

62. Edwards, Mathes, "Facial transplantation."

63. Benatar D, Hudson DA, "A tale of two novel transplants not done: The ethics of limb allografts," *British Medical Journal* 2002;324: 971–73.

64. Washington KM, Zanoun RR, Cadogan KA, Afrooz PN, Losee JE, "Composite tissue allotransplantation for the reconstruction of congenital craniofacial defects," *Transplantation Proceedings* 2009; 41 (2): 523–27.

65. Agich, Siemionow, "Facing the ethical questions."

66. Edwards, Mathes, "Facial transplantation."

67. Ross LF, "Donating a second kidney: A tale of family and ethics," *Seminars in Dialysis* 2000;13: 201–3.

68. Ibid.

69. Elson J, *Am I still a woman? Hysterectomy and gender identity* (Philadelphia: Temple University Press, 2004), as cited by Catsanos, Rogers, Lotz, "Ethics."

70. Fox R, Swazey JP, *Spare parts: Organ replacement in American society* (New York: Oxford University Press, 1992), 36.

71. OPTN/UNOS Vascularized Composite Allograft Transplantation Committee Report to the Board of Directors, Richmond, June 23–24, 2014, 6, http://optn.transplant.hrsa.gov/CommitteeReports/board_main_VascularizedCompositeAllograftTransplantation_6_16_2014_16_21.pdf.

72. Ibid.; see the briefing paper titled "Proposal to implement the OPTN's oversight of vascularized composite allografts (VCAs)," 7–36.

73. Ibid., 3.

INDEX